Non-Invasive Instrumentation and Measurement in Medical Diagnosis

Second Edition

Biomedical Engineering Series
Donald R. Peterson, Series Editor

Published Titles

*Please visit our website **www.crcpress.com** for a full list of titles*

Non-Invasive Instrumentation and Measurement in Medical Diagnosis

Second Edition

Robert B. Northrop

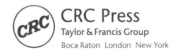

CRC Press
Taylor & Francis Group
Boca Raton London New York

CRC Press is an imprint of the
Taylor & Francis Group, an **informa** business

CRC Press
Taylor & Francis Group
6000 Broken Sound Parkway NW, Suite 300
Boca Raton, FL 33487-2742

First issued in paperback 2019

© 2018 by Taylor & Francis Group, LLC
CRC Press is an imprint of Taylor & Francis Group, an Informa business

No claim to original U.S. Government works

ISBN-13: 978-1-4987-4990-9 (hbk)
ISBN-13: 978-0-367-87563-3 (pbk)

Visit the Taylor & Francis Web site at
http://www.taylorandfrancis.com

and the CRC Press Web site at
http://www.crcpress.com

I dedicate this text to my former teachers and students.

Contents

Preface

This book is about the instruments, and sometimes the procedures, which are used for noninvasive medical diagnosis (NIMD) and therapy. Why stress "noninvasive (NI)"? NIMD is preferred whenever possible to avoid the risks and expenses attendant to surgically opening the body surface, for example, infections, adverse systemic reactions to anesthesia, dye injection, antibiotics and other medications, as well as surgical error. In many instances, NIMD is less expensive than equivalent invasive procedures, in other cases (e.g., imaging) it is the *only* practical means of diagnosis, and in some cases (e.g., imaging) it is the most expensive diagnostic modality because of the complex technologies involved.

This text was written based both on the author's experience in teaching EE 370, *Biomedical Instrumentation I*, for over 35 years in the Electrical & Computer Engineering Department (now Biomedical Engineering Department) at the University of Connecticut, and on his personal research on certain prototype, NI medical instrumentation systems. The contents of EE 370 have evolved with instrumentation technology and our knowledge of human diseases, physiology, biochemistry, and cell biology.

As NIMD is a rapidly growing, interdisciplinary field, a number of the systems described in this text are prototypes that are currently in the research phase of their development. In the author's opinion, these systems will probably be effective, and given Food and Drug Administration (FDA) approval, we will eventually see their general acceptance and use by the medical community. I have seen photonics and photonic means of measurement play an increasingly important role in modern NIMD instrument design. As the reader will see, the diagnostic photon is becoming increasingly important.

This book is intended for use in an introductory classroom course on *Noninvasive Medical Instrumentation and Measurements* taken by juniors, seniors, and graduate students in biomedical engineering. It will also serve as a reference book for medical students and other health professionals interested in the topic. Practicing physicians and nurses interested in learning the state of the art in this important field will also find this text valuable. Physicists, biophysicists, and physiologists working in the biomedical field will also find it of interest.

Reader background: Readers are assumed to have had introductory, core courses in human (medical) physiology, biomedical engineering, engineering systems analysis, and in electronic circuits. Their mathematical skills should include an introductory course on differential equations, as well as college-level algebra and calculus. As the result of taking these courses, the readers should be skilled in understanding systems block diagrams, simple electronic circuits, the concepts of frequency response and transfer functions, and the use of ordinary differential equations to describe systems' dynamics. It is also important to have an understanding of how the physiological parameters being measured figure in human health. Much of the material in this text is descriptive. However, many systems are analyzed in detail. The teacher who considers adopting this text for classroom use should be advised that there are no chapter home problems.

In writing the second edition of this text, I have been amazed at the depth, breadth, and quality of the information available on the topic of NIMD and all its modalities on the Internet. I can be criticized for using and citing Internet sources because they are often ephemeral in the purest sense. I estimate the half-life of a web resource as being about 5 years. However, web resources are a window on cutting-edge medical technologies. Sometime, the view begins with university press releases on new medical research. A good search engine, such as Google.com, is invaluable. Obviously, I have also relied on standard texts and referred journal references in my writing.

Non-Invasive Instrumentation and Measurements in Medical Diagnosis, 2nd edition, is organized into 18 chapters, and includes an *Index*, an extensive *Bibliography*, and a comprehensive *Glossary*. Below are the summarized chapter contents:

In Chapter 1, *Introduction to Noninvasive Medical Measurements,* I define what is meant by NI measurements and give many examples. (Some persons might argue that use of a colonoscope or a bronchoscope is in fact an invasive procedure; however, I classify their use as minimally invasive.) Also provided is an overview and history of the use of simple, NI procedures to diagnose disease as practiced in the nineteenth century and earlier, and I explain their importance in modern medicine.

Chapter 2, *Visual Inspection of Tissues with Endoscopes and Other Optical Devices,* describes the simple, modern, NI optical instruments that allow the medical practitioner to directly inspect tissues for foreign objects, infections, polyps, tumors, etc. Attention is given to the use of ophthalmoscopes and slit lamps to inspect the retina, the cornea, and internal structures of the eye. Various types of endoscopes are described that allow direct inspection of a variety of tissues and organs accessible from without the body (e.g., the lungs, colon, stomach, urethra, bladder, and renal pelvis). Modern, coherent fiber-optic bundles are used in some applications with miniature, high-resolution, digital TV cameras.

Chapter 3, *Noninvasive Diagnosis Using Sounds Originating from within the Body*, treats the medically important sounds arising from within the body (the fetal heart, heart, lungs, joints, blood vessel bruits, and otoacoustic emissions). Basic instrumentation is described, including the stethoscope, microphones, filters, and the use of FFT frequency analysis. The growing importance of time–frequency spectrograms in the description of sounds, and in NIMD is stressed.

In Chapter 4, *Measurement of Electrical Potentials and Magnetic Fields from the Body Surface*, we first describe the sources of skin-surface electrical potential from electrically active internal organs (heart, brain, muscles, retina, cochlea, nerves). The signal-coupling properties of various bioelectrodes are treated, followed by sections on the medical significance of each of the potentials (ECG, EMG, EEG, ERG, EOG, ECoG). Differential and medical isolation amplifiers are covered in detail, as are low-noise amplifier analysis and design. The SQUID, and biomagnetic measurements with SQUID arrays are also described.

In Chapter 5, *Noninvasive Measurement of Blood Pressure*, the use of the sphygmomanometer is described (manual and automatic) in measuring systolic and diastolic blood pressure. Blood pressure estimates can also be made from finger plethysmographs.

Chapter 6, *Body Temperature Measurements*, considers the basic thermometer (mercury and electronic) and its importance in detecting fever or hypothermia. Basic heat flow relations are used to describe thermometer response time. The design and physics of the no-touch, LIR thermometer that reads body temperature from the eardrum is elaborated.

Chapter 7, *Noninvasive Blood Gas Sensing with Electrodes*, describes the use of electrochemical electrodes on heated skin used to transcutaneously measure tissue pCO_2 and tissue pO_2.

In Chapter 8, *Tests on Naturally Voided Body Fluids*, we review a number of analytical instrumental techniques that can be used on body fluids (urine, saliva, and breath) to measure the concentrations of certain ions, glucose, urea, drugs, VOCs, etc. Various analytical instruments used in laboratory medicine are described, including dispersive and nondispersive spectroscopy, surface plasmon resonance, ion-selective electrodes, flame photometers, gas chromatography, and mass spectrometry. We then go on to review what can be found of diagnostic significance in urine, feces, saliva, and breath.

Chapter 9, *Plethysmography*, describes the applications of plethysmography in quantifying body volume changes due to breathing, muscle contraction, blood flow, etc. Body and limb volume changes can be measured by water displacement, pneumatically, or electronically.

Chapter 10, *Pulmonary Function Tests*, first describes the volume displacement spirometer, then the use of turbines and pneumotachs to electronically measure respiratory flow and volumes. Spirometers are used to quantify mechanical respiratory functions with such parameters as lung tidal volume, forced expiratory volumes, etc. Their use is critical in detecting obstructive lung diseases and plotting their progress. Also covered is the use of inhaled inert gases in the measurement of respiratory function.

The *Measurement of Basal Metabolism* is described in Chapter 11. The physiology behind the measurement protocol is explained, and the apparatus and protocol are given. Basal metabolism measurement is a basic NI means of assessing thyroid function.

Chapter 12, *Ocular Tonometry*, discusses the importance to monitor the intraocular pressure of healthy vision. The designs of various tonometers including the no-touch air-puff applanation system are described.

Chapter 13, *Noninvasive Tests Involving the Input of Audible Sound Energy*, treats measurements in which low-frequency acoustic energy (generally 2–2000 Hz) is used to characterize the respiratory system, or the ear canal and eardrum. We first describe the concepts of acoustic resistance, capacitance, and inertance (inductance), and show how a complex acoustic impedance (**Z**) can be simply measured.

The RAIMS system devised by the author is described for the measurement of the acoustic **Z** of the lungs and bronchial tree. Acoustic **Z** is also shown to be useful in characterizing the compliance of the eardrum and the tympanal reflex. Finally, a means of measuring the acoustic transfer function of the chest cavity and lungs with transmitted white noise is described. The measurement and acoustic **Z** of the lungs have application in detecting and quantifying obstructive lung disease.

In Chapter 14, *Noninvasive Tests Using Ultrasound (Excluding Imaging)*, we begin by describing the physics and mathematics associated with the Doppler effect. Next covered is the use of CW and pulsed Doppler ultrasound to measure blood velocity, and its diagnostic utility. Another application is the use of air-coupled ultrasound to measure the ocular pulse. The closed-loop, constant phase, NOTOPM system of Northrop and Nilakhe is described, and the uses of the ocular pulse in diagnosis are detailed. The same air-coupled, ultrasound ranging system was used by Northrop (1980) to design a prototype, no-touch infant apnea monitor.

A significant improvement on the NOTOPM system, the constant-phase, closed-loop, type 1, ranging system (CPRS), is presented and its possible future applications in the quantitative measurement of aneurisms, heart motion, and the shape of internal organs are described. (The CPRS system gives a simultaneous output of incremental distance and velocity.)

Chapter 15, *Noninvasive Applications of Photon Radiation (Excluding Imaging)*, covers a wide spectrum of topics (pun intended): x-ray bone densitometry by the DEXA method; tissue fluorescence spectroscopy; optical interferometric measurement of nanometer tissue displacements; Laser Doppler velocimetry; percutaneous IR spectroscopy; glucose measurement in the aqueous humor of the eye by polarimetry (the rotation of linearly polarized light); pulse oximetry; and applications of Raman spectroscopy in detecting cancer and dissolved glucose are also described.

Chapter 16, *A Survey of Medical Imaging Systems*, first considers the input modalities of coherent light, x-rays, ultrasound, and γ-rays from radioisotopes. The mathematical means for tomographic imaging are described, including the Radon transform and deblurring techniques. The production of x-rays and their use in flat imaging and CT scanners is treated. Also covered are magnetic resonance imaging (MRI), positron emission tomography (PET) imaging, radio-nuclide (isotope) imaging (SPECT), ultrasonic imaging, and passive, LIR thermal imaging in diagnosis. The present and future imaging capabilities of the emerging field of optical coherence tomography (OCT) are described. Also explored is the new use of coherent x-ray diffraction imaging in high-resolution mammography; all you need is a synchrotron.

In Chapter 17, *Innovations in Noninvasive Instrumentation and Measurements*, we consider possible modalities whereby medical professionals can noninvasively examine DNA for mutations, expediting the diagnosis of cancer and research on genetically caused diseases. The DNA microarray, or "gene chip" and the means of reading out probe hits on target molecules are described. We present the use of fluorescence tagging and laser scanning to read out gene chips, as well as electrical readouts. Biochips are also being designed that can test for specific antibodies to bacteria and viruses, as well as the pathogen coat proteins themselves. The detection of other, non-DNA molecules found in urine and saliva that may be associated with cancer growth is described.

Chapter 18, *Introduction to Noninvasive Therapies*, describes the therapeutic uses of externally applied electric currents, electric and magnetic fields, heat and percutaneous ultrasound energy to treat a variety of medical conditions, including but not limited to bone fractures, cancers, glioblastomas, osteoarthritis, etc. Interferential current therapy (ICT) has been shown to be effective in various degrees for the relief of chronic pain (TENS), stimulation of muscles, causing increased blood flow, reducing edema, and genera stimulation of tissue healing. Many claims exist for the therapeutic effects of externally applied, pulsed magnetic fields. These benefits have been observed in various clinical studies in various degrees. In Section 18.15, we examine the exciting new field of gene editing with CRISPR-Cas and CRISPR-Cpf1 endonucleases in potential therapies for certain genetic diseases.

Robert B. Northrop
Chaplin, Connecticut

MATLAB® is a registered trademark of The MathWorks, Inc. For product information, please contact:

The MathWorks, Inc.
3 Apple Hill Drive
Natick, MA 01760-2098, USA
Tel: 508-647-7000
Fax: 508-647-7001
E-mail: info@mathworks.com
Web: www.mathworks.com

About the Author

Robert B. Northrop, PhD, was born in White Plains, NY, in 1935. After graduating from Staples High School in Westport, CT, he majored in electrical engineering at MIT, graduating with a bachelor's degree in 1956. At the University of Connecticut, he received a master's degree in electrical and systems engineering in 1958. As the result of a long-standing interest in physiology, he entered a PhD program at UCONN in animal physiology, doing research on the neuromuscular physiology of molluscan catch muscles. He earned his PhD in 1964.

In 1963, he rejoined the UCONN EE Department as a lecturer, and was hired as an assistant professor of EE in 1964. In collaboration with his PhD advisor, Dr. Edward G. Boettiger, he secured a 5-year training grant in 1965 from NIGMS (NIH), and started one of the first, interdisciplinary, biomedical engineering graduate training programs in New England. UCONN currently awards MS and PhD degrees in this field of study, as well as BS degrees in biomedical engineering.

Throughout his career, Dr. Northrop's research interests have been broad and interdisciplinary and have been centered on biomedical engineering and physiology. He has done sponsored research (by the AFOSR) on the neurophysiology of insect and frog vision, and devised theoretical models for visual neural signal processing. He also did sponsor research on electrofishing and developed, in collaboration with Northeast Utilities, effective, working systems for guidance and control of migrating fish in hydroelectric plant waterways on the Connecticut River at Holyoke, MA, using underwater electric fields.

Still another area of his sponsored research (by NIH) has been in the design and simulation of nonlinear, adaptive, digital controllers to regulate *in vivo* drug concentrations or physiological parameters, such as pain, blood pressure, or blood glucose in diabetics. An outgrowth of this research led to his development of mathematical models for the dynamics of the human immune system, which were used to investigate theoretical therapies for autoimmune diseases, cancer, and HIV infection.

Biomedical instrumentation has also been an active research area for Dr. Northrop and his graduate students: An NIH grant supported studies on the use of the ocular pulse to detect obstructions in the carotid arteries. Minute pulsations of the cornea from arterial circulation in the eyeball were sensed using a no-touch, phase-locked, ultrasound technique. Ocular pulse waveforms were shown to be related to cerebral blood flow in rabbits and humans.

More recently, Dr. Northrop addressed the problem of noninvasive (NI) blood glucose measurement for diabetics. Starting with a Phase I SBIR grant, he developed a means of estimating blood glucose by reflecting a beam of polarized light off the front surface of the lens of the eye, and measuring the very small optical rotation resulting from glucose in the aqueous humor, which in turn is proportional to blood glucose. As an offshoot of techniques developed in micropolarimetry, he developed a magnetic sample chamber for glucose measurement in biotechnology applications. The water solvent was used as the Faraday optical medium.

He has written numerous papers in refereed journals, and 14 textbooks: *Analog Electronic Circuits* (1990); *Introduction to Instrumentation and Measurements* (1997); *Endogenous and Exogenous Regulation and Control of Physiological Systems* (2000); *Dynamic Modeling of Neuro-Sensory Systems* (2001); *Noninvasive Instrumentation and Measurements in Medical Diagnosis* (2002); *Signals and Systems Analysis in Biomedical Engineering* (2003); *Analysis and Application of Analog Electronic Circuits in Biomedical Engineering* (2004); *Introduction to Instrumentation and Measurements*—2nd edition (2005); *Introduction to Molecular Biology, Genomics & Proteomics for Biomedical Engineers* (with Anne N. Connor) (2009); *Signals and Systems Analysis in Biomedical Engineering*—2nd edition (2010); *Introduction to Complexity and Complex Systems* (2011); *Analysis and Application of Analog Electronic Circuits in Biomedical Engineering*—2nd edition (2012); *Ecological Sustainability: Understanding Complex Issues* (with Anne N. Connor) (2013), *Introduction to Instrumentation and Measurements*—3rd edition (2014).

Dr. Northrop is a member of Sigma Xi, Phi Kappa Phi, Eta Kappa Nu, Tau Beta Pi, and a Founding Fellow, Connecticut Academy of Engineers (2003).

His current research interest lies in complex systems and sustainability.

Dr. Northrop was on the Electrical & Systems Engineering faculty at UCONN until his retirement in June 1997. Throughout this time, he was director of the Biomedical Engineering Graduate Program. As Emeritus Professor, he writes texts, sails, and travels. He lives in Chaplin, CT, with his wife and a barn cat.

Acronyms and Abbreviations

Aβ	Amyloid-β polypeptide
ANSI	American National Standards Institute
BAc	Blood alcohol
BBR	Blackbody radiation
[bG]	Blood glucose concentration
BPD	Bronchopulmonary dysplasia
BPF	Band-pass filter
BTE	Behind the ear (hearing aid)
C³ (in physiology)	Command, communication, and control (of biochemical and physiological processes)
CAT	Computer-assisted tomography; Computed axial tomography (X-ray); Computer of average transients
cfDNA	Circulating free DNA
CMOS	Complementary metal oxide semiconductor
CMRR	Common-mode rejection ratio
COLD	Chronic obstructive lung disease
CPAP	Continuous positive airway pressure (ventilation)
CPDRS	Constant-phase distance ranging system
Cpf1	A CRISPR-associated endonuclease
CRISPR	Acronym for Clustered regularly interspaced short palindromic repeats
CRT	Cathode ray tube
CSF	Cerebrospinal fluid
DA	Differential (difference) amplifier
DARPA	Defense Advanced Research Projects Agency
D-C	Direct coupled
DC	Direct current
DEI	Diffraction-enhanced imaging
DEXA	Dual energy X-ray absorption
DLCO	Diffusion capacity of the lungs for carbon monoxide
DR	Diffuse reflectance
DRIS	Diffuse reflectance imaging system
dsDNA	Double-stranded DNA
DSF	Directional sensitivity function
DSP	Digital signal processing
DVT	Deep vein thrombosis
DXA	Dual-energy, x-ray absorption (test)
EECP	Enhanced external counterpulsation
EM	Electron micrograph, electromagnetic (fields)
EMF	Electromotive force (in V)
EMG	Electromyogram
ERP	Event-related potential
EtG	Ethyl glucuronide
FEV1	Forced Expiratory Volume in 1 s
FISH	Fluorescence *in situ* hybridization
FVC	Forced vital capacity
GBP	Glycan-binding protein
GE	Genetically engineered
HA	Hearing aid
Hz	Hertz (cycles per second)
IC	Integrated circuit
ICT	Interferential current therapy (also IFT)
IFC	Interferential current (tissue stimulation)
[ifG]	Interstitial fluid glucose concentration
IFT	Interferential current therapy
INR	International normalized ratio

iOS	Apple's proprietary mobile operating system (OS) for its handheld devices, such as the *iPhone, iPad,* and *iPod Touch.* The OS is based on the *Macintosh OSX*
IPAP	Inspiratory positive airway pressure
IPPV	Intermittent positive pressure ventilation
IR	Infrared
ISCEV	International Society for Clinical Electrophysiology
ISE	Ion-selective electrode
ITC	In the (ear) canal (hearing aids)
IV	Intravenous
lacZ	A gene in the lac operon. The proteins from the lac operon are lacZ, lacY, and lacA. The lac operon, found in *Escherichia coli* and other enteric bacteria, is required for the transport and metabolism of lactose
LDV	Laser Doppler velocimetry
LF	Low-frequency AC band 30–300 kHz
LIA	Lock-in amplifier
LIFE	Light-induced fluorescent endoscopy
LIR	Long wave infrared
LN_2	Liquid nitrogen
LOD	Limit of detection (minimum concentration of an analyte that can be distinguished from the blank). See below
LOR	Line of response (in PET events)
MAST	Medical antishock trousers
MEG	Magnetoencephalogram
M-FISH	FISH with multiple fluors
MIR	Midrange infrared wavelength (e.g., 1010–1095 cm^{-10})
mL	Milliliter
MOS	Metal oxide semiconductor
MS	Multiple sclerosis
MSIF	Multispectral imaging in the frequency domain
MSIS	Multispectral imaging in the spatial domain
mT	MilliTesla
mtDNA	Mitochondrial DNA
NADH	(reduced) nicotinamide adenine dinucleotide
ND	Neutral density
nDNA	Nuclear DNA
NDS	Nondispersive spectrophotometer
NDW	Neutral-density wedge
NI	Noninvasive
NIMD	Noninvasive medical diagnosis
NIR	Near-infrared light
NIT	Noninvasive therapy
NOTOPM	No-touch ocular pulse measurement
OCT	Optical coherence tomography
OCV	Open-circuit voltage
OD	Right eye
ODE	Ordinary differential equation
OIP	Occlusive impedance phlebography
OLD	Obstructive lung disease
OP	Ocular pulse
OPD	Optical path distance
OS	Left eye
OT	Output transducer (the "receiver" in hearing aids)
PA	Power amplifier
PAT	Photoacoustic tomography
PD	Phase detector
PDS	Pulsed Doppler system; Power density spectrum
PEMF	Pulsed electromagnetic field
PENS	Percutaneous electrical nerve stimulation

PLSR	Partial least squares regression
PMF	Pulsed magnetic field
PPOF	Polarization-preserving optical fiber
pps	Pulses per second
PROP-Z	Programmable probiotics with lacZ
psi	Pounds per square inch (pressure) (1 psi = 70.3 g/cm^2)
PVDF	Polyvinylidene fluoride
QPMS	Quadrupole mass spectrometer
RAIMS	Respiratory acoustic impedance measurement system
RBC	Red blood cell (erythrocyte)
RC	Resistance-capacitance
RE	Reference electrode
RF	Radio frequency
RMS (or rms)	Root mean square
RNAi	RNA interference
RPOX	Reflectance pulse oximetry
RTD	Resistance temperature detector
RV	Residual volume of lungs
SAMHSA	The (U.S.) Substance Abuse and Mental Health Services Administration
SCC	Short-circuit current
siRNA	Small interfering RNA
[SG]	Salivary glucose concentration
SKY	Spectral karyotyping of a nucleic acid
SLD	Superluminescent diode
SMU	Single motor unit
SPECT	Single-photon emission tomography
SPL	Sound pressure level
SPP	Surface plasmon polariton(s)
SPR	Surface plasmon resonance
SQUID	Superconducting quantum interference device
SRS	Stimulated Raman spectroscopy
ssDNA	Single-stranded DNA
STI	Sexually transmitted infection
SUS	Scanning ultrasound
tDCS	Transient DC (brain) stimulation
TEM	Transverse electromagnetic (waves)
Tempco	Temperature coefficient
THC	Tetrahydrocannabinol
THz	TeraHertz (1 THz = 10^{12} Hz)
TIR	Transcutaneous infrared
T_m	Melting (denaturing) temperature of a nucleic acid strand (Hydrogen bonds break)
TMS	Transcranial magnetic stimulation
tracrRNA	Transactivating CRISPR RNA
TUS	Therapeutic ultrasound
TV	Tidal volume
US	Ultrasound
VCCS	Voltage-controlled current source
VLF	Very low-frequency AC band (3–30 kHz)
VOC	Volatile organic compound
Wb	Weber: SI unit of magnetic flux. 1 Wb/m^2 = 1 T flux density (B)
0XD	Zero crossing detector

1 Introduction to Noninvasive Medical Measurements

1.1 DEFINITIONS OF NONINVASIVE, MINIMALLY INVASIVE, AND INVASIVE MEDICAL MEASUREMENTS

In this chapter, let us attempt to reach consensus about what we mean by noninvasive (NI) medical measurements. Any measurement system that does not physically breach the skin, or enter the body deeply through an external orifice is truly NI. Thus, the measurement of body temperature with a thermometer in the mouth, rectum, or ear canal is considered NI, as is the use of an otoscope to examine the outer surface of the eardrum. Similarly, the use of the ophthalmoscope and slit lamp which shine light in the eyes to examine the retina and the cornea and lens, respectively, is considered NI procedures. The transduction of sounds from the body surface (from the heart, breath, otoacoustic emissions, joint sounds, etc.) is truly NI, as is the recording of electric potentials on the skin from internal sources such as the heart (ECG), skeletal muscles (EMG), brain (EEG), etc. Medical imaging techniques such as x-ray, x-ray tomography (CAT scan), ultrasound, magnetic resonance imaging (MRI), positron emission tomography (PET), etc. are NI; they do involve the input of energetic radiation into the body, however, which generally carries low risk when proper energy levels and doses are observed.

Much can be learned from blood samples; namely, ion concentrations, red blood cell density, white blood cell density, the concentrations of certain hormones, antibodies, cholesterol, drug concentrations, DNA type, pathogens, chemical indicators of chronic diseases, etc. The drawing of small blood sample, say <1 cm^3, from a superficial vein by a needle and syringe or a lancet is considered to be a *minimally invasive procedure,* requiring sterile technique.

Endoscopy is a technique for visualizing tissues deep within the body yet topologically on the outer surface of the body. An example is bronchoscopy, where a bronchoscope is inserted through the mouth and larynx, into the trachea and bronchial tubes of the lungs to permit visualization of their surfaces and the surfaces inside larger alveoli. Another endoscope is the cystoscope which is inserted into the urethra to inspect the ureter, the prostate, and the inside of the bladder. Many other types also exist (Section 2.3). As a rule, endoscopes require sterile technique, and in most cases, local or general anesthesia; I consider them to be *moderately invasive instruments,* and *endoscopies moderately invasive procedures.*

Some endoscopes are used *invasively,* such as laparoscopes, which are inserted into the abdomen through a small incision in the wall of the abdomen, chest, or back. They are used to examine the *outsides* of the *internal* organs (bladder, gall bladder, intestines, kidneys, liver, lungs, spine, spleen, uterus, etc.) for tumors, infections, damage from trauma, etc. Another *invasive procedure*, for example, is cardiac catheterization with a fiber optic endoscope in order to view heart valves.

One can argue that there are fuzzy classification boundaries separating NI, minimally invasive, moderately invasive, and invasive diagnostic procedures. Anyone who has undergone a colonoscopy or proctoscopy may be quick to argue that they are more invasive than minimally invasive diagnostic procedures, considering the preparation, medication (analgesia or anesthesia), and discomfort involved. Thus, we argue that invasiveness should be assessed on a four-level (two-bit) scale, that is, levels 0–3.

This text is about the instruments and measurement systems used in making modern, noninvasive medical diagnoses (NIMDs). Some of the instruments and systems described are well-established, Food and Drug Administration (FDA)-approved systems; others are prototype systems that eventually may prove safe, medically and cost-effective. It is important for the reader to know where the field of NI diagnostic instrumentation is headed, as well as its present status. Its evolution is rapid, fueled by the advances in information processing and storage, as well as in the fields including photonics, molecular biology, and medical physics.

Throughout the history of medicine, up to the end of the nineteenth century, most medical diagnoses were necessarily NI. The physician used his or her eyes to observe skin lesions, and inflammation in the nose, throat, gums, ears, and skin. Tactile senses in the physician's hands were used to feel skin temperature, edema, swelling due to infection, lumps under the skin, etc. The physician's ear was used to listen to breath, bowel, and heart sounds. The odors of infection was sensed by the physician's nose. Exploratory surgery was seldom done because of the risk of shock due to pain and blood loss, and danger of infection.

Today, considerable emphasis is on the use of NI diagnosis in health maintenance and emergency medicine. Most of it can be carried out on an outpatient basis, and carries little risk of infection or complications which would add to the cost the patient's health maintenance organization (HMO) must pay. On the other hand, certain NI instruments, such as the various medical imaging systems, are very expensive to build and maintain and their use fee is commensurately large. Indeed, NI diagnostic procedures, including imaging systems, have been accused of driving up the cost of health maintenance and care. The effective but simple NI, level 0 instruments such as the electrocardiograph, the spirometer, and the slit lamp and their use certainly are not culprits in this respect. The advantage of being able to see tumors in the middle of soft tissues such as the brain, lungs, liver, spleen, and breasts will continue to drive the need to improve the resolution of expensive imaging systems, and to ensure their use where indicated.

1.2 MODALITIES OF NI INSTRUMENTATION

NI medical instruments can be broadly classified between those passive systems that put *no energy* into the body, and those that input some form of radiation energy, for example, microwaves, visible and UV light, x-rays, γ-rays, sound and ultrasound, and measure what energy is either absorbed, reflected, or transmitted at different wavelengths or frequencies. Among the purely passive systems, we have the well-known electrical measurements based on active nerve and/or muscle membranes. These include time-varying electrical potentials recorded from the skin surface from the heart (ECG), brain (EEG), muscles (EMG), ears (electrocochleogram [ECocG]), and eyes (EOG and ERG). Sounds from the body's interior can also be recorded from the skin surface, including sounds from the heart valves, pericardium (friction rub), blood vessels (bruit), lungs, bronchial system, pleural cavity, eardrums (spontaneous otoacoustic emissions), joints, etc. Body temperature can be sensed from the infrared radiation from the eardrum, or by physically measuring the temperature of the saliva and tissues under the tongue, or the temperature in the rectum by a liquid-in-glass thermometer, or a thermometer based on a thermistor or platinum resistance element (resistance temperature detector [RTD]). Tissue oxygen and carbon dioxide partial pressures (pO_2 and pCO_2) can be measured transcutaneously with special chemical electrodes. The only energy put in by endoscopes is white light required to visualize or photograph the tissue being inspected. Blood pressure can be measured noninvasively by Korotkoff sounds emitted by the brachial artery as the pneumatic pressure in a sphygmomanometer cuff is slowly reduced, allowing blood to surge into an artery.

Just about every other physiological modality that can be measured noninvasively requires some small input of energy. An important class of NI imaging systems uses pulsed ultrasonic energy. The energy level of the input ultrasound is made low enough to avoid tissue-destroying cavitation or heating. Other NI, nonimaging, diagnostic systems that use continuous-wave (CW) ultrasound include Doppler blood velocity probes and Doppler probes used to sense the fetal heartbeat or detect aneurisms.

Electromagnetic radiation includes radio-frequency electromagnetic waves, THz waves, infrared (IR), visible, and ultraviolet, as well as x-rays and gamma rays (Figure 1.1). The photons from UV radiation, x-, and gamma rays have sufficient photon energy (hν) to knock atomic electrons out of their inner orbits and rupture certain molecular bonds, causing DNA mutations, etc.; UVB, x-, and gamma rays are called *ionizing radiations* because of the potential destruction they can cause to biomolecules as the result of ionization of water and other molecules. Thus, the use of NI instruments that emit ionizing radiation is not without some small health risk. UVB photons do not penetrate the skin deeply; hence, UV damage to skin can include reddening (burns) and the initiation of various types of skin cancers. The corneas and lenses of eyes given excessive UVB radiation can develop cataracts. X- and gamma ray photons, on the other hand, can penetrate the body deeply, causing cell damage in the organs. A high-energy x-ray photon can directly damage a DNA molecule, leading to a cellular mutation if not internally repaired by the cell. If a photon-dislodged electron strikes a water molecule, it can create a *free radical*. The estimated lifetime of a free radical is ~10 μs, which means it can drift and encounter a DNA molecule, producing indirect damage as stable molecular configurations are restored. Note that we are mostly concerned with electromagnetic ionizing radiations in this text. Certain radioisotopes used in medical imaging and in cancer therapy emit energetic *alpha particles* (He nuclei), *beta particles* (electrons), or *neutrons*. These energetic particles can also generate free radicals and cause DNA damage, and initiate cell death by apoptosis.

X-ray machines of all sorts, bone densitometers, and CAT and PET scanners thus carry a small risk of inducing cancer, including leukemia, in the patient. However, most healthy persons absorb far more ionizing radiation in the form of 5.5 MeV alpha particles from the radioactive breakdown of inhaled, naturally occurring, *radon gas* (e.g., ^{222}Rn) than they do from x-rays. Note that

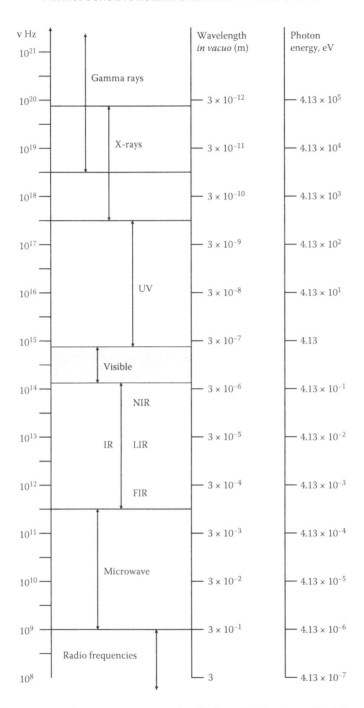

Figure 1.1 Electromagnetic spectrum ranges that find application in medical diagnosis. Photon energies in electron volts at a given wavelength are given in the right-hand column.

36 radioisotopes of ^{222}Rn have been characterized, with atomic masses ranging from 193 to 228. ^{210}Pb is formed from the decay of ^{222}Rn.

Other NI instrumentation systems such as impedance plethysmographs, pass low levels (in the microamp range) of alternating current (AC) in the frequency range from 25 to 100 kHz through the tissues being studied. The input of this current is apparently without risk; it is way below the level that will affect the heart, and there is no heating effect on the deep tissues.

1.3 CHAPTER SUMMARY

In this chapter, I have made the distinction between truly NI, minimally invasive, and invasive diagnostic instruments and procedures. NI instruments and procedures are important because most can be done in a doctor's office, or in a clinic to an outpatient. There are generally few side effects, and minimum risk from infection or other complications.

The following 17 chapters are about the design and application of the instruments used in NIMDs; their contents are outlined in the *Preface*. Certain signal processing algorithms, such as time–frequency analysis, are also described because of their importance in helping the diagnostician do his or her job. In *Chapter 17*, I indulge in speculation about where the field of NI diagnosis is heading, considering the on-going contributions from genetics, immunology, molecular biology, and biophotonics.

Chapter 18 treats NI therapies. That is, means of accelerating healing by externally applied electric currents (AC and direct current [DC]), externally applied electric and magnetic fields, externally applied ultrasound energy, externally applied aids to breathing (CPAP, IPAP), and even hearing aids.

2 Visual Inspection of Tissues with Certain Endoscopes and Other Optical Devices

2.1 INTRODUCTION

The oldest form of medical diagnosis is the direct visual observation of the patient's skin, tongue, gums, eyes, ears, and mucous membranes. Healthcare providers in the millennia before antibiotics were adept at diagnosing local infections, such as those resulting from cuts, abrasions, contusions (bruises), puncture wounds, etc., as well as bacterial skin infections called *carbuncles* (or *furuncles*) and *boils*. Swelling, skin color, and local heat are external signs of subcutaneous inflammation, which can be the result of bacterial infection, insect bites, or allergy. A fulminating tissue infection can be fatal if the pathogen spreads and attacks organs such as the heart, lungs, kidneys, or brain. A localized, or compartmented infection can produce pus, and in extreme cases, if the pathogen is anaerobic, gases can be produced including, but not limited to, H_2, N_2, and CH_4. Wound odors can come from anaerobic bacteria metabolizing necrotic tissues. Early physicians were adept at detecting sepsis in wounds from their gas odors (e.g., dimethyl sulfide [H_3CSCH_3], skatole [C_9H_9N], isovaleric acid [$(CH_3)_2CHCH_2CO_2H$], hydrogen sulfide [H_2S], cadaverine [$H_2N(CH_2)_5NH_2$], and putrescine [$H_2N(CH_2)_4NH_2$] gases). Breath sounds on inhalation, exhalation, or both were also important signs of respiratory infections and asthma.

Malignant melanoma skin lesions are identified by size, color, and texture. Touching and inspecting the skin allows an examiner to detect edema (pitting or nonpitting), and evaluate the general health of the peripheral circulation by the speed of capillary refill (return of skin color on removal of local pressure). Changes in skin and eye color (pallor, the yellowing of jaundice) are also diagnostic signs. Eye whites become yellowish in jaundice. The color of the skin on the palms of the hands is also a sign of liver health. Elevated skin temperature (as sensed by the examiner's hand) can indicate a fever; if the skin is cold and wet (diaphoretic), it may indicate shock.

General aspects of certain tissues are also diagnostic. A baggy face and puffy eyelids, indicative of nonpitting edema, can be the result of extreme hypothyroidism; the same swollen face can be the result of the systemic administration of steroids such as prednisone to control implant tissue rejection. Bulging eyes (exophthalmic condition) can be the result of hyperthyroidism, or severe meningitis. An abdomen swollen with fluid (*ascites*) can be a sign of *congestive heart failure*, as can swollen ankles, or be a result from a severe blood protein unbalance (low-serum oncotic pressure caused by hypoalbuminemia, and high-portal venous pressure) due to liver damage (e.g., from *alcoholic cirrhosis* or *hepatitis infection*). The color of the lips, gums, and tissues around the eyeballs, if pale, can indicate anemia; if blue, cyanosis; if deep red, CO poisoning. The same applies for the tissue under the fingernails and the fingertips.

Fortunately, a given medical condition is generally accompanied by several symptoms which often can lead to a fairly certain diagnosis. On the other hand, several medical conditions can share a symptom, making diagnosis more difficult. Perhaps today, many physicians pay less attention to outward signs than they do to blood and urine chemo-analyses, and various imaging readouts to make diagnoses. Still, direct observation is the place to begin any diagnosis. The following sections describe various instrumental enhancements for direct observation of various tissues. Note that certain endoscopic procedures are moderately invasive, and require sterile technique and sedation.

2.2 OPHTHALMOSCOPES, SLIT LAMPS, AND OTOSCOPES

2.2.1 Ophthalmoscopes

The ophthalmoscope is a simple optical instrument that permits the NI visualization of the front surface of the eye's retina (also known as the *fundus*), showing blood vessels, general color, surface smoothness, any tears or detachments, and the condition of the macula, etc. These features are normally viewed by the eye of the examining ophthalmologist, and in modern instruments can also be photographed or recorded as digital color images.

The progenitor of the modern, handheld ophthalmoscope was invented in 1851 by Herrmann von Helmholtz. von Helmholtz appreciated the need for the viewer's line of sight to be collinear with the illuminating beam from the light source. von Helmholtz made a primitive half-silvered mirror from four, thin, glass microscope slides stacked together. This design allowed the illumination source to be at right angles to the gaze axis of the examiner and patient's eyes (Keeler 2015). Within a year, in order to avoid the intensity losses inherent in partially reflective mirrors, a fully silvered mirror with a hole in it was used to direct the illumination source

5

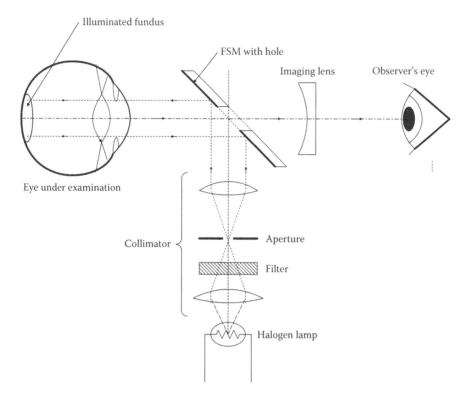

Figure 2.1 Schematic of the optical design of an ophthalmoscope. (Housing not shown.)

through the cornea and lens to the retina. The hole allowed the clinician an unobstructed view of the illuminated fundus. An *accessory lens* was placed in the viewer's sight path to bring the fundus into clear focus, regardless of the combined optical power of the eye's lens and cornea (Figure 2.1).

A modern ophthalmoscope uses a high-intensity halogen lamp as a light source; often certain colored filters are used over the illumination source to enhance the visibility of features of the fundus. The accessory viewing lens is selected by a turret or wheel. For example, the Neitz model BXα halogen ophthalmoscope has lenses with corrective powers ranging from +36 to −36 diopters, in 1-D steps; two lens wheels are used (Neitz Instruments Co., Ltd.). Although the optics of the ophthalmoscope are relatively simple, its design has been steadily improved since its invention 164 years ago. The current state of the art is the binocular ophthalmoscope in which the observer uses both eyes to visualize the fundus.

The *scanning laser ophthalmoscope* (SLO) and the confocal SLO (CSLO) have eliminated the need for direct human observation of the fundus. By rapidly scanning a finely focused, low-power laser beam over the retina in a precise pattern and collecting the backscattered light with a photosensor, it is possible to electronically image the fundus in good detail that is only limited by the optics of the eye under study (cornea, lens, and vitreous humor) (Webb et al. 1987, van de Velde 2006, Lima et al. 2011, Fromow-Guerra 2012, Bennett 2013, LaRocca et al. 2013).

In the CSLO, a pinhole lens is placed in front of the photodiode on a conjugate plane to the retina. Light reflected from different focal planes in the retina is selected by moving the pinhole, allowing tomographic (slice) images of the retina to be constructed over small areas. Using a 785 nm wavelength diode laser source and a novel, double-Gaussian fitting algorithm, it was possible to resolve 32 slices of the retina, 100 μm thick (Vieira et al. 1999). Very detailed, albeit monochrome, 3-D pictures of the optic disk in normal patients and those with macular edema were obtained. True color was sacrificed for fine textural detail. The use of near-infrared (NIR) light minimizes scatter in cloudy media, and lenses with beginning cataracts. SLO and CSLO make it possible to detect the signs of early age-related macular degeneration (ARMD), choroidal neoplasms, and retinas damaged by glaucoma (Kelley et al. 1997). The effectiveness of CSLO in diagnosing glaucoma has been evaluated by Yaghoubi et al. (2015).

One of the visible signs of ARMD is the presence of *drusen* in the retina. According to Cavallerano et al. (1994):

Drusen are yellow to yellowish white nodular deposits found in the deeper layers of the retina. Along with pigmentary abnormalities, drusen are often the earliest ophthalmoscopic signs of aging in the retina. Visual acuity may be normal at this stage. Drusen alone are not enough to satisfy the definition of ARMD when vision is normal. Several types of drusen have been described. The lesions are categorized by size, confluence, uniformity and sharpness of borders. Some form of drusen are found in the macular area in 50%–95% of persons over age 70. Among persons with drusen, 10%–15% may eventually develop exudative manifestations of ARMD.

Figure 2.2 illustrates a typical fundus showing macular drusen bodies. About 15% of the cases of ARMD are of the "wet" type, in which there is abnormal proliferation of leaky retinal blood vessels. These leaky vessels damage the macula and fovea (responsible for central, high-resolution, color vision), and are responsible for 90% of ARMD vision loss (Rowell 2000).

The reader will appreciate the tremendous diversity in the vascular anatomy of the fundus. Indeed, the unique, "retinal print" is used for biometric identification of individuals in security applications. (The retinal print has now been largely replaced by the use of the random patterns inherent in the iris for biometric identification purposes. The iris pattern is easier to acquire optically.) Thus, the use of the ophthalmoscope to detect retinal pathologies is not as simple as examining a chest x-ray for a broken rib. There is randomness and order in each fundus, and the challenge is to find features that are signs of disease in the image. Accordingly, there are many "fundus atlases" in print and online to guide diagnosis by example.

The modern, fixed-base, office ophthalmoscope allows the examining optometrist or ophthalmologist to inspect a fundus with binocular vision using a variety of light source wavelengths. The same instrument also allows the capture of colored digital images, or colored positive film images for archival purposes.

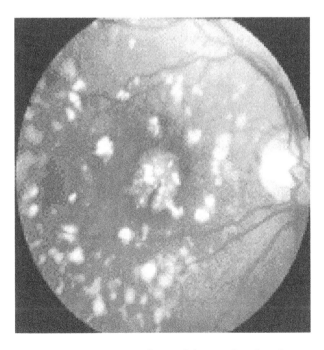

Figure 2.2 Ophthalmoscope camera image of retinal drusen. In color, drusen appear yellowish against the red retinal background. The fovea, containing drusen, is at the center of the image. The optic nerve entry is the light area on the right. (Image from Northrop, R.B. 2002. *Noninvasive Instrumentation and Measurement in Medical Diagnosis*. CRC Press, Boca Raton, FL. ISBN: 0-8493-0961-1.)

2.2.2 Slit Lamps

We have seen that the ophthalmoscope permits visualization of the features of inner surface of the retina, including signs of ARMD, damage from diabetes, and mechanical damage from trauma. The *slit lamp,* on the other hand, allows examination of the *optical structures of the eye* for pathologies, damage, and foreign objects, including the cornea, the lens, the iris, and the vitreous body. The components of a slit lamp consist of a long working distance, binocular microscope, normally directed in the horizontal plane at the eye under study. The microscope can be of the zoom type, giving magnification in the range of 5× to ~50×. The (azimuth) angle of the microscope axis with respect to the eye's gaze axis can be varied in the horizontal plane. The slit lamp also has a flexible light source based on a high-intensity halogen lamp. The lamp filament is projected onto a slit (adjustable in width, height, and angle with the vertical). The slit's image is in turn, directed to the desired part of the eye by a focusing lens. A cobalt blue filter can be inserted into the slit beam (pass peak at ~400 nm) to selectively excite the 550 nm green fluorescence of the vital stain, *fluorescein sodium.* Fluorescein is used to identify corneal abrasions, cuts, etc. where it selectively concentrates. A longwave-pass filter is used over the microscope objective to cut the blue light and to improve contrast of the fluorescent images.

The microscope and slit illuminator systems of a slit lamp are coupled around a common center of rotation so that the microscope will always be focused where the slit beam is projected. The slit source and microscope can also be independently directed for applications such as viewing sclerotic scatter in the cornea. The slit lamp must also have a head and chin rest to restrain the patient's head (and eyes) from moving during observation. Some slit lamps allow the slit source beam to be moved out of the horizontal plane; that is, be directed at the eye from above or below the horizontal plane (Riley 2007). To see a comprehensive summary of diagnostic procedures that can be done with a slit lamp, visit the NorthShore (2015) web site. Figure 2.3 illustrates schematically a plan (top) view of the basic components of a slit lamp.

2.2.3 Otoscopes

The otoscope allows the examining physician to observe the condition of the outer surface of the eardrum and the lining of the external auditory canal. Like the basic ophthalmoscope, it is a handheld instrument viewed by one eye of the clinician. Figure 2.4a shows a cross-sectional view of a conventional otoscope. A miniature, high-intensity halogen lamp with a built-in lens is used as the source, and a convex (magnifying) lens is used by the operator to enlarge the view of the eardrum. The earpieces are disposable, and come in various sizes to fit the patient's ear canal diameter. In Figure 2.4b, we see an otoscope with coaxial illumination (analogous to an ophthalmoscope); the rays from the halogen lamp are collected by a concave mirror and focused on the eardrum by

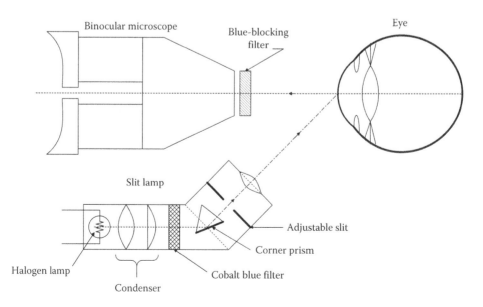

Figure 2.3 Schematic top view of the optics of a slit lamp.

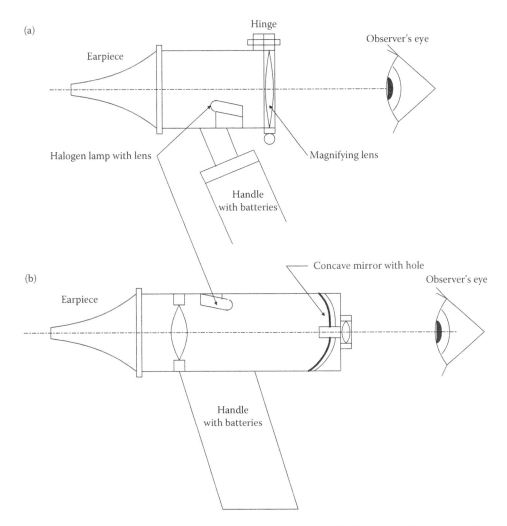

Figure 2.4 (a) Cutaway side view of a conventional otoscope. (b) Cutaway side view of a direct-view otoscope of the Hotchkiss type.

lens L_1. L_1 and L_2 form a microscope, enlarging the normally illuminated object. Such a coaxial illumination system is used in the Hotchkiss™ otoscope, as described on the Preferred Products web site brochure, accessed 3/18/16 at: www.preferredproduct.com/hotchkiss-otoscope/

An otoscope can be used to locate impacted *cerumen* (earwax) in the ear canal, as well as foreign objects (insects, Q-tip heads, beans, etc.). The otoscope is also useful in diagnosing middle ear infection through eardrum color. Convexity can mean fluid pressure in the middle ear, and of course tears and perforations can signify trauma and/or infection. The coaxial design of the Hotchkiss otoscope is particularly well suited for observation of ear canal procedures as they are done (e.g., removing cerumen or foreign objects).

Many otoscopes are easily converted to ophthalmoscopes. The handle holds the batteries, switch, and rheostat to control the lamp brightness, and has a universal bayonet-type fitting that enables either a conventional otoscope head or an ophthalmoscope to be powered.

2.3 ENDOSCOPES

An endoscope is an optical instrument that allows a physician to visually inspect the surfaces of certain body organs, internal cavities and tubes, or the surfaces of joints (Artyomov et al. 2007). Some endoscopes permit the surgeon to collect biopsies, such as colon polyps. Endoscopy is a minimally invasive (or invasive) procedure which requires sterile technique, and in most cases local or general anesthesia (Kimura 2010).

There are two major categories of endoscope: the rigid (straight tube) and the flexible (fiber optic [FO] bundle) type. The following "-scopys" are common to modern medical practice:

Arthroscopy: Invasive examination of the surface of joints for diagnosis and treatment of injury or joint diseases.

Bronchoscopy: Examination of the trachea and bronchial tubes of the lungs to reveal foreign objects, lesions, infections, cancer, tuberculosis, alveolitis, etc., and guide the taking of biopsy samples.

Colonoscopy: Examination of the interior of the large intestine to reveal polyps, diverticula, cancer, lesions, etc. Also, guide the taking of biopsy samples (Wayne et al. 2003, Olympus 2015).

Colposcopy: Visualization of the lining of the vagina and the cervix to detect infection, lesions, cancer, etc., also biopsies.

Cystoscopy: The endoscope is inserted through the urethra to examine the urethra, bladder, and prostate (men) for lesions, infection, and cancer.

Endoscopic retrograde cholangio-pancreatography (*ERCP*): A highly invasive procedure used to examine the liver's biliary tree, the gallbladder, the pancreatic duct, etc. to check for stones, lesions, cancer, etc.

Esophogastroduodenoscopy aka gastroscopy (*EGD*): Invasive examination of the upper GI tract; the esophagus, stomach, pyloric valve to reveal ulcers, hemorrhage, hiatal hernia, duodenal ulcers, cancers, etc.

Laparoscopy: Visualization of the exterior of abdominal organs such as the uterus, ovaries, bladder, intestines, pancreas, liver, etc. The laparascope is inserted through a small incision in the abdomen; the abdomen is inflated with sterile CO_2 gas for better visualization. (Perhaps helium would be a better gas to use for abdominal inflation because it is absorbed rapidly by tissues and body fluids, and is chemically inert [Northrop 1994].)

Laryngoscopy: Examination of the larynx.

Proctoscopy: Examination of the rectum and sigmoid colon (see *Colonoscopy*).

Thorascopy: A flexible FO endoscope is inserted invasively between the ribs to view the pleural cavity between the outer wall of the lungs and the inner wall of the chest in this invasive procedure. The pericardium can also be visualized. Inflating gas is used for better visual resolution. Thorascopy is used to detect infections, cancer, and pneumothorax (a ruptured alveolus allows breathed air to enter the pleural cavity, which may collapse a lung).

In the early 1900s, endoscopes were lighted with incandescent lamps, and had straight tubes. Although crude by today's standards, straight-tube endoscopes permitted the introduction of hand-manipulated instruments to take biopsies and to remove foreign objects, polyps, etc. Magnifying lenses could be used to see tissue details. Semiflexible *gastroscopes* were introduced in the 1930s which used multiple, cylindrical rod lenses. The optical quality of their images was of low quality. The first FO endoscope was developed at the University of Michigan in 1957 by Basil Hirschowitz; their widespread use began in the 1960s (Imaginis 2015). More recently, miniature, digital, charge-coupled device (CCD) cameras have been adapted to both straight tube and FO endoscopes. In some models, the CCD camera is located at the tip of the endoscope, and is optically coupled to the object by a short length of coherent FO cable. Illumination light is coupled to the tip of the endoscope by a coherent FO cable from a 150–300 W xenon light source. Some CCD cameras use an automatic exposure control to preserve image contrast over a wide range of illumination conditions.

Modern endoscopes now use real-time video recording. An example is the Pentax EC-3490TLi Video Colonoscope. This instrument features a 210° short turn radius at the tip for retroflex scope positioning that provides visualization and accessibility of the distal side of colon folds and flexures. The EC-3490TLi has a working length of 1700 mm, a 140° angle of view, an optical focal range of 3–100 mm, tip angle extremes of: up/down = 210°/180°, right/left = 160°/160°, outer diameter = 11.6 mm, and a forward water jet (Pentax Medical 2015).

Ultrathin FO endoscopes called *needlescopes* have diameters of 0.2–0.5 mm that contain 2000–6000 pixels. Such needlescopes have been inserted into mammary glands to try to detect breast cancer at early stages, and also inserted into the eye to view the back side of the iris, and the posterior chamber. They also have been used to visualize heart valves in action, and plaque in coronary arteries (Nanoptics 2000).

A coherent FO bundle is effectively a spatial sampling array that operates on the object. Because each optical fiber has an acceptance cone for input rays, a spatial low-pass filter is introduced in series with the 2-D spatial sampler. Generally, the smaller the diameter of individual optical fibers, the higher the spatial resolution, with some limits. According to Nanoptics (2000):

> For a [coherent] fiber optics bundle, the resolution can be defined by about half a line pair per fiber core. For example, if the individual fiber diameter is 50 μm, cores could resolve 10 line pairs per millimeter (10 lp/mm). Generally, the smaller the fiber core diameter, the greater the image resolution in a unit area of image fiber bundle. However, there are some phenomena which lead to reduced resolution such as cross-talk between individual [adjacent] fibers, and leaky rays from individual fiber[s]. These phenomena may deteriorate image quality and can be the main reason for reduction in spatial resolution. These phenomena become more important as the core diameter is increased. Therefore, the optimum core diameter for a given desired resolution depends on parameters such as cladding thickness, refractive index of the core and cladding and the wavelength of the incident ray.

The *packing fraction* of a FO bundle is defined as the total FO core surface area divided by the total area of optical fibers (core plus cladding). The packing fraction is proportional to the light gathering efficiency of the FO bundle because all light entering the cladding is lost. In practice, the minimum cladding thickness is about 1 μm. Thus, if the core diameter is 4 μm, the fiber end area is $\pi(3 \, \mu m)^2 = 28.27 \, \mu m^2$, and the core area is $\pi (2 \, \mu m)^2 = 12.57 \, \mu m^2$. Thus, the packing fraction is: $12.57/28.27 = 0.445$.

Another optical engineering trade-off in the design of FO endoscopes with CCD cameras involves matching the discrete fiber outputs to the discrete pixel inputs of the CCD chip. Because of optical interference effects between adjacent optical fibers, fiber outputs can be viewed by individual CCD pixel sensors, and a phenomenon known as *Moiré patterning* can occur in the received image. A wave of colors and lines flows through the image as the endoscope is moved. Often the Moiré effect can be suppressed by defocusing the CCD camera and rotating it with respect to the FO bundle, or by the use of a special *anti-Moiré filter* between the camera and the end of the FO bundle.

An important figure of merit for any imaging system is its *modulation transfer function* (MTF), S(u), also called its *contrast transfer function*. The MTF concept can be applied to any component of, or an entire imaging system; x-ray systems, endoscopes, CCD cameras, film, etc. can all be characterized by an MTF. The MTF is a normalized spatial sinusoidal frequency response comparing the amplitude response of the image to a spatial sinusoidal (+dc) object. In the x-dimension, the object's sinusoidal intensity is given by

$$I(x) = (I_o/2)[1 + \cos(2\pi ux)], \tag{2.1}$$

where the maximum intensity is I_o and u is the spatial frequency in cycles/mm.

The dc component is required because light intensity is nonnegative. Figure 2.5 shows a gray-scale, approximate, spatial, (1-D) sinusoidal object pattern, and Figure 2.6a shows a graph

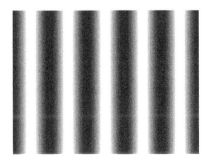

Figure 2.5 Photograph of an 8-bit, 1-D spatial sinewave MTF test pattern object for endoscopes, cameras, etc. (Image from Northrop, R.B. 2002. *Noninvasive Instrumentation and Measurement in Medical Diagnosis.* CRC Press, Boca Raton, FL. ISBN: 0-8493-0961-1.)

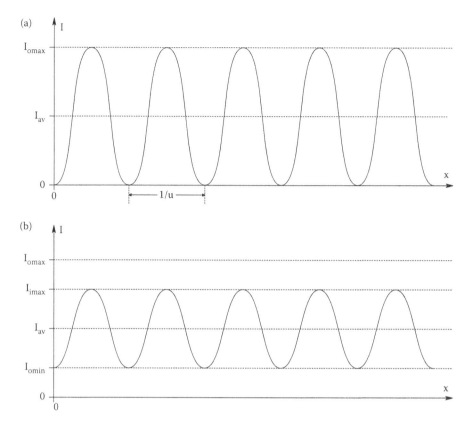

Figure 2.6 (a) Graph of the intensity in the x-direction of the test object of Figure 2.5. (b) A graph of the intensity of the image, given the test object as the image. Note that the average intensity is the same for both object and image, and there is no phase shift.

of the pattern's reflected intensity as a function of x. The object can also be characterized by its *contrast*, M_o.

$$M_o = \frac{I_{o\,max} - I_{o\,min}}{I_{o\,max} + I_{o\,min}},$$ (2.2)

where for maximum contrast, $I_{omin} \equiv 0$.

Figure 2.7 shows a typical 1-D sinusoidal image as processed by an optical system. A plot of the x-axis intensity of Figure 2.7 is shown in Figure 2.6b. Note that the average intensity is the same

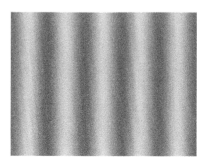

Figure 2.7 Simulated optical system's output (image), given the sinusoidal test object of Figure 2.5 as the input. Note that the spatial sinewave input is attenuated by the system's MTF. Peak contrast is also reduced. (Image from Northrop, R.B. 2002. *Noninvasive Instrumentation and Measurement in Medical Diagnosis*. CRC Press, Boca Raton, FL. ISBN: 0-8493-0961-1.)

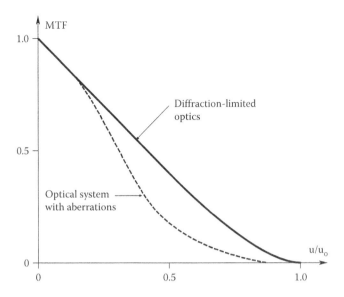

Figure 2.8 Examples of a modulation transfer function (MTF) of an ideal lens system (upper curve) and a nonideal imaging system (lower curve).

for both input and output graphs. Also note that the image contrast, M_i, is generally lower than the object contrast, M_o, especially at high-spatial frequencies. M_i is given by

$$M_i(u) = \frac{I_{i\,max} - I_{i\,min}}{I_{i\,max} - I_{i\,min}}. \tag{2.3}$$

The MTF of the optical system is defined by

$$S(u) \equiv \frac{M_i(\nu)}{M_o}. \tag{2.4}$$

The MTF response of an optical system at dc ($\nu = 0$) is generally 1 (or 100%), even though there may be a neutral density attenuation of the average intensity of the object. At very low-spatial frequencies (in radians/mm), the image contrast is basically that of the object. As the spatial frequency, ν, of the object is increased, the general spatial low-pass nature of diffraction-limited optics causes the image contrast to decrease, causing $S(\nu) \to 0$ as $\nu \to \infty$. Figure 2.8 illustrates the MTF of an ideal, diffraction-limited lens system along with the MTF of a practical imaging system. Note that high-spatial frequencies are lost in a practical imaging system from a variety of conditions, including the spectral distribution of the light, the system's numerical aperture, f-stop, the angle of the axis along which the test sine object is displayed, and nonlinear optical effects such as various aberrations, coma, astigmatism, distortion (barrel vs pincushion), and spatial sampling by packed optical fibers.

In many imaging systems, it is inconvenient to generate a sinusoidal (+dc) object; instead, a 1-D square wave object is used of the form:

$$I(x) = (I_o/2)\big[1 + SGN\{\sin(2\pi x/\lambda)\}\big] = I(x+\lambda). \tag{2.5}$$

This periodic object can be represented by the Fourier series:

$$I(x) = B_o + \sum_{n=1, n\,odd}^{\infty} A_n \sin(n\nu_o x), \tag{2.6}$$

where the *fundamental spatial frequency* in radians/mm is given by $\nu_o = 2\pi/\lambda$. B_o is the average value of the object's intensity, equal to $I_o/2$. The sine term (odd) Fourier series coefficients, A_n, are given by

$$A_n = (1/\pi)\int_{-\pi}^{\pi} I(x)\cos(n\nu_o x)d(\nu_o x). \tag{2.7}$$

13

For example, the third harmonic coefficient, A_3, can be calculated as

$$A_3 = (1/\pi)\int_0^\pi (I_o/2)\sin(3\nu_o x)d(\nu_o x) - (1/\pi)\int_\pi^{2\pi}(I_o/2)\sin(3\nu_o x)d(\nu_o x)$$

$$\downarrow$$

$$= (I_o/2)/(3\pi)\left\{[-\cos(3\nu_o x)]_0^\pi - [-\cos(3\nu_o x)]_\pi^{2\pi}\right\} = 4(I_o/2)/(3\pi). \tag{2.8}$$

Thus, the Fourier series for the square wave object can be written out in terms of its odd harmonics:

$$I(x) = (I_o/2) + [4(I_o/2)/\pi]\sin(\nu_o x) + [4(I_o/2)/(3\pi)]\sin(3\nu_o x)$$
$$+ [4(I_o/2)/(5\pi)]\sin(5\nu_o x) + \cdots. \tag{2.9}$$

The relation for the MTF (Equation 2.4) can still be used to characterize the optical system when a square wave object is used, but obviously the MTF derived is the result of the superposition of the responses to all of the harmonics making up the "sine" square wave. As the period of the spatial square wave object is made smaller, the optical image responds to fewer and fewer of the high-spatial harmonics; the image becomes a rounded square wave. At limiting spatial resolution, the optical system responds only to the dc + fundamental frequency term in the series, and the image is basically a low-contrast, intensity sine wave.

We have seen that endoscopes can be guided to and focused on specific tissues. They also can be used to guide the taking of tissue samples for biopsy (to determine whether certain cells are cancerous). In some endoscopes, tissue is actually cut off and sucked into the endoscope for collection. Another method is to dislodge the targeted cells by abrasion with a brush operated through the endoscope. The loose cells are then sucked into the end of the endoscope for collection and examination.

2.4 CCD AND CMOS ACTIVE PIXEL IMAGE SENSORS

2.4.1 CCD Image Sensors

In many medical imaging applications, the CCD camera or the complementary metal oxide semiconductor (CMOS) active pixel sensor chip have replaced photographic film, including x-ray film. CCD cameras come in various styles and sizes. Some CCD sensors are responsive to colored objects, others produce monochrome images. Color is of paramount interest in medical imaging applications because, in the case of endoscopy, the physician is looking for color changes indicating inflammation, infection, tumors, etc. When fluorescence techniques are used to detect tumors, bacterial infections, etc., the operator needs to see the colored, fluorescent object against an otherwise normal background.

Figure 2.9 illustrates a typical CCD camera chip. A rectangular array of photodiode photosensors forms the basic transducer matrix. Depending on application, there can be as few as 180 (H) × 120 (V) photodiodes in the CCD array, to well over 1280 (H) × 1024 (V) sensors. (The image aspect ratio

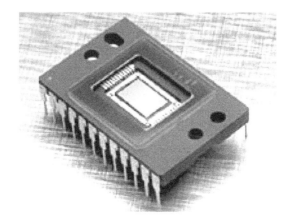

Figure 2.9 Basic Kodak CCD array IC. The photosensor matrix is on the inner rectangle. (Used with permission of Kodak.) (Image from Northrop, R.B. 2002. *Noninvasive Instrumentation and Measurement in Medical Diagnosis*. CRC Press, Boca Raton, FL. ISBN: 0-8493-0961-1.)

is generally 4:3 in camera chips.) For example, the 1999 Kodak KAF-3000CE CCD color camera chip has 3 megapixels arranged in a 2016 (H) × 1512 (V) array, a 6 MHz nominal clock rate, and a nominal readout time of 590 ms. The active sensor array is about 0.8″ × 0.584″, a 4:3 aspect ratio. The KAF-3000CE color CCD imager uses three color filters in a repeating pattern over adjacent pixels. The filters pass red, green, and blue light. The blue filter's transmission peaks at about 450 nm, and is about 100 nm wide. The green filter peaks at ~530 nm, and is ~100 nm wide. The red filter peaks at ~625 nm and is ~100 nm wide. How the outputs from the various color pixels are combined to create a color image on a digital monitor or cathode ray tube (CRT) display is beyond the scope of this section.

The 2010, super high-resolution, Kodak KAF-39000 color CCD image sensor chip has a 7216 (H) × 5412 (V) (39 M) array of square pixels, occupying a 49 mm (H) × 36.8 mm (V) photosensitive array with a 4:3 aspect ratio. The presence of antiblooming circuitry gives a 4 ms, 1000× saturation exposure protection. Maximum data rate is given as 24 MHz. The nominal readout time is given as 1077 ms. The KAF-39000 is the "Cadillac" of CCD imaging chips.

Light from the object is focused on the flat surface of the CCD array. Photons striking the *pn* junction of a pinned photodiode cause photoelectrons to be generated. These photoelectrons are collected in "storage wells" in the proximity of each of the illuminated *pn* junctions. The number of electrons in a given well is proportional to the light intensity times the *integration time* or *exposure* (generally ~1/60 s). At frame readout time, the charge in each photodiode's storage well is sequentially shifted out to a charge-to-voltage converter circuit by a system of vertical shift registers (one for each vertical column of sensors) that feed into a common, horizontal shift register. As each pixel's voltage is generated, it goes to a track and hold circuit that feeds an analog-to-digital converter (ADC). The ADC sequentially generates a 14 bit or 16 bit word for each pixel, for each frame. The CCD camera's digital output is fed to a computer for further image processing and image display generation. Figure 2.10 illustrates the organization of the CCD camera's shift

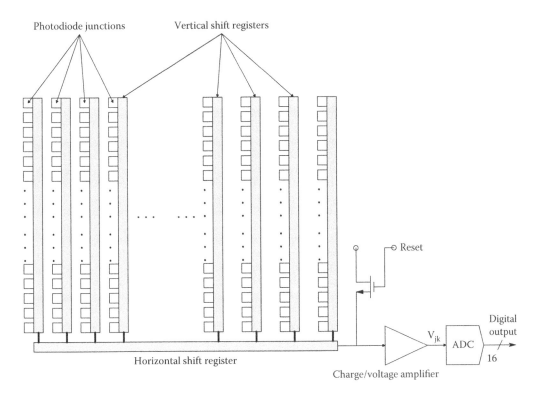

Figure 2.10 Functional organization of a basic CCD imaging IC. The photosensor elements are organized into N columns, each of M sensors. The sensors load the N analog, charge-coupled shift registers in parallel, then each shift register is sequentially downloaded in parallel, one pixel at a time, into the horizontal output shift register where each pixel is output, one at a time, until all N × M pixels have been digitized and downloaded to the image-processing and storage computer. Early designs had maximum frame rates of 30–60 fps (to download and digitize all N × M pixels).

registers and ADC. Not shown are the complex clock waveforms necessary to effect readout and reset the wells to zero charge at the beginning of the next frame cycle (Kodak 2015).

If the exposure (time × intensity) of a given *pn* junction is too large, a phenomenon known as *blooming* occurs. The overexposure causes so many photoelectrons to be produced that they exceed the capacity of the well to hold them, and they leak out into neighboring wells, corrupting the image. There are two ways to avoid blooming; one is to incorporate electron "gutters" that surround each well and carry off the electron overflow into the CCD chip design. This method costs about 30% of the effective pixel area and reduces both well depth and sensitivity. Another method to reduce blooming is to limit exposure, take multiple frames, and use signal averaging on the image to improve the signal-to-noise ratio.

CCD cameras are available as integrated packages with lenses, board-level do-it-yourself systems, and as chips. Some integrated CCD cameras are configured as 30 frame/s, TV cameras using the IEEE1394-1995 standard interface. Some, like the now obsolete Sony DFW-V300 camera, give VGA (640 × 480) resolution (8 bits/ch) with 30 fps and a 200 Mbps data transfer rate. A wide variety of CCD cameras and systems are made by: Adimec Electronic Imaging Inc., Basler AG, CohuHD, Edmund Optics Inc., Framos GmbH, Toshiba Imaging Systems, Crystal® (Cirrus Logic®), EG&G Reticon, Hamamatsu, Horiba Scientific, Matrix Vision GmbH, Spectral Instruments, Inc., Kodak, Optronics, Ophir-Spiricon LLC, Panasonic, Teledyne DALSA, QUINTUS®, Sony, etc. The *Photonics Buyer's Guide* lists 165 companies manufacturing and/or selling CCD cameras for biomedical applications. (See www.photonics.com/category.aspx?CatID=13650 Accessed 5/06/15.)

Some cameras are suitable for fluorescence microscopy, and all forms of endoscopy. The wide popularity and application of CCD imaging systems stems from their ability to produce high-resolution images almost instantaneously (e.g., in 1/30 s) in high-resolution digital format which can then be stored compactly in that form, and manipulated by various picture processing algorithms to improve picture quality and to extract image features.

One way of characterizing the resolution of CCD imaging systems is by the MTF, described in Section 2.3. Another way, analogous to transient testing of a temporal signal processing system, is to examine the camera's resolution of line pair objects, and pairs of dots. This is analogous to seeing how narrow and how close together two input pulses have to be before they cannot be resolved at an amplifier's output. The line and dot test objects are generally made black on white (or white on black), with 100% contrast.

2.4.2 CMOS Active Pixel Image Sensors

Active pixel image (API) sensors are replacing CCD imaging chips in many applications. They have the advantage of being less expensive than a CCD chip of equivalent resolution. They also have less pronounced "blooming effects" when an object source intensity has overloaded the sensor, causing the sensor to "bleed" the charge from the light source into other pixels. There is a major disadvantage of API sensors in capturing moving images: An API sensor typically captures a pixel row at a time within 16.7–20 ms; (depending on the refresh rate) this may result in a "rolling shutter" effect, where the image is skewed (tilted to the left or right), depending on relative camera-to-object movement. However, CCD image sensors capture the entire image at one sampling time as a single frame (all pixels). The CCD frame rate limits the dynamic performance of CCD movie chips. API chips also have reduced quantum efficiency because their active circuitry takes more area/pixel on the chip than that for a CCD device.

Each sensor pixel in an API device uses a *pinned photodiode* image photodetector (see Glossary), a floating diffusion, a transfer gate, reset gate, selection gate, and source-follower readout transistor; this is the so-called, *4T cell*. Figure 2.11 illustrates a schematic of the noble, active, three-transistor (3T) pixel circuit. When the reset transistor, Q_{rst}, is turned on, the photodiode is connected to the power supply, V_{RST}, clearing all integrated charge in the diode's "well." Since Q_{rst} is *n*-type, the pixel operates in soft reset. The source-follower readout transistor, Q_{sf}, acts as a buffer which allows the pixel voltage, V_p, to be sensed without removing the accumulated diode charge. Its power supply, V_{DD}, is typically tied to the power of the reset transistor. The select transistor, Q_{sel}, allows a single row of the pixel array to be read by the readout electronics. Note that by adding more metal oxide semiconductor (MOS) transistors, functions such as *global shutter* (as in CCD chips), as opposed to the more common *rolling shutter*, can be realized.

Color sensing using modified API technology is found in the Foveon X3 sensor invented by D. Merrill. In this device, three photodiodes are stacked on top of each other using planar fabrication techniques, each photodiode has its own 3T readout circuit. Each successive layer acts as an optical filter for the diode below it, shifting the spectrum of absorbed light in the successive layers.

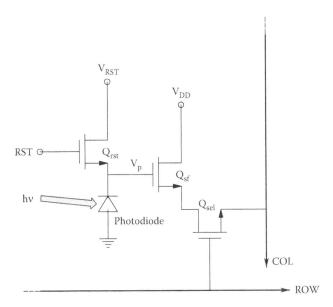

Figure 2.11 Schematic of a noble, three-transistor, active-pixel sensor circuit module. Note that other two- and four-transistor active-pixel sensor circuit designs exist.

By deconvolving the response of each layered detector, red, green, and blue signal components can be reconstructed (Foveon 2010). A recent Foveon X3 Fx17-78-F13 model image sensor chip has 14.1 Megapixels in an $2652 \times 1768 \times 3$ detector array in a 3:2 aspect ratio. The effective area is 20.7 mm $\times$ 13.8 mm. Full frame readout speed ≥ 5 fps, with capability to read out VGAx3 VPS video at 30 fps.

Another, solid approach to API color imaging is found in the use of the Bayer color filter mosaic arrays (Olympus 2012). Named after Kodak engineer Bryce Bayer, the Bayer filters consist of a rectangular array of tiny, colored polymer filters that cover every photodiode (pixel) in the array. Each photodiode in the array is covered with a red, green, or blue filter, giving it a broad-band wavelength sensitivity in red, green, or blue bands of the input spectrum, respectively. The total number of green filters in the array is equal to the number of red and blue filters combined. The emphasis on green filters is due to human visual response, which reaches a peak sensitivity in the 550 nm (green) wavelength region of the visible spectrum. Each colored plastic microlens in the Bayer filter has a square border, and covers not only the individual photodiode but also its associated three transistors (Olympus 2012).

2.5 NI DIAGNOSIS OF SKIN LESIONS

2.5.1 Introduction

Skin lesions, and lesions on the surface of internal tissues viewed with endoscopes are indicative disease conditions. In the case of skin lesions, the cause can be inflammation caused by a lodged foreign object, an infection, an insect bite, a benign growth, or a cancer. A lesion is detectable by eye because it generally involves some sort of swelling, a color change from the surrounding tissues, and it has a different texture. NI diagnosis of the type and cause of the lesion is the challenge. Diagnoses of lesions of this type are traditionally experience-based personal observations. In the case of skin melanomas, a physician with more than 10 years of experience can diagnose correctly ~80% of the time. The diagnostic accuracy rate for physicians with 3–5 years of diagnostic experience and 1–2 years of experience is 62% and 56%, respectively. As you will see, some work has been done to devise machine-vision-based expert systems to diagnose malignant melanomas versus benign nevi and other lesions (Grin et al. 1990).

2.5.2 Malignant Melanoma

Melanocytes are nondermal cells derived embryologically from the tissue matrix for the brain and medullary spine; they migrate during fetal development into the skin, where they settle within the epidermal layer. Melanocytes are characterized by the ability to produce the pigment melanin in response to UV radiation in order to protect the skin from sunburn damage (tanning). Melanocytes also respond to other biochemical signals (e.g., certain hormones).

There are three major categories of *skin cancer*: (1) *melanoma*, (2) *squamous cell carcinoma*, derived from malignant keratinocytes, and (3) *basal cell carcinoma*, derived from malignant basal keratinocytes (WebMD 2014). According to the Skin Cancer Foundation (2015), skin cancer of various types affects ~5 million persons in the United States per year. In 2006, 3.5 million cases were diagnosed in 2.2 million people. An estimated 73,870 new cases of invasive melanoma were diagnosed in the United States in 2015. An estimated 9940 persons died of melanoma in 2015. Melanoma accounts for less than 2% of skin cancer cases, but the vast majority of skin cancer deaths.

Friedman et al. (1985) set forth an "ABCD Rule of Visual Melanoma Diagnosis." This can be stated:

A = Asymmetry in lesion in 0, 1, or 2 axes.

B = Border irregularity. Abrupt cutoff of pigment pattern at the border in up to 8 segments.

C = Number of colors present (white, red, blue-gray, light and dark brown, black).

D = Number of dermatoscopic structural elements: Areas without any structures, network, branched streaks, dots, and globules.

The dermatoscopy score, S, is calculated from the single values for A, B, C, and D by the following formula: $S = 1.3A + 0.1B + 0.5C + 0.5D$. If S > 5.45, a melanoma can be highly suspected (specificity ~75%, sensitivity ~90%). Melanocytic lesions with S < 4.75 are probably benign nevi, while those with 4.74 < S < 5.45 are suspicious and should be removed and be checked histoscopically. *Example*: A = 2, B = 0, C = 3 (light brown, dark brown, black), D = 4 (network, branched streaks, structureless areas, globules); so S = 6.1.

The real challenge is accurate, differential diagnosis of melanomas from large moles (nevi), seborrheic keratosis lesions, etc. The gold standard is biopsy, where the lesion is surgically removed and its cells examined microscopically. Some workers have designed prototype, machine vision-based, computer programs to extract the common features of melanomas. The input device is generally a high-resolution, color, CCD camera focused on the lesion which is well illuminated with white light. One such system, described by Ercal et al. (1994), used a modified ABCD rule with a multilayered, *feed-forward neural network* trained using the generalized delta rule (back-propagation training algorithm) to obtain better than 80% differential success on digitized, real, melanoma images. The neural network was given the following 14 inputs: irregularity index (1), percent asymmetry (1), R, G, and B color variances (3), relative chromaticity (R, G, and B) (3), spherical color coordinates (L, α, β) (3), and (L*, a*, b*) color coordinates (3).

A review of detection methods for melanomas from digital color images can be found in the paper by Cila Herman (2012). Table 2.1 lists eight melanoma detection technologies described in her review.

Note that the first three available NI methods in Table 2.1 are *qualitative*, as is OCT, that is, they rely on the experience and knowledge of the examiner. However, quantitative data are available from the multispectral imaging in the frequency domain (MSIF), multispectral imaging in the spatial domain (MSIS), THzI, and IRSD methods. Herman (2012) concluded: "Every year, around 2.5–3 million skin lesions are evaluated in the US, and over 100,000 are diagnosed as melanoma. The objective is to develop automated diagnostic instruments for the [NI] screening of individual

Table 2.1: Summary of Melanoma Detection Methods

NI Method	Radiation Type	Technology Readiness
Digital photography	White light	Available
Dermoscopy	Polarized light	Available
Confocal scanning laser microscope	Near-IR	Available
MSIS-multispectral imaging in the spatial domain	Different wavelengths	Premarket approval
MSIF-multispectral imaging in the frequency domain	Different wavelengths	Research phase
THz imaging (ThzI)	THz EM radiation	Research phase
IR in spatial domain (IRSD)	Naturally emitted IR	Research phase
OCT-optical coherence tomography	Near-IR	Research phase

lesions and full-body screening, as well as sophisticated instruments that can provide dermatologists with fine detail regarding the structure of a lesion and staging information *in vivo.*"

Another approach to quantifying skin melanomas uses the optical reflectance characteristics at different wavelengths of the components of these lesions. Wallace et al. (2000) described a spectrophotometric approach to skin tumor classification. An area 1.5 mm in diameter was illuminated with broadband white light from a 75 W xenon arc lamp passed through 18 quartz fibers, each with a 200 μm core diameter and an NA = 0.2. Twelve quartz fibers in the same 30-fiber bundle traveled from the common object (skin) end to a monochromator with an output wavelength that could be scanned between 320 and 1100 nm. Wallace et al. measured reflectance spectra for normal skin, skin near the lesions, and various types of lesions, including malignant melanoma. The reflectance fraction, R(λ), was defined as:

$$R(\lambda) = \frac{S(\lambda) - D}{S_{ref}(\lambda) - D},$$ (2.10)

where S(λ) is the sensor current from the measured, reflected intensity at wavelength λ, D is the dark current, and $S_{ref}(\lambda)$ is the sensor output at λ when the probe is directed at a white calibration object.

The following number of spectra were obtained for the following types of pigmented skin lesions: malignant melanoma (15 cases, 55 spectra), melanoma *in situ* (9, 33), dysplastic nevus (11, 36), compound nevus (32, 98), seborrheic keratosis (14, 42), basal cell carcinoma (5, 15), and "other" (37, 120). In summary, following the application of a statistical classification rule, the authors claimed results comparable with an expert dermatologist; the sensitivity was 100%, and the specificity was 84.4%. *Note that lesion size, shape, and fine structure did not enter into the analysis of* Wallace et al. (2000).

2.5.3 Discussion

In the future, we expect to see improvements in automated detection of malignant melanoma lesions. Combining spectral analysis with the ABCD method may hold promise. Also it is known that the metabolisms of malignant melanocytes differ from normal cells, so it is possible that tagging malignant cells with fluorescent antibodies or radioactive metabolites may yield good results. Raman spectroscopy of the malignant cells is another approach that may be tried. (See Section 15.9 of this text for a description of some applications of Raman spectroscopy to medical diagnosis.)

2.6 CHAPTER SUMMARY

Diagnosis by direct visual inspection of tissue surfaces has been used by physicians since earliest times. The medical importance of a lesion lies in its color(s), swelling, size, texture, any exudate, etc. Such diagnosis is experience based; an inexperienced person can easily differentiate between a wart, a boil, or an impetago lesion, but diagnosis of suspect skin cancers by eye is not easy. Fortunately, there are comprehensive data bases available for various skin lesions and retinal pathologies. Visual inspection is generally just the beginning of diagnosis of skin cancer; initial impressions are verified by biopsy and DNA analysis.

We have seen that there are a number of optical aids that have been developed in the past 150 years or so for visual inspection of various body parts. The least invasive are the ophthalmoscope, slit lamp, and the otoscope. Recently, the development of FO endoscopes has permitted the inspection of the surfaces of internal mucous membranes that are contiguous with the body's surface. Such procedures are generally semi-invasive, because sterile technique is required, and the patient is generally given local or general anesthesia. It was discovered recently that there is differential fluorescence between normal and tumorous tissues, and near-UV light can be delivered by the endoscope to the target lesion. Other spectrophotometric techniques can also be used with endoscopes. For example, Raman spectroscopy may prove useful in differentiating between normal and cancerous tissues (Section 15.9).

Computers have made it easy for diagnosticians to download digital photographs of suspect lesions from color CCD cameras, and compare them with known figures in a database. CCD images have also expedited data storage to track the course of an infection or lesion being treated, giving an objective measure of progress.

3 Noninvasive Diagnosis Using Sounds Originating from within the Body

3.1 INTRODUCTION

3.1.1 Background

There are many endogenous sources of acoustic energy that have diagnostic significance. These include, but are not limited to, heart sounds (valves leaking, blood turbulence, pericardial friction rub), the lungs (rales, rhonchi, squeaks, crepitations, gurgling, pleural friction rub, silence), arteries (*bruit*, also known as turbulence sounds caused by a *stenosis*, or narrowing of a blood vessel), stomach and intestines (sounds of digestion, borborygmi), joints (arthritic friction rub, tendon snap, etc.), and the inner ear (*otoacoustic emissions* [OAEs]). The absence of sounds can also have diagnostic significance. Most of these sounds have acoustic spectral energy in the lowest range of human hearing as well as at audible low frequencies. Some of these sounds have origin in the elastic vibrations of dense connective tissues, or vibrations induced in elastic artery walls by blood turbulence, or vibrations induced by blood passing through small apertures. All such sound vibrations propagate through the body's tissues with losses, reflections, and refractions to the skin, in which perpendicular vibrations are introduced.

Stethoscopes and microphones respond to the sound waves that the vibrating skin radiates into the air. Surface vibrations can be measured directly by accelerometers on the skin surface, or laser Doppler sensors in which the Doppler shift in a laser beam reflected from the skin is detected. The Doppler frequency shift is proportional to skin velocity, so this signal must be integrated to obtain a signal proportional to vibration amplitude.

To make an effective, NI diagnosis, the medical professional listening with a stethoscope must: (1) be able to hear the tones of the sound and (2) have stored in his or her memory the acoustic patterns of many normal versus abnormal sounds for the source of sound being heard. As an alternative, the sound can be picked up electronically by an accelerometer, low-frequency microphone, or laser Doppler microphone, then amplified, digitized, processed by computer into a *time–frequency spectrogram* (TFS) which can be compared visually to normal and pathological exemplar spectrograms stored in the computer's memory.

3.1.2 Stethoscopes

Aside from the white lab coat, probably the symbol the public associates most with physicians and nurses is the stethoscope worn around the neck. The modern acoustic stethoscope has evolved from its original format invented in 1816 by the French physician R.T.H. Laennec. Laennec invented the stethoscope to improve the perception of endogenous sounds, and also that the physician would not have to place his ear directly on the chest of the patient. To quote Laennec: "Direct auscultation was as uncomfortable for the doctor as it was for the patient, disgust in itself making it impracticable in hospitals. It was hardly suitable where most women were concerned and, with some, the very size of their breasts was an obstacle to the employment of this method" (Ferns 2007).

Laennec's original stethoscope was a hollow wooden cylinder with a funnel-like termination (a bell, or inverse horn) at the end that touched the patient. The distal end fitted into the doctor's ear canal. In its modern form, the stethoscope has two types of chest pieces: A shallow bell (for acoustic impedance matching), and a stiff, vibrating diaphragm (over a small bell chamber) that makes direct contact with the skin. The latter form is called a cardiology stethoscope. The chest piece (at the apexes of the bells) is attached to two, flexible tubes, 25–30 cm in length, which, in turn, connect to two metal ear tubes that insert into the clinician's ears. The ear tubes are spring-loaded to hold them in the ears. The flexible tubes can be neoprene, plastic, or even latex. Their material and dimensions will affect the frequency response of acoustic transmission from the body surface to the ears. The frequency response of the acoustic transmission of modern, acoustic stethoscopes has been measured by several workers (Jacobson and Webster 1977, Korhonen et al. 1996, Riederer and Backman 1998). Figure 3.1 illustrates the magnitude of the acoustic transmission in dB: $20 \log_{10}$ (rms sound pressure out/rms sound pressure in). The trace with one major peak is for the diaphragm-type, cardiology chest piece alone (no tubes or earpieces). The single peak at ~800 Hz may be due to diaphragm mechanical resonance, or a series Helmholz resonance involving the bell chamber. The acoustic transmission of the same chest piece, given tubes, and earpieces shows multiple peaks due to transmission line-type resonances of the tubes. Note that the peaks do not appear to be related as simple harmonics.

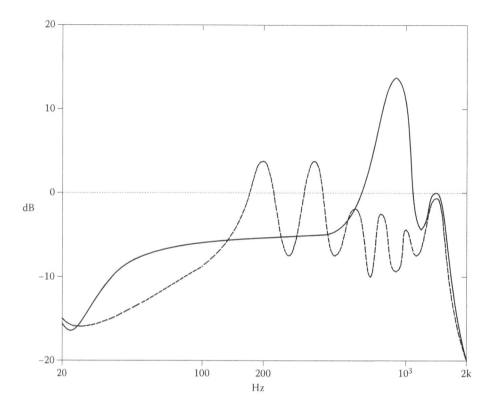

Figure 3.1 Measured acoustic transmission sound pressure level versus frequency for a modern diaphragm-type stethoscope chest piece (one large peal at ~900 Hz). The transmission frequency response of the complete stethoscope is shown on the same axes; note the many peaks and nulls caused by the tubes. (Adapted from Figure 3.1 in Northrop, R.B. 2002. *Noninvasive Instrumentation and Measurement in Medical Diagnosis.* CRC Press, Boca Raton, FL. ISBN: 0-8493-0961-1.)

Figure 3.2 shows the difference in transmission between a conventional bell-type chest piece, and one with a diaphragm. The simple bell shows more than 15 dB attenuation relative to the diaphragm stethoscope in the frequency range from 15 to 60 Hz.

Thus, what clinicians hear through modern, acoustic stethoscopes is "flavored" by the complex frequency transmission caused by its acoustic elements. Interns learn to recognize certain sounds associated with a healthy body as well as pathologies using acoustic stethoscopes. Thus when a broadband, electronic, acoustic sensor is used, its output amplified linearly and presented through high-fidelity headphones, a person trained with an acoustic stethoscope may find the sounds unrecognizable. Surely Laennec's original tube had a flatter frequency response than a modern acoustic stethoscope because it had no 30 cm lengths of elastic tubing to resonate.

Available now are electronic stethoscopes that avoid the worst of the tube resonance problem. The chest piece contains a broadband microphone, amplifier power supply, and frequency bandwidth adjustment and volume control. The conditioned amplifier output is sent to a miniature loudspeaker, or headphones. The loudspeaker is coupled directly to the spring-loaded, metal earpieces; the headphones are worn directly over the ears. For example, the 3M™ Littmann® electronic stethoscope, model 3100, offers electronic ambient noise reduction up to 85%, amplification gain of 24X, and wide frequency response.

The Cardionics® E-scope® has a selectable, 45–900 Hz bandwidth for heart sounds, and a 50 Hz to 2 kHz bandwidth for breath (lung) sounds. For the E-scope II, the maximum amplitude or sound pressure level without distortion is 120 dB at 100 Hz, about 30 times louder than an acoustic stethoscope. Its conditioned electrical output can power a speaker feeding the metal earpieces, headphones, and a tape recorder. It has a variable volume control, and a selection of diaphragms and bells to couple sound from the skin to the microphone. Because of its good acoustic isolation, the manufacturer claims it is useful in noisy environments, such as medivac helicopters and ambulances.

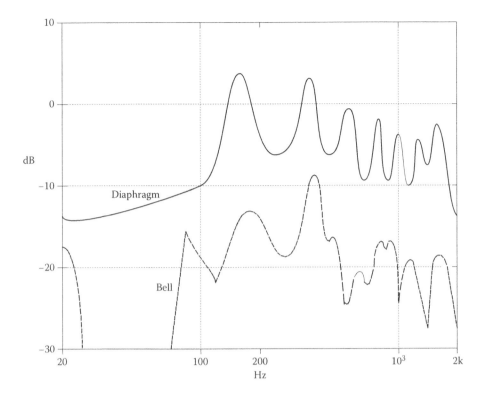

Figure 3.2 Measured acoustic transmission frequency response of two complete stethoscopes: one with a simple bell chest piece (*lower curve*), the other with a diaphragm chest piece (*upper curve*). Note the bell chest piece stethoscope rejects low frequencies from ~15 to 60 Hz. (Adapted from Figure 3.2 in Northrop, R.B. 2002. *Noninvasive Instrumentation and Measurement in Medical Diagnosis*. CRC Press, Boca Raton, FL. ISBN: 0-8493-0961-1.)

3.1.3 Microphones

There are several types of microphones suitable for picking up air-coupled body sounds from the skin. These include the following: *capacitor microphones,* where the induced vibration of a metalized Mylar film forming one plate of a capacitor changes the capacitance between it and a fixed plate, inducing a change in the capacitor voltage under conditions of constant charge; *crystal* or *piezoelectric microphones,* in which air-coupled sound pressure vibrates a piezo-crystal, directly generating a voltage proportional to dp/dt, where p is the sound pressure at the microphone; and *electret microphones* are variable capacitor sensors in which one plate has a permanent electrostatic charge on it; the moving plate varies the capacitance, inducing a voltage which is amplified. Electret microphones are small in size, and found in hearing aids, tape recorders, cell phones, laptop computers, etc.

Microphones generally have a high-frequency response that is quite adequate for endogenous body sounds. It is their low-frequency response that can be lacking. Indeed, some heart sounds are subsonic, ranging from 0.1 to 20 Hz (Webster 1992). The range 0.1–10 Hz is generally inaudible, while sound with energy from 10 to 20 Hz can be sensed as subsonic pressure by some listeners. To record body sounds, the author modified a pair of B&K Model 4117 piezoelectric microphones to cover down to <1 Hz by inserting a fine, stainless-steel wire into the pressure relief hole that vents the space in back of the piezo-bender element. The wire increased the acoustic resistance of the vent hole and thus increased the low-frequency time constant of the microphone from about 0.05 s (corresponding to a −3 dB frequency of ~3 Hz) to >0.15 s, giving a −3 dB frequency <1 Hz. The high, −3 dB frequency of the Model 4117 microphone was ~10 kHz. The voltage sensitivity of the B&K Model 4117 microphone at mid-frequencies is about 3 mV/Pa, or 3 mV/10 μbar.

Another, high-quality, B&K microphone used by the author is the B&K Model 4135, ¼″ condenser microphone. This research-grade device had a high frequency, −3 dB frequency in excess of 100 kHz, a total capacitance of 6.4 pF with a diaphragm-to-plate spacing of 18 μm. For body sounds, the low-frequency end of the 4135's frequency response is of interest. Three factors affect the Model 4135 microphone's frequency response: (1) The acoustic time constant formed by the acoustic capacitance (due to the volume between the moving [front] diaphragm and the insulator supporting the fixed plate), and the acoustic resistance of the small-pressure equalization tube venting this volume. As in the case described above, the acoustic resistance can be increased by inserting a fine wire in the tube; this raises the acoustic time constant, and lowers the low −3 dB frequency. (2) The low −3 dB frequency is affected by the electrical time constant of the parallel RC circuit shunting the microphone capacitance (Figure 3.3). (3) The mechanical resonance frequency of the vibrating membrane and its mass generally set the high-frequency end of the microphone's response. The smaller and thinner the diaphragm, the higher will be its upper −3 dB frequency.

In the circuit of Figure 3.3b, C_o is the 6.4 pF microphone capacitance, C_{in} is the signal-conditioning amplifier's input capacitance plus any wiring (stray) capacitance, R_{in} is the input resistance of the amplifier (greater than 10^{12} Ω), and R_s is the Thevenin source resistance of the source charging the capacitor to its fixed polarizing voltage. Olson (1940) analyzed the electrical circuit of a capacitor microphone; he showed that under certain assumptions, it could be reduced to one, simple series

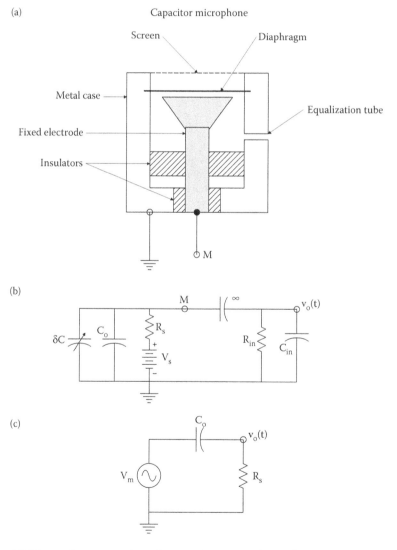

Figure 3.3 (a) Schematic cross section of a capacitor microphone. (b) Equivalent circuit of the capacitor microphone. δC is caused by the sound pressure waves. (c) Simplified linear circuit of the capacitor microphone.

loop containing the DC polarizing voltage source, V_s, in series with the average value of the microphone's capacitance, C_o, plus C_{in} (Figure 3.3c). (Normally, $C_o \gg C_{in}$ so we will call the capacitance, C_o.) The amplifier's R_{in} is normally $\gg R_s$, so the AC output voltage of the microphone is assumed to be developed across R_s. Let us write a loop equation for the simplified loop:

$$V_s - iR_s - C^{-1} \int i \, dt = 0. \tag{3.1}$$

Now the sound pressure vibrates the capacitor's diaphragm; we assume that it modulates the capacitance sinusoidally. Thus:

$$C(t) = C_o + \delta C \sin(\omega t). \tag{3.2}$$

This expression for C(t) is substituted in Equation 3.1, and the resulting equation is differentiated with respect to time. This results in a first-order, nonlinear, ODE in the loop current, i(t), which is solved to yield a frequency response function, from which we can write:

$$i(t) = \frac{V_s[\delta C/C_o]}{\sqrt{R_s^2 + 1/(\omega C_o)^2}} \sin(\omega t + \varphi_1) - \frac{V_s R_s \delta C/C_o^2}{\sqrt{[4R_s^2 + 1/(\omega C_o)^2]}\sqrt{[R_s^2 + 1/(\omega C_o)^2]}} \sin(2\omega t + \varphi_1 - \varphi_2)$$

$$+ \text{ Other higher-order harmonics.} \tag{3.3}$$

Note that $\varphi_1 = \tan^{-1}[1/(\omega R_s C_o)]$ and $\varphi_2 = \tan^{-1}[1/(\omega 2R_s C_o)]$. When $\delta C/C_o \ll 1$, the fundamental frequency term dominates, and the AC, small-signal output of the microphone (superimposed on the DC voltage), V_s, can be written as a frequency response function:

$$\frac{V_o}{\delta C}(j\omega) = \frac{V_s R_s \omega}{\sqrt{1 + (\omega C_o R_s)^2}} \angle \varphi_1. \tag{3.4}$$

Olson pointed out that this is the same result obtained if we place an open-circuit (Thevenin) voltage of $v_{oc} = V_s (\delta C/C_o) \sin(\omega t + \varphi_1)$ in series with C_o and R_s in the loop, and observe $v_o(t)$ across R_s. From Equation 3.4, we see that the low-corner frequency is $f_{Lo} = 1/(2\pi R_s C_o)$ Hz. For example, if $C_o = 7$ pF, and $R_s = 10^{10}$ ohms, then $f_{Lo} = 2.3$ Hz.

3.1.4 Acoustic Coupling

Whatever kind of sensor is used to detect endogenous sounds over the skin, there is a problem in efficiently coupling the sound vibrations from within the body to the microphone (or the eardrum). Since the days of Laennec and his first stethoscope, a bell-shaped or conical interface has been used to effectively couple a relatively large area of low-amplitude acoustic vibrations on the skin to a small area of larger amplitude vibrations in the ear tube(s). This bell-shaped interface is in fact an *inverse horn*. Inverse horns (literally, cow horns) were used pre-twentieth century as hearing aids. Note that the pinna of the human ear is an effective, inverse horn, matching the low-acoustical impedance of open space to the higher impedance of the ear canal and eardrum. Like all horns, the pinna exhibits comb filter properties, attenuating certain high frequencies in narrow bands around 8 and 13 kHz (Truax 1999).

Regular horns were first used as speaking trumpets, later as acoustic output devices for early mechanical record players (Victrolas); here the lateral displacement of the needle on the disk vibrated a mica diaphragm (~2″ diameter). A *horn* was used to couple those vibrations to a room and listeners. Most acoustics textbooks describe horns in the role of coupling sound from a small-diameter, vibrating piston to a large-diameter opening into free space (the room). In examining endogenous body sounds, the opposite events occur. A large area of small-amplitude acoustic vibrations on the skin is transformed by the *inverse horn* to a small area of large-amplitude vibrations (at the eardrum or microphone). It is beyond the scope of this section to mathematically analyze the acoustics of direct and inverse horns. However, we will examine them heuristically. Basically, horns and inverse horns are acoustic impedance-matching systems. They attempt to couple the acoustic radiation impedance of the source to the acoustic impedance of the horn termination. The termination in the case of a stethoscope is the rather complex input impedance of the coupling tubes (or tube, in Laennec's instrument); in the case of a microphone, it is the moving diaphragm. If impedances are not matched, sound transmission will not be efficient because there will be reflections at interfaces between any two media with different *characteristic acoustic impedances*; for example, at the skin–air interface, and at the air–microphone interface. The characteristic acoustic impedance of a medium is a real number defined simply by (Truax 1999):

$$Z_{ch} = \rho/c \text{ cgs ohms.} \tag{3.5}$$

For air, the density, ρ, is a function of atmospheric pressure, temperature, and relative humidity.

The velocity of sound, c, in air not only is a function of atmospheric pressure, temperature, and relative humidity, but also of frequency. Thus the Z_{ch} of air can vary over a broad range, varying from ~40 to 48 cgs ohms (43 is often taken as a compromise or "typical" value). An average Z_{ch} for body tissues (skin, muscle, fat, connective tissue, organs, blood) is ~2×10^5 cgs ohms. Thus we see that there is an enormous impedance mismatch in sound going from the body to air, and much intensity is reflected back internally. Clearly, there will be better sound transmission through the skin when the skin "sees" a much larger acoustical impedance looking into the throat of the inverse horn. As far as the author knows, there has been no scientific attempt to optimize the shape of the inverse horn used with the acoustic stethoscope, or, for that matter, any attempt to design the most efficient pressure microphone pickup.

The complex acoustic impedance on one side of a vibrating piston set in an infinite baffle has been shown to be (Olson 1940):

$$\mathbf{z_A}(kR) = [\rho c/(\pi R^2)]\left[1 - \frac{J_1(2kR)}{kR}\right] + \mathbf{j}\omega[\rho/(2\pi R^4 k^3)]K_1(2kR) \text{ cgs acoustic ohms,} \tag{3.6}$$

where ρ is the air density ($\cong 1.205 \times 10^{-3}$ g/cm^3), c is the speed of sound in air ($\cong 2.877 \times 10^4$ cm/s), R is the piston radius (cm), $k \equiv 2\pi/\lambda = \omega/c$, $J_1(2kR)$ is the first-order Bessel function of the first kind, $K_1(2kR)$ is a first-order, modified Bessel function of the second kind. (Bessel function values can be found from tables or calculated from infinite series.) Note that πR^2 is the piston area.

Figure 3.4 shows plots of the normalized real and imaginary parts of $\mathbf{z_A}(kR)$. Note that Re{$\mathbf{z_A}(kR)$} and Im{$\mathbf{z_A}(kR)$} increase with frequency until $\omega > c/R$. The Bessel functions contribute to the ripples at high ω.

Horns can be classified as conical, parabolic, exponential, catenoidal, or hyperbolic, depending on how their cross-sectional area varies with z, the distance from the throat (smaller end). For regular (output) horns, A(z) *increases* monotonically with z, such as used in early phonographs. A(z) *decreases* monotonically with z for inverse horns. Leach (1996) developed a closed-form, mathematical analysis for a class of horns known as *Salmon's family* (these include conical, catenoidal, exponential, and hyperbolic forms). Leach's analysis employs the formalism of two-port circuit analysis; he used PSpice™ for his simulations. Leach gave expressions for: $\mathbf{Z}_{11}(\omega)$, $\mathbf{Z}_{12}(\omega)$, $\mathbf{Z}_{21}(\omega)$, and $\mathbf{Z}_{22}(\omega)$, in terms of the horn's two-port propagation constant, $\gamma(\omega)$, the horn area at the throat (input, or z = 0) end, A_0, the horn area at its output end (z = L), A_L, and dA(z)/dz evaluated at z = 0 and z = L (A_0' and A_L', respectively). He also gave expressions for the transfer functions, $\mathbf{T}_1(\omega)$ and $\mathbf{T}_2(\omega)$. Figure 3.5 shows the equivalent controlled source, analog circuit for horn input and output pressures ($\mathbf{P}_1$ and $\mathbf{P}_2$) (analogous to sinusoidal voltages $\mathbf{V}_1$ and $\mathbf{V}_2$). The volume velocities, $\mathbf{U}_1$ and $\mathbf{U}_2$, are analogous to the AC currents $\mathbf{I}_1$ and $\mathbf{I}_2$ in the two-port. Note that normally a load impedance, $\mathbf{Z}_L$, must appear across the output terminals of the two-port circuit to represent the impedance the horn is driving. Without belaboring the details of Leach's analysis, the reader can appreciate its complexity. The utility of Leach's analysis is that one can analyze inverse horns, that is, ones in which the throat (input end) is larger than the output end.

3.1.5 Discussion

We have stressed that to sense endogenous sounds from the body, air-coupled, sound pressure waves must be coupled to the sound sensor (microphone or eardrum) using some type of an inverse horn as an acoustic impedance-matching device. The price paid for using an inverse horn is that it inserts a comb filter-type of frequency response into the sound air transmission path. Typically, the pressure transfer function for a horn is poor at low frequencies (e.g., below 100 Hz), then rises abruptly with increasing signal frequency. The high-frequency part of the transfer function generally has a comb filter ripple on it, giving enhanced transmission at frequencies determined by the Bessel functions inherent in $\mathbf{z_A}(2\pi f)$.

To overcome the low-frequency loss in transmission inherent in horns, some workers have placed vibration sensors directly on the skin in order to record subsonic (and LF sonic) vibrations efficiently. Such sensors can be piezoelectric accelerometers which respond to the second

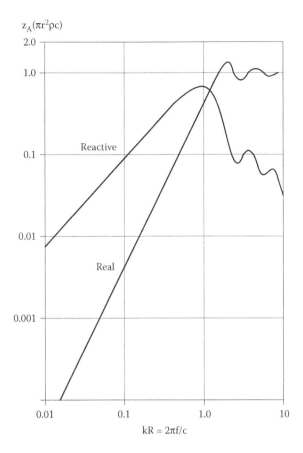

Figure 3.4 Plot of the scaled real and imaginary parts of the acoustic driving point impedance of a vibrating cylindrical piston. (Adapted from Olson, H.F. 1940. *Elements of Acoustical Engineering.* D. Van Nostrand Co., Inc., NY.)

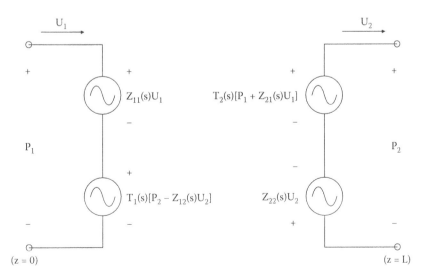

Figure 3.5 Two-port equivalent analog circuit describing the transmission behavior of acoustic horns.

derivative of the skin displacement, $\ddot{x}(t)$. A double integration is required to recover $x(t)$, which produces the sound. If the peak vibration, δx, is $< \lambda/4$ of the laser used, an *interferometer* such as a Fizeau or a Michelson can be used to directly measure $x(t)$ of the skin. When a laser Doppler technique is used on the skin (Hong 1994), then the output signal is proportional to $\dot{x}(t)$.

3.2 MEANS OF ANALYSIS FOR ACOUSTIC SIGNALS

3.2.1 Introduction

There are several ways that an audio-frequency signal from an endogenous body sound can be processed. On the qualitative side, we can observe a microphone output voltage on an oscilloscope versus time. Very little useful information is gained by doing this. Another way is to listen to it, either with a stethoscope, or using headphones. The amplitude, pitch, and rhythm of a complex physiological sound are features that the brain can store, identify, and compare. Clearly, some individuals are inherently better at this than others. Persons with "trained ears" such as musicians are better at making diagnoses with acoustic stethoscopes than others. Recall that the stethoscope in its earliest, nineteenth-century form was probably less distorting to body sounds that the modern instrument. As we have seen, all stethoscopes impose a transfer function on the input sound that has low transmission at low frequencies, and a comb filter-type response at higher frequencies.

To remove the problem of inverse horn and tube transfer functions, plus human psychoacoustics, body sounds may be better sensed directly from skin vibrations by laser interferometry. The signal so derived is proportional to the skin displacement, hence is at the endogenous sound frequency. The signal so derived can then be displayed in the frequency domain after digital processing as its average *root power density spectrum* (the spectrum must be averaged over several cardiac cycles, or breath cycles if the lungs are involved). Interferometric signals tend to be noisy, however, and the apparatus is expensive and delicate.

When the laser Doppler technique is used on skin, the resulting (mixed) output signal's frequency is given by $f_D = 2|\dot{x}|/\lambda$ Hz. Note that the frequency of the Doppler signal is proportional to the *magnitude of the skin velocity*, and *is not* the sound originating in the patient's body. A simple laser Doppler system cannot differentiate between a positive versus a negative frequency shift (due to $\dot{x} > 0$ and $\dot{x} < 0$, respectively).

Probably the two best ways to sense body sounds are as follows: (1) Use a well-designed, inverse horn to couple the skin vibrations through the air to a capacitor microphone's diaphragm. The signal, so acquired, after amplification and filtering to improve the signal-to-noise ratio, can be listened to with headphones (a high-fidelity electronic stethoscope), or processed by a computer to form an average, *root power density spectrogram* or a TFS. (2) Miniature, IC accelerometers can be attached to the skin to measure vertical (sound) vibrations. Variations of the fast Fourier transform (FFT) are used to calculate the sound (average) spectrogram and the TFS. Diagnostic information about the heart can be obtained by examining anomalies in the cardiac power spectrogram or the TFS. The TFS shows how sound frequencies and intensity are distributed in time over the events that produce the sound.

3.2.2 Discrete Fourier Transform and the Power Density Spectrum

The power density spectrum (also known as autopower spectrum) is used to characterize the spectral (frequency) content of *stationary signals* in the frequency domain. A stationary signal is the one in which the physical processes and environmental conditions giving rise to the signal do not change with time. Another way to view stationarity is to note that the statistics governing the production of the signal are constant. Signals derived from physiological systems are, in general, nonstationary. In a physiological system, an approximation to stationarity may exist for the short time over which data is recorded.

When we digitize and calculate an estimate to the power spectral density of heart sounds over many cardiac cycles, the spectrum will contain a peak at the mean heartbeat frequency, plus peaks at all the frequencies of all the sounds in the cardiac cycle. Information is lost on the spectral content of individual sounds (such as from mitral valve closing), and when in the cardiac cycle these sounds occur. One way to examine the spectra of individual sounds as they occur is to synchronize the sampling of the cardiac sound signal with the ECG waveform to gate only those sounds of interest. The display of the phonocardiogram spectrum is usually presented as a root power density spectrogram (a spectrogram is computed from finite length data). Because many spectrograms are averaged to reduce noise, the display generally shows *mean* rms volts/$\sqrt{\text{Hz}}$.

To gain an understanding of the theory behind the calculation of a power density spectrum, we will first review the basics of the continuous Fourier transform (CFT) and the autocorrelation function. The CFT pair for a stationary signal is well known:

$$X(j\omega) \equiv \int_{-\infty}^{\infty} x(t)\exp[-j\omega t]dt \tag{3.7}$$

$$x(t) \equiv (1/2\pi)\int_{-\infty}^{\infty} X(j\omega)\exp[+j\omega t]d\omega. \tag{3.8}$$

The autocorrelation of a stationary signal, x(t), is defined as

$$r_{xx}(\tau) \equiv (1/2T)\int_{\substack{-T \\ \lim T \to \infty}}^{T} [x(t)x(t+\tau)]dt. \tag{3.9}$$

The autocorrelation function has many interesting properties; the most important here is the fact that it is real and even in τ. The autopower *spectrum* is simply the CFT of the autocorrelation function:

$$S_{xx}(2\pi f) \equiv S_{xx}(f) = \int_{-\infty}^{\infty} r_{xxf}(\tau)\exp[-j2\pi f\tau]d\tau. \tag{3.10}$$

$S_{xx}(f)$ is a *two-sided, even, positive-real function of frequency*. It has the units of mean squared volts/ Hz. Depending on the form of x(t), there are many mathematical models for power density spectra, for example: white noise, 1/f noise, Gaussian, exponential, Markov, etc. (Lee 1960).

In the real world, the power density spectrum is approximated by the use of finite data. It is also calculated using periodic samples of the time function. The calculation of a root power density spectrogram begins with acquiring a long analog record of the sound under study. This signal is often analog bandpass-filtered to improve its signal-to-noise ratio. The high-frequency filter cut-off is adjusted to prevent *aliasing*. That is, the conditioned analog signal is low-pass filtered to remove any spectral energy at or above one-half the sampling frequency (i.e., the Nyquist frequency, f_N). The signal is then digitized (sampled) periodically; a total of N samples are taken, spaced T_s seconds apart. Each sample is converted to a digital number by an ADC, and the samples are stored in computer memory. Thus a *signal epoch* of duration $T_E = (N-1)T_s$ is required (sample 0 is taken at t = 0, sample (N − 1) is taken at t = T_E). For computational convenience, N is always made a power of 2, that is, $N = 2^B$, in order to be able to use an FFT algorithm. Typically, B might be 12, so N = 4096 samples. In the frequency domain, the spectrogram will have data values spaced at $\Delta f = 1/[(N-1)T_s]$; the maximum useful frequency of the spectrogram will be $f_s/2 = f_N$, the Nyquist frequency.

The discrete Fourier transform (DFT) of a sampled, finite-length signal is given by

$$X(k\Delta f) = X(k) = (1/N)\sum_{n=0}^{N-1} x(n)\exp\left[-jk(2\pi/N)n\right], \tag{3.11}$$

k = 0, 1, 2…(N − 1). n is sample number.

or:

$$X(k) = (1/N)\sum_{n=0}^{N-1} x(n)\cos(kn2\pi/N) - j(1/N)\sum_{n=0}^{N-1} x(n)\sin(kn2\pi/N). \tag{3.12}$$

Note that X(k) is in general complex, with a real and imaginary part for every k. X(k) is generally calculated using one of the efficient FFT algorithms. Calculation of the *discrete power density spectrogram* can proceed by several methods. First, an array of N samples of x, $[x_N]$, is made and stored (N even). The array elements (samples) are renumbered so they extend from $-(N/2-1)$ to $+N/2$. Next, the *discrete autocorrelogram* of x(n), $r_{xx}(k)$, can be calculated in the time domain by the following function (Papoulis 1977):

$$r_{xx}(k) = \frac{1}{N-k}\sum_{n=[-(N/2-1)+|k|/2]}^{(N/2-|k|/2)} x(n+k/2)x(n-k/2). \tag{3.13}$$

Note that ideally $r_{xx}(k)$ is even in k. Papoulis (1977) showed that $r_{xx}(k)$ is an unbiased estimator of the discrete autocorrelation, $R_{xx}(k)$. The *discrete autopower spectrogram*, $S_{xx}(q)$, is simply the DFT of $r_{xx}(k)$. That is:

$$S_{xx}(q) = (1/N) \sum_{k=-N/2}^{N/2-1} r_{xx}(k)\exp\left[-jq(2\pi/N)k\right], \quad (q = 0, \pm 1, \dots, \pm N/2) \text{ msV/Hz.} \tag{3.14}$$

where $S_{xx}(q)$ is positive-real and even in q.

$S_{xx}(q)$ is computed M times (e.g., M = 16) from M epochs of N samples of x(t) (sound) data, and corresponding points are averaged to form $\overline{S_{xx}(q)}$ with reduced noise. The *root power spectrogram* is simply:

$$s_{xx}(q) = \sqrt{|\overline{S_{xx}(q)}|} \text{ rms volts}/\sqrt{Hz}. \tag{3.15}$$

The autopower spectrogram of x(t) can be computed using a number of algorithms. In the Blackman–Tukey method, the sample autocorrelogram is *windowed* before the autopower spectrogram is computed. A *windowing function,* w(n), weights the sampled data array to form the product:

$$z(n) = x(n)w(n), \quad -N/2 \le n \le (N/2 - 1). \tag{3.16}$$

Windowing functions are used on finite-length, sampled data before DFTing in order to minimize some function of the spectral error, $\mathbf{E}(q) = \mathbf{X}(q) - \mathbf{X_w}(q)$, where $\mathbf{X}(q)$ is the DFT of x(t) as $N \to \infty$, and $\mathbf{X_w}(q)$ is the DFT of x(n)w(n). There is a trade-off between spectral resolution and spectral smoothness for windows other than rectangular. One way to appreciate what a window does is to take the DFT of a pure sine wave given a rectangular window. We see a sharp peak at the fundamental frequency of the sine wave, and also smaller side-lobe peaks on either side of the main peak. The side-lobe peaks are artifactual; no such frequencies exist in the analog signal. The use of a windowing function reduces the side-lobe artifacts, but generally at the expense of broadening the fundamental frequency peak and thus decreasing spectral resolution.

The simplest windowing function is, of course, the *rectangular window*, which is inherent in all finite data arrays, $[x_N]$. Here $w_r(n) = 1$ for $-N/2 \le n \le (N/2 - 1)$, and 0 for $|n| > N/2$. Other windows include the *Bartlett* or *triangular window:* $w_b(n) = [1 - |n|/(N/2 + 1)]$ for $-N/2 \le n \le (N/2 - 1)$, and 0 for $|n| > N/2$. The *Hanning window* is also widely used: $w_h(n) = \frac{1}{2}[1 + \cos(2\pi n/N)]$ for $-N/2 \le n \le (N/2 - 1)$, and 0 for $|n| > N/2$. Many other types of windows exist, including the *Parzen, Hamming, Tukey, Kaiser,* and *Parabolic* (Papoulis 1977, Williams 1986).

The *Blackman–Tukey spectrogram function* can be written as

$$S_{xx}(q) = \sum_{k=-N/2}^{N/2} r_{xy}(k)w(k)\exp\left[-jq(2\pi/N)k\right] \quad q = 0, \pm 1, \dots, \pm N/2, \tag{3.17}$$

where w(k) can be one of the window functions described above.

In summary, there are many ways to compute the power density spectrogram of a recording of body sounds. For example, the Matlab® Signal Processing Toolbox™ has a utility, P = spectrum (x,m) that uses the *Welch method* (Proakis and Manolakis 1995) to calculate the autopower spectrogram of a sampled (discrete) signal array, $[x_N]$. The Hanning window is used on each epoch of m samples before the calculation; m is also the number of points in the FFT. Note that N = km, where k is the (integer) number of epochs in $[x_N]$ FFTd, and $m = 2^B$. The routine automatically averages the k spectrograms. Other Matlab spectrum functions calculate the cross-power spectrogram of two time signals, $[x_N]$ and $[y_N]$. A root spectrum is calculated by

$$\sqrt{S_{xy}(q)} = \sqrt{[\text{Re}\{\mathbf{S_{xy}}(q)\}]^2 + [\text{Im}\{\mathbf{S_{xy}}(q)\}]^2}. \tag{3.18}$$

That is, it is the square root of the mean-squared real part of $\mathbf{S_{xy}}(q)$ plus the mean-squared imaginary part of $\mathbf{S_{xy}}(q)$. $S_{xx}(q)$ is positive-real, that is, it has no imaginary terms.

Many stand-alone, digital sampling oscilloscopes (DSOs) not only allow data capture and visualization, but they also come with utilities that compute root power spectrograms of signals. The operator can choose the sampling rate, the window, the number of samples, and the number of spectra to be averaged together to reduce noise. National Instruments' Lab View® data acquisition and signal-processing software for PCs and laptop computers will also compute spectrograms.

Because heart sounds occur sequentially, each is associated with a physical event in the cardiac cycle, and information is lost if we pool these periodic events in a common spectrogram. In the following section, we examine the interesting DSP algorithms associated with time–frequency analysis (TFA), first used to analyze speech and animal sounds.

3.2.3 Time–Frequency Analysis for Transient Sounds

In this section, we will examine the techniques used to make a TFS. The first use of TFSs was to characterize the frequency content versus time in human speech (also known as the "voice print"). This application was soon extended to the analysis of animal sounds used for navigation, prey location, and communication (e.g., whales, dolphins, bats, birds). The original speech spectrograph was an all-analog system. In the earliest sound spectrographs, the sound signal was recorded on analog magnetic tape. The tape was passed over a rapidly spinning drum containing the playback head (one rotation defined the time window). The resulting analog signal from the rotating head was sent to a narrow-bandpass filter whose center frequency was proportional to the height of the recording stylus on the spectrogram chart. The higher the peak voltage at the BPF output, the darker the data point on the spectrogram. This procedure was time-consuming, and there is an obvious trade-off on filter rise time, which is inversely related to filter bandwidth.

TFSs are the preferred form of spectral analysis when the sounds being studied are short-term, nonstationary, or transient, in nature. As TFA displays a signal recorded in time in both time *and* frequency, it can be shown that there is an ultimate trade-off between the time-resolution and frequency-resolution of any TFS. This trade-off is analogous to Heisenberg's uncertainty principle in quantum physics. It can be stated simply as $(\Delta f\ \Delta t) \geq 1$. Δf is the frequency resolution in Hz, and Δt is the length of signal used to calculate the TFS in seconds (National Instruments 2014).

There are a number of discrete algorithms for calculating TFSs, including, but not limited to: the *short-term Fourier transform* (STFT), the *Wigner transform* (WT), the *Wigner–Ville transform* (WVT), the *binomial transform* (BT), the *Choi–Williams transform* (CWT), the *Gabor transform* (GT), and the *adaptive Gabor transform* (AGT). Each transform has its advantages and disadvantages, however, for sources which contain overlapping (additive) sound sources in time. Wood et al. (1992) remarked that the BT "provides higher joint resolution of time and frequency than the spectrograph and spectrogram [STFT] and better interpretability than other time–frequency transforms such as the Wigner-Ville." The BT evidently is an efficient algorithm with very good cross-term suppression properties (Wood and Barry 1995).

We will first examine properties of certain TFS algorithms. For pedagogical purposes, we will first treat them in integral rather than discrete forms. The complex CFT of a time signal, x(t), is given by the well-known integral:

$$X(jf) = \int_{-\infty}^{\infty} x(t)\exp[-j2\pi ft]dt, \quad (X(jf) \text{ is in general complex}). \tag{3.19}$$

The first TFS algorithm to be considered here is the STFT which has been used since the 1950s to calculate spectrograms to characterize human speech and was first applied to the TFS analysis of heart sounds by McCusik et al. (1959). The STFT spectrogram is calculated by

$$STFT(t,f) = \left| \int_{0}^{\tau} x(t)g(t-\tau)\exp[-j2\pi ft]dt \right|^2, \tag{3.20}$$

where x(t) is the audio signal and g(t) is a *windowing* or *gating function*. g(t) is slid along x(t) by fixing τ.

If the gating function is Gaussian, then the STFT is called a *Gabor transform* (some workers have used a Hanning gating function in their discrete data realization of the STFT TFS).

The discrete form of the STFT can be written as

$$STFT(n,q) = \left| \sum_{m=-L/2}^{(L/2)-1} x(m)g(n-m)\exp\left[-j(2\pi/L)mq\right] \right|^2, \tag{3.21}$$

where L is the length of the sliding window, g(n), and g(n) is an even function around $(n − m) = 0$.

The STFT is positive and has no problem with cross-term interference. However, its frequency resolution is inferior to the WV and CW TFSs.

The WT is given by a CFT of the time-shifted product:

$$W(t,f) = \int_{-L/2}^{L/2} \left[x(t + \mu/2)x^*(t − \mu/2) \right] \exp[−j2\pi f\mu] d\mu, \tag{3.22}$$

where $\mu/2$ is the shift, L is the duration of the integration, and x^* is the complex conjugate of x (x is real, so this notation is meaningless in this case).

The integral is computed many times for $t = k\Delta t$, k = 1, 2, 3, …, M. There is an equivalent definition of WV(t, f) in the frequency domain as a continuous, inverse Fourier transform (CIFT).

$$WV(t,f) = \left(\frac{1}{2\pi} \right) \int_{-\infty}^{\infty} X(f + \nu/2)X^*(f − \nu/2)\exp[+j\nu t] d\nu, \tag{3.23}$$

Note that the WVT is real, although it can go negative. As the WVT depends *quadratically* upon the signal, a signal composed of sums of frequencies will produce a WVT containing cross-terms from the sums and differences of the component frequencies. This means that certain signals that are the sums of several frequencies occurring at the same time will produce "fuzzy" WVTs. If the signal is statistical, instead of sums of sinusoids, then the signal's autocorrelation function, $R_{xx}(\tau_1 − \tau_2)$, can replace the product, $[x(t + \mu/2)x^*(t − \mu/2)]$, in the CFT integral, with the τs replaced by $R_{xx}[(t + \mu/2), (t − \mu/2)]$, or $R_{xx}(\mu)$ (Bastiaans 1997).

When x(t) in the WT is replaced with the *analytical signal*, $Ax(t) \equiv x(t) + j[HX(t)]$, the WT is called the *Wigner–Ville transform* (WVT). HX(t) is the *Hilbert transform* (HT) of x(t), defined as (Papoulis 1977):

$$HX(t) \equiv (1/\pi) \int_{-\infty}^{\infty} \frac{x(\tau)}{\pi(t − \tau)} d\tau = (1/\pi)x(t) \otimes (1/t). \tag{3.24}$$

It can be shown that the HT filters out the negative frequencies in the analytical signal. The discrete form of the WVT is given by

$$WVT(k,q) = 2 \sum_{m=-L/2}^{(L/2)-1} Ax(k + m)Ax^*(k − m)\exp\left[−j(2\pi/L)mq\right]. \tag{3.25}$$

Here, L is the block length over which the DFT is calculated, and Ax(k) is an analytical sequence computed from a discrete HT.

The WVT possesses the highest resolution of the TF algorithms; however, it suffers the most serious interference problems, and can go negative.

Finally, let us examine the CFT version of the BT TFS. First, we find the running estimate of the signal's autocorrelation at various times, t: $r_{xx}(t, \tau)$. This autocorrelation function is then convolved in the time domain with a binomial smoothing function, given by

$$R_{cxx}(t, \tau) = r_{xx}(t, \tau) \otimes h_{bin}(t, \tau). \tag{3.26}$$

Hence:

$$BT(t,f) = \int_{-\infty}^{\infty} R_{cxx}(t, \tau)\exp[−j2\pi ft] dt. \tag{3.27}$$

$$\text{In discrete form, } h_{bin}(m,k) = \left(\frac{|k|}{m + |k|/2} \right)^{2-|k|} \tag{3.28}$$

According to Wood et al. (1992), "The Binomial Transform uses a binomial approximation to the exponential [Gaussian], and is particularly efficient because the convolution in Equation 3.26 may be implemented using shift and add operations alone, avoiding floating point multiplication."

In summary, the choice of algorithm for TFA of a nonstationary time signal will depend on the desired resolution in the time and frequency domains, and the presence of superimposed frequencies and/or noise in the signal. In summary, there is no one, good, universal method.

3.2.4 Discussion

Body sounds are nonstationary in nature, and generally periodic. If we take the Fourier transform of the sound over several cycles, the resultant spectrogram contains all the spectral energy in the sound, but tells us nothing about when a given spectral component occurred. TFA had its origin in the early analog spectrograms used for "voice-print" analysis. Today, TFA is done digitally with a wide choice of algorithms and display modalities. TFA is particularly useful in aiding the analysis of heart and breath sounds. It provides a visual, quantitative record of what spectral components occurred when. TFA algorithms are included in Matlab's Signal Processing Toolbox, and in the national instruments signal-processing software. Expect to see an increasing reliance on TFA as a signal descriptor in medical diagnosis.

3.3 HEART SOUNDS

3.3.1 Introduction

One of the earliest, NI measures of health in humans was the sounds made by the beating heart. After Laennec's invention of the stethoscope, it became apparent that heart sounds could be more complex than a simple "lub-dub." By observing the action of a beating heart in surgically opened animal chests, early workers could correlate features in the heart sounds with specific events in the cardiac cycle. For example, the "lub" sound comes from the closing of the tricuspid and mitral (A-V) valves at the beginning of systole. The "dub" is associated with the sudden closure of the aortic and pulmonary (semilunar) valves at the end of systole. The sounds are now known not to come from the valves alone, but from kinetic energy stored in moving blood being transformed into elastic stretch of the valves and the heart's walls, causing them to vibrate when the valves abruptly stop the moving blood. In the case of the first heart sound (lub), the initial contraction of the ventricles forces the tricuspid and mitral valves to close and then bulge toward the atria until their leaves are snubbed by the *chordae tendineae*. The elastic tautness of the valves then causes the moving mass of the blood, which is incompressible, to cause the ventricular walls and closed valves to vibrate. There is also vibrating turbulence in the blood. These vibrations have a low-frequency content; they are transmitted through the chest tissues to the chest wall, where they cause the skin to vibrate perpendicularly. The second heart sound (dub) occurs at the end of systole when the aortic and pulmonary (semilunar) valves close. At this point, the pressure in the aortic arch exceeds that in the left ventricle, even though the blood is still moving in the aorta. Again, kinetic energy of the blood and potential energy of stretched blood vessels interact. The outward-moving blood in the aorta is forced back against the valves; their elastic stretch redirects the blood outwardly. The valves and the aorta walls are under tension, and so vibrate at subsonic and low-sonic frequencies when excited by the moving mass of the aortic blood. The timing of these events, the aortic blood pressure, and the ECG waveform are shown in Figure 3.6.

When heart sounds are recorded directly from the heart surface with miniature accelerometers, or with good acoustic coupling from the chest wall to a broadband microphone with good low-frequency response, further details of normal heart sounds can be heard, seen on a flat screen monitor, or viewed as TFSs. Interestingly, the best points to listen to or record specific heart sounds are not directly over direct projections to the chest surface from the valve involved. For example, the auscultation point for sounds associated with the opening and closing of the aortic semilunar valve is at the second intercostal space at the right edge of the sternum. The sounds from the pulmonary semilunar valve are best heard at the left side of the sternum at the second intercostal junction. Listen at the lower left tip of the sternum for sounds from the tricuspid valve (between the right atrium and right ventricle). To best hear the sounds from the bicuspid valve (between the left atrium and left ventricle), listen at the fifth intercostal space on the left, mid-clavicular line.

In Figure 3.6, the first (normal) heart sound, S_1, has several components. Vibrations were introduced by the closure of the tricuspid and mitral valves between the atria and ventricles when the ventricles begin their forceful contraction. There may also be turbulence sounds as blood is forced into the aorta. The sound originating with the closure of the mitral valve is generally louder than the tricuspid sound. This difference is because the pressure in the left ventricle is higher than that in the right, and the mitral valve and heart walls are under more tension. Under conditions of inspired air (expanded lungs), it is sometimes possible to hear a "split" between the two A-V valve

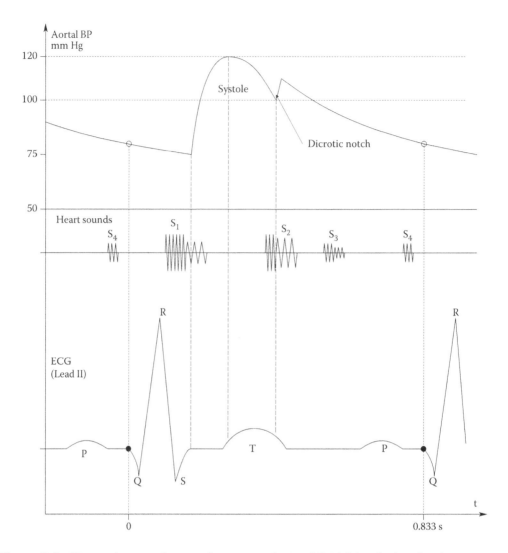

Figure 3.6 Timing diagram showing the times in the Lead II ECG (cardiac) cycle when various normal heart sounds occur, and a typical aortic blood pressure waveform.

sounds. That is, the louder sound caused by the mitral valve precedes the softer sound caused by the tricuspid valve.

The second heart sound, S_2, is associated with the closure of the aortic valve between the left ventricle and the aorta, and the closure of the pulmonary valve between the right ventricle and the pulmonary artery. The frequency content of S_2 is higher because there is greater elastic tension on the associated valves, the ventricles, and the walls of the aorta and pulmonary artery. S_2 can also exhibit a split between the sounds associated with the two valves. The louder aortic valve closes slightly before the pulmonary valve when the chest is inflated. The sounds are virtually coincident with an expired chest.

The third heart sound, S_3, is a weak, very low-frequency sound caused by atrial blood being forced into the ventricles. It is considered normal in children and young adults, but can indicate left-ventricular hypertrophy or ventricular dysfunction in adults over 40. S_3 occurs in the last third of diastole (Tilson-Chrysler 1994).

The S_4 sound or "atrial gallop" precedes S_1, and is due to vigorous atrial contraction forcing blood into the ventricles. It contains frequencies no higher than about 20 Hz and is therefore almost inaudible. It can be seen on oscilloscope displays and by TFSs. S_4 is found in patients with hypertension, aortic stenosis, acute myocardial infarction, or left-ventricular hypertrophy (Guyton 1991).

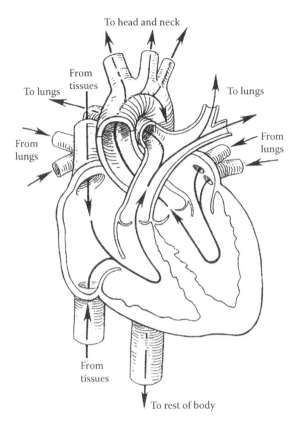

To head and neck

From tissues

To lungs

To lungs

From lungs

From lungs

From tissues

To rest of body

Figure 3.7 Cutaway view of the anatomy of a human heart and blood vessels showing the valves.

3.3.2 Abnormal Heart Sounds

There are many cardiac defects that can lead to the production of additional or modified heart sounds. Some of these will be discussed below. The reader should be aware that there are many web sites where one can download and listen to electronically recorded heart sounds as *.wav files. Also McGill University's Physiology and Music Departments in Canada have a unique Medical Informatics web site at which the viewer can listen to various cardiac sounds (normal and abnormal) at various chest recording sites, in addition, the viewer can download 3-D, colored, mesh, TFSs covering several cardiac cycles of a particular sound, as well as read text about the source and significance of the sound (Zhang et al. 1998, Falk et al. 2010).

A major source of anomalous heart sounds is damaged heart valves. Heart valves, in particular the left heart valves, can either fail to open properly (i.e., they are *stenosed*) or they cannot close properly, causing a backflow of blood, or *regurgitation*. A major source of heart valve damage can be infection by a group A hemolytic streptococcus, such as scarlet fever, sore throat, or middle ear infection. A serious complication of group A streptococcus infections is *rheumatic fever,* one of the characteristics of which is *carditis* and valve damage. The streptococcus bacteria manufacture a protein called the "M-antigen," to which the immune system forms antibodies. Unfortunately, these antibodies also attack certain body tissues, notably the joints and the heart valves. Guyton (1991) stated: "In rheumatic fever, large hemorrhagic, fibrinous, bulbous lesions grow along the inflamed edges of the heart valves." The scarring from this autoimmune inflammation leaves permanent valve damage. The valves of the left heart (aortic and mitral) are the most prone to damage by antibodies.

In *aortic valve stenosis,* the valve cannot open properly; there is an abnormally high-hydraulic resistance against which the left ventricle must pump. Thus, the peak left intraventricular pressure can rise as high as 300 mmHg, while the aortic pressure remains in the normal range. The exiting blood is forced through the small aperture at very high velocity, causing turbulence and enhanced

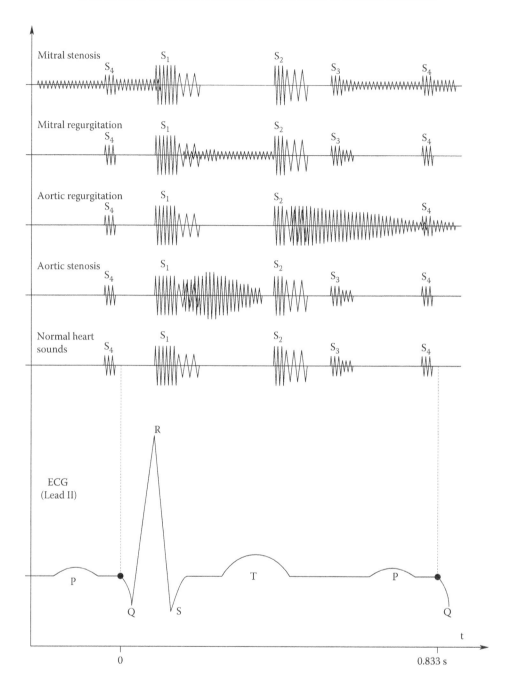

Figure 3.8 Schematic timing diagram of normal and abnormal heart sounds caused by certain heart pathologies referenced to the Lead II ECG waveform.

vibration of the root of the aorta. This vibration causes a loud murmur during systole that is characteristic of aortic stenosis.

Aortic regurgitation, on the other hand, occurs because the damaged aortic valve does not close completely. Again, there is a high-velocity jet of blood forced back into the left ventricle by aortic back pressure during diastole (when the left ventricle is relaxed). This back pressure makes it difficult for the left atrium to fill the left ventricle, and of course, the heart must work harder to pump a given volume of blood into the aorta. The aortic regurgitation murmur is also of relatively high pitch, and has a swishing quality (Guyton 1991).

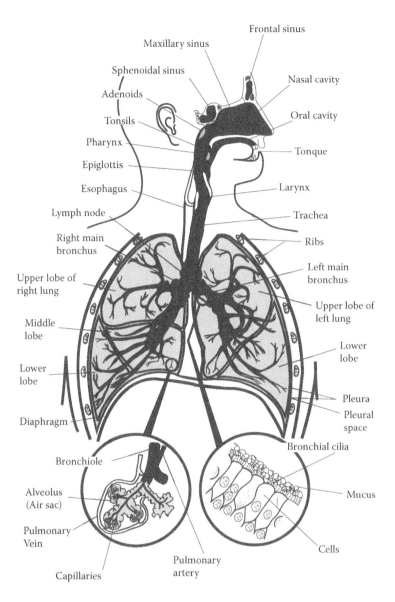

Figure 3.9 Anatomy of the lungs, trachea, and bronchial tubes. (Figure is in public domain.)

In *mitral valve stenosis,* the murmur occurs in the last two-thirds of diastole by blood jetting through the valve from the left atrium to the left ventricle. Owing to the low-peak pressure in the left atrium, a weak, very low-frequency sound is produced. The mitral stenotic murmur often cannot be heard; its vibration must be felt, or seen on an oscilloscope from a microphone output. Another audible clue to mitral stenosis is an "opening snap" of the mitral valve, closely following the normal S$_2$.

Mitral valve regurgitation takes place during systole. As the left ventricle contracts, it forces a high-velocity jet of blood back through the mitral valve, making the walls of the left atrium vibrate. The frequencies and amplitude of mitral valve regurgitation murmur are lower than aortic valve stenosis murmur because the left atrium is not as resonant as is the root of the aorta. Also, the sound has to travel further from the left atrium to the front of the chest.

Another cardiac defect that can be diagnosed by hearing the S$_2$ sound "split" is a left or right *bundle branch block.* The synchronization of the contraction of the muscle of the left and right ventricles is accomplished by the wave of electrical depolarization that propagates from the AV node, down the *bundle of His,* which bifurcates into the left and right bundle branches which run down on each side of the *ventricular septum.* Near the apex of the heart, the bundle branches branch extensively into the *Purkinje fibers* which invade the inner ventricular cardiac muscle syncytium, carrying the electrical activity that triggers ventricular contraction. See Figure 3.7 for a schematic, cut-away view of the heart, and Figure 3.8 for a time-domain schematic of where certain heart sounds occur in the cardiac cycle.

If the bundle branch fibers on the *right* side of the septum are damaged by infection, the contraction of the right ventricle will lag that of the right, and the sound associated with the aortic valve closing will lead that caused by the pulmonary valve. This split in sound S_2 is heard regardless of the state of inhale or exhale. A *left* bundle branch block will delay the contraction of the left ventricle; hence, delay the aortic valve sound with respect to that of the pulmonary valve. This condition causes reverse splitting of S_2 during expiration, but is absent on inspiration. Other causes of the reverse split include premature right-ventricular contraction (as opposed to a delayed left-ventricular systole), or systemic hypertension (high-venous return pressure).

3.3.3 Discussion

Owing to the subtlety of the patterns and timing of cardiac sounds, and the fact that some of their frequencies are too low to be heard by a typical human ear, there is an increased reliance on either observing the sound waveforms on an oscilloscope, or using a TFS to observe the fine frequency structure of the component sounds as they occur. There is certainly more information in the latter class of display.

3.4 BREATH SOUNDS

3.4.1 Introduction

As air passes in and out of the normal respiratory system during normal breathing, certain sounds can be heard by auscultation of the back and chest over the lungs, trachea, and bronchial tubes with an acoustic or electronic stethoscope. As in the case of heart sounds, it requires a good ear and much experience to use breath sounds effectively for NI diagnosis. The normal sounds perceived are due in part to air turbulence, air turbulence exciting damped mechanical resonances in connective tissues, and alveoli stretching open on inspiration, and shrinking on expiration. Normal breath sounds are classified as *tracheal, bronchial, bronchovesicular,* and *vesicular.* Tracheal sounds are heard over the trachea; they have a harsh quality and sound like air moving through a pipe. Heard over the anterior chest over the sternum and at the second and third intercostal spaces, the bronchial sounds originate in the bronchial tubes (Figure 3.9) and have a more hollow quality, not as harsh as tracheal sound. They are generally louder and higher in pitch; expiratory bronchial sounds last longer than inspiratory sounds, and there is a pause at peak inspiration. Bronchovesicular sounds are heard in the posterior chest, between the scapulae, and also in the center of the anterior chest. They are softer than bronchial sounds and also have a tubular quality. Vesicular sounds are soft, breezy or rustling in nature, and can be heard throughout most of the lung fields. Heard throughout inspiration, they continue with no pause through the beginning of expiration, and fade away about one-third of the way through expiration.

Several web sites for medical and nursing students have online, audio samples of normal and abnormal breath (and heart) sounds that can be played on your computer's audio system. The R.A.L.E. (2008) and UWashington (2015) web sites offer online samples of lung sounds and heart sounds and murmurs, respectively.

3.4.2 Abnormal Breath Sounds

Almost all diseases of the lungs are characterized by certain classes of abnormal breath sounds. Also certain systemic conditions can affect lung sounds, such as congestive heart failure, or high-altitude disease. The challenge is to use the abnormal sounds (plus other information) to diagnose the disease and to evaluate its severity.

Abnormal breath sounds include the following:

The absence of sounds over a certain lung volume. This generally means that air is not entering the bronchioles and alveoli in that lung volume; this can be due to fluid filling the volume, a tumor, etc.

Adventitious sounds, including:

1. Crackles (or rales)

2. Wheezes (or rhonchi)

3. Stridor

4. Pleural friction rub

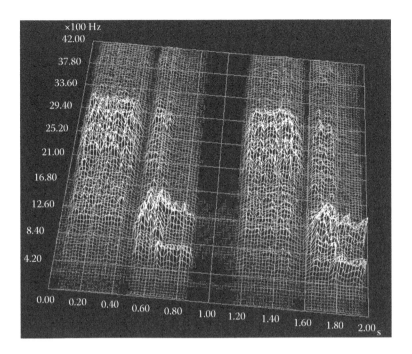

Figure 3.10 Time–frequency spectrogram of the bronchial system for lungs producing sonorous rhonchi; two breaths are shown. (Figure adapted from Figure 3.10 in Northrop, R.B. 2002. *Noninvasive Instrumentation and Measurement in Medical Diagnosis.* CRC Press, Boca Raton, FL. ISBN: 0-8493-0961-1.)

Crackles or rales are caused by air being forced past respiratory passages that are narrowed (but not blocked) by fluid, mucus, or pus. These sounds are intermittent, nonmusical and transient; they can be heard on inspiration and/or expiration. Crackles are often associated with inflammation or infection of the small bronchi, bronchioles, and alveoli. Crackles that do not clear with coughing can indicate pulmonary edema. Crackles can be subdivided into fine, medium, and coarse.

Wheezes can be heard continuously through inspiration and/or expiration. They are produced when air moves through airways narrowed by constriction or swelling. Squeaky wheezes are called *sibilant rhonchi*, lower-pitched wheezes with a moaning or snoring quality are referred to as *sonorous rhonchi*. A cause of sonorous rhonchi is secretions in the larger airways that occur with bronchitis, asthma, bronchial pneumonia, etc.

Stridor is a high-pitched, harsh sound heard during breathing. It is caused by an obstruction in an upper airway (trachea, bronchial tubes), which can be an inhaled foreign object which requires emergency attention.

A *pleural friction rub* is a low-pitched, grating or creaking noise that only occurs mostly when the lungs are expanding during inspiration, although some rubbing sound is heard on expiration. Its cause is the rubbing of the inflamed outside surface of the lung with the inflamed inner surface of the chest wall. (Normally the pleural surfaces are well lubricated, and make no discernable noise.)

Figures 4 through 6 in the paper by Taplidou et al. (2003) illustrate T-F spectrograms used to detect rhonchi. Sonorous rhonchi are a symptom of bronchitis or asthma.

Figure 3.10 illustrates a TFS of lungs producing gurgling breath sounds (Northrop 2003, Figure 7.2). Three breathing cycles are shown. Note that the band of significant sound power density is from 600 Hz to 2.25 kHz on inspiration, while when exhaling, the frequencies of the rhonchi having significant sound power are ~1.3 kHz. We can also see that the dominant frequencies on exhale tend to die out. (A graph of tracheal air velocity (or volume) vs time would be useful in interpreting this diagram.)

3.4.3 Discussion

Diagnosis of respiratory diseases and conditions by their sounds is an art. Clearly, the listener must be able to discriminate different frequencies, that is, have a musician's ear, for best effect. It goes without saying that the diagnostician/listener must have extensive clinical experience on which to base his or her judgment. Viewing a T-F spectrogram of the sound can aid in the diagnostic decision, but interpretation of the T-F spectrogram by itself also requires an extensive experience database with this modality, as well. The comb filter properties of the traditional stethoscope would appear to complicate this diagnostic process.

3.5 OTOACOUSTIC EMISSIONS

3.5.1 Introduction

Traditionally, the human hearing mechanism had been viewed as a purely passive process with no efferent feedback from the central nervous system (CNS). Sound waves impinging on the ear drum vibrate it, causing the three ossicles in the middle ear to vibrate in turn the oval window of the cochlea. The vibrations in the cochlea act in a complex manner to stimulate regions of hair cells under the tectorial membrane; the hair cells in turn send neural signals along the eighth cranial nerve to the CNS. As it has developed, the hearing process may also involve efferent neural signals from the CNS.

OAEs, first described by Kemp (2002), are narrowband acoustic signals generated in the inner ear by certain motile outer hair cells. Presumably, these hair cells vibrate in response to some sort of local, active, nonlinear, feedback mechanism. There are three classes of OAEs: (1) spontaneous, CW emissions; (2) click or tone-burst, transient-evoked emissions (TEOAEs); (3) distortion product emissions ($[2f_1 - f_2]$ DPOAEs) in response to CW stimuli of two sinusoidal frequencies. Spontaneous, CW emissions are pure tone, and occur in about 68% of infants under 18 months, decreasing to 35% in adults under 50, and are down to 20% in persons over 50 having normal hearing (Redhead 1998). All normal human ears emit reflex TEOAEs to clicks and tone bursts, and DPOAEs to CW, two-frequency stimuli. Spontaneous OAEs have also been found in such diverse animals as frogs (*Rana* sp.), bats, gerbils, barn owls, opossums, mice, kangaroo rats, lizards, chinchillas, dogs, cats, guinea pigs, monkeys, and horses (Robinette and Glattke 2011). Kemp (2002) stated: "… an eardrum oscillation of only 10^{-10} m (the diameter of an atom of hydrogen) will create a 'large' OAE of intensity 34 dB(SPL) (1 mPa) in a 1-mL ear canal volume."

Most hearing impairment is associated with a decrease or loss of OAEs. Thus, several companies have developed NI instruments to test the OAE reflex. Such tests are particularly useful in diagnosing hearing impairment in neonates and infants too young to talk. OAE testing is also applicable to detect the effects of ototoxic drugs (e.g., tetracycline) on hearing, to detect early signs of loud noise-induced deafness in teenagers and industrial workers, to check hearing following episodes of Meniere's disease, and to detect lesions affecting the eighth nerve or cochlea (Cunningham 2011).

To perform a DPOAE test, a probe is inserted into the end of the ear canal, much like a hearing aid earpiece. The probe contains a miniature microphone and two miniature earphones. In a typical DPOAE test, the CW sound stimuli from the headphones are $f_1 = 2.0$ kHz and $f_2 = 2.5$ kHz, at 70 dB (SPL). Thus, the DPOAE is at $(2f_1 - f_2) = 1.5$ kHz, typically at $\sim$8 dB (SPL), or 62 dB weaker that the stimuli's sound pressure (less than 1/1000 the sound pressure of the stimuli) (Leonard et al. 1990).

Leonard et al. showed that the $(2f_1 - f_2)$ CW, DPOAE follows the input dB(SPL) with a sigmoid curve. There is a threshold input dB(SPL) below which no DPOAE is produced. This threshold is frequency-dependent and individual-dependent; covering a wide range from 35 to 58 dB. The threshold is higher in ears with hearing loss, and the dB level of the DPOAEs is lower. The loudest stimuli used were 80 dB (SPL); these typically produced an OAE as loud as $\sim$15 dB (SPL) in normal ears.

3.5.2 Otoacoustic Testing

There are many different scientific parameters that can be used to characterize OAEs. In the case of click-evoked, transient emissions, an obvious analysis modality is the TFS; the response latency as a function of stimulus amplitude is also of interest. The click is basically the impulse response of the miniature loudspeaker used to stimulate the ear. Its pressure waveform can be approximated as the impulse response of an underdamped, second-order, low-pass system. That is: $p(t) = P_o \exp(-\xi \omega_n t) \sin [\omega_n \sqrt{1 - \xi^2})t]$. ξ is the loudspeaker's damping factor, and $\omega_n = 2\pi f_n$ is the natural resonant frequency of the loudspeaker in r/s. f_n is made as high as possible, and $\xi \rightarrow 0.5$, so the frequency content in p(t) is high, as seen from its Fourier transform, $\mathbf{P}(j\omega)$. The click is thus a broadband, transient stimulus.

DPOAEs are the result of steady-state, f_1 and f_2 stimulation. Thus, the power density spectrogram of the DPOAE is of interest; it will show not only the established $2f_1 - f_2$ product but also any other residual terms such as $2f_1 + f_2$, $2f_2 \pm f_1$, $3f_1$, $3f_2$, $f_2 \pm f_1$, $2f_1$, and $2f_2$. (The last three terms can be the result of a square-law nonlinearity, the others are from a cubic nonlinearity operating on the $p_{in} = A \sin(2\pi f_1 t) + B \sin(2\pi f_2 t)$ input.)

An example of a commercially available, TOAE testing system is the Otoport™ and Otocheck AE + ABR™ transient emission testers, made by *Otodynamics, Ltd.*, Hertfordshire, UK. In one testing mode, 260 repetitions of 80 dB clicks at 4 clicks/s, each lasting 1 ms, are given and the TOAEs are recorded. The first 20 ms of each, alternate TOAE is averaged to form two alternate arrays, each made from the average of 130 responses. The testing machine then computes a correlation coefficient between the two data arrays. If the TOAE response is 100% consistent, the correlation will be 1.00, or 100%. Variability between successive TOAEs will cause a lower correlation called the *Waverepro%*. The Waverepro% needs to be below ~35% before hearing loss is detectable by conventional audiometry. Redhead (1998) showed how the Waverepro% declines with age, and also how it decreases with cumulative exposure to industrial noise and loud, personal stereo use.

Intelligent Hearing Systems of Miami, FL, markets the *SmartOAE™*, a computer-based, CW OAE testing system. This is a research-grade instrument that displays the root power density spectrogram of the DPOAE. It also displays the DPOAE signal-to-noise ratio, noise statistics, testing parameters, etc. The input dB SPL can be set from 0 to 75 dB SPL, and input frequencies can be varied from 500 Hz to 8 kHz.

3.5.3 Discussion

The measurement of the $(2f_2 - f_1)$ OAE has found use in the NI diagnosis and quantification of hearing loss from various causes, including Meniere's disease, tetracycline toxicity, lesions affecting the eighth nerve or cochlea, etc., or ideopathic causes. Otoacoustic testing is particularly valuable in testing the hearing of infants too young to speak. The $(2f_2 - f_1)$ product is "hard-wired" into the auditory system; it does not habituate or fatigue, and thus provides a valuable, objective test of the closed-loop auditory system.

3.6 CHAPTER SUMMARY

One of the basic, low-cost modalities of NIMD is the analysis of sounds originating from within the body. It is well known that the sound transmission properties of the body act as a low-pass filter to internal sound sources as they propagate to the body surface. In addition, the traditional physician's stethoscope imposes a comb filter-type transmission on sounds it couples from the skin to the listener's ears. Even with these handicaps, an experienced cardiologist or respiratory specialist can recognize abnormal sounds and correlate them with suspect pathologies.

The modern approach to analyzing heart and breath sounds is to use an electronic stethoscope which eliminates the spectral distortions caused by the acoustics inherent to a conventional stethoscope's coupling tubes. We have seen that a great *visual* aid in analyzing nonstationary body sounds is the TFS. We reviewed several ways of computing TFSs, and their relative merits. The TFS plots the spectral components of sounds versus time, providing a quantitative, graphical description of sounds to complement the subjective impression of the listener.

This chapter has considered heart and breath sounds, and the pathologies that can be diagnosed from them. OAEs were also covered, and their potential importance in diagnosing hearing problems was described. Several medical school web sites provide audio clips of body sounds and their corresponding TFSs.

4 Measurement of Electrical Potentials and Magnetic Fields from the Body Surface

4.1 INTRODUCTION

It has long been known that electric fields generated by action potentials accompanying the conduction of nerve impulses, and from the depolarization of muscle membranes, can propagate through the various volume conductor layers of body tissues and be sensed on the skin surface. Such potentials are given names according to their sources: From muscles, we have the *electromyogram* (EMG); from the brain, the *electroencephalogram* (EEG) and *evoked cortical potentials* (ECPs), from the eyes we have the *electrooculogram* (EOG) and the *electroretinogram* (ERG), the *electrocochleogram* (ECoG) from the ear, and from the heart, the *electrocardiogram* (ECG or EKG).

All of these potentials have frequency spectra that basically span the audio range of frequencies, and in some cases, very low, subsonic frequencies as well. Their amplitudes are basically in the range of 10s of microvolts to 10s of millivolts. All bioelectric signals are noisy, that is, they are recorded with bioelectric background noise, as well as random measurement noise from electrodes, amplifiers, and the surrounding electrical environment. (For a comprehensive treatment of noise in biomedical amplifiers, see Northrop (2014)). Signal averaging is often used to improve the signal-to-noise ratio (SNR) of evoked transient signals such as ECPs and ERGs (Northrop 2010).

Probably, the most widely used bioelectric signal for diagnostic purposes is the ECG. It is relatively large, easy to record, and can be displayed in 3-D, vector form to aid diagnosis. Changes in the ECG vector display can occur when an area of heart muscle is starved for oxygen, necrotic because of a previous infarct, or a pathology in the right sinus node and/or the Purkinje fiber conduction system. The reason ECG analysis is so effective is that the cardiac pumping cycle involves the synchronized, spatiotemporal spread of electrical activity through the volume of the heart muscle. Thus, a region of damaged muscle shows up as a reduced potential when the wave of activity reaches that region. Another sign of damage is the inability of damaged heart muscle membranes to electrically repolarize in a normal manner after contraction (depolarization) has occurred.

The following sections describe the electrodes and amplifiers used to record bioelectric potentials, the sources of the potentials, and what they tell us. Along with the section on signal conditioning, sources of noise and low-noise amplifier design are treated. Special medical isolation amplifiers (MIAs) are described.

Also covered is the recording of the very small, transient magnetic fields resulting from the transient flow of ionic currents accompanying nerve and muscle action potentials. The *superconducting quantum interference device* (SQUID) is introduced, and we show how it is used to monitor brain and heart electrical activity, etc. SQUIDS are generally used experimentally, and as in the case of MRI, the cost of running a SQUID array is considerable (it requires a magnetically shielded room, a source of liquid helium, and extensive electronics). On the plus side for magnetoencephalography (MEG) is that it truly is a no-touch, NI recording method. From multiple SQUID recordings, volumes of magnetic activity in the brain can be generated by computer, and colored according to their intensity. Magnetic voxel resolution is highest in the cortex, and decreases with increasing depth into the brain.

4.2 ELECTRODES

4.2.1 Introduction

The NI measurement of bioelectric potentials from the body surface (skin) generally makes use of electrochemical electrodes to couple the electrical potentials at points on the skin surface to the copper wires that connect to the signal-conditioning amplifier/recorder. A good electrochemical electrode must have as low impedance as possible in the range of frequencies occupied by the signal. The reason for needing low-electrode impedance is that thermal noise is produced by the real part of the electrode's impedance. A high impedance electrode is in general, noisier than a low-impedance electrode, and can limit signal resolution. The input impedance of a modern MIA used to condition the biomedical signal is generally so high ($>10^9$ Ω) that a few tens of kilohms of electrode impedance has little effect on attenuating the open-circuit bioelectric signal. In the late nineteenth century and early twentieth century, before the invention of high-gain, high-input impedance amplifiers, ECG measurement was done with sensitive galvanometers that were driven by ECG currents from the body. Thus, early ECG electrodes had to have really low impedances. The patient placed a foot into a large jar of salt water that was connected to the galvanometer by a wire attached to a large carbon rod electrode also in the jar. The other contact with the body was a hand placed in a jar of salt water and similarly connected to the galvanometer. A roving electrode was made from a saline-soaked sponge.

With modern electrode systems, a water-based, electrolyte paste, cream, or gel containing sodium, potassium, and chloride ions is used to galvanically couple the skin to the electrode's metal–salt surface. The electrolyte may also contain an organic gelling agent to prevent it from running, and a preservative to inhibit mold and bacteria growth. Synapse® conductive electrode cream and spray made by Kustomer Kinetics, Inc., Arcadia, CA, lists the following ingredients: water, sodium chloride, propylene glycol, mineral oil, glyceryl monostearate, polyoxyethelene stearate, stearyl alcohol, calcium chloride, potassium chloride, methylparaben, butylparaben, propyl paraben, perfume, and D&C Red #19 dye. The electrolyte gel is largely responsible for maintaining low-electrode impedance, hence low-thermal noise, and also for reducing electrical motion artifacts from relative motion of the electrode with the skin. Some of its ingredients keep it from drying out. Early body surface electrodes were held in place by elastic rubber straps. A modern recording electrode has a self-adhesive "skirt" surrounding the electrolyte gel-filled center cup which contains the silver chloride contact electrode. Some of the newer, disposable electrodes, such as the Burdick CardioSens/Ultra® II, and the Nikotabs EKG electrodes (NIKOMED 0315) use a conductive, latex adhesive over the entire 1″ × 1″ active area of the electrode to attach it to the skin.

Nearly all modern, stick-on, skin electrodes interface the current-carrying electrons in the copper wire to a thin layer of silver chloride deposited on a thin layer of silver metal attached to the copper wire. The principal ions carrying charge through the skin are sodium, potassium, and chloride. These ions are in serum (extracellular fluid) and sweat. These ions have different mobilities, that is, they travel at different speeds in a given medium in the same electric field. The electrolyte paste or adhesive couples these ions to the Ag|AgCl layer where the half-cell reaction that involves electrons occurs. Note that there are no free electrons in the electrolyte, and no anions and cations in the solid phase (metal, metal salt) of the electrode. Charge transfers at electrode surfaces make 1/f noise, so it is important that very little current flows in the connecting wire and at the electrode interface (Northrop 2012).

4.2.2 Electrode Half-Cell Potential

Two different electrodes coupled by a common electrolyte form an *electrochemical cell.* This cell has a measurable *DC, electrochemical, open-circuit EMF* associated with it which is a function of the ion activities in the electrolyte and on the electrode surfaces. The cell EMF is also a function of the Kelvin temperature. The cell EMF is the algebraic sum of the *DC half-cell potentials* of the two electrodes. Half-cell potentials are found by measuring the EMF of a cell consisting of a so-called, *hydrogen electrode* half-cell, *defined* to have 0 V, fixed *standard half-cell potential* ($E_H^0 = 0$). The other half-cell is the one under measurement. By convention, a hydrogen half-cell electrode is made by bubbling H_2 gas at p = 1 atmosphere over a platinum screen electrode covered with platinum black. The Pt screen is immersed in an aqueous electrolyte having temperature T°K and some pH. Note that pH is defined as: $pH \equiv -\log_{10}(a_{H+})$, where a_{H+} is the hydrogen ion *activity* in the electrolyte of the hydrogen half-cell. It can be shown (Maron and Prutton 1958) that if the gas pressure is 1 atmosphere, the hydrogen electrode's half-cell potential varies with temperature and pH according to:

$$E_H = -\frac{RT}{F}\ln(a_{H+}) = -\frac{2.303\,RT}{F}\log_{10}(a_{H+}) = \frac{2.303\,RT}{F}\,pH \text{ Volts,} \tag{4.1}$$

where F is the Faraday number (96,500 Cb/equivalent), T is the kelvin temperature, and R is the SI gas constant (8.31446 J/(mole °K)).

Standard half-cell potentials have been tabulated for many metal|metal salt half-cells, including the ubiquitous silver|silver chloride electrode; several are shown in Table 4.1.

The half-cell potential of a silver|silver chloride electrode can be shown to be given by

$$E_{Ag/AgCl} = E^0_{Ag|AgCl} + \frac{RT}{F}\ln(a_{Cl-}). \tag{4.2}$$

That is, it depends on the electrochemical activity (concentration) of the chloride ions surrounding the electrode. The concentration of chloride ions is held relatively constant by the electrode gel between the silver chloride surface and the skin. Because two identical silver chloride electrodes are used to measure biopotentials, their nearly identical half-cell potentials oppose each other,

Table 4.1: Oxidation Half-Cell Potentials versus a Standard Hydrogen Electrode

Electrode	Oxidation Electrode Reaction	Standard Half-Cell Potential, E^0, at 25°C
$H_2 \mid H^+$	H_2 (g, 1 atm.) $= 2H^+ + 2e^-$	0.0000 V
$Ag \mid AgCl$	$Ag(s) + Cl^- = AgCl(s) + e^-$	-0.22233
$Ag \mid Ag^+$	$Ag(s) = Ag^+ + e^-$	-0.7991
$Hg \mid HgCl_2(s), Cl^-$	$2\,Hg(l) + 2Cl^- = Hg_2Cl_2 + 2e^-$	-0.2680
$Pb \mid PbSO_4(s), SO_4^=$	$Pb(s) + SO_4^= = PbSO_4(s) + 2e^-$	$+0.3546$

Source: When the reactions are written as reductions, the standard potentials have reversed signs.

giving a DC "skin cell" potential of a few microvolts. Most biopotentials recorded from the skin (e.g., ECG, EEG, EMG) do not require direct coupling; however, hence the small DC potential unbalance between a pair of silver chloride electrodes is not important. What is important is that the electrodes have low impedance, and not generate excessive motion artifact noise. A major component of motion artifact noise is low-frequency in nature, and arises when the electrode suddenly "sees" a change in chloride ion concentration, modulating $E_{Ag|AgCl}$.

4.2.3 Equivalent Circuits for AgCl Skin Electrodes

One should never try to measure an electrochemical electrode's DC resistance with an ohmmeter. An ohmmeter passes a direct current through the electrode which causes ions to migrate toward or away from the AgCl/electrolyte interface, altering the local concentration of chloride which affects the electrode's half-cell potential. In addition, if the potential imposed across the electrode's interface by the ohmmeter is large enough, oxidation or reduction reactions can occur at the electrode's surface, further altering the passage of current and the electrode's half-cell potential. Thus, we see that if any direct current is forced through the electrode by an ohmmeter, or by an amplifier's DC bias current, irreversible chemical changes can occur at the electrode's interface, altering its half-cell potential and generally increasing its resistance. An electrode's DC resistance is in general nonlinear; it does not obey Ohm's law. Thus the electrical characterization of electrodes is best done by using small AC voltages with varying frequency and measuring the magnitude and phase of the small currents that flow. The use of AC voltage avoids the problems of net ion migrations in the electrolyte, and irreversible oxidation/reduction reactions at the interface.

The electrical impedance of a silver|silver chloride skin electrode used to record bioelectric potentials consists of frequency-dependent real and imaginary parts. Take two, identical AgCl electrodes with electrolyte gel and place them face-to-face, as shown in Figure 4.1a. Thus, the impedance measured with a low alternating current will be $2\,\mathbf{Z_e}(f)$. A plot of the electrode's impedance magnitude versus frequency, $|\mathbf{Z_e}(f)|$, follows the shape shown in Figure 4.1b. The shape suggests a simple parallel RC circuit in series with a second resistor as shown in Figure 4.1c. Parameter constancy in this model is a gross approximation because C_i, R_i, and R_G are all functions of frequency and AC current density. Nevertheless, at frequencies above 10 kHz, $\mathbf{Z_e}$ is relatively constant and, in this example, is approximated by $R_G \cong 65$ ohms. At very low frequencies, C_i is basically an open-circuit, and $\mathbf{Z_e} = R_i + R_G \cong 2000$ ohms. Thus $R_i \cong 1935$ ohms. The first break frequency occurs at $f_b \cong 300 = 1/(2\pi R_i\,C_i)$ Hz, so $C_i \cong 0.274\ \mu F$.

When two AgCl electrodes are attached to the skin, the equivalent circuit becomes more complex. Each input of the recording amplifier sees the series-parallel RC circuit describing the AgCl/electrolyte interface, in series with another parallel RC circuit modeling the interface between the conductive gel and the *stratum corneum* of the epidermis. The dermis and subcutaneous layer of the skin, plus the complex, subcutaneous tissues are modeled electrically by a simple resistance, R_T. Figure 4.2 illustrates the simplified Thevenin impedances seen by a differential biomedical amplifier used to record a biopotential such as an ECG, EMG, or EEG. A major source of the resistive component of this Thevenin impedance is the natural oil and dead skin cells in the skin's *stratum corneum*. When the oil is removed by rubbing with a solvent such as ethanol or acetone, and the surface cells are debrided with an abrasive such as fine sand-paper, a considerable reduction in R_s occurs.

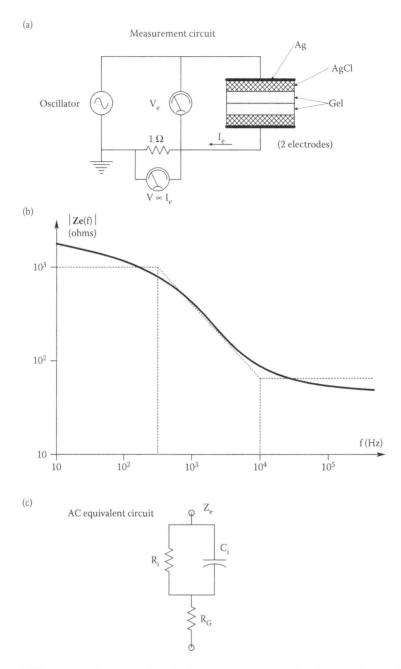

Figure 4.1 (a) Test circuit for measuring the impedance magnitude of silver|silver chloride skin electrodes. The voltmeter-ammeter method is used with a sinusoidal VFO. (b) Plot of a typical impedance magnitude of a silver|silver chloride skin electrode. Bode plot asymptotes are shown. (c) Lumped-parameter, equivalent circuit model for the electrode.

4.2.4 Dry Electrodes

Instead of galvanically coupling the internal biopotential to the amplifier through the skin with a pair of reversible, electrochemical electrodes, it is possible to coat a metal electrode with a micron-thin, insulating layer of oxide (e.g., SiO_2), or use a high-dielectric constant film over the electrode to conductively isolate it from the skin and body. The equivalent input circuit of a dry electrode amplifying system is shown in Figure 4.3. The insulated, dry electrode appears as a capacitor,

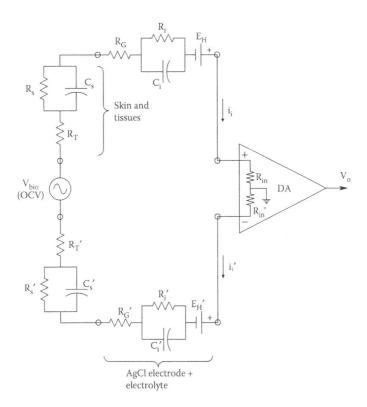

Figure 4.2 Complete equivalent input circuit for a differential amplifier connected to two silver|silver chloride skin electrodes, showing the CGR equivalent circuits for the skin, and the Thevenin open-circuit voltage of a biopotential, V_{bio}.

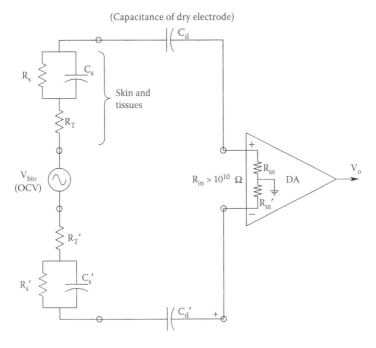

Figure 4.3 Equivalent circuit for a DA connected to two "dry" skin electrodes. Note that the dry electrodes are modeled by simple capacitors, while the skin and biopotential OCV have the same models as shown in Figure 4.2.

C_d, on the order of 1 nF. Because of the very high-input impedance of the amplifier's headstage ($R_{in} > 10^{10}$ Ω, $C_{in} < 1$ pF) and dry electrodes, this system is very subject to electrode motion artifacts, for example, triboelectric artifacts from lead motion, and also to static electricity in the space around the electrodes. To minimize these effects, the amplifier's headstages are mounted directly over each electrode. In spite of their simplicity, dry electrodes are generally not used in clinical practice because the system is very noisy, and their expense precludes throwing away electrode/amplifiers after use. It is much easier to use disposable, film-type, AgCl/electrolyte electrodes.

4.2.5 Invasive Electrodes

Since this text is about NI measurements, we will only mention some of the electrode types that penetrate the skin that can be used in medical diagnosis. Needle electrodes and wire hook electrodes are inserted through the skin into muscle fibers to record from single motor units (SMUs), small groups of motor units, and motor neurons. Their purpose is to record muscle action potentials and verify motor innervation. These electrodes are made from a mechanically tough, chemically inert or relatively inert material such as platinum–10% iridium alloy, tungsten, or stainless steel. A small hook in the end holds the wire in place, but the wire is thin and flexible enough so that the electrode can be pulled out with minimum tissue damage.

Many other types of invasive electrodes are used in *in vivo* electrophysiological research, including wick electrodes and suction electrodes used to pick up nerve fibers without damaging them. Pairs of hook electrodes are used for the same purpose. For extracellular recording of neuron action potentials in the brain or spinal cord, glass-insulated, metal microelectrodes are used. Their tips are bare and generally coated with platinum black to reduce their impedance. Saline-filled, glass micropipette electrodes are used to record the transmembrane potential from single neurons and other cells; they penetrate the cell wall which seals around them. Glass micropipette electrodes can have equivalent Thevenin resistances ranging from 10^7 to over 10^{10} ohms, depending on tip diameter and the filling electrolyte composition (3 M KCl is often used). Tip diameters can be made a fraction of a micron in order to penetrate axons and small cells. An Ag|AgCl wire is generally used to interface with the electrolyte in the lumen of a glass micropipette electrode.

4.3 BIOPOTENTIAL AMPLIFIERS

4.3.1 Introduction

In this section, we will examine the systems properties of biopotential amplifiers while giving minimum attention to the electronic circuit details of their innards. Specifically, we will describe them by the equivalent circuits of their inputs, including input resistance, input capacitance, DC input bias current, DC input offset voltage, equivalent short-circuit input voltage noise source, and the equivalent input current noise source. At the output, we will either use the Thevenin model (open-circuit voltage and Thevenin series resistance) or the Norton model (short-circuit current source in parallel with the Norton conductance). The Thevenin or Norton sources are related to the input voltage by a transfer function (generally a Laplace rational polynomial), or a frequency response function used for steady-state sinusoidal input voltages.

Amplifiers used for biopotential recording fall into two categories: those with a single-ended inputs, and those with differential (or differencing) inputs. Both types will be considered including special-purpose instrumentation and biopotential amplifiers, as well as amplifiers made with op-amps as building blocks. Single-ended and differential amplifiers (DAs) can be further subdivided into those that are reactively coupled (R-C) and do not pass DC, and direct-coupled (D-C) amplifiers that amplify DC signals. For example, op-amps are D-C, DAs, while ECG amplifiers are generally R-C DAs.

As the noise performance of an amplifier system is generally set by the noise injected by the first stage of amplification, that is, the headstage, we will also discuss the factors contributing to low-noise amplifier design at an electronic systems level.

4.3.2 Single-Ended Input Amplifiers

A single-ended input amplifier can be characterized by the equivalent circuit shown in Figure 4.4. It can easily be made up from an op-amp, as shown in Figure 4.5. When the op-amp is operated in the noninverting mode, the equivalent input circuit is that of the op-amp itself, and the transfer function is given approximately by

$$\frac{V_o}{V_{in}}(s) \cong \frac{(1 + R_F/R_1)}{(1 + s\tau_a)}, \tag{4.3}$$

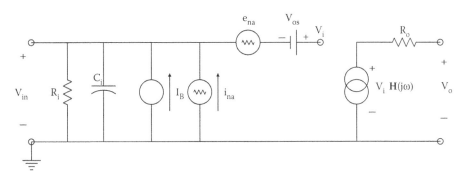

Figure 4.4 Equivalent circuit of a single-ended amplifier, showing DC offset voltage (V_{os}) and bias current (I_B), as well as the equivalent short-circuit input noise voltage root power spectrum (e_{na}) and input noise current root power spectrum (i_{na}). A Thevenin output model is shown. The OCV is $V_i\,\mathbf{H}(j\omega)$. The Thevenin resistance is R_o.

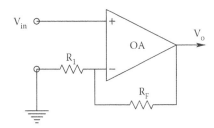

Figure 4.5 Noninverting op-amp circuit. Ideally, $V_o/V_{in} = 1 + R_F/R_1$.

where $\tau_a = (1 + R_F/R_1)/(2\pi f_T)$ seconds; f_T is the op-amp's Hz *gain-bandwidth product,* also known as *unity gain frequency, a figure of merit* (Northrop 2012).

Most bioelectric signals (with the exception of EMGs) have little spectral energy above 1 kHz, so amplifier f_T is generally not critical, as long as it is above 1 MHz. Single-ended amplifiers are used as interstages in multistage amplifiers, and as headstages for applications where the biosignal's SNR is good. That is, where there is little interference picked up by the recording electrodes and wiring connecting them to the amplifier. This is generally not the case, however, and DAs are generally used for headstages in recording low-level bioelectric signals from the skin, such as EEG, ECG, EMG, EOG, etc.

If one is measuring DC or very low-frequency biopotentials, such as EEG, body surface or bone potentials, the D-C headstage amplifier used must be free from temperature-caused, DC drift. *Chopper stabilization* is one technology used to achieve high DC drift stability. Reactive coupling avoids the DC drift problem when DC and very low-frequency potentials are not being measured. Reactive coupling is generally used with EEG and EMG signals because of their higher bandwidths and lack of DC signal information. In R-C amplifiers, successive gain stages are coupled with capacitor-resistor high-pass filters.

4.3.3 Differential Amplifiers

DAs are widely used for biopotential recording because of their ability to reduce or cancel common-mode interference and noise (Northrop 2012, Chapter 3). A D-C DA has a frequency response function that can be approximated by

$$\mathbf{V}_o = \frac{K_1}{(1+j\omega\tau_1)}\mathbf{V}_i - \frac{K_2}{(1+j\omega\tau_2)}\mathbf{V}_i'. \tag{4.4}$$

Ideally, K_1 is made $= K_2$, and $\tau_1 = \tau_2$, thus any interference signal that appears simultaneously at input V_i and V_i' is cancelled by vector subtraction. Such interference and noise can include capacitively coupled 60 Hz hum, magnetically induced 60 Hz and 120 Hz hum, ignition noise from gasoline engines, noise from fluorescent lights, etc. A voltage that is common to both DA inputs is called a *common-mode signal*. The *common-mode input signal* is defined formally as

$$V_{ic} \equiv (V_i + V_i')/2. \tag{4.5}$$

The difference mode input signal is similarly defined:

$$V_{id} \equiv (V_i - V_i')/2. \tag{4.6}$$

The amplifier output can be written in terms of V_{ic} and V_{id}:

$$\mathbf{V_o} = \mathbf{V_{id}A_D} + \mathbf{V_{ic}A_C}. \tag{4.7}$$

In general, the complex common-mode gain, $\mathbf{A_C}$, is very small, and *increases* at high frequencies. The difference-mode gain can be approximately modeled by $\mathbf{A_D} = 2K_1/(1 + j\omega\tau_1)$. A figure of merit for all DAs is the *common-mode rejection ratio* (CMRR), usually given in dB, defined by

$$\text{CMRR} \equiv 20 \log_{10}|\mathbf{A_D}/\mathbf{A_C}| \text{dB}. \tag{4.8}$$

Note that the CMRR is a function of frequency. It is very large at low frequencies, for example, >100 dB, and generally decreases steadily for $f > f_T/K_1$. An *ideal DA* has $\mathbf{A_C} \to 0$. Manufacturers generally specify the CMRR at a low frequency where it is maximum, such as 60 Hz. Another, more general way to define CMRR is

$$\text{CMRR} \equiv 20 \log_{10}\left\{\frac{V_{ic} \text{ to produce a certain } V_o}{V_{id} \text{ to produce the same } V_o}\right\}. \tag{4.9}$$

We will use the definition of Equation 4.9 to show how unbalances in Thevenin source resistance can affect the CMRR of the amplifier connected through electrodes to a biopotential source. The numerical argument of CMRR is always taken as a positive number.

As you can see from Figure 4.6, the input impedance for DAs is lower for difference-mode (DM) input signals than it is for common-mode (CM) input signals because R_{id} carries current for DM inputs. This is ordinarily not a problem because the Thevenin source resistances are generally several orders of magnitude less than either the DM or CM input resistances. In situations where the bioelectrode impedances approach the input impedances of the amplifier, it is shown below that the effective CMRR of the amplifier *as connected* can be significantly lower than (or higher than) the CMRR specified by the manufacturer for the basic DA alone. Figure 4.7 illustrates the simplified input circuit of a DA connected to a generalized, two-source biosignal. When the two sources are equal and add, there is a DM, open-circuit input voltage, v_{sd}. When the two sources are equal and oppose each other, there is a nonzero, CM, open-circuit input voltage, v_{sc}. If the input circuit is perfectly balanced, that is, $R_{ic} = R_{ic}'$, and $R_s = R_s'$, then the CMRR of the system is the same as that of the amplifier, that is, $\text{CMRR}_{sys} = \text{CMRR}_A$. If one of the Thevenin source resistances

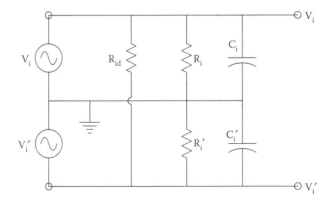

Figure 4.6 Equivalent input impedance model for a difference amplifier. R_{id} conducts no current for a pure common-mode input giving a higher CM input impedance than for DM input.

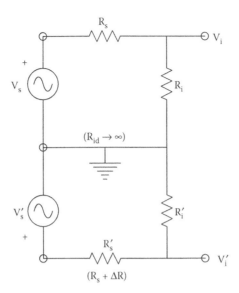

Figure 4.7 Simplified input circuit of a DA showing two unequal Thevenin sources.

is larger or smaller than the other, that is, $R'_s = R_s + \Delta R$, then a purely CM v_{sc} will produce a DM component, V_{id}, at the DA's input nodes, as well as a CM component, V_{ic}, and a purely DM v_{sd} will produce a CM component at the DA's input nodes, as well as a DM component. These unwanted components affect the CMRR of the overall system, as shown below. The overall or system CMRR is then defined as

$$\text{CMRR}_{\text{sys}} \equiv 20 \, \log_{10} \left\{ \frac{V_{sc} \text{ to produce a certain } V_o}{V_{sd} \text{ to produce the same } V_o} \right\} \text{dB.} \tag{4.10}$$

To calculate the CMRR_{sys}, we first let $V_s = V'_s$, so the input is pure CM, that is, $V_{sc} = V_s$. Now from Figure 4.7, we see that:

$$V_i = V_{sc} \, R_i/(R_i + R_s), \tag{4.11}$$

$$V'_i = V_{sc} \, R_i/(R_i + R_s + \Delta R). \tag{4.12}$$

V_{ic} and V_{id} can be found for the V_{sc} input:

$$V_{ic} \equiv (V_i + V'_i)/2 = (V_{sc}R_i/2)\left\{ \frac{1}{R_i + R_s} + \frac{1}{(R_s + R_i)[1 + \Delta R/(R_i + R_s)]} \right\}. \tag{4.13}$$

Because $R_i \gg R_s$, the $\Delta R/(R_i + R_s)$ term is $\ll 1$, and we can finally write:

$$V_{ic} \cong \frac{V_{sc}R_i}{R_i + R_s}. \tag{4.14}$$

Similarly, we can find $\mathbf{V_{id}}$ given $\mathbf{V_{sc}}$:

$$\mathbf{V_{id}} \equiv (\mathbf{V_i} - \mathbf{V'_i})/2 = \frac{\mathbf{V_{sc}}R_iR_s}{(R_i + R_s)^2} \frac{\Delta R}{R_s}. \tag{4.15}$$

Now the amplifier output is

$$\mathbf{V_o} \cong \mathbf{A_D} \frac{\mathbf{V_{sc}}R_iR_s}{(R_i + R_s)^2} \frac{\Delta R}{R_s} + \mathbf{A_C} \frac{\mathbf{V_{sc}}R_i}{(R_i + R_s)}. \tag{4.16}$$

Now we let $\mathbf{V'_s} = -\mathbf{V_s}$ to create pure $\mathbf{V_{sd}}$. In the manner used above, we find:

$$\mathbf{V_i} = \mathbf{V_{sd}} \, R_i/(R_i + R_s), \tag{4.17}$$

$$V_i' = -V_{sd}\ R_i/(R_i + R_s + \Delta R). \tag{4.18}$$

The DA's DM input is approximately:

$$V_{id} \cong V_{sd}\ R_i/(R_i + R_s). \tag{4.19}$$

And the CM input is

$$V_{ic} \cong \frac{V_{sd}R_iR_s}{(R_i + R_s)^2} \frac{\Delta R}{R_s}. \tag{4.20}$$

Using Equation 4.7, we can write the expression for V_o in terms of V_{sd}:

$$V_o \cong A_D \frac{V_{sd}R_i}{(R_i + R_s)} + A_C \frac{V_{sd}R_iR_s}{(R_i + R_s)^2} \frac{\Delta R}{R_s}. \tag{4.21}$$

Now in Equations 4.21 and 4.16, we let $V_o = 1$, and solve for V_{sd} and V_{sc}, respectively, and substitute these expressions into Equation 4.10 for the log argument. After some algebra, the log argument (numerical value of the $CMRR_{sys}$) is found to be:

$$argCMRR_{sys} \cong \left| \frac{argCMRR_A}{(argCMRR_A)\ \Delta R/(R_i + R_s) + 1} \right|, \tag{4.22}$$

where $argCMRR_A \equiv |A_D/A_C|$. Note that $argCMRR_{sys}$ can go to ∞ (i.e., make an ideal DA) if

$$\frac{\Delta R}{R_s} = \frac{-(1 + R_i/R_s)}{argCMRR_A}. \tag{4.23}$$

Figure 4.8 is a plot of $|argCMRR_{sys}|$ versus $\Delta R/R_s$. As a numerical example, assume that $CMRR_A = 100$ dB, so $argCMRR_A = 10^5$. Let $R_i = 10^8\ \Omega$, and $R_s = 10^4\ \Omega$. To get $argCMRR_{sys} \to \infty$, ΔR must $= -10^3\ \Omega$. Note that it is more practical to add 1 k externally in series with R_s, instead of subtracting 1 k from R_s'. Also note from Figure 4.8 that when $\Delta R \to 0$, $CMRR_{sys} = CMRR_A$.

The lesson the development above teaches us is that even if we spend extra money to buy a DA with a very high $CMRR_A$, hidden source impedance unbalance can significantly reduce its actual,

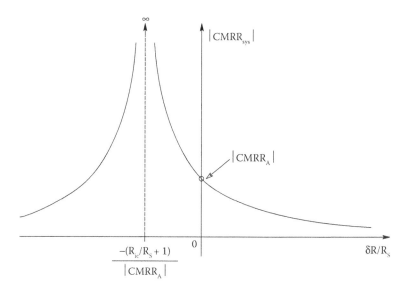

Figure 4.8 Plot of the magnitude of the numerical common-mode rejection ratio versus the fractional unbalance in the sources' Thevenin resistors. Note that in theory, it is possible to manipulate $\Delta R/R_s$ to make the CMRR $\to \infty$.

effective CMRR value. On the other hand, it is possible to make a silk purse out of a sow's ear; an inexpensive DA with a modest $CMRR_A$ can be made to have a very high $CMRR_{sys}$ by manipulating the apparent source resistances by adding a fixed, external resistor in series with one electrode and the corresponding amplifier input. In practice, the shunt capacitances associated with the input leads, and the DA's input capacitances can further unbalance the input circuit and can reduce the CMRR at high frequencies.

4.3.4 Op-amps Used for Signal Conditioning

The well-known, noninverting op-amp configuration shown in Figure 4.5 generally has a very high-input impedance (set by the op-amp), and its −3 dB frequency f_b is given by

$$f_b = f_T/(1 + R_F/R_1).\tag{4.24}$$

That is, the higher the DC gain, the smaller the amplifier's bandwidth. This trade-off of bandwidth for gain is a general property of conventional op-amps.

Another op-amp property that can figure in the choice of a given type of op-amp for a given application is the op-amp's *slew rate,* η. The units of η are V/ms or V/s. η is a large-signal parameter that gives the maximum magnitude of the rate of change of the output voltage. η is determined by the internal electronic circuitry of the op-amp, typically ranging from ~10 to over 1000 V/µs in really fast op-amps. Op-amps that have high ηs also generally have high f_Ts.

Op-amps can be used to make DAs suitable for recording biopotential signals. Such circuits are called *instrumentation amplifiers* (IAs). A common, 3-op-amp IA circuit design is shown in Figure 4.9. In this circuit, high CMRR is obtained by *precisely* matching the primed and nonprimed resistor pairs. If they are made equal, and the op-amps are assumed ideal, then pure CM excitation $\left(V_i = V_i' = V_{ic}\right)$ will make $V_2 = V_2' = V_{ic}$, and zero current will flow in R_1 and R_1'. Thus R_1 and R_1' can be removed, and it is clear that $V_3 = V_3' = V_{ic}$, hence the ideal op-amp, OA3, connected as an ideal DA gives $V_o = 0$. Thus $A_C = 0$. When $V_i' = -V_i$, there is ideal DM excitation with $V_{id} = V_i$. Hence $V_2 = V_i$ and $V_2' = -V_i$; thus there is $2V_{id}$ across $R_1 + R_1'$. Since $R_1 + R_1'$, using superposition it is easy to see that $V_c = 0$, effectively at ground potential. Now $V_3 = V_{id}(1 + R_2/R_1)$, and $V_3' = -V_{id}(1 + R_2/R_1)$. V_o is found from superposition:

$$V_o = V_3 \frac{R_4}{(R_4 + R_3)}(1 + R_4/R_3) + V_3'\left(-\frac{R_4}{R_3}\right),$$
$$\downarrow \tag{4.25}$$
$$V_o = V_{id} \frac{2\,R_4(R_1 + R_2)}{R_3 R_1}.$$

Thus $A_D = 2R_4\,(R_1 + R_2)/(R_3\,R_1)$ for this op-amp IA circuit. In practice, the op-amps are not ideal, they have finite $CMRR_A$s, and the resistors will not be perfectly matched, so the IA will have a

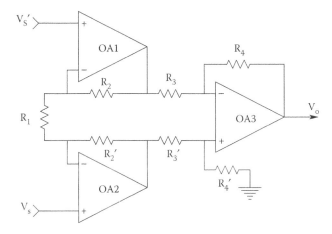

Figure 4.9 Well-known, three-op-amp instrumentation amplifier circuits. The resistors must be accurately matched to maximize the IA's CMRR.

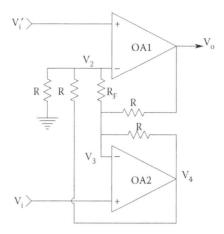

Figure 4.10 Two-op-amp IA circuits. Resistors, R, must be precisely matched for highest CMRR.

finite $CMRR_{sys}$. To maximize the $CMRR_{sys}$, it is possible to deliberately introduce a small amount of asymmetry into the circuit, for example, by making R_1' variable around the fixed R_1 value.

Another IA architecture uses only two op-amps and matched resistors. The circuit is shown in Figure 4.10. To analyze this circuit, we will use superposition. First, we let $V_i' > 0$ and $V_i = 0$. By the ideal op-amp assumption, $V_2 = V_i'$ and $V_3 = 0$. Node equations are written for the V_2 and V_3 nodes:

$$V_2(2G + G_F) - V_4G - V_3G_F = 0, \tag{4.26}$$

$$V_3(2G + G_F) - V_4G - V_2G_F - V_oG = 0. \tag{4.27}$$

From the ideal op-amp assumptions,

$$V_i'(2G + G_F) - V_4G = 0 \tag{4.28}$$
$$-V_4G - V_i'G_F - V_oG = 0$$
$$\downarrow$$
$$-V_i'(2G + G_F) - V_i'G_F = V_oG$$
$$\downarrow$$
$$V_o = -V_i'2(1 + R/R_F). \tag{4.29}$$

Next, we let $V_i > 0$ and set $V_i' = 0$. Thus by the ideal op-amp assumption, $V_3 = V_i$ and $V_2 = 0$. Again, we write the node equations for the V_2 and V_3 nodes and solve for V_o:

$$V_o = +V_i2(1 + R/R_F). \tag{4.30}$$

By superposition, we can finally write:

$$V_o = (V_i - V_i')\,2(1 + R/R_F) = V_{id}\,4(1 + R/R_F). \tag{4.31}$$

Thus $A_D = 4(1 + R/R_F)$, with a minimum of 4, and due to resistor matching and ideal op-amps, $A_C = 0$.

One advantage of using op-amps to make IAs is that the final cost is generally lower than a commercial, single-chip, IA. Another benefit is that there are available some very low-noise op-amps so that the op-amp IA can often be designed to have a better output SNR than a commercial counterpart. A small disadvantage is that in addition to two or three op-amps, five to seven discrete resistors are needed (usually one or two are needed for a commercial IC IA to set the gain).

Op-amps can also be used to make active filters (AFs) to improve the output SNR of recorded biopotentials (cf. Northrop 2012, Chapter 7). A typical noise root power density spectrum (PDS), such as might be found at the output of a D-C bioamplifier, is shown in Figure 4.11; note that at low frequencies, the spectrum has a 1/f component that is present in all amplifiers at low frequencies,

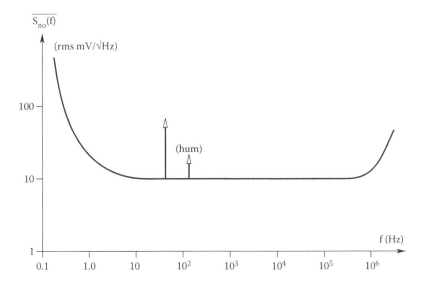

Figure 4.11 Typical, one-sided, noise voltage root power density spectrum seen at the output of a high-gain amplifier. The root spectrum's units are rmsVolts/√Hz.

and often arises with the signal because of ion reactions at electrode wet interfaces. The root PDS also has spikes from coherent interference from power lines at 60 Hz and 120 Hz. The center part of the root PDS remains flat to frequencies well above the normal biomedical range. Thus, as a biopotential signal has a root PDS that lies within the noise root PDS, the output SNR can be improved by passing only the signal spectral bandwidth, excluding high- and low-frequency noise, where applicable. Thus, the amplified biopotential signal plus noise can be band-pass or low-pass filtered by op-amp AFs, and notch AFs can be used to remove coherent interference. The spikes shown in Figure 4.11 are from coherent interference (e.g., 60 Hz and 120 Hz power line fields).

4.3.5 Noise and Low-Noise Amplifiers

An unfortunate property of all electronic amplifiers is that they introduce noise into the amplified signal. This noise provides a fundamental limitation to the resolution of very small signals, as determined by the SNR at the amplifier's output. In this section, we will examine how amplifier noise can be described, and how SNR at the amplifier's output can be maximized.

First, let us make a distinction between *noise* and *interference,* both of which degrade output SNR. Interference is generally *coherent,* that is, periodic in nature, and generally comes from some man-made source, such as power lines, fluorescent lights, or automobile ignitions. Noise, as we define it, is completely random; it is the result of the random motion of many, many electrons in resistors and semiconductor devices (diodes, BJTs, and FETs). The descriptor of noise that we will use in this section is the *one-sided* PDS. The significance of a PDS can be interpreted heuristically by referring to Figure 4.12. A random noise voltage source, $e_N(t)$, is connected to an *ideal low-pass*

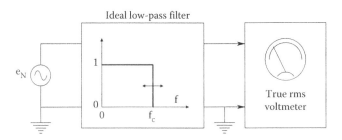

Figure 4.12 Basic set-up for measuring the one-sided mean-squared power density spectrum of a noise source.

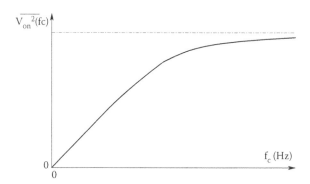

Figure 4.13 Representative plot of the cumulative mean-squared noise voltage obtained with the circuit of Figure 4.12 as f_c is increased from zero.

filter whose cut-off frequency, f_c, is variable between 0 and ∞. A broadband, true RMS (TRMS) voltmeter is connected to the filter output. We slowly increase the filter's cut-off frequency from zero and plot the squared meter reading versus the cut-off frequency. Figure 4.13 shows the plot of the cumulative mean-squared volts versus f_c. Note that this plot *is not* the PDS. To find the PDS, we must find the slope of the cumulative msV plot. That is

$$S_n(f) = \frac{d\, v_{on}^2(f)}{df} \text{ mean-squared volts/Hz.} \qquad (4.32)$$
$$f_c \rightarrow f$$

where $S_n(f)$ is the one-sided PDS of the noise source: it is nonnegative. The *root PDS* is simply $\sqrt{S_n(f)}$.

Electrical engineers like to work with idealized components, amplifiers, voltage sources, etc. Noise is no exception. One type of idealized noise source makes *white noise*. A white noise PDS is constant over $0 \le f \le \infty$. That is, its PDS is $S_{Wn}(f) = \eta$ msV/Hz. A 1/f noise PDS is of the form: $S_{n/f}(f) = b/f$ msV/Hz. When a real noise PDS has a long, flat region, we say it is "white" in that range. White and 1/f PDSs can be added together to form a composite PDS. Note that superposition of noise PDSs *can only be done using mean-squared quantities*. It is not technically correct to add root spectra; the PDSs must be added, then the square root taken to get the combined root PDS.

A large source of noise in circuits is from resistors (capacitors and ideal inductors do not make noise, although they can contribute to the shaping of a PDS). Resistors make white, *thermal* (or Johnson) noise; statistical thermodynamics tells us that the PDS for a resistor's thermal noise is given by

$$S_{Rn}(f) = 4kTR \text{ msV/Hz}, \qquad (4.33)$$

where k is Boltzmann's constant (1.38×10^{-23} J/°K), T is the kelvin temperature, and R is the resistor value in ohms. (At VHF, resistor lead inductance and shunt capacitance cause the real thermal noise spectrum from a resistor to drop off to zero.)

If two resistors are in series at different temperatures, the total voltage PDS across them is: $S_{Rn}(f) = 4k(T_1R_1 + T_2R_2)$ msV/Hz. If the two resistors are in parallel, the voltage PDS is

$$S_{Rn}(f) = 4kT_1R_1\left[R_2/(R_1 + R_2)\right]^2 + 4kT_2R_2\left[R_1/R_1 + R_2\right]^2 \text{ msV/Hz} \qquad (4.34)$$

See Figure 4.14 for a summary of how thermal noise from resistors combines.

Note that when an average or DC current, I, passes through a resistor, it also emits 1/f noise in addition to its thermal noise. That is,

$$S_{Rn}(f) = 4kTR + A I^2/f \text{ msv/Hz.} \qquad (4.35)$$

Certain resistor materials have lower A's than others, for example, wire-wound resistors have a lower A coefficient than do carbon composition resistors.

Circuit	Noise equivalent circuit with noisless R's	Power density spectrum (white)

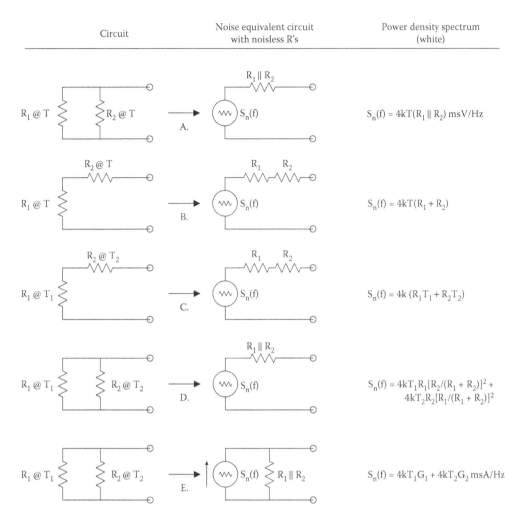

A. $S_n(f) = 4kT(R_1 \| R_2)$ msV/Hz

B. $S_n(f) = 4kT(R_1 + R_2)$

C. $S_n(f) = 4k\,(R_1T_1 + R_2T_2)$

D. $S_n(f) = 4kT_1R_1[R_2/(R_1 + R_2)]^2 + 4kT_2R_2[R_1/(R_1 + R_2)]^2$

E. $S_n(f) = 4kT_1G_1 + 4kT_2G_2$ msA/Hz

Figure 4.14 Five examples of how the white thermal noise power spectrums from pairs of resistors combine. In the Thevenin noise-equivalent circuits, the resistors are noiseless.

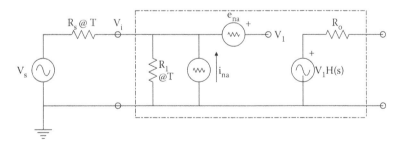

Figure 4.15 Two-source noise models for amplifiers and transistors. $e_{na}(f)$ is the equivalent input short-circuit voltage, noise root power spectrum in rmsV/$\sqrt{}$Hz. $i_{na}(f)$ is the equivalent input noise current root power spectrum in rmsA/$\sqrt{}$Hz.

The bad news is, every resistor, transistor, and diode in IC op-amps, DA's, and IA's makes noise. As you will see, the good news is that components in the first stage (input, or headstage) of an amplifier are mostly responsible for the overall amplifier's output noise. The total output noise from an amplifier is always referred to its input terminals with the *two noise source model*, shown in Figure 4.15. e_{na} is really $e_{na}(f)$. e_{na} is the *equivalent, short-circuited input noise voltage root PDS*.

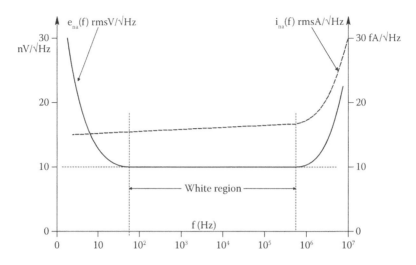

Figure 4.16 Plots of $e_{na}(f)$ and $i_{na}(f)$ for a typical FET input amplifier. Note that in the midband range of frequencies, e_{na} and i_{na} can be considered "white." Amplifiers having BJT headstages typically have a lower e_{na} and a larger i_{na}. Also, i_{na} has a $1/\sqrt{f}$ component at low frequencies generally not seen in FET-input amplifiers.

$e_{na}(f)$ has the units of $\mathrm{rmsV}/\sqrt{\mathrm{Hz}}$. A typical $e_{na}(f)$ plot is shown in Figure 4.16. Note that it has a $1/f$ region, a white region, and increases again at high frequencies. e_{na} accounts for the amplifier's output noise when its input is short-circuited; when open-circuited, two other sources must be considered: the thermal noise from the input resistance, R_1 at T, and the *equivalent input current source root PDS*, $i_{na}(f)$, in $\mathrm{rmsA}/\sqrt{\mathrm{Hz}}$. The value of i_{na} depends on the amplifier's input DC bias current, I_B, because most of i_{na} comes from input device shot noise. FET input headstages generally have very low i_{na}s, while BJT headstages which have much larger bias currents have larger i_{na}s. The output voltage noise PDS of the amplifier is shaped by the amplifier's frequency response function, $\mathbf{H}(j\omega)$. For an *open-circuited input* amplifier, the PDS at the V_i node can be written (assuming white spectra):

$$S_{Vin}(f) = e_{na}^2 + 4kTR_1 + i_{na}^2 R_1^2 \; \mathrm{msV/Hz}. \tag{4.36}$$

It can be shown that the noise PDS at the amplifiers output is (Papoulis 1977):

$$S_{Von}(f) = S_{Vin}(f) \, |\mathbf{H}(j2\pi f)|^2 \quad \mathrm{msV/Hz}. \tag{4.37}$$

Note that the square of the absolute value of the frequency response vector, $\mathbf{H}(j2\pi f)$, is used. Now the total mean-squared noise voltage at the amplifier output is found by

$$\overline{v_{on}^2} = \int_0^\infty [e_{na}^2 + 4kTR_1 + i_{na}^2 R_1^2] \, |\mathbf{H}(j2\pi f)|^2 \, df \; \mathrm{msV}. \tag{4.38}$$

That is, the output noise PDS is integrated with respect to Hz frequency from 0 to ∞. If we include the amplifier's input capacitance in parallel with R_1, a low-pass filter is formed for the thermal noise current from R_1, and from i_{na}. The output PDS is then:

$$S_{Von}(f) = e_{na}^2 \, |\mathbf{H}(j2\pi f)|^2 + \left[i_{na}^2 + 4kTG_1\right] \frac{R_1^2}{|1 + j2\pi f C_1 R_1|^2} \, |\mathbf{H}(j2\pi f)|^2. \tag{4.39}$$

Note that the low-pass filter's frequency response magnitude squared must be included as a factor for the noise currents with the amplifier's frequency response magnitude squared. The integral of $S_{Von}(f)$ over $0 \le f \le \infty$ gives the total output ms noise voltage for this open-circuited model.

When the amplifier is connected to a Thevenin signal source, as shown in Figure 4.15, R_s is in parallel with R_1. We can generally assume that $R_1 \gg R_s$, so R_1 can be set equal to ∞

(an open-circuit), and we can neglect C_1. We also assume that e_{na} and i_{na} are white to simplify calculations. The ms output noise is then given by

$$\overline{v_{on}^2} = \left[e_{na}^2 + 4kTR_s + i_{na}^2 R_s^2 \right] \int_0^\infty |H(j2\pi f)|^2 \, df \text{ msV}. \tag{4.40}$$

The integral in Equation 4.40 is called the *noise gain² bandwidth* (G²BW) function of the frequency response function. It can be expressed, in general, as $K_v^2 B$, where K_v is the amplifier's low-frequency gain if it is a D-C amplifier, or the amplifier's midband gain if it is an R-C (AC) amplifier. B is the *equivalent noise bandwidth* in Hz. A table of G² BW functions for common amplifier transfer functions can be found in Northrop (2012, Table 9.1). For example, a simple band-pass amplifier, such as used for ECG recording, has a frequency response which can be modeled by

$$H(j2\pi f) = \frac{K_V 2\pi f_L}{(1 + j2\pi f \tau_L)(1 + j2\pi f \tau_H)}. \tag{4.41}$$

The G²BW function for this amplifier can be shown to be:

$$G^2BW = K_V^2 \left[\frac{1}{4\tau_H(1 + \tau_H/\tau_L)} \right], \tag{4.42}$$

where the term in brackets is the *noise bandwidth*, B, in Hz, K_v^2 is the midband gain squared, τ_L is the time constant of the low-frequency pole, and τ_H is the time constant of the high-frequency pole, in seconds.

Now let a sinusoidal signal of V_s peak volts be applied to the amplifier [$v_s(t) = V_s \sin(2\pi fs\, t)$]. Assume its frequency, f_s, is in the mid-frequency or passband range of $H(j2\pi f)$, so it gets multiplied by the midband gain, K_V. Thus the *mean-squared output signal* is simply:

$$\overline{V_{os}^2} = \left(V_s^2/2 \right) K_V^2 \text{ msV}. \tag{4.43}$$

The mean-squared output SNR is then:

$$SNR_o = \frac{\left(V_s^2/2 \right) K_V^2}{\left[e_{na}^2 + 4kTR_s + i_{na}^2 R_s^2 \right] K_V^2 B}. \tag{4.44}$$

Examining Equation 4.44, we see that decreasing the noise bandwidth, B, around the frequency of the signal, f_s, will raise the SNR_o.

A noise figure-of-merit for an amplifier is its *noise factor*, F, defined as

$$F \equiv \frac{SNR_{in}}{SNR_o}. \tag{4.45}$$

Its *noise figure* is given in dB:

$$NF \equiv 10 \log_{10}(F) \tag{4.46}$$

For the case of the sinusoidal input at f_s, the output SNR is given by Equation 4.44. The input mean-squared SNR is defined as

$$SNR_{in} \equiv \frac{\left(V_s^2/2 \right)}{4kTR_s B}. \tag{4.47}$$

In this case, the only noise assumed to accompany the signal is the thermal white noise from its Thevenin resistor, R_s. This noise must be given the noise bandwidth of the amplifier, B. Using the definition for noise factor, we find the well-known result (Northrop 1997):

$$F = 1 + \frac{e_{na}^2 + i_{na}^2 R_s^2}{4kTR_s}. \tag{4.48}$$

Manufacturers of low-noise amplifiers typically specify an NF in dB. Along with this number, the R_s, B, and T must also be given. An ideal, noiseless amplifier has F = 1. The larger F is, the poorer the noise performance of the amplifier.

The bottom line in designing signal conditioning systems, however, is not the minimization of amplifier F, but the maximization of amplifier SNR_o.

One way SNR_o can be maximized for AC (band-pass) signals is through the use of a precision, low-noise, impedance-matching transformer to couple the Thevenin circuit of the source to the amplifier. The transformer circuit is shown schematically in Figure 4.17. The mean-squared (MS) signal at the output is

$$S_o = \overline{v_s^2} n^2 K_V^2 \text{ msV.} \tag{4.49}$$

Note that the open-circuit source voltage is multiplied by the turns ratio, n, of the transformer on the amplifier side. The MS noise at the output is given by (Northrop 2012):

$$N_o = \left[e_{na}^2 + i_{na}^2 (n^2 R_s)^2 + n^2 4kTR_s \right] K_V^2 B \text{ msV.} \tag{4.50}$$

Note that the resistance i_{na} "sees" looking back into the transformer can be shown to be $n^2 R_s$. Thus, the msSNR$_o$ of the circuit is

$$SNR_o = \frac{\overline{v_s^2} n^2 K_V^2}{\left[e_{na}^2 + i_{na}^2 \left(n^2 R_s \right)^2 + n^2 4kTR_s \right] K_V^2 B}, \tag{4.51}$$

$\downarrow$

$$SNR_o = \frac{\overline{v_s^2}}{\left[e_{na}^2 / n^2 + i_{na}^2 n^2 R_s^2 + 4kTR_s \right] B}. \tag{4.52}$$

The SNR_o clearly has a *maximum* when its denominator has a *minimum*. When the denominator is differentiated with respect to n^2 and set equal to zero, we find that maximum SNR_o occurs when the transformer's turns ratio is

$$n = n_o = \sqrt{e_{na}/(i_{na}R_s)}. \tag{4.53}$$

The *maximum* SNR_o is thus:

$$SNR_{omax} = \frac{\overline{v_s^2}/B}{4kTR_s + 2e_{na}i_{na}R_s}. \tag{4.54}$$

Because real transformers are noisy (their windings have resistance that makes thermal noise, and their magnetic cores make Barkhausen noise), the actual SNR_o never reaches the value given by Equation 4.54. In practice, transformer maximization of SNR_o is justifiable only if (Northrop 2012):

$$\left[e_{na}/(i_{na}R_s) i_{na}R_s/e_{na} \right] > 20. \tag{4.55}$$

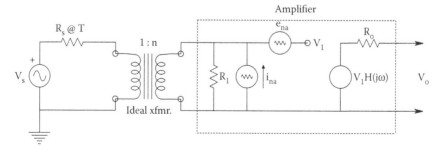

Figure 4.17 Equivalent circuits for an amplifier using an ideal transformer to maximize its output SNR at the same time it minimizes its noise figure (NF). The transformer's turns ratio, n, is varied to maximize the SNR_{out}. See text for analysis.

In all the developments above, we have assumed that both e_{na} and i_{na} are white, that is, they have the values seen in the flat range of their plots versus frequency. For example, if an Analog Devices' AD6251 IA is used, $e_{na} = 4nV/\sqrt{Hz}$ in the white region, and $i_{na} = 0.3\ pArms/\sqrt{Hz}$. Let the $R_s = 5000$ ohms.

Thus $[4 \times 10^{-9}/(3 \times 10^{-13} \times 5 \times 10^3) + (3 \times 10^{-13} \times 5 \times 10^3)/4 \times 10^{-9}] = 3.042 < 20$, and the use of a transformer would not be practical. Note that $e_{na}/i_{na} = 13.3\ k\Omega$ for this amplifier. Now let us use an FET input IA, the Burr–Brown INA1102 which has $e_{na} = 10\ nVrms/\sqrt{Hz}$ and $i_{na} = 1.8\ fArms/\sqrt{Hz}$. Again, let $R_s = 5\ k\Omega$. Thus $[1 \times 10^{-8}/(1.8 \times 10^{-15} \times 5 \times 10^3) + (1.8 \times 10^{-15} \times 5 \times 10^3)/1 \times 10^{-8}] = 1.11 \times 10^3 \gg 20$, and the use of a transformer is justified. Its turns ratio should be: $n_o = \sqrt{1 \times 10^{-8}/(1.8 \times 10^{-15} \times 5 \times 10^3)} = 33.3$, and $e_{na}/i_{na} = 5.56 \times 10^6\ \Omega$. It should be stressed that low-noise, impedance-matching transformers are expensive, and their low-frequency, -3 dB frequencies are ~ 3 Hz, limiting their usefulness for certain, low-frequency bioelectric signal conditioning.

When a high-gain amplifier is designed with two or more, separate, cascaded, noisy amplifier stages, as shown in Figure 4.18, the output ms SNR can be found. Assuming scalar gains, we have:

$$SNR_o = \frac{\overline{v_s^2}K_{V1}^2K_{V2}^2K_{V3}^2}{\left[\left(4kTR_s + e_{na1}^2 + i_{na1}^2R_s^2\right)K_{V1}^2K_{V2}^2K_{V3}^2 + e_{na2}^2K_{V2}^2K_{V3}^2 + e_{na3}^2K_{V3}^2\right]B}. \tag{4.56}$$

Dividing by the overall gain^2 gives us an instructive expression for the SNR_o:

$$SNR_o = \frac{\overline{v_s^2}/B}{\left(4kTR_s + e_{na1}^2 + i_{na1}^2R_s^2\right) + e_{na2}^2/K_{V1}^2 + e_{na3}^2/\left(K_{V1}^2K_{V2}^2\right)}. \tag{4.57}$$

Thus as long as $K_{V1} > 5$, the SNR_o of the amplifier cascade is approximately that of the headstage alone. *That is, importantly, the headstage sets the noise performance of the cascaded amplifier.* If, for some reason, a unity gain buffer stage is used as the headstage, the e_{na} of the second stage also becomes significant, and then that and the headstage *both* have to be chosen for low e_{na}s.

As an example of calculating the output SNR of an amplifier, consider the noninverting op-amp shown in Figure 4.19. The MS output signal is

$$S_o = \overline{v_s^2}\left(1 + R_2/R_1\right)^2\ msV. \tag{4.58}$$

The ms output noise is

$$N_o = B\left[\left(4kTR_s + e_{na}^2 + i_{na}^2R_s^2\right)\left(1 + R_2/R_1\right)^2 + 4kTR_1\left(R_2/R_1\right)^2 + 4kTG_2R_2^2\right]. \tag{4.59}$$

Putting these expressions together and doing some algebra, we find:

$$SNR_o = \frac{\overline{v_s^2}/B}{4kTR_s + e_{na}^2 + i_{na}^2R_s^2 + 4kTR_1R_2/(R_1 + R_2)}. \tag{4.60}$$

The expression is similar to the SNR_o for the amplifier of Figure 4.15, except there is an extra term derived from the thermal noise in R_1 in parallel with R_2. For high gain, we make $R_2 \gg R_1$; however, low-absolute values should be used so $R_1R_2/(R_1 + R_2)$ will be small.

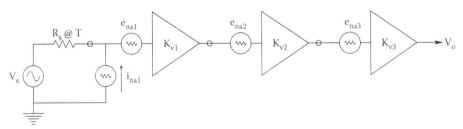

Figure 4.18 Three cascaded noisy stages used to make a high-gain amplifier. The stage with the lowest e_{na} and a gain >5 should be the headstage.

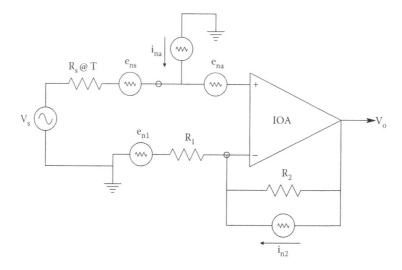

Figure 4.19 Noninverting op-amp amplifier showing the five noise sources contributing to the output noise. The resistors R_s, R_1, and R_2 all contribute white thermal noise to the net ms input noise. Note that negligible noise arises in the OA's output resistance.

As we have seen, DA's have two active inputs, and thus can be assigned an independent i_{na} and e_{na} for both inputs. While two sources at each input are technically correct, it is more expedient to use only one, equivalent e_{na} and i_{na} *at one input.* These are the parameters that manufacturers in fact give us in IA specs. Because, in general, the amplifier's $|A_D| \gg |A_C|$ in the operating range of interest, we can neglect the CM noise components resulting from using single sources at either the + or − inputs. Inspection of Figure 4.20 allows us to write an expression for the ms signal output,

$$S_o = \overline{v_{sd}^2} A_D^2 \text{ msV} \tag{4.61}$$

given pure DM signal in. That is, $v_s' = -v_s$. The ms noise output is found from finding the MS value of $v_{id} = (v_i - v_i')/2$ for the noise voltages.

$$\overline{v_{id}^2} = 1/4[\overline{v_i^2} - \overline{2v_i v_i'} + \overline{v_i'^2}] \rightarrow 1/4[\overline{v_i^2} + \overline{v_i'^2}]. \tag{4.62}$$

The mean cross-term $\rightarrow 0$ because the thermal noise sources from R_s and R_s' are uncorrelated. $\overline{v_i'^2} = 4kTR_s'B$, and $\overline{v_i^2} = [e_{na}^2 + 4kTR_s + i_{na}^2 R_s^2]B$. Assuming that $R_s = R_s'$, the total mean-squared noise voltage at the output is

$$N_o = A_D^2 B[e_{na}^2 + 8kTR_s + i_{na}^2 R_s^2]/4 \text{ msV}. \tag{4.63}$$

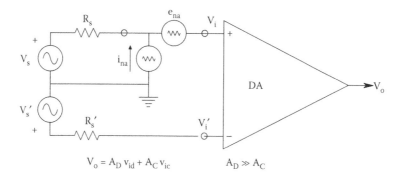

$$V_o = A_D v_{id} + A_C v_{ic} \qquad A_D \gg A_C$$

Figure 4.20 Differential amplifier's input noise can be approximated as coming from only one input. A high CMRR is assumed.

And the DA's ms output SNR is

$$SNR_o = \frac{\overline{v_{sd}^2}(4/B)}{\left[e_{na}^2 + 8kTR_s + i_{na}^2 R_s^2\right]}. \tag{4.64}$$

The "4" factor in the numerator comes from the definition of v_{id}.

As a numerical example, let us calculate the rms v_{sd} required to give an ms $SNR_o = 9$ (the same as an rms $SNR_o = 3$). Assume the noise sources are white and the noise bandwidth is 400 Hz, also, $e_{na} = 4$ nVrms/$\sqrt{Hz}$, $i_{na} = 0.3$ pArms/$\sqrt{Hz}$, $R_s = R_s' = 4000\ \Omega$, and $T = 300$ K. Thus:

$$9 = \frac{\overline{v_{sd}^2}(4/400)}{[1.6 \times 10^{-17} + 8 \times 1.38 \times 10^{-23} \times 300 \times 4 \times 10^3 + 9 \times 10^{-26} \times 1.6 \times 10^7]}.$$
$$\qquad\qquad\downarrow\qquad\qquad\qquad\downarrow\qquad\qquad\qquad\qquad\downarrow \tag{4.65}$$
$$1.3248 \times 10^{-16}\quad [1.499 \times 10^{-16}]\qquad 1.44 \times 10^{-18}$$

Solving for $\sqrt{\overline{v_{sd}^2}}$, we find that an rms, DM input of 0.3673 μV will give an rms $SNR_o = 3$. In practice, this voltage may be significantly higher because $e_{na}(f)$ and $i_{na}(f)$ will have 1/f spectral components in the low end of the signal's band-pass region. We ignored the 1/f problem in this example for mathematical simplicity.

To examine how the 1/f spectrum of e_{na} should be treated, let us return to the example illustrated in Figure 4.19. We will assume that $e_{na}^2(f) = b/f + e_{naw}^2$; i_{na} and all resistor noises will be assumed to be white. The noise bandwidth, B, will be defined over the interval, $\{f_L, f_H\}$, that is, $B = f_H - f_L$. Thus, the output ms noise is

$$N_o = \int_{f_L}^{f_H} \left[\left(b/f + e_{naw}^2 + 4kTR_s + i_{na}^2 R_s^2\right)\left(1 + R_2/R_1\right)^2 + 4kTR_1\left(R_2/R_1\right)^2 + 4kTG_2R_2^2\right] df$$
$$\downarrow \tag{4.66}$$
$$N_o = \left(1 + R_2/R_1\right)^2 \left\{b \ln\left(f_H/f_L\right) + \left[e_{naw}^2 + 4kTR_s + i_{na}^2 R_s^2\right](f_H - f_L)\right\}$$
$$+ [4kTR_1\left(R_2/R_1\right)^2 + 4kTR_2](f_H - f_L).$$

The ms output SNR is then:

$$SNR_o = \frac{\overline{v_s^2}/B}{(b/B)\ln(f_H/f_L) + e_{naw}^2 + 4kTR_s + i_{na}^2 R_s^2 + 4kTR_1R_2/(R_1 + R_2)}. \tag{4.67}$$

The first term in the denominator of Equation 4.67 is the extra ms noise from the 1/f part of the e_{na}^2 spectrum. Good resolution of threshold, low-frequency, bioelectric signals requires the use of amplifiers with low e_{na}^2 1/f noise; not only should the parameter b be small (b has the units of ms volts), but also the white component of e_{na}^2 should be small as well.

A low-noise amplifier is one which has $e_{na} < 10$ nV/$\sqrt{Hz}$ in its white region. The best, low-noise amplifiers use BJT headstages in which the transistor DC biasing can be optimized to give the least e_{na}. In some low-noise, BJT-input amplifiers, such as the LT1028 op-amp, $e_{na} = 1.1$ nVrms/$\sqrt{Hz}$ at 1 kHz, and a minimum of 0.85 nVrms/$\sqrt{Hz}$ at 1 kHz, and $i_{na} = 4.7$ pArms/$\sqrt{Hz}$ at 10 Hz, and 1.0 pArms/$\sqrt{Hz}$ at 1 kHz. The input impedance of the LT1028 is 20 MΩ (DM) and 300 MΩ (CM) and its input bias current is $I_B = 25$ nA. (Most JFET-input amplifiers have I_Bs on the order of picoamps, and corresponding i_{na}s on the order of fArms/$\sqrt{Hz}$. JFET op-amps also have R_{in}'s on the order of 10^{13} ohms to 10^{14} ohms. A short table of low-noise amplifiers and their properties [op-amps, IA's and isolation amps] can be found in Northrop (2014, Table 3.2).

4.3.6 Medical Isolation Amplifiers

All amplifiers used to record biopotential signals from humans must meet certain standards for worst-case voltage breakdown and maximum leakage currents through their input leads which are attached to electrodes on the body, and maximum current through any driven output lead attached to the body. A variety of testing conditions or scenarios to ensure patient safety have been formulated by various regulatory agencies (cf. Northrop 2012, Section 8.3). The conservative leakage current and voltage breakdown criteria set by the *National Fire Protection Association* (NFPA) (Quincy, MA), and the *Association for the Advancement of Medical Instrumentation* (AAMI) have generally been adopted by medical equipment manufacturers in the United States and by U.S. hospitals and other healthcare facilities. There are a number of other regulatory agencies that also are involved in formulating and adopting the electrical medical safety standards: These include: The *International Electrotechnical Commission* (IEC), the *Under-writers Laboratories* (UL), the *Health Industries Manufacturers' Association* (HEMA), the *National Electrical Manufacturers' Association* (NEMA), and the *U.S. Food and Drug Administration* (FDA). Most of the standards have been adopted to prevent patient electrocution, including burns, the induction of fibrillation in the heart, muscle spasms, etc.

Space does not permit us to go into the effects of electroshock, and the many of scenarios by which it can occur. Nor can we explore the technology of safe grounding practices and ground fault interruption. The interested reader should consult Chapter 14 in Webster (1992) and Chapter 8 in Northrop (2012) for these details.

If the threshold, AC, surface current required to induce cardiac fibrillation in 50% of dogs tested is plotted versus frequency, it is seen that the least current is required between 40 and 100 Hz; note that this includes power line frequencies. From 80 to 600 μA rms of 60 Hz current will induce cardiac fibrillation when applied directly to the heart, as through a catheter (Webster 1992). Thus, the NFPA-ANSI/AAMI standard for ECG amplifier lead leakage is that *isolated* input lead current (at 60 Hz) must be <10 μA between any two leads shorted together, <10 μA for any input lead connected to the power plug ground (green wire) with and without the amplifier's case grounded. A more severe test is that isolation amplifier input lead leakage current must be <20 μA when any input lead is connected to the high side of the 120 Vac mains. To meet these severe tests for leakage, the MIA has evolved (cf. Section 8.3 in Northrop 2012).

Isolation is accomplished by electrically separating the input stage of the MIA from the output stage. That is, the input stage has a separate, floating power supply and a "ground" that are connected to the output side of the MIA by a resistance of over 1000 megohms, and a parallel capacitance in the low picofarad range. The signal output of the input stage is also isolated from the MIA's output by a similar very high impedance, although the Thevenin output resistance of the MIA can range from milliohms to several hundred ohms.

There are three major means of effecting the galvanic isolation of the input and output stages of MIAs. *The first means* is to use a high-quality, toroidal transformer to magnetically couple regulated AC power from the output side to the isolated input stage where it is rectified and filtered, and also is coupled to rectifiers and filters serving the output amplifiers. Frequencies in the range of 100–750 kHz are typically used with transformer isolation MIAs. The output signal from the isolated headstage modulates an AC carrier which is magnetically coupled to a demodulator on the output side. *A second means of isolation* is to use photo-optic coupling of the amplified signal; usually pulse-width or delta-sigma modulation of the optical signal is used, although direct, linear, analog, photo-optic coupling can be used. In the optical type of MIA, a separate, isolated, DC/DC converter must be used to power the input stage. *A third means of isolation* is to use a pair of small (e.g., 1 pF) capacitors to couple a pulse-modulated signal from the isolated input to the output stage. A separate, isolated power supply must be used with the differential capacitor-coupled MIA, too. Some of the critical specifications of five types of medical-grade MIAs are listed in Table 4.2.

In the Burr–Brown, ISO121, differential capacitor-coupled MIA is used with a separate, isolated clock to run its duty cycle-modulator. The clock frequency can be from 5 to 700 kHz, giving commensurate bandwidths, governed by the Nyquist criterion.

A simplified schematic of an Analog Devices AD289, magnetically coupled MIA is shown in Figure 4.21. Note that this MIA has a single-ended input. The clock power oscillator drives a toroidal core, T1, on which are wound coils for the input and output isolated power supplies, and for the synchronizing signals for the double-sideband, suppressed-carrier (DSBSC) modulator and demodulator. A separate toroidal transformer, T2, couples the modulated output signal to the output side of the MIA. This is basically the architecture used in the Intronics 290 and the Burr–Brown BB3656 MIAs.

An unmodulated, feedback-type, analog, optical isolation system is used in the Burr–Brown BB3652, differential, optically coupled, linear IA. This IA still requires a transformer-isolated power supply for the input headstage, and for the driver for the linear optocoupler. A feedback-type linear optocoupler, similar to that used in the BB3652, is shown in Figure 4.22. (In the BB3652, OA1 is replaced with a high-input impedance DA headstage.) The circuit works in the following manner: The summing junction of OA2 is at 0 volts. The DC bias current through R_{B1}, I_{B1} drives the OA2 output negative, biasing the LED, D2, on at some I_{D20}. D2's light illuminates photodiodes D1 and D3

Table 4.2: Comparison of Properties of Some Popular Medical Isolation Amplifiers

Amplifier	IA294	IA296	BB 3652	BB ISO121	AD210
Isol/Type	Transformer/ MIA	Transformer/ MIA	Optical/MIA	Capacitor/ MIA	Transformer/ MIA
Manufacturer	Intronics	Intronics	Burr–Brown	Burr–Brown	Analog Devices
CMV isolation	±5000 V cont. ±6500 V 10 ms pulse	±5000 V cont ±6500 V 10 ms pulse	±2000 V continuous ±5000 V, 10 s	3500 Vrms	2500 Vrms contin. 3500 Vpk contin.
CMRR at 60 Hz	120 dB at 60 Hz	160–170 dB	80 dB at 60 Hz	115 dB IMR at 60 Hz	100 dB
Gain range	10 (fixed)	1–100	1 to >100, by formula	1 V/V (fixed)	1–100 V/V
Leakage to 120 Vac mains	10 μA max	0.5 μA	0.5 μA 1.8 pF leakage capacitance	$I_{ac} = V2\pi fC$ $C \cong 2.21$ pF	—
Noise	8 μV ppk 0.05–100 Hz	0.3 μV ppk 10–100 Hz BW	4 μV ppk 0.05–100 Hz BW	4 μVrms/√Hz	18 nV/√Hz at 1 kHz
Bandwidth	0–1 kHz	0–1 kHz, −3 dB	0–15 kHz, ± 3 dB	0–60 kHz (c. 200 kHz clock)	20 kHz −3 dB
Slew-rate	—	—	1.2 V/μs	2 V/μs	—

Source: Northrop, R.B. 2012. *Analysis and Application of Analog Electronic Circuits to Biomedical Instrumentation,* 2nd Ed. CRC Press, Boca Raton, FL. ISBN: 978-1-4398-6669-6.

equally; the reverse photocurrent through D1 drives OA2's output positive, reducing I_{D2}. It thus provides a linearizing, negative feedback around OA2, acting against the current produced by the input voltage, V_{in}/R_1. As D1 and D3 are matched photodiodes, the reverse photocurrent in D3 equals that in D1, that is, $I_{D10} = I_{D30}$, and $V_o = R_3 (I_{D30} - I_{B3})$. The bias current I_{B3} makes $V_o \to 0$ when $V_{in} = 0$. Now when $V_{in} > 0$, the input current, V_{in}/R_1, makes the LED D2 brighter, increasing $I_{D1} = I_{D3} > I_{D10} = I_{D30}$, thus increasing V_o. Thus $V_o = K_V V_{in}$. Note that analog optoisolation eliminates the need for a high-frequency carrier, modulation, and demodulation, while giving a very high degree of galvanic isolation. Unfortunately, the isolated headstage still must receive its power through a magnetically isolated power supply. It could use batteries, however, which would improve its isolation.

The third type of isolation uses high-frequency, *duty-cycle modulation* to transmit the signal across the isolation barrier using a differential, 1 pF capacitor coupling circuit. This type of IA also needs an isolated power supply for the input stages, the clock oscillator, and the modulator. Figure 4.23 illustrates schematically a simplified version of how the Burr–Brown ISO121, capacitively isolated MIA works. The signal V_{in} is added to a high-frequency, symmetrical triangle wave, V_T, with peak height, V_{pkT}. The sum of V_T and V_{in} is passed through a comparator which generates a variable-duty-cycle square wave, V_2. Note that the highest frequency in V_{in} is $\ll f_c$, the clock frequency, and $|V_{inmax}| < V_{pk}$. The state transitions in V_2 are coupled through the two, 1 pF capacitors as spikes to a flip-flop on the output side of the IA. The flip-flop's transitions are triggered by the spikes. At the flip-flop's output, a $\pm V_{3m}$, variable duty-cycle square wave, V_3, is then averaged by low-pass filtering to yield V_o.

The duty cycle of V_2 and V_3 can be shown to be:

$$\eta(V_{in}) \equiv T_+/T = (1/2 + V_{in}/2V_{pkT}), |V_{in}| < V_{pkT}. \tag{4.68}$$

The average of the symmetrical flip-flop output is

$$V_o = \overline{V_3} = V_{in}(V_{3m}/V_{pkT}). \tag{4.69}$$

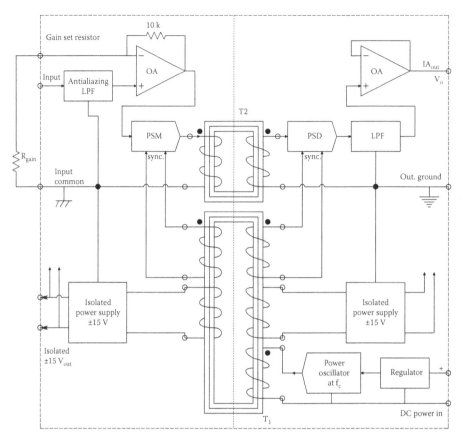

Figure 4.21 Simplified schematic circuit of an Analog Devices' magnetically coupled isolation amplifier (AD289). A transformer is used to couple power to the isolated headstage, and also to couple the isolated, acquired analog signal back to the output.

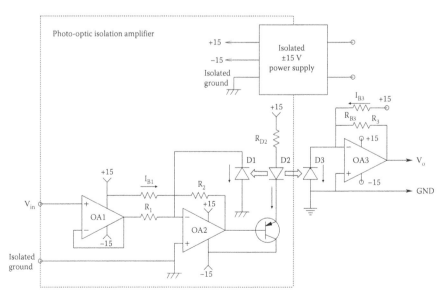

Figure 4.22 Simplified schematic of an isolation amplifier in which the isolated acquired signal is coupled to the output using a linearized analog photocoupler. Power must be coupled to the headstage through an isolation transformer (not shown).

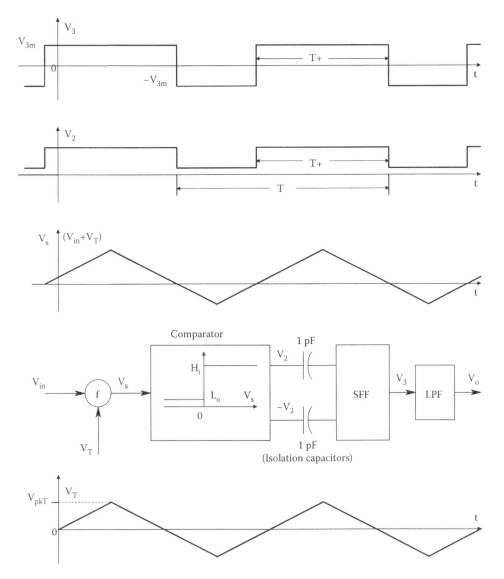

Figure 4.23 Duty cycle modulation system is used to couple the isolated acquired signal back to the output of a capacitively coupled IA. Power for the isolated headstage's subsystems (triangle wave generator, comparator, input preamplifier) must again be coupled to it by an isolation transformer.

Thus, the output signal is proportional to V_{in}. The actual circuitry of the Burr–Brown, ISO121 is more complex than described above, but the basic operating principle remains the same.

Certified isolation amplifiers *must* be used in surgery and intensive-care hospital environments where cardiac catheters are used. While the scenarios for direct cardiac electroshock do not generally exist for outpatients, IAs are still used for ECG, EEG, and EMG applications to limit liability in the unlikely event of an electroshock incident.

4.3.7 Driven-Leg ECG Amplifiers

In this section, we will examine the driven-leg ECG amplifier architecture and demonstrate that it acts to raise the overall ECG amplifier's CMRR, making the ECG DA less sensitive to common-mode hum and interference. Figure 4.24 illustrates the schematic of a 3-op-amp DA connected as a lead I ECG amplifier to the right and left arms. As we defined in Section 4.3.3,

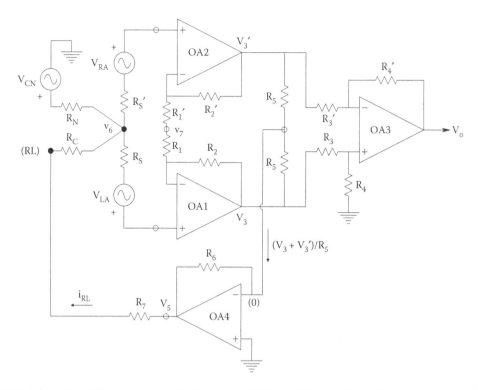

Figure 4.24 Simplified schematic of a driven-leg ECG amplifier similar to the system invented by Hewlett-Packard. Note that a three-op-amp DA is used from which it is easy to derive and amplify a common-mode signal between the two R_s's. The amplified CM signal, V_5, injects a current into the v_6 common node through the right leg (RL) which has resistance R_C. The net effect of the driven leg is to reduce output sensitivity to the CM noise, v_{CN} by common-mode negative feedback (CMNF).

the ECG amplifier's output voltage can be written in terms of its DM and CM gains and input signals.

$$V_o = v_{id}A_D + v_{ic}A_C. \tag{4.70}$$

(We will use scalar gains and voltages to simplify the analysis.) The DM and CM input voltages are given as before:

$$v_{id} \equiv (v_i - v_i')/2, \quad v_{ic} \equiv (v_i + v_i')/2. \tag{4.71}$$

When the input to the 3-op-amp DA is *pure DM*, the current into the summing junction of OA4 is zero, hence $v_5 = 0$. In the DA, we assume that $R_{in} \gg R_S, R_S', R_N$, and R_C. Also, the corresponding circuit resistors are matched ($R_s = R_s'$, etc.). Thus, any CM gain is the result of OA3's finite CMRR. Consider first the two ECG input voltages, v_{LA} and v_{RA}, with v_{CN} and $v_5 = 0$. By definition, lead I voltage, $v_I \equiv (v_{LA} - v_{RA})$, and

$$V_o = \left[(v_{LA} - v_{RA})/2\right]2A_D + \left[(v_{LA} + v_{RA})/2\right]2A_C$$
$$\downarrow \tag{4.72}$$
$$V_o = v_I A_D + \left[(v_{LA} + v_{RA})/2\right] 2A_C.$$

There is a small, unwanted, component of output voltage due to the input signal's CM component. If $v_{CN} \neq 0$, then there is a CM input component equal to v_{CN}. Thus, V_o is now:

$$V_o = v_I A_D + \left[(v_{LA} + v_{RA})/2\right] 2A_C + v_{CN}A_C. \tag{4.73}$$

With V_5 connected to the patient's right leg through resistor R_7, the ECG DA is given *common-mode negative feedback* (CMNF) which has the effect of raising the amplifier's CMRR (Northrop 1990).

The numerical CMRR of the DA *without* CMNF is simply $\text{CMRR}_{DA} = A_D/A_C$. The CMNF only affects the overall A_C, making it smaller; A_D is unchanged.

The current into OA4's summing junction, which is effectively at ground potential, is simply $i_{4sj} = (V_3 + V_3')/R_5$. This same current flows through R_6, so by Ohm's law,

$$V_5 = -(V_3 + V_3')(R_6/R_5). \tag{4.74}$$

As the DM DA output with CMNF is unchanged, we will examine only the CM output:

$$V_o = v_{ic}A_C = [(v_{LA} + v_{RA})/2]\, 2A_C + v_{CN}A_C(R_C + R_7)/(R_C + R_7 + R_N) + V_5A_CR_N/(R_C + R_7 + R_N)$$

$$\downarrow$$

$$v_{ic}A_C = [v_{Ic}]\, 2A_C + v_{CN}A_C(R_C + R_7)/(R_C + R_7 + R_N) - (v_{ic})2(R_6/R_5)A_CR_N/(R_C + R_7 + R_N)$$

$$\downarrow$$

$$v_{ic}[1 + 2(R_6/R_5)R_N/(R_C + R_7 + R_N)] = [v_{Ic}]\, 2 + v_{CN}(R_C + R_7)/(R_C + R_7 + R_N)$$

$$\downarrow$$

$$v_{ic} = \frac{2[v_{Ic}] + v_{CN}(R_C + R_7)/(R_C + R_7 + R_N)}{[1 + 2(R_6/R_5)R_N/(R_C + R_7 + R_N)]}. \tag{4.75}$$

Thus, the CMNF reduces not only the CM interference, but also the CM component of V_1. Clearly, we want to make $2(R_6/R_5)R_N/(R_C + R_7 + R_N) \gg 1$ to reduce the effective v_{ic}. To do this, (R_6/R_5) can be made $\gg 1$. We have little control of R_C, and no control of R_N.

For safety reasons, the current from OA4 into or out of the right leg must not exceed 1 μA. In other words,

$$10^{-6}\,A \geq i_{cmf} = \frac{|V_5|}{(R_C + R_7)}. \tag{4.76}$$

Let us make $R_7 = 10^6\ \Omega$; then if we limit $|V_5| < (10^{-6}R_C + 1)$ volts, the $\pm 1\ \mu$A limit is met.

While the driven-leg ECG amplifier was an innovative solution to the problem of unwanted CM signals, its extra complexity is generally not warranted today. Modern ECG isolation amplifiers have CMRRs that are 140–160 dB. Such high, inherent CMRRs are the result of laser trimming internal components during manufacturing in order to give component symmetry, which causes $A_C \to 0$. In some medical DA designs, CMNF is used internally in the circuit to reduce A_C.

4.3.8 Discussion

Biopotentials recorded noninvasively from the body surface have a range from single microvolts to over ten mV, depending on the source. Skeletal muscles and the heart are the stronger potential sources; the brain, the ECoG, ERG, and EOG have the weaker signals. For safety reasons, the amplifiers used clinically to record biopotentials are generally the isolation type. Many biopotential amplifiers are also R-C, DA's. They have low-noise, high-input impedance front-ends, and adjustable bandwidths to suit the signal being recorded and minimize output noise. Signals from the brain and heart generally require a high frequency, -3 dB frequency of little over 100 Hz; amplifiers used to condition EMG signals require more high-frequency bandwidth, generally $\sim$5 kHz at the most.

In this section, we have stressed the sources of amplifier noise and ways to calculate the output SNR for an amplifier system. Many EEG measurements have poor output SNR, and signal averaging must be used to recover an event-evoked brain potential. In the future, we can expect to see a continued slow improvement in low-noise amplifier headstage noise. Twenty years ago, a "low-noise" amplifier's short-circuit input noise was $e_{na} = 12\ \text{nV}\sqrt{\text{Hz}}$. Today, amplifiers are available with about 1/10th that e_{na}, and better. Often it is possible to design an IA from low-noise op-amps that exceeds the noise specs of commercial units, and costs less as well.

4.4 ECG

4.4.1 Introduction

Over 150 years ago, the Italian physicist, Carlo Matteucci, showed that an electric current accompanies each heartbeat. The next year, in 1843, the German physiologist, Emil Dubois-Reymond, confirmed Matteucci's findings in frogs (Jenkins 2009). A preparation was used called the "rheoscopic frog." Before the invention of the galvanometer to measure minute currents, the "action potentials" (a term invented by Dubois-Reymond) of muscles, including the heart, could be detected by placing a frog muscle on the contracting muscle and seeing it also contract with the stimulated muscle, or by placing a motor nerve innervating a frog muscle on an exposed heart ventricle, for example, and observing the muscle contract slightly in advance of the heart (Fye 1999).

The first, effective device that was used to measure the action potentials of the beating heart was the *mercury capillary electrometer*, invented by the French physicist, Gabriel Lippmann, in 1872. A thin capillary tube was partially filled with mercury, with a layer of sulfuric acid above it. When the cardiac action potential was applied across the capillary column, the mercury column moved up and down with the potential. This displacement was so small that it had to be observed with a microscope. For the next 25 years or so, the capillary electrometer was the only means of measuring the ECG. In 1895, the Dutch physiologist, Willem Einthoven, had refined the capillary electrometer and developed a correction formula to compensate for its poor frequency response so he could visualize the P, Q, R, S, and T inflections seen in ECG waveforms recorded with modern instrumentation.

Einthoven went on to modify a *string galvanometer*, previously invented to receive telegraph signals in 1897 by a French engineer, Clement Ader. In 1901, Einthoven used his string galvanometer to measure the ECG. His first string galvanometer had a huge, heavy magnet, in the airgap of which ran a thin silk string under tension, made conductive by rubbing with powdered silver. The ends of the string were connected to wires that led to two, saline-filled jars in which the patient immersed either two hands, or a hand and a foot. The low impedance of the saline jar electrodes allowed a relatively large action current to flow through the galvanometer string. The solenoidal magnetic field surrounding the current-carrying string interacts with the linear magnetic field in the magnet's air gap, and the string experiences a differential force along its length given by the vector cross-product:

$$\mathbf{dF} = I\,\mathbf{dl} \times \mathbf{B} \text{ newtons.} \tag{4.77}$$

$\mathbf{dF}$ tries to force the string out of the airgap, as shown in Figure 4.25. A light beam is projected on the string, which casts a shadow, the displacement of which is proportional to the galvanometer current. Note that a string under tension will tend to vibrate at a resonant frequency given by

$$f_r = \frac{1}{2L}\sqrt{(s/\rho)} \text{ Hz,} \tag{4.78}$$

where L is the string length in meters, s is the stress on the string in N/m^2, and ρ is the density of the string material in kg/m^3.

Evidently, Einthoven's string galvanometer's resonant frequency was high enough, and its damping coefficient was large enough not to cause excessive artifacts on his recordings. Einthoven went on with his pioneering work to characterize heart pathologies from the *ECG leads I, II,* and *III*. He was a pioneer in this area of NI diagnosis, for which he earned the 1923 Nobel Prize in medicine. A picture and description of an Einthoven string galvanometer made by "The Cambridge and Paul Instrument Co., Ltd." may be found in the paper by Rivera-Ruiz et al. (2008). This particular ECG galvanometer used a huge electromagnet. Its deflection sensitivity was 1 mm/0.1 μA, and its period was ~0.005 s ($f_r = 200$ Hz).

Vacuum tube amplifiers were first applied to the measurement of the ECG in 1928 by Ernstine and Levine, and all subsequent ECG recordings have involved amplification of ECG voltages, rather than the direct use of ECG current which activated the string galvanometer (Jenkins 1997).

Modern ECG amplifiers are R-C, and have standard corner (−3 dB) frequencies of 0.05 and 100 Hz (Rawlings 1991). The recording medium is generally moving paper, and robust galvanometer movements with bandwidths from DC to over 100 Hz move the writing element, making a graph of the ECG voltage versus time. The ECG can be written with a pressurized ink pen, or a moving hot stylus (on special heat-sensitive paper), or a fixed, hot stylus matrix (special paper moves past it), or a UV light beam (on special photosensitive paper). The ECG record can also be digitized and stored in computer memory, and then displayed on a monitor in a moving display (seen in hospital operating rooms [ORs] and intensive care units [ICUs]), or as a static display. Such computer-processed displays can then be printed out by a laser printer.

4.4.2 Electrode Placements

The original lead I, II, and III ECG electrode placements were defined by Einthoven in 1912. The electrode placement was called *Einthoven's triangle*; it is still used today for routine ECG

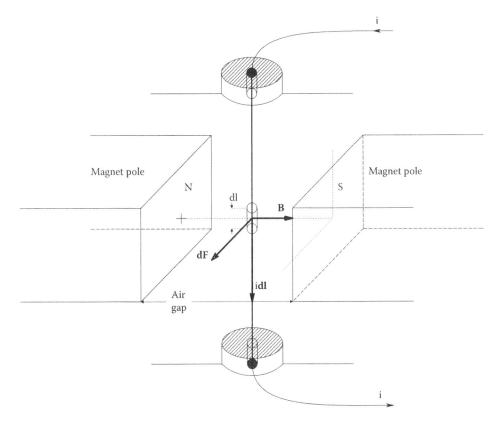

Figure 4.25 Schematic of a string galvanometer. The downward-flowing current causes the steady **B** field to force the string out of the airgap in the direction shown. String deflection is approximately proportional to I; it is generally sensed optically.

measurement. Electrodes are placed on the left leg (on the shin above the foot), on the right arm (about one-quarter of the way from the wrist on the medial surface), and on the left arm in the same location. The potentials at these body locations will be denoted: v_{LL}, v_{RA}, and v_{LA}, respectively. To avoid muscle EMG artifacts, electrodes are purposely located away from large muscle groups on the calf or upper arm. ECG lead I is the potential between the left arm (+) and the right arm (−), that is, $v_1 = v_{LA} - v_{RA}$. Lead II is taken between the left leg (+) and the right arm (−), that is, $v_2 = v_{LL} - v_{RA}$, and lead III is between the left leg (+) and the left arm (−), that is, $v_3 = v_{LL} - v_{LA}$. These sites are remote from the heart, but they were determined originally in the nineteenth century as the only practical locations for the saline-filled jar electrodes in which the limbs were immersed. *Einthoven's law* is basically a statement based on the (now) well-known Kirchhoff's voltage law of electrical circuits. Basically, it says that if any two of the three, bipolar limb lead ECG voltages are known at any instant, the third voltage can be found by summing the known two with appropriate attention to algebraic sign.

The three *augmented unipolar leads* are called aVR, aVL, and aVF. Circuit connections needed to record these ECG voltages are shown in Figure 4.26. These voltages resemble Einthoven's lead I, lead II, and lead III voltages, respectively, except the aVR waveform appears like an inverted lead I waveform.

To focus on possible local defects in ventricular muscle, or conduction problems, recordings are also made from *six precordial leads*. The recording set-up is shown in Figure 4.27. The resistances, R, are typically 5 kilohms. By writing a node equation on the v_T node, it is easy to show that the reference voltage, v_T, is

$$v_T = (1/3)[v_{RA} + v_{LA} + V_{LL}]. \tag{4.79}$$

Thus, the DA output is actually "v_k" = $[v_k - v_T] K_A$, $k = 1, ..., 6$.

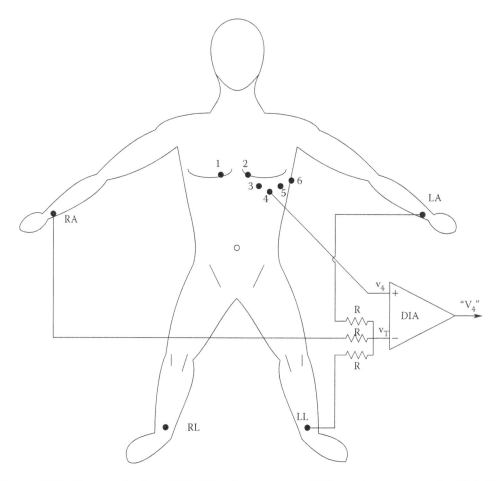

Figure 4.26 How are the three ECG AV leads are measured? The resistors are equal, ~5 kΩ. The amplifiers are differential medical isolation amplifiers.

By using pairs of electrodes at various nonstandard locations on the chest, abdomen, and back, it is possible, at any point in time in the cardiac cycle, to make a map of isopotential contours on the body. These contours describe how the skin surface potential varies in time during the cardiac cycle, and underscores the fact that electrically, the heart is not a simple, fixed dipole voltage source embedded in a homogeneous volume conductor, but rather a superposition of time- and space-varying dipoles embedded in an inhomogeneous volume conductor. As the lungs fill with air, the ECG decreases in amplitude and can change shape. Although ECG signals are voltages in time, they are recorded at different sites on the body surface (defining an internal volume), and so offer an opportunity to investigate the *volume variation* of cardiac potential in time.

The normal, temporal features of a lead II ECG waveform are shown in Figure 4.28. Because of the tremendous variability in individual anatomy, cardiac conditioning, and conditions under which an ECG is measured, there is considerable variability in *normal* lead II ECGs. The P wave occurs as the atrial muscle is depolarizing; its mean peak amplitude is ~0.107 mV. There is a large variability in P waves seen; some individuals have no visible P wave, in others it is as high as 0.3 mV. The duration of the P wave can range from 0 to 100 ms. This variability in amplitude and duration can be seen in normal individuals.

The *P–R interval*, I_{PR}, in Figure 4.28 relates to the depolarization of the atria, the AV node, the AV bundle and its branches, and the Purkinje system. The normal range of the P–R interval is 120–200 ms. Sinus tachycardia can reduce I_{PR} to ~110 ms (Rawlings 1991). The duration of the Q *wave* is normally <30 ms. The amplitude of the Q wave can range from 0% to −25% of the R wave peak. The *R wave* amplitude can range from 0.05 to 2.8 mV and still be considered normal. The duration of the R wave (rise time) is usually <70 ms. The fall time of the S *wave* is from 0 to 50 ms. The duration of the entire QRS complex in lead II is 50–100 ms.

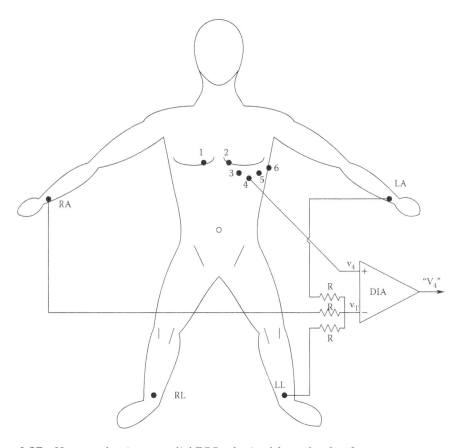

Figure 4.27 How are the six precordial ECGs obtained from the chest?

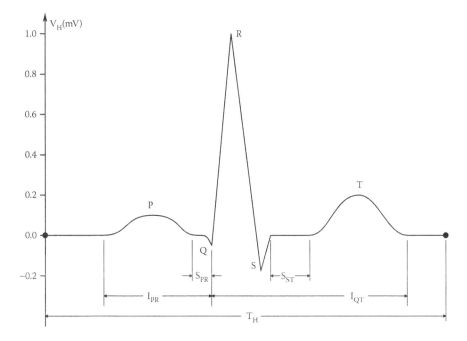

Figure 4.28 Schematic of a normal Lead II ECG waveform showing intervals and amplitudes used in diagnosis.

The duration of the *S-T segment*, S_{ST}, is from the end of the QRS complex to the onset of the T wave. *The Q-T interval*, I_{QT}, is the time it takes for the ventricles to depolarize, contract, relax, and repolarize. There are several formulas to predict its normal range from other intervals in the ECG cycle, but in general, it should be shorter than 425 ms. The *T wave* occurs during ventricular muscle repolarization, and is normally positive, having a duration of from 100 to 250 ms. Its normal, mean, peak amplitude is 0.267 mV, with a minimum of 0 and a maximum of 0.8 mV. In some individuals, a small *U wave* is seen following the T wave. Its origin is uncertain (Rawlings 1991). Figure 4.29 illustrates one, normal, typical, ECG cycle of leads I, II, and III, V_1, V_3, and aV_R. Note the inverted QRS spike in leads V_1 and aVR (also seen in V_2; not shown).

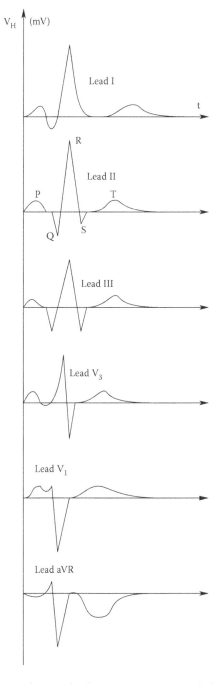

Figure 4.29 Summary of typical normal ECG waveshapes recorded from various defined leads.

4.4.3 Vector Cardiography

Picture the human body described by three, orthogonal axes: The **y**-axis is the vertical axis running from head to feet. The **z**-axis is the dorsal axis; it runs from the chest to the back. The **x**-axis is the horizontal axis, running from the right hand to the left hand through the chest. Also consider three orthogonal planes that meet in the center of the chest: The *sagittal* or *median plane* is defined by the **y** and **z** axes; it passes vertically through the center of the body. The *coronal or horizontal plane* contains the **x** and **z** axes; it is parallel to the ground. The *frontal plane* contains the **x** and **y** axes; it also runs from the head to the ground.

Vector cardiography can be used to describe the electrical activity of the heart as ECG vector tip projections versus time in the three planes described above. ECG vector projections in the frontal plane are probably more common, however. Naturally, the frontal ECG vector tip locus depends on the state of the cardiac cycle. The ECG leads I, II, and III, *or* aVR, aVL, and aVF define a set of three vector axes, spaced 60° apart, lying in the frontal plane. The three ECG voltages are treated as three vectors which at any time are resolved by vector addition to a vector or point at the vector positive tip in the frontal plane. An example of a vector sum of V_I, V_{II}, and V_{III} in the frontal plane at some time t_1 is shown in Figure 4.30. This is $\mathbf{V}(t_1) = \mathbf{V_I}(t_1) + \mathbf{V_{II}}(t_1) + \mathbf{V_{III}}(t_1)$. The vector axes are at 0°, −60°, and −120°. The (positive) tip of the vector $\mathbf{V}(t_1)$ defines a point. If the voltage vectors $\mathbf{V_I}$, $\mathbf{V_{II}}$, and $\mathbf{V_{III}}$ are sampled throughout the cardiac cycle, we can generate a closed curve connecting the points at the end of $\mathbf{V}(t_k)$. This curve is the *frontal plane vector cardiogram* (VCG). This type of VCG is easily calculated by computer. The voltages V_I, V_{II}, and V_{III} are sampled, and converted into **x** and **y** components:

$$\mathbf{V_x}(t_k) = V_I(t_k) + V_{II}(t_k)\cos(60°) + V_{III}(t_k)\cos(120°) \tag{4.80}$$

$$\mathbf{V_y}(t_k) = V_{II}(t_k)\sin(60°) + V_{III}(t_k)\sin(120°) \text{ (Note that positive } \mathbf{y} \text{ is downward.).} \tag{4.81}$$

Next we put the net vector into polar form. Its magnitude is

$$V(t_k) = \sqrt{V_x^2(t_k) + V_y^2(t_k)}. \tag{4.82}$$

The angle of $\mathbf{V}(t_k)$ is

$$\gamma(t_k) = \tan^{-1}\left\{V_y(t_k)/V_x(t_k)\right\}. \tag{4.83}$$

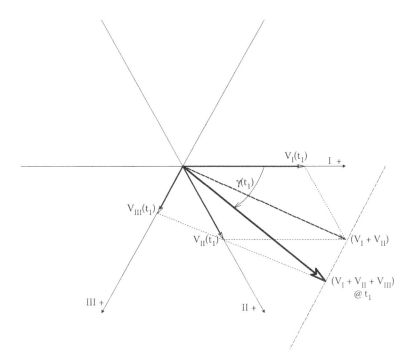

Figure 4.30 Vector addition of ECG waveforms from Leads I, II, and III in the frontal plane. Notice the three, fixed vector axes are spaced 60° apart.

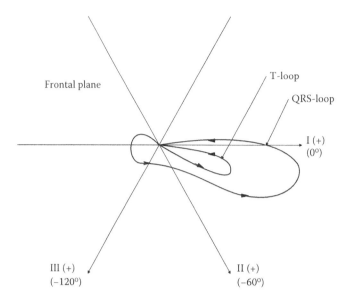

Figure 4.31 Typical frontal vectorcardiogram derived from Lead I, II, and III voltages. Note that there are two loops, both traversed counterclockwise, one from the QRS complex, and the smaller one from the T-wave.

So the VCG voltage at $t = t_k$ can be written:

$$\mathbf{V}(t_k) = V(t_k) \angle \gamma(t_k). \tag{4.84}$$

Note that in this vector convention, positive $\gamma(t_k)$ is measured clockwise from the positive **x**-axis.

Actually, there are three loops in the VCG, a very small one for the P wave, another large one for the QRS complex, and a third small one for the T wave. Representative vector loops for the QRS and T waves in the frontal plane are shown in Figure 4.31. The large VCG loop from the QRS complex has great utility in diagnosing a multitude cardiac of problems, ranging from conduction blocks (bundle branch blocks), ventricular hypertrophy, various ventricular myopathies, coronary artery ischemia, localization of infarctions, etc. (Guyton 1991). VCG loops vary from beat-to-beat, and a cardiologist must take this small, normal variability into consideration in making a diagnosis.

By recording from suitable electrodes lying in the median and horizontal planes, VCG plots can be created as closed curves lying in those planes, as well as in the frontal plane. From these three vector projections, a 3-D view of how the ECG vector varies in time can be constructed. The length of the resultant vector tip at $t = t_k$ in **xyz** space is given by the Pythagorean theorem, and its angles can be resolved by trigonometry. Figure 4.32 illustrates a representative, 3-D, VCG for one cardiac cycle.

The *Frank VCG System* using seven electrodes is shown in Figure 4.33. Note the Frank axis convention where the positive **x**-axis points left, positive **y** is down, and positive **z** points dorsad. The Frank system uses a resistive summing circuit to resolve the three orthogonal components of the VCG with 13% error, compared with a "gold standard" system that summed the outputs of 150 electrodes. The nine-electrode, precordial system had 10% error compared with the 150-electrode system, and an experimental 30-electrode system gave only 1% error (Rawlings 1991).

4.4.4 ECG Analysis, Feature Extraction, and Diagnosis

An experienced cardiologist can read a standard set of ECG traces or a VCG and make a diagnosis based on education and experience. When one considers the many things that can go wrong with the heart, this diagnostic ability is remarkable. Biomedical engineers, computer scientists, and cardiologists have tried since the days of the venerable DEC PDP-series computers in the 1970s to design pattern recognition software that could diagnose common cardiac pathologies, given various ECG lead voltages as inputs. Early ECG diagnostic programs would measure waveform features such as the various intervals and segment lengths associated with the PQRST elements of

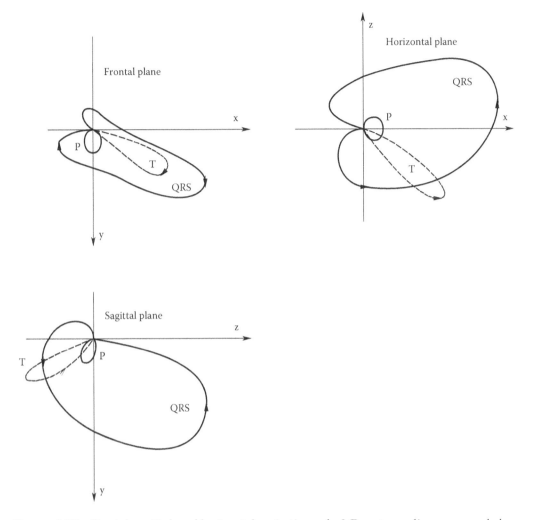

Figure 4.32 Frontal, sagittal, and horizontal projections of a 3-D vectorcardiogram recorded using a multiple 3-D electrode array such as the Frank system.

the lead II ECG waveform, and also examine peak heights and slopes, and then compare them to a standard database for statistical analysis. Certain sets of out-of-range ECG features could then be assigned probabilities for various cardiac diseases. Such programs were good for gross screening, but were nothing you would want to bet your life on.

More sophisticated techniques have now emerged for ECG analysis, including the use of Fourier-transformed ECGs, time–frequency (TF) analysis of ECGs (Clayton et al. 1998), and 2-D, frequency-domain analysis of VCG loops (Lei et al. 1997). Work has also been done with trainable artificial neural networks (ANNs) for the diagnosis of cardiac pathologies, applying the trainable ANN to recognizing anomalies in the time-domain, QRS complex (Barro et al. 1998).

4.4.5 Discussion

As NI diagnostic modalities, the ECG and VCG are probably among the more cost-effective diagnostic modalities presently available. The electrodes are simple and inexpensive, and the ECG signals are conditioned by inexpensive, differential isolation amplifiers, and their digitized outputs are easily processed by computer to form moving chart recorder displays, or vector displays. Much can be learned from the various waveforms of the different ECG leads, and from the VCG about the state of the heart muscle over its surface, and the state of the internal, excitation conduction system of the heart.

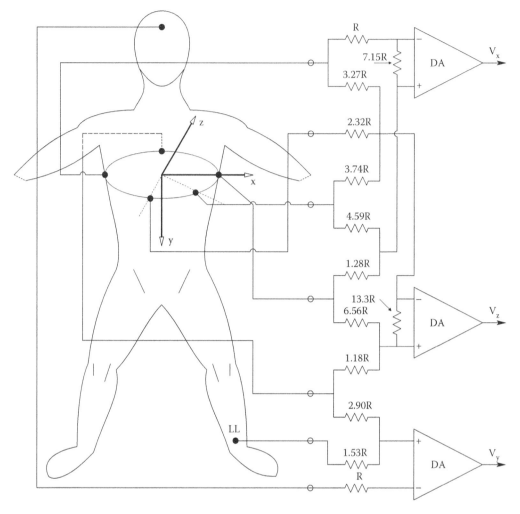

Figure 4.33 Schematic of the Frank VCG electrode system. The DAs are medical isolation amplifiers. The three analog voltages V_x, V_y, and V_z are used to generate the 3-D VCG display.

4.5 EMG

4.5.1 Introduction

An important bioelectric signal that has diagnostic significance for many neuromuscular diseases is the EMG, which can be recorded from the skin surface with electrodes identical to those used for electrocardiography, although, in some cases, the electrodes generally have smaller areas than those used for ECG (<1 mm²). To record from SMUs, or even individual muscle fibers (several of which comprise an SMU), needle electrodes that pierce the skin into the body of a superficial muscle can also be used. (This semi-invasive method obviously requires sterile technique.) EMG recording is used to diagnose some causes of muscle weakness or paralysis, muscle or motor problems such as tremor or twitching, motor nerve damage from injury or osteoarthritis, and pathologies affecting motor end plates (MEPs).

Many of the problems associated with the motor system that can be diagnosed using EMGs arise from autoimmune causes (e.g., myasthenia gravis, the Eaton–Lambert syndrome), others come from genetic disorders (e.g., the dystrophies: Duchenne, Becker, limb-girdle, Landouzy–Dejerine), and still others come from motoneuron problems that can be genetic in origin, or from virus infection (Polio, coxsackievirus, and other enteroviruses). For a more detailed description and classification of motoneuron disorders, see Rubin (2015).

4.5.2 Origin of EMGs

There are several types of muscle in the body, for example, cardiac, smooth, and striated. Striated muscle in mammals can be further subdivided into *fast* and *slow muscles* (Guyton 1991). Fast muscles are used for fast movements; they include the two *gastrocnemii*, laryngeal muscles, the extraocular muscles, etc. Slow muscles are used for postural control against gravity; they include the *soleus*, abdominal muscles, back muscles, neck muscles, etc. EMG recording is generally carried out on both slow and fast skeletal muscles. It can also be done on less superficial muscles such as the extraocular muscles that move the eyeballs, the eyelid muscles, and the muscles that work the larynx.

Most striated muscles are innervated by motor neurons that have origin at various levels in the spinal cord. That is, motor neurons receive excitatory and inhibitory inputs from motor control neurons from the CNS, as well as excitatory and inhibitory inputs from local feedback neurons from muscle spindles (responding to muscle length x and dx/dt) and the Golgi tendon organs (responding to muscle tension) and the Renshaw cells (inhibitory interneurons in the gray matter of the spinal cord) (Guyton 1991). Individual motor neuron axons controlling the contraction of a particular striated muscle innervate small groups of muscle fibers called SMUs. Many SMUs comprise the entire muscle. The synaptic connections between the terminal branches of a single motor neuron axon and its SMU are called *motor end plates* (MEPs). MEPs are chemical synapses in which the neurotransmitter, acetylcholine (ACh), is released presynaptically and then diffuses across the synaptic cleft or gap to ACh receptors on the subsynaptic membrane. A schematic drawing of an MEP at different magnifications is shown in Figure 4.34. When a motor neuron action potential arrives at the MEP, it triggers the exocytosis or emptying of about 300 presynaptic vesicles containing ACh. (There are $\sim 3 \times 10^5$ vesicles in the terminals of a single MEP; each vesicle is about 40 nm in diameter.) Some 10^7 to 5×10^8 molecules of ACh are needed to trigger a muscle action potential (Katz 1966). The ACh diffuses across the 20–30 nm synaptic cleft in ~ 0.5 ms, where some ACh molecules combine with receptor sites on the protein subunits forming the subsynaptic, ion-gating channels. Five, high-molecular weight protein subunits form each ion channel. ACh binding triggers a dilation of the channel to ~ 0.65 nm. The dilated channels allow Na^+ ions to pass inward; however, Cl^- is repelled by the fixed negative charges on the mouth of the channel. Thus, the subsynaptic membrane is depolarized by the inward J_{Na} (i.e., its transmembrane potential goes positive from the ca. -85 mV resting potential), triggering a *muscle action potential.* The local subsynaptic, transmembrane potential can go to as much as $+50$ mV, forming an *end plate potential* (EPP) spike fused to the muscle action potential it triggers, having a duration of ~ 8 ms, much longer than a nerve action potential.

The ACh in the cleft and bound to the receptors is rapidly broken down (hydrolized) by the enzyme *cholinesterase* resident in the cleft, and its molecular components are recycled. A small amount of ACh also escapes the cleft by diffusion, and is also hydrolyzed.

Once the postsynaptic membrane under the MEP depolarizes in a superthreshold EPP spike, a *muscle action potential* is generated that propagates along the surface membrane of the muscle fiber, the *sarcolemma*. It is the muscle action potential that triggers muscle fiber contraction and force generation. Typical muscle action potentials, recorded intracellularly at the MEP and at a point 2 mm from the initiating MEP, are shown in Figure 4.35. The muscle action potential propagates at 3–5 m/s, its duration is 2–15 ms, depending on the muscle, and it swings from a resting value of ca. -85 mV to a peak of ca. $+30$ mV. At the skin surface, it appears as a triphasic spike of 20–2000 μV peak amplitude (Guyton 1991).

To ensure that all of the deep contractile apparatus in the center of the muscle fiber is stimulated to contract at the same time and with equal strength, many transverse, radially directed tubules penetrate into the center of the fiber along its length. These *T-tubules* are open to the extracellular fluid space, as is the surface of the fiber, and they are connected to the surface membrane at both ends. The T-tubules conduct the muscle action potential into the interior of the fiber in many locations along its length.

Running longitudinally around the outsides of the contractile myofibrils that make up the fiber are networks of tubules called the *sarcoplasmic reticulum* (SR). The T-tubules and SR are shown schematically in Figure 4.36. Note that the terminal *cisternae* of the SR butt against the membrane of the T-tubes. When the muscle action potential penetrates along the T-tubes, the depolarization triggers the *cisternae* to release calcium ions into the space surrounding the myofibrils' contractile proteins. The Ca^{++} binds to the protein troponin C, which triggers contraction by the actin

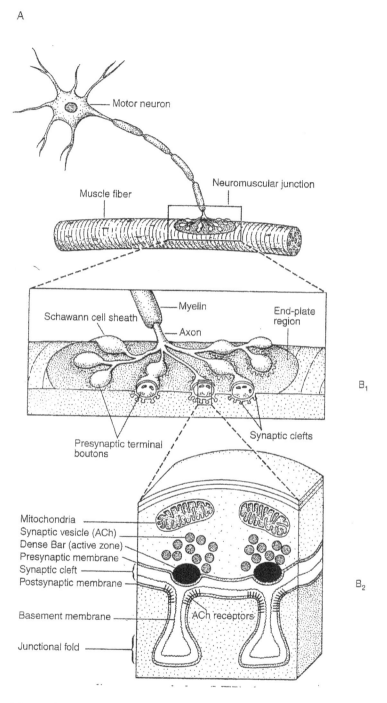

Figure 4.34 Mammalian motor end plate (MEP) shown at different magnifications. At low-magnification, we see a myelinated motor neuron leaving the spinal cord and synapsing on a muscle fiber. In the middle panel, at medium magnification, we see how the presynaptic boutons from the motoneuron ending make contact with the postsynaptic membrane region of the muscle fiber. At the highest (EM) magnification at the bottom of the figure, the ultrastructural details of the MEP and the basement membrane are shown. (From Kandel et al. (1991), *Principles of Neural Science, 3rd ed.* Appleton & Lange, Norwalk, CT. With permission from the McGraw-Hill companies.) (Image from Northrop, R.B. 2002. *Noninvasive Instrumentation and Measurement in Medical Diagnosis*. CRC Press, Boca Raton, FL. ISBN: 0-8493-0961-1.)

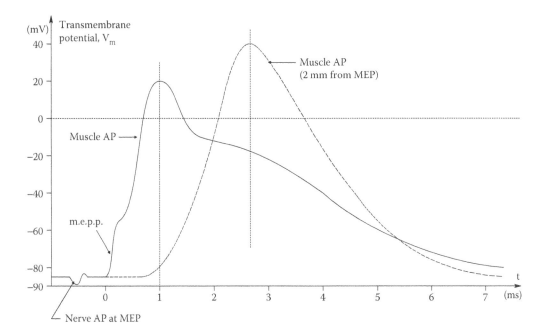

Figure 4.35 Representative intracellularly recorded muscle action potentials.

and myosin proteins. (We will not go into the molecular biophysics of the actual contraction process here.)

A synchronous stimulation of all of the motor neurons innervating a muscle produces what is called a *muscle twitch*, that is, the tension initially falls a slight amount, then rises abruptly, then falls more slowly to zero again. Sustained muscle contraction is caused by a steady (average) rate of (asynchronous) motoneuron firing. When the firing ceases, the muscle relaxes. Muscle relaxation is actually an active process. Calcium ion pumps located in the membranes of the SR longitudinal tubules actively transfer Ca^{++} from outside the tubules to back inside the SR system. It is the lack of Ca^{++} in proximity to troponin C that allows relaxation to occur. In resting muscle, the concentration, $[Ca^{++}]$, is about 10^{-7} M in the myofibrillar fluid (Guyton 1991). In a twitch, $[Ca^{++}]$ rises to $\sim 2 \times 10^{-5}$ M, and in a tetanic stimulation, the $[Ca^{++}]$ is about 2×10^{-4} M. It takes about 50 ms for the Ca^{++} released by a single motor nerve impulse to be taken up by the SR pumps to restore the resting $[Ca^{++}]$ level.

The Ca^{++} pumps require metabolic energy to operate; *adenosine triphosphate* (ATP) is cleaved to the diphosphate form to release the energy needed to drive the Ca^{++} pumps. The pumps can concentrate the Ca^{++} to $\sim 10^{-3}$ M inside the SR. Inside the SR tubules and cisternae, the Ca^{++} is stored in readily available ionic form, and, as a protein chelate, bound to a protein, calsequestrin.

So far, we have described the events associated with a single muscle fiber. As noted above, small groups of fibers innervated by a single motoneuron fiber are called an SMU. In muscles used for fine actions, such as those operating the fingers or tongue, there are fewer muscle fibers in a motor unit, or equivalently, more motoneuron fibers per total number of muscle fibers. For example, the laryngeal muscles used for speech have only two or three fibers per SMU, while large muscles used for gross motions, such as the gastrocnemius, can have several hundred fibers per SMU (Guyton 1991). To make fine movements, only a few motoneurons fire out of the total number innervating the muscle, and these do not fire synchronously. Their firing phase is made random in order to produce smooth contraction. At maximum, tetanic stimulation, the mean frequency on the motoneurons is higher, but the phases are still random to reduce the duty cycle of each SMU.

4.5.3 EMG Amplifiers

The amplifiers used for clinical EMG recording must meet the same stringent specifications for low-leakage currents as do ECG amplifiers (see Section 4.3). EMG amplifier gains are typically $\times 1000$, and their bandwidths reflect the transient nature of the SMU action potentials. Typically, an EMG

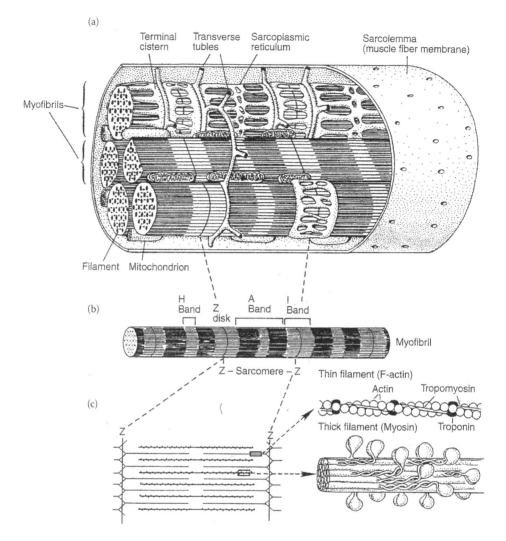

Figure 4.36 (a) Schematic 3-D structure of a striated muscle fiber. (b) Structure of an individual myofibril showing bands. (c) Schematic cross-section of an individual sarcomere. The thick filaments are made up of arrays of myosin molecules. The myosin molecule has a stem region and a globular double head that protrudes from the stem. Thin filaments are composed of polymerized actin molecules. Note the molecular complexity of this system. (From Kandel et al. 1991. *Principles of Neural Science, 3rd ed.* Appleton & Lange, Norwalk, CT. With permission from the McGraw-Hill companies.) (Image from Northrop, R.B. 2002. *Noninvasive Instrumentation and Measurement in Medical Diagnosis.* CRC Press, Boca Raton, FL. ISBN: 0-8493-0961-1.)

amplifier is R-C, with low- and high-frequency −3 dB frequencies of 300 Hz and 3 kHz, respectively. With an amplifier having variable low- and high-frequency −3 dB frequencies, one generally starts with a wide pass bandwidth, say 100 Hz to 10 kHz, and gradually restricts it until individual EMG spikes just begin to round up and change shape. Such an ad hoc-adjusted bandwidth will give a better output SNR than one that is too wide or too narrow.

4.5.4 What EMGs Can Tell Us

There are many diseases and conditions that can alter the normal operation of striated muscle. The problem can be in the CNS, or the spine where motoneuron activation occurs. Abnormal muscle action can also be due to a problem with the MEP, the ACh receptors, or the biochemical mechanisms coupling the MEP spike to muscle contraction. The major objective of EMG analysis is to sort out whether the problem lies with the motor nerve activation, the synaptic coupling from

MEP to SR, or the contractile process itself. Often a superficial motor nerve (e.g., the *ulnar nerve* in the forearm) is stimulated electrically using skin surface electrodes, and needle electrodes are used to record SMU activity in a superficial muscle in the hand (e.g., the *hypothenar muscle*). This type of recording allows the neurologist to see if the synaptic coupling mechanism is normal from the latencies and amplitudes of the SMU action potentials.

When investigating the EMGs of large skeletal muscles such as the biceps or gastrocnemius, the motor nerves are not available for superficial, external stimulation. EMG skin surface electrodes are commonly used, so the firing of many SMUs is picked up simultaneously. During a strong muscle contraction, their amplitudes and firing phases are superimposed to give an EMG that looks like a burst of noise. In addition, if the muscle is allowed to shorten under load, the active SMUs at muscle length L_o can move away from the recording electrodes (fixed on the skin) and other SMUs will contribute to the net EMG at $L = L_o - \Delta L$. If the behavior of certain SMUs is required, then the patient must do an *isometric muscle contraction* to minimize SMU motion relative to the recording electrodes.

Single motor fiber recording done on potentials from superficial hand muscles, such as the *extensor digitorum communis,* can be used to diagnose diseases of the neuromuscular junction, including myasthenia gravis, the Eaton–Lambert syndrome, botulism, etc. Twenty-five micrometer diameter wires are inserted into the muscle mass through the skin using hypodermic needles. The fine wire electrodes contact one or two single muscle fibers from a common SMU. By measuring the "phase jitter" between two fibers, and comparing it to the jitter of a normal, reference muscle with the same load (level of contraction), diagnosis can be made (Kandel et al. 2012).

The frequency, amplitude, and duration of SMU triphasic spikes recorded with larger, percutaneous wire electrodes can also be used to diagnose such conditions as: anterior horn cell (motoneuron soma and dendrite) disease, demyelinating neuropathy, axonal neuropathy, neuromuscular transmission disorder, and certain myopathies. Figure 4.37 illustrates EMGs from an SMU in a partially denervated muscle.

A problem in recording from SMUs or single muscle fibers with wire electrodes is interference from action potentials on neighboring SMUs and fibers. These artifactual EMG spikes are generally smaller in amplitude than the desired spikes. It is possible to improve the SNR of the desired spikes by passing the recorded EMG signal, e(t), through an odd nonlinearity of the form:

$$y(t) = K \, \text{sgn}[e(t)]\{\exp[a \, | \, e(t) \, | \,] - 1\}. \tag{4.85}$$

The slope of this nonlinearity for e > 0 is

$$\frac{dy}{de} = K \, a \, \exp[a \, e]. \tag{4.86}$$

Thus, the larger values of e(t) get proportionally more amplification, suppressing noise and small EMG spikes recorded with the desired spikes. This type of nonlinearity distorts the desired spikes, but does not affect the timing or phase jitter, which is of main interest.

EMGs can be viewed in the *time domain* (most useful when single fibers or SMUs are being recorded), in the *frequency domain* (the FFT is taken from an entire, surface-recorded EMG burst under standard conditions), or in the time–frequency (T–F) domain (cf. Section 3.2.3 of this book). In the latter case, the T–F display shows the frequencies in the EMG burst as a function of time. In general, a higher frequency content in the T–F display indicates that more SMUs are being

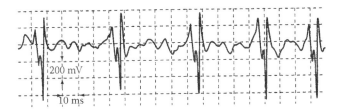

Figure 4.37 Surface EMG recorded from a rapidly firing, partially denervated SMU. Note the curious multiple peaks on the EMG. (Image from Northrop, R.B. 2002. *Noninvasive Instrumentation and Measurement in Medical Diagnosis.* CRC Press, Boca Raton, FL. ISBN: 0-8493-0961-1.)

activated at a higher rate (Hannaford and Lehman 1986). T–F analysis can show how agonist–antagonist muscle pairs are controlled to do a specific motor task.

Still another way to characterize EMG activity in the time domain is to pass the EMG through a TRMS conversion circuit, such as an AD637 IC. The output of the TRMS circuit is a smoothed, positive voltage proportional to the square-root of the time average of $e^2(t)$. The time averaging is done by a single time constant, low-pass filter. For another time domain display modality, the EMG signal can be full-wave rectified and low-pass filtered to smooth it.

4.5.5 Discussion

In this section, we have seen that the EMG when recorded along with motor neuron activity, or by itself, can be processed in the time–frequency or T–F domains to reveal evidence pointing to various neuromuscular diseases. Electrodes used for EMG recording from the skin surface are generally small Ag|AgCl types, similar to those used for ECG and EEG recording. Percutaneous wire electrodes, inserted into a superficial muscle mass by hypodermic needles, are used to record action potentials from SMUs and single muscle fibers. These electrodes are removable, and constitute a mildly invasive procedure that carries a small risk of infection.

4.6 ELECTROENCEPHALOGRAM

4.6.1 Introduction

The EEG is a relatively low-frequency, spontaneous, electrical potential recorded from an electrode on the scalp. (The second electrode can be on an earlobe or also on the scalp.) The peak amplitude of the EEG can be as large as 150 µV peak-to-peak (delta waves), but more typically, it is less than 50 µV ppk (alpha rhythm). The EEG was discovered by the German psychiatrist and electrophysiologist, Hans Berger. Berger's initial discovery of EEG activity was made using a string galvanometer and surface electrodes on his son's scalp. At Jena, Berger went on to study EEGs in relation to brain diseases in the 1920s. In 1929, he published a paper entitled *Über das Electrenkephalogramm des Menschen.*

EEGs can be used to diagnose organic brain abnormalities such as abscesses, various forms of epilepsy, focal seizures, arteriovenous malformations (e.g., aneurisms, infarcts), tumors, hemorrhages, physical injury to brain tissue from head trauma, etc. Often abnormal EEG results point to the need for detailed imaging studies such as dye-injection/x-ray fluoroscopy, CAT, or MRI. EEGs are also used in brain research to localize brain volumes responsible for certain mental activities.

4.6.2 Sources and Classification of the EEG

Owing to its low-frequency nature, it is evident that fast action potentials on the axons of brain neurons contribute little to the EEG potential. The spiking axons run in various directions, and their very small, external potentials tend to average out in the volume conductors of the brain, the CSF, the meninges, and the skull and scalp. The generation of EEG potentials requires a neural source close to the inside surface of the skull that is coherent, that is, all the neurons must be aligned similarly and act together electrically. It turns out that the pyramidal cells in the center layers of the cerebral cortex are, in fact, the major source of the EEG potentials. Figure 4.38 illustrates schematically the various cells found in a radial slice through the cerebral cortex, including the pyramidal cells. Note that the apical dendritic branches of the pyramidal cells lie in the outermost layer of the cortex, next to the skull. These dendrites receive excitatory and/or inhibitory inputs from surrounding neurons and ascending axons. If the apical dendrites are receiving excitatory inputs, some positive ion current carried by an ion such as Na^+ enters them, depolarizing the pyramidal cell toward firing. The inward, apical J_{Na} is supplied by an extracellular current flowing outward from deeper layers in the cortex. This current flow is in response to the apical portions of the stimulated pyramidal cell going negative, while the deep portions are positive, creating an effective dipole on the cortex around the stimulated cell. If the apical dendrites of a pyramidal cell receive inhibitory inputs, there is a net outward flow of positive ions (or a net inward flow of negative ions such as J_{Cl}). Thus, inhibition of a pyramidal cell causes its apex to go positive, reversing the external current flow, and making the outer surface of the cortex positive around the inhibited cell. Many pyramidal cells in a region of cortex surface must be excited or inhibited together to create a local dipole large enough to be sensed through the skull by electrodes on the scalp.

EEG potentials on the scalp are generally no more than 150 µV peak-to-peak. They are generally classified in the frequency domain by their power spectral content. The *spectrum* of *alpha waves* lies between 7.5 and 13 Hz; it is produced in adults when a person is in a conscious, relaxed state with

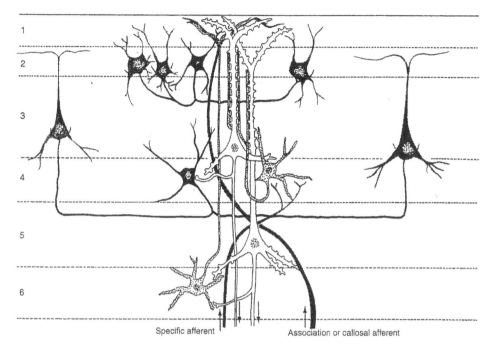

1

2

3

4

5

6

Specific afferent   Association or callosal afferent

Figure 4.38   Representative silver-stained section through the human cerebral cortex showing the principal types of neurons. (From Kandel et al. 1991. *Principles of Neural Science, 3rd ed.* Appleton & Lange, Norwalk, CT. With permission from the McGraw-Hill companies.) (Image from Northrop, R.B. 2002. *Noninvasive Instrumentation and Measurement in Medical Diagnosis.* CRC Press, Boca Raton, FL. ISBN: 0-8493-0961-1.)

the eyes closed. It disappears when attention is focused on a task and the eyes are opened. *Alpha waves* are best recorded from the posterior lateral parts of the scalp.

Beta waves have spectral energy of 14 Hz and greater. They are best recorded frontally. Beta activity is present when a person is alert or anxious, with their eyes open.

Theta potentials are abnormal in alert adults but are seen during sleep, and in prepubescent children.

Delta waves have the largest amplitudes and the lowest frequency ($\leq$3.5 Hz). It is a normal rhythm found in infants $\leq$1 year, and in adults in deep sleep (stages 3 and 4). Delta activity may also occur when the patient has a subcortical brain lesion. Normal delta waves occur in bursts in adults, called *frontal intermittent rhythmic delta activity* (FIRDA). All EEG waveforms are nonstationary and can be characterized in the frequency domain by short-term Fourier analysis.

4.6.3 EEG Recording Systems

As we have mentioned above, electrodes for EEG recording are generally small AgCl types that use a conductive coupling gel. In some cases, small, saline-saturated sponges are used to couple the AgCl electrodes to the scalp. The hair is parted and pushed aside for good, low-resistance, electrode contact. EEG potentials can be recorded between pairs of electrodes on the scalp, or between a scalp electrode and a "remote" electrode attached to an earlobe. The voltage difference between any single electrode and the electronic average of the potentials from the rest of the electrodes can also be viewed.

A standard placement of EEG electrodes was adopted in 1958 called the *International 10–20 Electrode System* (Webster 1998). This arrangement is shown schematically in Figure 4.39. Note that the odd electrode numbers are on the left side of the head. Electrodes C_3 and C_4 are placed to overlay the region of the central sulcus of the brain. The oval electrodes in the figure are on the vertical sides of the head (forehead, temples, etc.).

Neurophysiologists, wishing to further localize the sources of EEG activity in the cortex, have gone to larger arrays of electrodes than in the standard 10–20 array. Such arrays can contain 32, 64, 128, and even 256 individual electrodes. They are used for medical diagnosis, research in physiological psychology, and biofeedback applications such as the EEG-controlled computer mouse. Figure 4.40

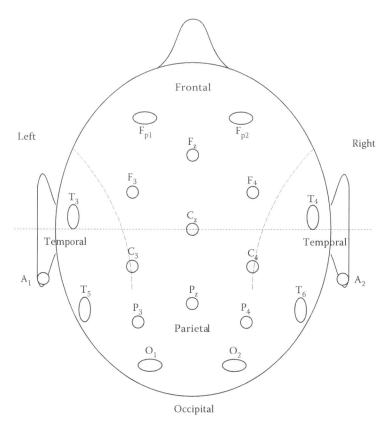

Figure 4.39 Top view of the head showing the standard electrode placements for the international 10–20 EEG electrode array.

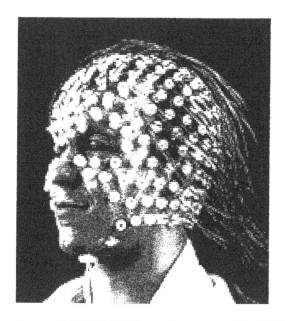

Figure 4.40 Geodesic Sensor Net© EEG 128-electrode array made by EGI, Inc. (Figure used with permission of EGI, Inc.) (Image from Northrop, R.B. 2002. *Noninvasive Instrumentation and Measurement in Medical Diagnosis*. CRC Press, Boca Raton, FL. ISBN: 0-8493-0961-1.)

illustrates a subject wearing an EGI 128-electrode, EEG "helmet" array. The Electrical Geodesics, Inc. (EGI), Geodesic EEG System (GES) 400, is a 256-electrode array (EGI 2015). Another company that makes multielectrode EEG arrays is Axion Biosystems (768 stimulating or recording electrodes).

4.6.4 2-D Spatial Sampling of Scalp EEG Potentials by Electrode Arrays

The *sampling theorem,* as originally derived, deals with the analog reconstructability of periodically sampled *time* signals by ideal low-pass filtering. The sampling theorem is easily extended to the periodic sampling of 1-D signals in space (x-dimension), the periodic spatial sampling of 2-D, spatial signals (e.g., pictures) in (cartesian) **x** and **y**-dimensions, and finally, the spatial sampling of 2-D signals on the surface of a sphere (θ and ϕ dimensions). At a given point in time, the scalp-recorded EEG can be treated as a 2-D signal mapped on the surface of an idealized *hemisphere* (the scalp). Clearly, evenly spaced electrodes on the scalp can be thought of as representing a spatial, voltage-sampling array on the surface of a hemisphere. Figure 4.41 illustrates one quadrant of the hemisphere with the potential at time t_o at a point, $V(t_o, \rho, \theta, \phi)$, shown. What we are interested in is the maximum spacing (hence minimum number) of electrodes on the hemisphere surface required to accurately estimate a continuous, analog distribution of the EEG voltage, $V(t_o, \rho, \theta, \phi)$.

To begin with, we will review the sampling theorem in 1-D linear space: Assume an analog voltage, $V(x)$, exists. This voltage is periodically sampled along the **x**-axis, forming a number sequence, $V^*(x)$. The sampling process can be thought of mathematically as being an *impulse modulation* of the continuous signal. That is $V(x)$ is multiplied by a train of unit impulses, $P_T(x)$, along the x-axis:

$$V^*(x) = V(x) \cdot P_T(x) = V(x) \sum_{n=-\infty}^{n=\infty} \delta(x - nX_s), \tag{4.87}$$

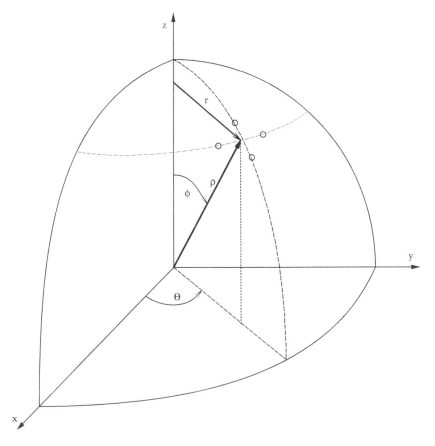

Figure 4.41 Quadrant of a hemisphere (model for the skull) showing the spherical coordinate system used to define the spatial distribution of electrical activity on the scalp at any time t. $\rho = R$ in this simplified model (R is the hemisphere's radius).

where X_s is the spatial sampling period, that is, the spacing between the unit impulses. In the spatial frequency domain, this multiplication is equivalent to complex convolution. $F\{\cdot\}$ is the Fourier transform operator.

$$F\{V*(x)\} = \mathbf{V}*(ju) = \mathbf{V}(ju) \otimes \mathbf{P}_T(ju). \tag{4.88}$$

As $P_T(x)$ is periodic, it can be expressed as an exponential form discrete *Fourier series* in distance, x.

$$P_T(x) = \sum_{n=-\infty}^{n=\infty} \delta(x - nX_s) = \sum_{n=-\infty}^{n=\infty} C_n \exp(-jnu_sx), \tag{4.89}$$

where u_s is the spatial sampling frequency in radians/mm. $u_s \equiv 2\pi/X_s$. The Fourier coefficient, C_n, is given by

$$C_n = (1/X_s) \int_{X_s/2}^{X_s/2} P_T(x) \exp(+jnu_sx) \, dx = (1/X_s), \text{ all n}. \tag{4.90}$$

Thus, the output of the spatial sampling process can be written:

$$V*(x) = V(x) \left[(1/X_s) \sum_{n=-\infty}^{n=\infty} \exp(-jnu_sx) \right] = (1/X_s) \sum_{n=-\infty}^{n=\infty} V(x) \exp(-jnu_sx). \tag{4.91}$$

Finally, we use the Fourier transform theorem for complex exponentiation:

$$F\{y(x) \, e^{-jax}\} \equiv \mathbf{Y}(ju - ja). \tag{4.92}$$

Now in the *spatial frequency domain*, the spatially sampled voltage can be written:

$$F\{V*(x)\} = \mathbf{V}*(ju) = (1/X_s) \sum_{n=-\infty}^{n=\infty} \mathbf{V}(ju - jnu_s). \tag{4.93}$$

Equation 4.93 is called the *Poisson sum* form of the spatially sampled signal. Figure 4.42a shows the spatial frequency spectrum of $V*(x)$ when the *baseband spectrum*, $\mathbf{V}(ju)$, contains no spatial frequencies in excess of the *spatial Nyquist frequency*, defined as: $u_N \equiv u_s/2 = \pi/X_s$. Theoretically, $V(x)$ can be recovered from $\mathbf{V}*(ju)$ by ideal, spatial low-pass filtering. In Figure 4.42b, $\mathbf{V}(ju)$ contains spatial frequencies in excess of $u_s/2$, and the overall, repeating, spectrum, $\mathbf{V}*(ju)$, is said to be *aliased*. There is overlap between the upper and lower portions of adjacent, repeated spectral components which creates lost information when $\mathbf{V}*(ju)$ is ideal low-passed filtered in an attempt to recover $V(x)$.

Thus, in order to avoid aliasing and lost information in sampling the EEG distribution, $V(t_o,\rho,\theta,\phi)$, on the scalp "hemisphere," the electrodes which constitute a spatial sampling array should be spaced closely enough together so that the highest spatial frequencies in $F\{V(\theta,\phi)\}$ are less than the spatial Nyquist frequencies, π/Θ_s and π/Φ_s radians/radian, where Θ_s is the electrode spacing in radians in the θ dimension, and Φ_s is the electrode spacing in radians in the ϕ dimension. Normally, Θ_s is made equal to Φ_s for ease in constructing the array. Note that in the hemispheric head model, the radius ρ is considered constant.

It is easy to meet the *temporal* Nyquist criterion for the EEG signals at all the N electrodes when they are sampled and digitized for computer input. Each of the N, $V(t,\rho,\theta,\phi)$ signals is passed through a temporal, sharp cut-off, low-pass, antialiasing filter, and then sampled (digitized) at a rate at least 2.5 times the filter's -60 dB frequency. For practical purposes with the EEG, the time sampling frequency is generally made ~300 samples/s.

Justification for the large (e.g., N = 128 electrode) array is found in a key paper by Srinavasan et al. (1998), titled *Estimating the Spatial Nyquist* [frequency] *of the EEG*. In this paper, the authors considered the head to be part of a sphere with about a 9 cm radius. They examined visual, event-related EEG potentials (ERPs) using the International 10–20 Electrode System (19 electrodes on

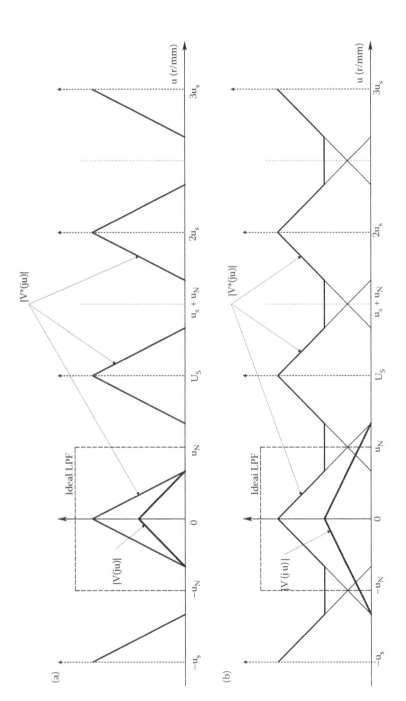

Figure 4.42 (a) With no spatial aliasing. (b) With spatial aliasing. Illustration of spatial aliasing in a 1-D distribution of voltage in x. u is the spatial frequency of the signal V(x) and its spatially sampled array, V*(nX_s), where X_s is the distance between samples and u has the dimensions of radians/cm. In (a), the bandwidth of V(ju) is low enough to prevent aliasing; all of the high-frequency information in V*(ju) can be recovered. When the bandwidth of V*(ju) is increased so that its maximum spatial frequency exceeds the spatial Nyquist frequency, $u_N = \pi/X_s$ r/cm, then aliasing occurs, as shown in (b).

the scalp and a reference electrode on an earlobe), and also, the 32, 64, and 128 geodesic electrode arrays (a geodesic is the shortest distance between two points on the surface of a sphere). Thus, the electrodes are equidistant in geodesic arrays on the head; spaced less than 5 cm on centers in a hexagonal pattern in the 32 electrode array, less than 4 cm for a 64 array, and slightly less than 3 cm for the 128 array (Srinavasan et al. 1998).

Srinavasan et al. defined spatial frequencies on the sphere in terms of the *orthogonal basis functions* for spherical surfaces, the spherical harmonics $Y_{mn}(\theta, \phi)$. They consider the $Y_{mn}(\theta, \phi)$ to be analogous to the sine and cosine basis functions used in the Fourier time series representation of EEG signals. They stated: "Just as any time series of EEG signal can be described by its power spectrum (coefficients applied to each of a the [sic] series of sine waves), any potential field defined on a sphere can be represented as a weighted sum of spherical harmonics."

Srinivasan et al. concluded that the 128-electrode geodesic electrode array was capable of resolving spherical harmonics up to degree n = 7 without aliasing. They concluded: "... we found that spherical harmonics of degree n = 9 are visibly distorted. With 64, 32, and the 19 [scalp] electrodes corresponding to the International 10–20 System the highest spherical harmonics that can be sampled without [spatial] aliasing are n = 6, 4 and 3, respectively."

A heuristic way to visualize the n = 8 case is to consider the circumference of the sphere at its "equator" being divided into eight, equal "cycles" of sinusoidal potential activity. These waves are shown in Figure 4.43 in which we are looking down at the top of the head. The equation describing these waves is

$$V_8(\theta, \phi) = V_8\left(\theta, \pi/2\right) = V_{o8}\,\sin(8\theta). \tag{4.94}$$

θ is measured in radians, and V_8 is shown as a radial displacement from the circle's circumference. The angular period of the V_8 equatorial wave is $\Theta = 2\pi/8$ radians, and its spherical spatial

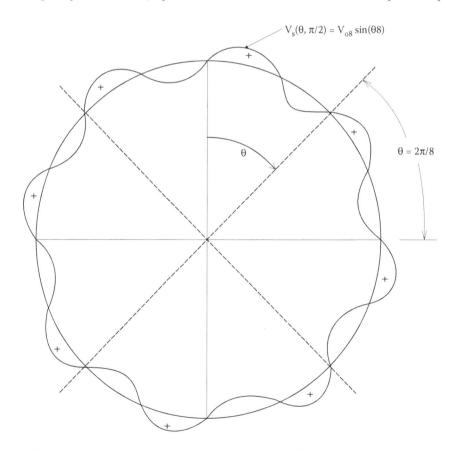

Figure 4.43 Spatial sinusoidal distribution of voltage (radially) on the "equator" of the head hemisphere model. Instead of x, we use the angular coordinate, θ.

frequency is 8 radians/radian. Note that the electrode spacing for the 128-electrode array is ~2.9 cm, which subtends an angle of $\theta = \tan^{-1}(2.9/9) = 0.312$ radians. The angular period of the $n = 8$ spherical harmonic is 0.785 radians. The spatial Nyquist period for the $n = 8$ wave is 0.393 radians, so while theoretically not aliased, the reconstruction fidelity of the $n = 8$ spherical sinewave is poor, giving credibility to the authors' observation that the $n = 9$ spherical harmonic was badly aliased.

Srinavasan et al. pointed out that the four volume conductor layers formed by the meninges, the cerebrospinal fluid, the skull, and the scalp act as a spatial low-pass filter to spatial waveforms present on the surface of the cortex (the electrocorticogram). This low-pass filter has an approximately Gaussian shape. Its transfer function magnitude is down to ~50% of the attenuation at the first spherical harmonic at the second spherical harmonic ($n = 2$), and is down to 5% of the first harmonic attenuation at $n = 6$. For $n \geq 7$, the spatial filter transmission is <5%. Thus, the four head layers act as a built-in, spatial antialiasing filter with gradual high-spatial frequency attenuation.

The 128-electrode, scalp array allows a 2-D computer interpolation and reconstruction of the EEG potentials at all points on the head. This allows researchers to localize local sites of activity (or inactivity) on the underlying cerebral cortex which are task- or situation-specific. It should make the localization of CNS pathologies easier.

4.6.5 EEG Amplifiers, Interfaces, and Signal Processing

Modern EEG signal conditioners used on human subjects generally use very high-gain, low-noise, and high-input impedance R-C amplifiers which have adjustable high-pass and low-pass filters to define the system band-pass. For example, the signal conditioners in the Teledyne Electronic Technologies TET-MD S3200 32-electrode EEG system have the following properties (Table 4.3).

The EGI Clinical EEG System 400 amplifiers intended for use with the Geodesic Net®, multielectrode EEG systems have the following specifications (Net Amps 2015): 32, 64, 128, or 256 channels; input impedance, >1 G ohm; sampling rate, adjustable up to 8 kHz per channel; input dynamic range, ±200 mV; bandwidth, DC to 2000 Hz; input noise, <0.9 μVrms at 1 ksps; CMRR >90 dB; IMR, 120 dB; adjustable high-pass and low-pass filters.

Table 4.3: Properties of the Teledyne 32-Channel, EEG Signal Conditioning System

Parameter	Minimum	Maximum	Units	Notes
Dynamic range	2.0	5000	μV ppk	
DC input impedance	100		Megohms	
Electrode DC offset		400	mV	
Input DC bias current		10	nA	
Input voltage noise		3	μV ppk	
Input resolution	0.25		μV	
Amplifier CMRR	90		dB	at 60 Hz
Saturation recovery time		7	s	
Low-pass filter		75	Hz (fixed)	6th-order Bessel (no ringing)
High-pass filter	0.3	0.5	Hz (variable)	First-order passive
Programmable gain/channel:		10^4, 5000, 10^3, 902		
Number of channels:		32		
ADC				
Resolution		16 bit		
Sampling rate		250	samples/s	
Sample and hold		32		One per channel
Communication port				
RS485 protocol	0.5	1.0	Mbps	Baud rate
Double isolation		4000	Vac	System with primary isolation transformer

Researchers and clinicians recording multielectrode EEG responses have traditionally examined raw data in the time domain, much the same as cardiologists view multitrace ECG records. However, the prospect of dealing with 128 individual traces in the time domain is daunting. Using a computer, 128-electrode, spontaneous EEG data can be color mapped onto the surface of a sphere or phantom head by various Matlab routines developed by EGI. Colors can be chosen so deep red represents areas having high, positive, instantaneous EEG voltage, orange is for less positive scalp voltage, through yellow, green, blue to purple for high-negative voltage. 2-D, T–F analysis can also be done in which a 2-D, discrete, root PDS is calculated from the spatio temporal sampled EEG, $V(t, \theta, \phi)$, that is, $\sqrt{S_V(t, u, v)}$ in $rmsV/\sqrt{rad/rad}$. Also, simple, 1-D cross-correlation, cross power spectra and coherence functions can be calculated from signals from pairs of electrodes to demonstrate functional connectivity between different parts of the brain.

It is also theoretically possible to calculate a *Vector EEG* (analogous to a vector ECG) by adding the potentials recorded at each electrode vectorially. Here i_k is a unit vector projecting from the center (origin) of the equivalent head hemisphere to the kth electrode site on the hemisphere surface at $\{\theta_k, \phi_k\}$. There are a total of N = 128, equally spaced electrode sites on the hemisphere's surface. Thus, the net EEG (dipole) vector can be written as

$$\mathbf{V}_v(t, \rho, \theta, \phi) = \sum_{k=1}^{N} \mathbf{i}_k V(t, \theta_k, \phi_k). \qquad (4.95)$$

The positive tip of vector $\mathbf{V}_v(t, \rho, \theta, \phi)$ is scaled to appear inside the sphere as a point of light at some radial distance $\rho = |\mathbf{V}_v|$ from the origin. As the EEG changes in time, the point of light will move around inside the sphere, its distance from the origin will be proportional to its magnitude and its direction from the origin will point toward the region of maximum surface positivity. Unfortunately, unlike the heart, the EEG is composed of the superposition of the electrical activity of millions of pyramidal cells distributed evenly over the volume cerebral cortex. The cortex itself is convoluted and folded. Only a fraction of the pyramidal cells are oriented radially toward the inside of the skull. Pooling all of this diverse activity in one vector sum loses all the details unique to cortical electrical activity. A vector EEG is probably a bad idea; in this case, it is a misapplication of reductionism. The brain is far more complex electrophysiologically than the heart.

Another approach to interpretive viewing of the EEG is to use the 128-electrode array to plot the electroencephalographic *energy density surface* on the surface of the skull hemisphere. First, 2-D splines or another interpolation algorithms are used to find an algebraic approximation to $V(t, \theta, \phi)$ on the hemisphere. Next, the computer calculates an effective, *charge density* surface, $\rho(t, \theta, \phi)$, at time t from Poisson's equation (Sears 1953, Chapter 3):

$$\rho(t, \theta, \phi) = -\varepsilon_o \nabla^2 V(t, \theta, \phi) = -\varepsilon_o \left[\frac{\partial^2 V}{\partial \theta^2} + \frac{\partial^2 V}{\partial \phi^2} \right], \qquad (4.96)$$

where ε_o is the permittivity of space (8.854×10^{-12}). Now the *product* of $\rho(t, \theta, \phi)$ and $V(t, \theta, \phi)$ is the desired *EEG energy density surface*, Ψ:

$$\Psi(t, \theta, \phi) = \rho(t, \theta, \phi) \, V(t, \theta, \phi) J/m^2, \qquad (4.97)$$

where $\Psi(t, \theta, \phi)$ can be calculated over the hemisphere for any type of EEG voltage distribution, but then so can the 2-D Fourier transform of $V(t, \theta, \phi)$. Perhaps 2-D, T–F analysis will prove useful in interpreting EEGs as well.

4.6.6 Event-related Potentials and Signal Averaging

Another diagnostic and scientific tool in physiological psychology is the evoked transient EEG response to periodic sensory stimulation. The stimulation can be *visual* (periodic flashes of light, or presentation of a figure), *auditory* (periodic clicks or tones can be used), or *tactile* (transient pressure applied periodically to body parts). Other sensory modalities can also be used (pain, heat, cold, odor). Such periodically applied, transient stimuli evoke transient electrical activity from the brain; initially from the sensory nerve input nuclei, then from the brainstem, and lastly from the sensory cortex. These EEG transients, also called event-related potentials (ERPs), are generally small, often around 1 µV peak. Thus, ERPs are generally of the same order of magnitude as amplifier noise, and noise from muscles (EMGs) picked up by the EEG electrodes. Also, ERP voltages are generally smaller than other unrelated EEG activity seen at the same electrode.

Synchronous signal averaging is used to extract the ERP transient out of its additive noise environment. In synchronous averaging, every time the stimulus is given, a short record of ERP plus noise is periodically digitized and each sample is stored in an array of memory registers. Let us assume that k = M = 2048 samples are taken following each input stimulus. As each successive stimulus is given, the sampling process is repeated, and corresponding new samples are added to the summed contents of each array element. This process continues until N stimuli have been given, and N records have been sampled. Then the sum in each of the M registers is divided by N, creating an average in the array. The sample mean for the kth sample of ERP + noise is simply:

$$m_N(k) = (1/N)\sum_{j=1}^{N}[e_k + n_k]_j = (1/N)\sum_{j=1}^{N}e_{kj} + (1/N)\sum_{j=1}^{N}n_{kj} \quad (k = 1,\ldots, M). \tag{4.98}$$

Now we assume that the noise has zero mean and some MS value, sic:

$$E\{n_{kj}\} \equiv 0 \tag{4.99}$$

$$E\{n_{kj}^2\} \equiv \sigma_{nk}^2, \quad \text{(the noise is nonstationary).} \tag{4.100}$$

Also, the signal is characterized by

$$E\{s_{kj}\} \equiv \overline{s_k} \tag{4.101}$$

$$E\{s_{kj}^2\} \equiv \sigma_{sk}^2 + \left(\overline{s_k}\right)^2 \tag{4.102}$$

The two Equations, 4.101 and 4.102, tell us that the ERP differs slightly from stimulus to stimulus. We are now interested in the improvement in SNR between the averager's output and its input. The MS SNR at the averager input is

$$\text{SNR}_{in} = \frac{\text{MS Signal}}{\text{MS Noise}} = \frac{\sigma_{sk}^2 + \overline{s_k^2}}{\sigma_{nk}^2}, \quad k = 1,\ldots, M. \tag{4.103}$$

It is easy to show that the *MS signal output* is

$$S_o = \sigma_{sk}^2/N + \overline{s_k^2} \quad \text{mean-squared volts.} \tag{4.104}$$

The *MS noise output* can be shown to be:

$$N_o = \left[\sigma_{sk}^2 + \sigma_{nk}^2\right]/N \quad \text{mean-squared volts.} \tag{4.105}$$

Thus the MS output SNR is

$$\text{SNR}_{out} = \frac{\sigma_{sk}^2/N + \overline{s_k^2}}{\left[\sigma_{sk}^2 + \sigma_{nk}^2\right]/N} = \frac{\sigma_{sk}^2 + N\overline{s_k^2}}{\left[\sigma_{sk}^2 + \sigma_{nk}^2\right]} \tag{4.106}$$

Also, if the signal is deterministic, $\sigma_{sk}^2 \to 0$, the MS SNR_{out} increases linearly with N. Life is not that simple though. All signal averagers have some inherent, built-in noise which we can assume appears at their output such that $N_o = \left[\sigma_{sk}^2 + \sigma_{nk}^2\right]/N + \sigma_A^2$. With averager noise present, the best $\text{SNR}_{out} \to \overline{s_k^2}/\sigma_A^2$ as $N \to \infty$.

Figure 4.44 illustrates an ERP recorded using a vertex scalp electrode. An auditory cognition task was used in which a subject was asked to count 2 kHz tone bursts that occurred infrequently (15% of tones presented) and to ignore 500 Hz tones presented 85% of the time. The tones were binaurally presented at random times at 85 dB for 50 ms. The large ERP at ~300 ms was evoked by the 2 kHz tones to be counted, and the 500 Hz tones gave rise to the lower peak at ~250 ms. (It is not known how many responses were averaged.)

ERPs are frequently used in evaluating the effects of psychotropic drugs on the parts of the brain giving rise to the ERPs. That is, ERPs are averaged from each of the electrodes in the array for a normal patient, and for the same patient taking the drug, and comparisons are made. Data can be given as individual ERP time waveforms, or as a 2-D, color-coded, voltage map on the surface of the hemisphere model of the skull (Boeijinga 2002, Gilles et al. 2002).

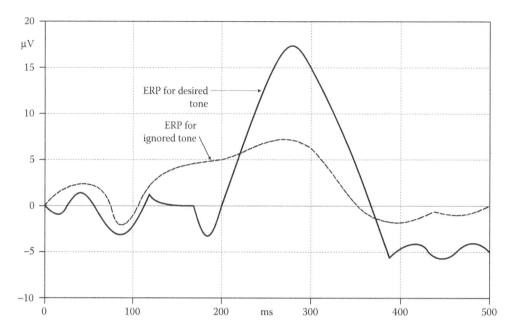

Figure 4.44 Example of an averaged ERP recorded from the vertex. The dark trace with the peak at ~280 ms is evoked by the test tone to be noted; the dashed trace with the smaller peak is evoked by a tone to be ignored. Random presentation was used. (Adapted from Figure 4.44 in Northrop, R.B. 2002. *Noninvasive Instrumentation and Measurement in Medical Diagnosis.* CRC Press, Boca Raton, FL. ISBN: 0-8493-0961-1.)

4.6.7 Discussion

In this section, we have seen that the EEG is an indirect sign of brain activity. The amplitude and frequency of spontaneous EEG change with the state of consciousness of the subject. By recording EEG over the entire head with a dense electrode array, it is possible to have a computer make a spatial map of the continuous, instantaneous EEG over a hemispherical model of the scalp. The spatial EEG map is generally coded by color, for example, large positive regions are deep red, with decreasing positive amplitudes becoming orange, then yellow. White is zero. Negative potentials range from light green through blue to purple for large negative potentials. These colors provide a heuristic, three- to four-bit quantization of the EEG potentials on the scalp surface; very qualitative.

ERPs provide a useful tool for the investigation of the brain's processing of sensory information. Signal averaging must be used to extract the ERP from the random background noise recorded with it. ERPs are used to test neonates' hearing and vision noninvasively. Other display modalities for EEG signals are also finding favor: The energy density plot over the skull surface versus time is one such mode. Another is the use of T–F analysis on individual electrode signals. Pairs of EEG signals can be cross-correlated, and the FFT can be used to calculate their cross-power spectrum and coherence to identify causal connections (Ding et al. 2000). EEGs cannot be used to construct a unique map of brain activity (the inverse problem), because many internal patterns of neural activity can give rise to the same scalp surface potentials (functional ambiguity).

There is a whole laundry list of diseases and conditions that can be diagnosed noninvasively by recording ERPs and spontaneous EEG signals. Some of these include *epilepsy* (grand mal, petite mal, and temporal lobe), *abscesses, tumors, vascular lesions* (cerebral infarcts and intracranial hemorrhages), *sleep disorders, ingestion of psychoactive drugs, and depth of anesthesia.* ERPs can be specifically used to investigate how workload affects attention and task performance in the human operator (Goldman 1987).

4.7 OTHER BODY SURFACE POTENTIALS

4.7.1 Introduction

The functioning of both nervous tissue and muscle is accompanied by electrical phenomena involving both the generation of electric potentials and the existence of current densities in the surrounding volume conductors. Current density is due to the movement of mobile, low-molecular-weight ions such as Cl^-, K^+, Na^+, Ca^{++}, and Mg^{++} in electric fields and concentration gradients. Electrons, in general, are not involved (they are in mitochondrial and chloroplast metabolisms, however). The physical and biochemical origins of bioelectric phenomena are more complex than can be covered here. However, it is safe to assert that nerves and muscles exhibit electric (and magnetic) behavior because of the controlled, selective passage of ions through gating and "pump" proteins in cell membranes. The control of transmembrane ionic currents can be chemical, physical, or electrical in nature (Kimball 2014). In addition, all nerve and muscle cells possess ion pumps, which are specialized, transmembrane proteins that expend metabolic energy to transfer specific ions through cell membranes (either in or out, as the case may be) against electric field forces and/or concentration gradients. In the steady state, the pumps establish resting, steady-state ion concentration gradients across membranes and some electric potential difference as well (Lodish et al. 2000). The insides of resting nerve and muscle cells are always negative with respect to the outside of these cells. The action potentials that electrophysiologists record are caused by gated, transient, transmembrane ion currents (ions moving in response to local electric fields and concentration gradients). The transmembrane currents and pump currents give rise to the observed, extracellular current densities and electric fields.

In this section, we will discuss the sources, medical and physiological significance, and measurement of the EOG, ERG, and the ECoG.

4.7.2 EOG

The EOG is used to test the integrity of the retinal epithelium at the back of the retina, as well as certain mid-retinal layers. Active ion transport in the retinal pigment epithelium creates a net DC potential (an effective dipole) from the cornea to the pigment layer; the cornea is normally positive. The EOG is on the order of single mV, and so can be measured with a standard ECG amplifier with gain of 10^3, and bandwidth of 0.1–30 Hz. (Actually, what is measured is not the DC potential, but the *change in potential* caused by having the eyes move laterally rapidly from center to left and right.) Special, small, AgCl|AgCl electrodes are used, located at the corners of the eye (nasal and lateral *canthi*) being studied. A reference (ground) electrode is attached to some remote site such as the forehead or an earlobe (Figure 4.45). The differential voltage between the corners of the eye follows the approximate rule:

$$V_{EOG} \cong V_o \sin(\theta), \tag{4.107}$$

where θ is the lateral gaze angle measured from the eye's centered position. V_o depends on the state of dark- and light-adaptation of the eye, and the light level. The patient is asked to generate gaze saccades of $\pm 30°$ in response to fixation LEDs that are switched (C, L, R, L, R, etc.) every 1–2.5 s. The EOG waveform appears as a rounded square wave.

Clinical EOG data can be presented in two forms: (1) the *Arden ratio* (ratio of light peak to dark trough) and (2) *ratio of light peak to dark-adapted baseline*. The *light peak* is the peak-to-peak EOG waveform for L → R → L saccades with a light-adapted eye given a general, uniform, background illumination of 35–75 lx. The *dark trough* is the peak-to-peak EOG amplitude in response to the same amplitude saccades recorded in the dark for an eye having been in the dark 15 min. The *dark-adapted baseline* is the saccadic EOG measured for an eye that has been dark-adapted at least 40 min. The International Society for Clinical Electrophysiology of Vision (ISCEV) sets the standards for EOG measurement (Marmor et al. 2011, ISCEV Standards 2015).

Figure 4.46 illustrates a typical record of EOG peak-to-peak amplitudes for dark adaptation and then returns to light. $\pm 30°$ saccades are used. The responses of a typical, normal eye are shown by the open circles. The values used to compute the Arden ratio are circled. The dark circles illustrate the typical responses of an eye with severe, inherited, retinal dystrophy. EOG may also be used in the diagnosis of toxicity affecting vision; toxic substances such as *methanol, ethanol, toluene, ethambutol,* and *phenothiazine* can be causal in retinal dysfunction.

A major disadvantage of the EOG is that the test takes so long (30 min to an hour). The ERG, which measures the eye's transient electrical response to flashes of light with no eye movements involved, can often provide more detailed diagnostic information in far less time.

4.7.3 Electroretinogram

Figure 4.47 illustrates a horizontal section through the right eye showing how the ERG recording electrodes are applied (ISCEV Standards 2015). The positive electrode is held on the corneal

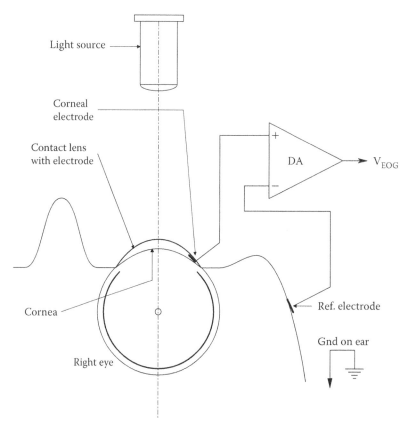

Figure 4.45 Schematic coronal section through the right eye and skull showing electrode placement for EOG recording.

surface by a saline-filled contact lens. It can be a noble metal such as gold or platinum, or be a small, flat AgCl electrode. An AgCl reference electrode is placed on the side of the head, near the stimulated eye. A ground electrode is attached to the ear or forehead. In ERG recording, the gaze is fixed to avoid picking up EMG artifacts from the extraocular muscles that move the eyeball. The stimulus is switched on and off (typically on for 5 ms, off for various intervals depending on the test) and the ERG voltage is recorded using an R-C amplifier. Use of a D-C amplifier is indicated if long flashes are used and long-term ERG behavior is of interest. (Direct coupling means that the amplifier will be subject to long-term, DC drift and is unnecessary when using short flashes.)

Generally, the pupil is dilated with mydriatic eyedrops, and parameters such as the flash intensity, wavelength (if cones are being tested), and the state of the dark- or light-adaptation of the eye are varied. The ISCEV gives standards for five types of ERG test (McCulloch et al. 2015): (1) rod receptor response in dark-adapted eye (the eyes are considered dark-adapted after 30 min in total darkness), (2) maximal response of the dark-adapted eye, (3) oscillatory potentials (in a dark-adapted eye given a short, 5 ms flash), (4) cone receptor response in light-adapted eye, and (5) flicker fusion response to periodic stimuli (5 ms flashes at 30/s). The ISCEV also gives standards for electrodes and illumination levels. They also recommend that the minimum recording amplifier band-pass be 0.3–300 Hz, and be adjustable for oscillatory potential recordings and special requirements; the amplifier's input resistance should be in excess of 10 MΩ. When recording very low-amplitude ERG waveforms, dynamic signal averaging is recommended; the average ERG is displayed to the operator as it is collected.

A representative 7000°K, white-light, whole-retina, D-C-recorded ERG is shown in Figure 4.48. In reality, there would be noise on the recorded waveform; also, a long duration (250 ms) flash is shown here. Note that like the ECG, the ERG waveform has labeled segments which can be related to distinct electrophysiological events among various classes of retinal neurons. The

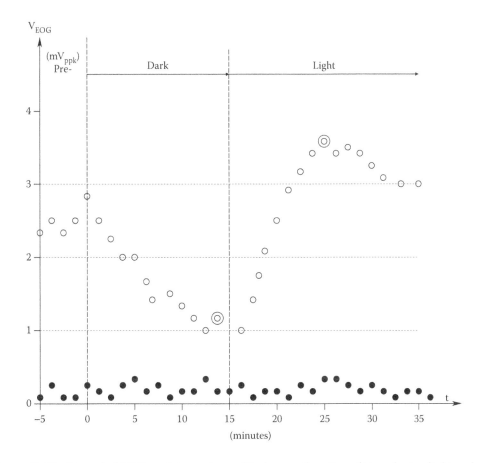

Figure 4.46   Record of EOG peak-to-peak amplitudes as a function of time during light and dark adaptation. *Circles*: normal eye. *Dots*: eye with severe retinal dystrophy.

peak-to-peak amplitude of the ERG is lower than the EOG, typically 400–500 µV. The fast, cornea-negative, *a-wave* of the ERG is probably due to the mass hyperpolarization response of the rods and cones to the test flash of light. The a-response is measured from the baseline to the first (negative) peak of the ERG. The positive, *b-wave* amplitude is due to the activity of second-order retinal neurons in the middle of the retina, and involves the ionic currents around the Müller (glial) cells. The *b*-wave amplitude is measured from the negative *a*-peak to the positive *b*-peak. The *b*-wave time to peak is measured from the beginning of a flash to the *b*-peak. Small, *oscillatory potentials* are sometimes seen on the rising edge of the *b*-wave. Oscillatory potentials most likely originate from the *amacrine cells* for stimulus conditions (mesopic vision) that elicit both rod and cone responses (Niemeyer 1995). Parameters used in making clinical evaluations of vision from ERG tests include the *a*- and *b*-amplitudes and the *b* time to peak.

When recording *oscillatory potentials,* the eye is generally dark-adapted. The amplifier band-pass is reset to 75–100 Hz at the low end (high-pass filter), and 300–1000 Hz at the high end (low-pass filter). The ISCEV recommends that flashes be given every 15 s to dark-adapted eyes, and 1.5 s apart for light-adapted eyes when studying oscillatory ERG potentials. Peak oscillatory potentials are generally less than 25 µV ppk, so signal averaging can be useful. Flicker fusion studies are usually done on light-adapted eyes at 30 flashes/s.

In order to test *macular cones* for areas of dysfunction, such as from laser damage, infection, parasites, or Best's juvenile vitelliform macular dystrophy (Best's disease), a *multifocal ERG* is done by flashing a spot a few microns diameter on and around the macula (e.g., from a laser) in several hundred contiguous locations, and recording the ERG at each location. Signal averaging has to be used because of the very small amplitude of the multifocal ERG responses. The responses from the multifocal ERG are used to make a retinal contour map of ERG performance

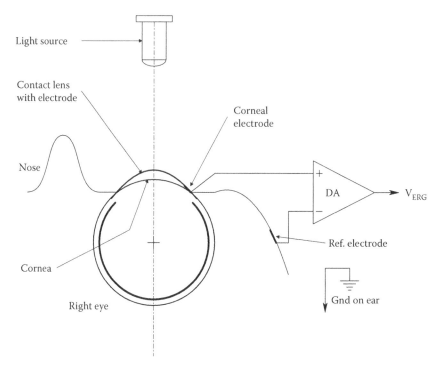

Figure 4.47 Schematic coronal section through the right eye and skull showing electrode placement for ERG recording.

(see Figures 4.49 and 4.50). The high density of normal cones at the center of the macula gives a peak in the averaged response surface, and a pit at the center of a macula damaged by toxoplasmosis (Verdon 2000).

It should be stressed that the ERG and EOG *do not test vision*, they are used as a measure of the functional integrity of the cells in the layers of the retina being illuminated. Some of the

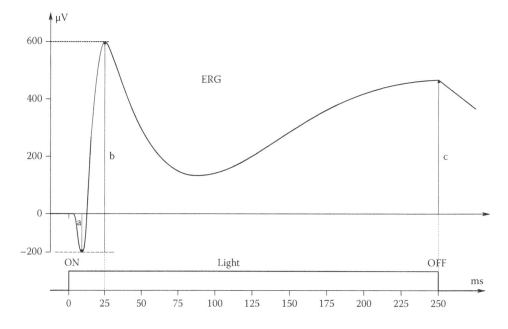

Figure 4.48 Typical normal ERG waveform recorded in response to a 250 ms flash.

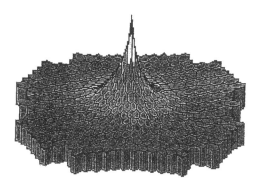

Figure 4.49 Contour map of averaged peak ERG responses to flashes of a focused spot of laser light directed at the macula of the retina. The spot was a few microns in diameter. The peak response at the center of the macula is from the high density of cones there. (Figure from Northrop, R.B. 2002. *Noninvasive Instrumentation and Measurement in Medical Diagnosis*. CRC Press, Boca Raton, FL. ISBN: 0-8493-0961-1.)

retinal diseases that give abnormal ERG results are *retinitis pigmentosa, achromatopsia, cone (Best's) dystrophy, cone-rod dystrophies, congenital amaurosis,* and *night blindness.*

4.7.4 Electrocochleogram

ECoG is an NI, electrophysiological test of cochlear function that is used in the diagnosis of *Ménière's disease* (MD), *endolymphatic hydrops,* and in the differential diagnosis of eighth nerve neuroma (Ferraro 2000). The ECoG is a transient electrical potential produced by neurons in the cochlea in response to a repeated, audio click stimulus. The audio "click" can be a short, high-frequency, sinusoidal tone burst of about 5 ms in duration; different frequencies are used from 1 kHz or above. For example, a 5 ms burst at 2 kHz will contain 10 sound pressure cycles. Another way to produce clicks is to stimulate the transducer (usually a miniature headphone) with a narrow, DC pulse. The sound produced follows the headphone's electromechanical impulse response; it is a damped sinusoid at the resonant frequency of the headphone. If the pulse polarity is such that the initial displacement of the transducer's diaphragm is toward the head, a *condensation* or compression wave stimulus is said to be produced. A *rarefaction* stimulus occurs when the initial diaphragm movement is away from the head. The ECoG responses are slightly different for each type of stimulus, as shown in Figure 4.51 (Ferraro and Tibbils 1999). These averaged waveforms were from a patient with MD.

The positive electrode for recording the ECoG can be a small, spherical electrode of silver or a noble metal (i.e., Pt or Au) inserted down the ear canal to gently contact the edge of the tympanal membrane (TM). In some ECoG procedures, a fine wire is inserted through the TM and middle ear space to make contact with the round window membrane of the cochlea. Certainly the electrode that touches the outer surface of the TM is less invasive and carries far less risk of infection. The ECoG signal is weaker at the TM than at the round window, however. The AgCl negative electrode is placed on the skin at the back of the ipsilateral pinna, and the ground electrode is placed

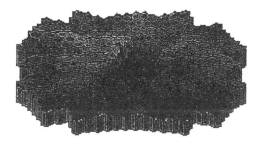

Figure 4.50 Contour map of averaged peak ERG responses to flashes of a focused spot of laser light directed at the macula of the retina. The lack of response at the center is from retinal damage from toxoplasmosis, a sporozoan intracellular parasite. (Figure from Northrop, R.B. 2002. *Noninvasive Instrumentation and Measurement in Medical Diagnosis*. CRC Press, Boca Raton, FL. ISBN: 0-8493-0961-1.)

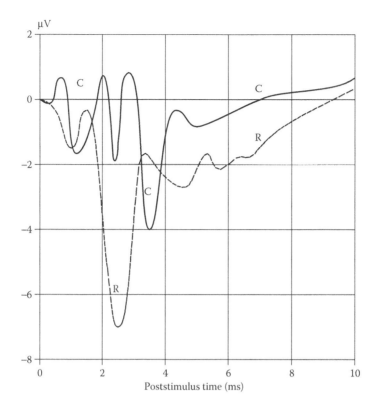

Figure 4.51 Averaged electrocochleograms. Trace C is the ECoG resulting from a click that starts with a condensation or compression of sound pressure. Trace R is the ECoG that results when the click starts with a rarefaction of sound pressure. (From Ferraro, J.A. and R. Tibbils. 1999. *Am. J. Audiol.* 8(1): 21–27.)

on the forehead. See Figure 4.52 for a vertical section through the outer, middle, and inner ear, and the recording electrode positions.

The normal ECoG amplitude recorded from the TM is about 5 µV ppk, so signal averaging is required to enhance the ECoG above uncorrelated amplifier and source noise. The ECoG amplifier is R-C and typically has a mid-band gain of 10^4. The −3 dB frequencies are typically 5 Hz and 3 kHz; 12 dB/octave (two pole) filters are used (Ferraro and Tibbils 1999). Figure 4.53 illustrates the key parameters used in evaluating the ECoG in the time domain. Perhaps a Fourier transform approach, including T–F analysis, might offer some new features that would aid diagnosis.

4.7.5 Discussion

That the eyes exhibit both a DC potential from the cornea to the rear of the eyeball under steady-state conditions of illumination, as well as transient potential changes for ON and OFF of illumination is not surprising, considering the density of retinal neurons and their physical alignment in the retinal neuropile. The DC or steady-state potential is difficult to measure accurately because of drift in the coupling electrodes' half-cell potentials. Also, the DC potential varies with the state of light- or dark-adaptation, and the intensity of the average illumination. To avoid the problem of DC drift, the DC potential is square wave-modulated by having the subject make precise, saccadic eye movements. This allows the measurement of a square-wave, EOG. Thus, an R-C amplifier can be used.

In the measurement of the ERG, the gaze is fixed, and the transient potential changes in response to flashes of light are recorded with an R-C amplifier. Both EOG and ERG are used to detect and quantify diseases of the retina.

The ECoG is another transient potential recorded with an R-C amplifier from electrodes on the eardrum and the pinna. Caused by the acoustic stimulation of sensory neurons (hair cells) in the cochlea, the peak ECoG is in the range of single microvolts, and like cortical-evoked responses,

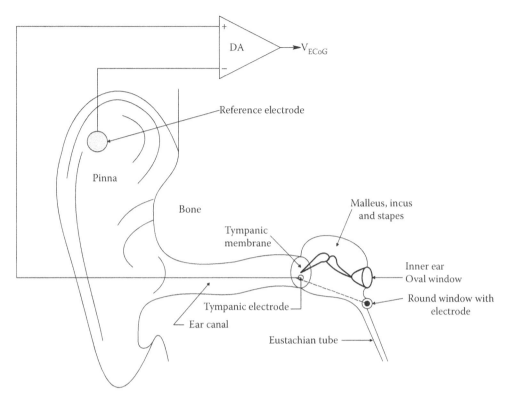

Figure 4.52 Schematic vertical (frontal) section through the outer and middle ear showing the positions of the ECoG recording electrodes.

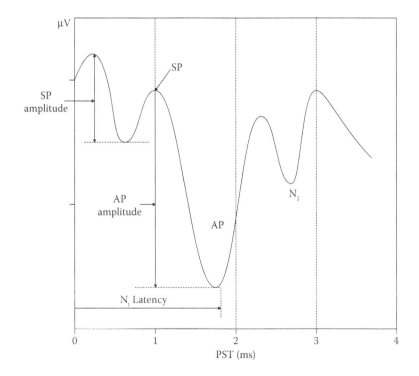

Figure 4.53 Key ECoG waveform parameters used in evaluating the ECoG response.

signal averaging must be used to visualize it. It is used primarily in the diagnosis of endolymphatic hydrops also known as Ménière's disease (MD). By recording the acoustic, evoked cortical potential at the same time, it is possible to separate the diagnosis of MD or other cochlear disease from problems with the eighth nerve and/or brain.

4.8 MAGNETOELECTRIC MEASUREMENTS

4.8.1 Introduction: SQUID and SQUID Arrays

A SQUID is basically a low-noise, ultrahigh-sensitivity, magnetic field-to-voltage sensor. "SQUID" is the acronym for **s**uperconducting **qu**antum **i**nterference **d**evice. SQUIDs permit *no-touch*, NI measurements of the transient, neuro-muscular ion flows in skeletal neurons, the brain, muscles, and the heart.

Figure 4.54a illustrates a basic DC SQUID. The SQUID is the most sensitive sensor for magnetic fields known, being noise-limited by broadband magnetic input noise equivalent to about $5fT$ rms/$\sqrt{Hz}$. At the heart of a low-temperature SQUID is a ring made from niobium (Nb), a period V_B metal which is superconducting at the 4.2°K temperature of boiling liquid helium. One property of superconductors is that they have zero resistance below their critical temperature. Hence, once a current starts to flow around a superconducting circuit, it will continue to flow if left undisturbed.

The ring's inductance is in the nanohenry range; its two halves are joined with two *Josephson junctions* (JJs). Physically, a JJ is a very thin (<3 nm) film of metal oxide (e.g., Al_2O_3) insulator sandwiched between two superconducting conductors. A JJ is a quantum effect device. Current flowing in the superconductor is carried by *Cooper pairs* of electrons; the Cooper pairs pass through the JJ by *tunneling* (strangely, a DC current can flow through the JJ with zero potential difference across it).

The SQUID is, in fact, a four-terminal device; two terminals are used to input a DC bias current, I_B, and the same two terminals are used to monitor the output voltage, V_o. V_o remains zero until the bias current reaches a critical value, I_o. Then the output voltage increases with current, and is also a function of the magnetic flux linking the SQUID ring. The DC bias current is made greater than I_o. The superconducting SQUID ring circuit undergoes the phenomenon of *fluxoid quantization* in which the magnetic flux linking the SQUID is given by $n\Phi_o$, where n is an integer, and Φ_o is the *flux quantum*, equal to $h/(2q) = 2.068 \times 10^{-15}$ Wb. If we apply an additional flux, Φ_i, through the SQUID ring, a supercurrent, $I_S = -\Phi_i/L$, is set up in the ring to create a flux which cancels Φ_i. In other words, $LI_S = -\Phi_i$. From Figure 4.54b, we see that at a constant bias current, the SQUID output voltage varies periodically as a function of Φ/Φ_o (Northrop 2014, Section 8.7). (Note L is the inductance of the SQUID ring.)

Figure 4.54c shows that an active, DC feedback current can be used to operate the SQUID as a null-flux detector, also called a *flux-locked SQUID*. The SQUID DC output voltage is integrated, amplified, and used to control a voltage-controlled current source with transconductance, G_M. The current in the feedback coil produces a flux equal and opposite to the input flux, Φ_i, nulling V_o. By adjusting I_B, the SQUID's operating point is located at one of the open circles in the V_o versus Φ/Φ_o plot. By using a feedback, null mode of operation, the SQUID is given a large, linear dynamic range; the flux-locked SQUID output is now $V_C = K\Phi_i$.

A second type of flux-locked SQUID, shown in Figure 4.55, uses a high-frequency oscillator to superimpose an AC flux on top of the net DC flux in its superconducting ring. Any DC deviation from the null operating point produces an AC component in the SQUID's output voltage which is detected by a phase-sensitive rectifier plus a low-pass filter (i.e., a lock-in amplifier). The DC output of the lock-in amplifier is integrated, and the integrator's DC output, V_o, is used to set the DC feedback current to the SQUID. The use of the integrator in the feedback path creates a Type 1 control loop which has zero steady-state error (Ogata 1970).

Note that all SQUIDs are operated with a superconducting pickup coil/transformer circuit that couples the flux from the $\mathbf{B_z}$ source to the SQUID ring. SQUIDs with first- and second-derivative gradiometer pickup coils (also superconducting) are shown in Figure 4.56. Gradiometer coils allow the SQUID pickup to discriminate against flux linkages common to both coils. The *first-order gradiometer* uses two pickup coils wound in opposition and spaced δz apart so that the Φ coupled to the SQUID ring is proportional to $\boldsymbol{\delta B_z}$. In effect, the first-order gradiometer responds to $\partial B/\partial z$, where the $\mathbf{i_z}$ unit vector is $\perp$ to the plane of the pickup coils. First-order gradients from a magnetic dipole fall off as $1/r^4$, so the first-order gradiometer coils discriminate against distant sources of magnetic interference in favor of local dipoles in the brain surface. It also responds more weakly to deep brain current dipoles. Figure 4.57 illustrates schematically how a first-order gradiometer

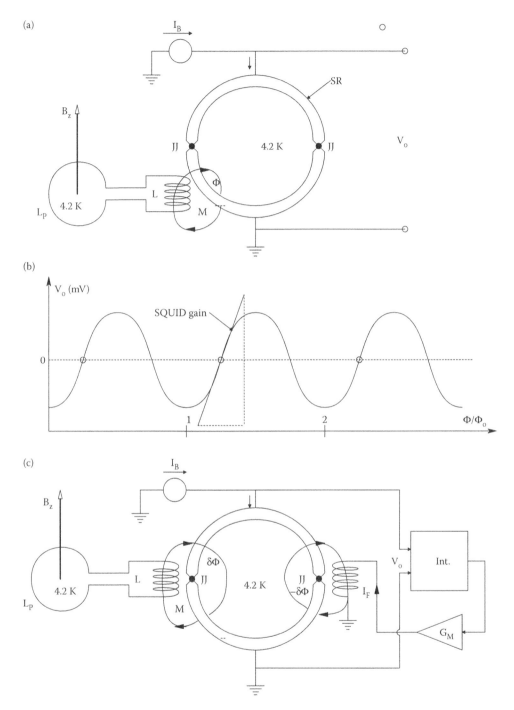

Figure 4.54 (a) Schematic of a basic SQUID circuit. (b) Plot of a SQUID's output voltage at constant input current showing the periodicity as a function of the ratio of the applied magnetic flux (Φ) to the flux quantum (Φ_o). (c) A flux-locked SQUID that uses feedback to stabilize its operating point.

input SQUID can sense the B field from a "current dipole" in the brain. The circle of constant **B** of radius a provides more flux to the gradiometer coil closest to the skull, hence produces a SQUID output. Flux cutting both coils equally, such as from the earth's magnetic field, produces no output. A three-coil gradiometer responds to $\partial^2 B/\partial z^2$, and is even better at discriminating against nonbrain, B noise. Note that there can be millions of current dipoles active at once, and because

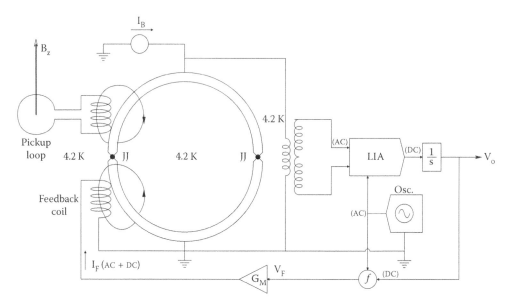

Figure 4.55 AC-modulated, flux-locked SQUID.

of the way the cortex is folded, some can be parallel to the surface of the skull, such as shown in the figure, and others may be directed radially. The B from the radial dipoles will only be sensed weakly with SQUID coils that are parallel to the skull surface.

4.8.2 Magnetoencephalogram

The MEG is the result of the minute magnetic fields produced when ionic currents flow inside the brain as the result of neural activity. The potential differences that produce these currents give rise to the EEG recorded from electrodes on the skin of the scalp. MEG is a true "no-touch," NI, recording method because the magnetic sensors used do not physically contact the head. They do need to be close to it, however. Large arrays of ultrasensitive SQUID magnetometers are used to measure the brain's magnetic fields arising from neural action potentials. In the following sections, we will describe the physical and neural origins of the MEG, how SQUIDs work, and how they are used.

All biomagnetic measurements are based on the physical principle that moving charges generate a magnetic field. Classical mathematical derivations of the magnetic field intensity generally assume some constant current, I, flowing in a long, straight wire. Current is simply the number of charges/s passing a plane though the wire's cross-sectional area. In metal wires, current is carried by mobile conduction band electrons. In biological systems, there are no wires, and current is best thought of as current density, $\mathbf{J}(\rho,\theta,\phi)$, in amps/m^2, in spherical coordinates. Current density is a vector quantity whose direction is the same as the velocity of the $\oplus$ ions drifting in an electric field and/or responding to a concentration gradient by movement from high to low concentration volumes. Current density is also related to the electric field distribution in the volume conductor: $\mathbf{J} = \sigma\mathbf{E}$, where σ is the effective conductivity of the biological medium (e.g., the brain). In biological tissues, conductivity is also a function of position, that is, $\sigma(\rho,\theta,\phi)$ S/m.

The major ions that contribute to extracellular current density around active neurons are chloride (Cl^-), sodium (Na^+), and potassium (K^+). To a lesser degree, other mobile ions such as calcium (Ca^{++}) and magnesium (Mg^{++}) can also contribute to a net ionic current density. In densely packed neural tissues, such as the cerebral cortex or the retina, when a volume of interneurons is activated by chemical synaptic inputs, the interneurons may be excited or inhibited. Both types of inputs cause certain ions to flow into or out of the postsynaptic neuron's dendrites or cell body, wherever the synapses make contact. The passage of these ions through the postsynaptic membranes causes local concentration differences in those ions in the extracellular fluid, and consequent electrical potential changes. These local potential changes and concentration gradients cause the $\oplus$ ions to move *en masse* in the same general direction, forming a *volume current density*, $\mathbf{J}(\rho,\theta,\phi)$. Thus, the local current density surrounding groups of active neurons is generally normal to the surface of the cortex (i.e., parallel to the axons of the pyramidal cells), and may have either

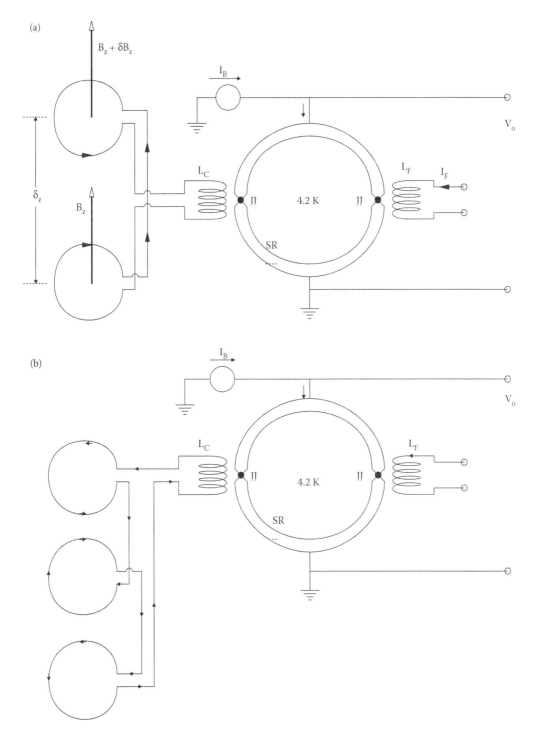

Figure 4.56 (a) A first-order gradiometer SQUID. (b) A second-order gradiometer SQUID.

sign. It is strongest in the neighborhood of the stimulated cells, and tapers off with distance from them. Note that there are about 10^7 neurons under each cm^2 of cortical surface, and 2/3 to 3/4 of them are perpendicular to the surface (Nuñez 1981a). Note also that the surface of the cortex is convoluted, so that in certain areas the pyramidal cell axes are perpendicular to a tangent plane to the skull; in other areas their axes are oriented parallel to the plane, and in still other areas, their

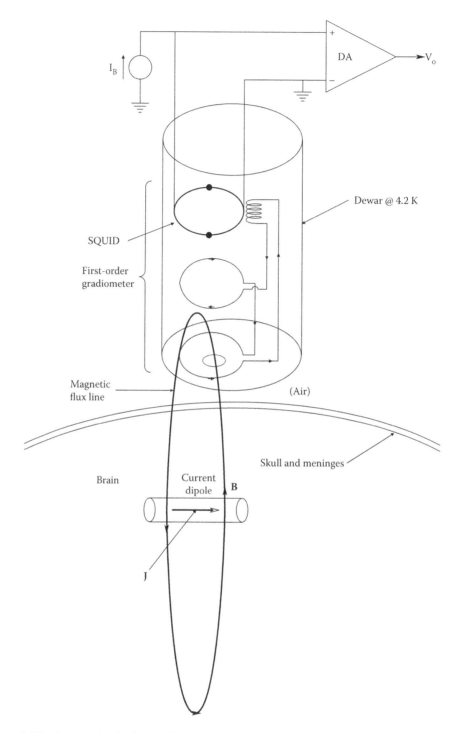

Figure 4.57 Schematic of a first-order gradiometer SQUID used to measure **B**(t) from neural activity at the skill surface.

axes are at various angles to the plane over them. Thus, the magnetic field source geometry is very complex.

Refer to Figure 4.58 to examine the geometry of magnetic field production by a solid "tube" (not a metal wire) of moving charges. We will assume that the charges are chloride, potassium, and sodium ions. The net current in the tube can be written as

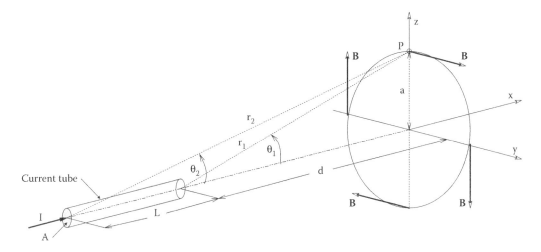

Figure 4.58 Diagram of the vectors relevant to calculating the magnetic flux density vector **B** at a point P due to a finite length current tube.

$$I = A \sum_{j=1}^{N} n_j q_j v_j, \tag{4.108}$$

where A is the cross-sectional area of the tube, n_j is the number of moving ions of species j per unit volume, q_j is the charge on each of the ions of species j, and v_j is the mean drift velocity of ions of species j. Note that for Cl⁻, both q *and* v are negative. Also the current density is just $J = I/A$. v_j is different for each type of ion.

A differential volume element of the tube is $dV = Adx$. Using the *Biot–Savart law*, we can write an expression for elements of the magnetic field intensity, dB, produced by dVs of moving charge (Sears 1953). Refer to the geometry in Figure 4.58.

$$dB = \frac{\mu_o \left[\sum n_j q_j v_j\right] Adx \sin(\theta)}{4\pi r^2}. \tag{4.109}$$

Note that $x = a/\tan(\theta)$, so $dx = -a\csc^2(\theta)\,d\theta = -a\,d\theta/\sin^2(\theta)$, and $\sin(\theta) = a/r$, so $r = a/\sin(\theta)$. Making substitutions for r and dx, we can finally write:

$$dB = -\frac{\mu_o \left[\sum n_j q_j v_j A\right] \sin(\theta)\,d\theta}{4\pi a}. \tag{4.110}$$

Integrating, we find the total magnetic field at point P is given by

$$B = \frac{\mu_o \left[\sum n_j q_j v_j A\right]}{4\pi a} [\cos(\theta)]\Big|_{\theta_1}^{\theta_2} = \frac{\mu_o [I]}{4\pi a}[\cos(\theta_2) - \cos(\theta_1)]. \tag{4.111}$$

Note that the tube of current density, **J**, is surrounded by concentric tubes of constant **B**. **B** at some point P near the current tube is always at right angles to a radial line drawn ⊥ from the tube's axis to P; its direction is given by the right-hand rule (the thumb points in the direction of **J**, and the fingers curl in the direction of **B**).

It will be obvious to the reader that by Kirchhoff's current law, current cannot flow in the tube and just stop; there must be a closed circuit. What we assume in the derivation above is that the current is concentrated in the tube (i.e., it has a high **J**), and that at the ends it fans out in all directions and disperses in volumes of very low **J**. Thus, the **B** field at a point P is largely due to the high **J** in the finite-length tube.

As an example, let us calculate **B** at point P given the dimensions: L = 2 mm = 0.002 m, d = a = 1 cm = 0.01 m, I = 100 nA. The angles are: $\theta_1 = 45°$, $\theta_2 = \tan^{-1}(0.01/0.012) = 39.81°$. Now

$$B = \frac{4\pi \times 10^{-7} \times 100 \times 10^{-9}}{4\pi \times 0.01} [\underbrace{\cos(39.81°)}_{0.7682} - \underbrace{\cos(45°)}_{0.7071}] = 61.1 \times 10^{-15} = 61.1 \text{ fT}. \qquad (4.112)$$

$$\underset{0.06111}{}$$

Now let us calculate B at a radius a = 1 cm = 0.01 m from the center of the current tube. Now $\theta_2 = \tan^{-1}(0.01/0.001) = 84.289°$, $\theta_1 = (180° - 84.289°) = 85.711°$. Thus, B = 1.99 × 10^{-13} T $\cong$ 200 fT. SQUIDs can resolve time-varying magnetic fields on the order of 5–10 fT.

In order to study the MEG in detail, a large array of SQUIDs and their super-conducting pickup coils, all cooled by liquid helium (or LN$_2$), are configured in a helmet-like structure that closely surrounds the patient's head but does not touch it. An MEG system must be used in a large, magnetically shielded room, generally made from layers of high-permeability metals (e.g., mu-metal) and electrically conductive metals (e.g., aluminum or copper). The MEG SQUID pickup coils are oriented parallel to the head surface in order to record deep brain activity. These coils respond to radial, **B**$_r$, from the brain. The SQUID signal voltages are processed to form a moving, 4-D display of brain neuronal activity. The software is able to localize source current dipoles to voxels (volume sample cells) a few millimeters on a side. The average noise level of the MEG system is several fT/$\sqrt{\text{Hz}}$. It is the noise level and the SQUID coil spatial density that determine the voxel resolution of an MEG system.

A helmet-shaped MEG system was developed at the Los Alamos National Laboratory which used 155 SQUID sensors. The LNL workers used photolithographically integrated, SQUID, first-order, superconducting gradiometer magnetometers with a base length distance (δz) of ~2 cm. The sensor bandwidth was DC to ~5 kHz, with 22-bit ADC resolution. The prototype system was tested with a phantom head containing 1.59 mm radius magnetic dipole coils at various locations and orientations throughout the phantom head volume. The system had SQUID sensitivities about 10 fT/$\sqrt{\text{Hz}}$. Details of the LANL MEG array and its performance can be found in Fishbine (2003) and Matlashov et al. (2002).

BioMag, the Low Temperature Laboratory at the Helsinki University of Technology, developed an MEG system using 61 dual-channel, planar gradiometer SQUIDs having a 16.5 mm baselength (δz) (see: www.biomag.hus.fi/meg.html Accessed 5/01/15). This system is being used to detect the onset of epilepsy not visible on scalp EEG, as well as a host of other brain studies. BioMag publications go back to 1994.

Many university centers and research hospitals around the world (e.g., the United States, the United Kingdom, Japan, Korea, Germany, Switzerland, etc.) are developing or have developed MEG array systems; too many to describe here. Three major goals of this research have been to reduce the cost, reduce the noise, and increase the voxel (volume) resolution.

One of the problems with SQUID arrays for MEG studies is that they are *very expensive*; typically (>US$3.36 million, plus operating costs of ~$240,000 annually), they are large, and generally not portable and they require expensive, magnetically shielded operating rooms. A squid array can consume up to 3 L of liquid helium/hour, and the patient must be thermally insulated from this cold. The thickness of this insulation forces the SQUIDs' input coils to be set back from the head, decreasing sensitivity. A SQUID MEG system also requires electronics to bias the SQUIDs, operate them under flux-locked conditions, convert the analog signals to digital form, and then process them by powerful computers for display and storage.

One advantage of MEG recording with a SQUID array is that it is truly a "no-touch," noninvasive measurement. As the data are presented as a shifting, color map of neural activity on either a spherical surface approximating the head, or as a color volume display in 3-D, interpretation can be subjective, requiring clinical experience, and generally simultaneous EEG recording for correlation. A disadvantage of using a SQUID MEG system is its complexity and cost. To justify its application, it must provide information about brain function and dysfunction that is unavailable from conventional EEG arrays.

4.8.3 Magnetocardiography Using SQUIDs

The currents associated with cardiac muscles active in the beating of a heart also produce time-varying magnetic fields that can be sensed with SQUID magnetocardiography (MCG) arrays. A question that must be asked is: Can SQUID-based MCG outperform conventional multielectrode ECG arrays in terms of providing diagnostic information?

One advantage that shrinks the cost/benefit ratio of an MCG system lies in measuring and characterizing the fetal heartbeat *in utero* (Cuneo et al. 2013). The fetus is covered with the *vernix caseosa* during the second and third trimesters of pregnancy (cf. Glossary). Waxy vernix has poor electrical conductivity (it acts as an insulator for ECG currents), hence real-time assessment of fetal heart arrhythmias by conventional ECG electrodes on the mother's abdomen is difficult (Strasburger et al. 2008).

An MCG requires no electrodes (unless signal averaging is used for noise reduction where each MCG cardiac cycle is synchronized with the corresponding ECG QRS spike). An MCG can be implemented quickly, for example, in an ER when a patient comes in complaining of chest pain. MCG can be used to distinguish between healthy subjects and patients with myocarditis and patients with ischemic heart disease without previous myocardial infarction with high sensitivity and specificity (Sosnytskyy et al. 2013).

MCG also has merit in the no-touch measurement of heart activity in animals used experimentally, or in veterinary practice (Koch 2004).

SQUID arrays that have sensitivities on the order $fT/\sqrt{Hz}$ have been widely used for low-level biomagnetic measurements. They, unfortunately, require a constant source of liquid helium for maintaining superconductivity of their JJs and the associated pickup coils. Newer, high-temperature SQUIDs use yttrium-barium-copper oxide (YBCO) junctions which superconduct at ~93 K, above the temperature of boiling LN_2 (77 K). (LN_2 is far less expensive to acquire and make than LHe.)

4.8.4 Other Magnetoelectric Measurements

While our focus on biomagnetic measurements and research has been on the MEG and the MCG, several other biomagnetic phenomena in the body have also been studied. These include the peripheral nerves (MNG), muscles (MMG), the retina (MOG), and the smooth muscle of the intestines. For comparison, the peak B field in the MCG is about 150 pT, about 1000 times larger than the MEG. The fetal MCG is smaller, no more than 12 pT. Large skeletal muscles produce about 50 pT when they contract, and the retina of the human eye radiates ~5 pT.

While the low level of the MEG requires recording in a magnetically shielded room, the relatively larger amplitude of the MCG often permits its recording without shielding, using a first-order gradiometer in which the farther pickup coil is located on the back over the heart, and the near coil is placed over the heart on the chest. Both coils and the SQUID are bathed in liquid helium. The economy of not using a shielded room is paid for by a background magnetic noise level that requires signal averaging (presumably synchronized with the ECG QRS spike) to obtain a "clean" MCG waveform. Multiple gradiometer SQUIDS can be used to visualize a vector MCG.

Rijpma et al. (1999) described work on the development of a portable, high-critical temperature (Hi-T_c) MCG system underway at the Department of Applied Physics, University of Twente, The Netherlands. An LN_2-cooled, second-order gradiometer was being developed to study the fetal MCG using minimum shielding. Another, Hi-T_c, SQUID gradiometer was described by workers at Friedrich Schiller University, Jena. The Hi-T_c SQUID is made from YBCO ceramic; and is cooled by a four-valve, pulse tube refrigerator, rather than LN_2. The gradiometer coils are mounted on a solid sapphire plate, used for a cold heat exchanger. Other nonmetallic materials are used in the construction of the measurement head (e.g., hardened paper) to eliminate magnetic artifacts. An MCG plot of dB/dx in pT/cm was shown. The QRS spike is about 14 pT/cm; 231 averages were used to reduce noise (Gerster et al. 1998).

Finally, we mention the success of a Korean research group in recording the MCG using a novel, Hi-T_c SQUID system (Lee et al. 2008). They developed a Double Relaxation Oscillation SQUID (DROS) in the form of a two-coil, second-order, planar gradiometer. The overall chip size was 3×4 cm; the coils were square, multiturn, 1 cm on a side, and 3 cm on centers. Sixty-four gradiometers were used. The DROS had a high-voltage transfer coefficient of 3 mV/Φ_o, a low, equivalent-field gradient noise of $2.6(fT/cm)/\sqrt{Hz}$ in the white region, and $4.4(fT/cm)/\sqrt{Hz}$ at 1 Hz. Inside their thin shielded room, the average noise was ~$7 fT/\sqrt{Hz}$ at 200 Hz. An MCG recorded with their DROS system is shown in Figure 4.59. Note that only 64 averaging cycles were used to obtain a very clean MCG that closely resembles a conventional lead I ECG. For details, the interested reader should visit the web site of the Superconductivity Group at the Korea Research Institute of Standards and Science.

4.8.5 Optical Atomic Magnetometers

For the past 51 years or so, SQUIDs, operating at 4°K (the temperature of boiling liquid helium), have been unique as the ultrahigh-sensitivity magnetic field sensors, with sensitivities extending

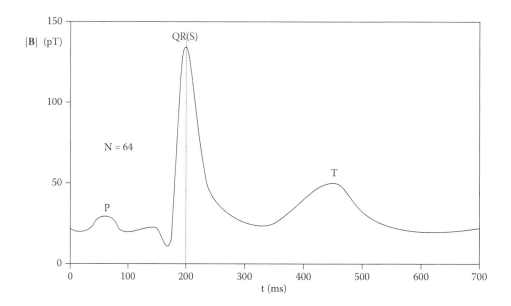

Figure 4.59 Typical magnetocardiogram (MCG) recorded with a double relaxation oscillation SQUID. Note that the waveform shows the P, Q, R, and T inflections, but is missing the S peak. About 64 averages were done.

down to $1\mathrm{fT}/\sqrt{\mathrm{Hz}}$ (1 fT = 10^{-15} T). We have described two of their applications in detail above in NI medical diagnosis in measuring the fetal MCG and the MEG.

In the past 15 years or so, researchers have developed a new class of sensitive magnetometer that does not require superconductors and the attendant liquid helium, and which can be microfabricated (Mhaskar et al. 2012, Sander et al. 2012). A schematic of a microfabricated, fiber-optically coupled optical magnetometer (OM) device is shown in Figure 4.60. Note that there are many designs for OMs: for example, see the dual beam designs by Patton et al. (2012) and Tiporlini and Alameh (2013). In a simple version of the OM, the pump and probe light beams are derived from the same laser source.

Tiporlini and Alameh (2013) described the design of a prototype OM using adaptive noise cancellation for unshielded, room-temperature magnetocardiography. Their system had a sensitivity as high as a conventional SQUID-based MCG system. Their optically pumped quantum magnetometer has the advantage of operating at room temperature, and has the potential of miniaturization in a volume of ~1 mm³. In 2010, Griffith et al. described an optically pumped, alkali atom (^{87}Rb) magnetometer with $5\mathrm{fT}/\sqrt{\mathrm{Hz}}$ sensitivity when operated in the spin-exchange relaxation-free (SERF) regime. The twin ^{87}Rb cells were each $3 \times 2 \times 1$ mm in dimension.

The principle of operation of a basic, optically pumped, quantum magnetometer requires that a circularly polarized laser beam be transmitted through a glass cell containing the vapor of an alkali metal such as cesium or rubidium. The need for a metal vapor means some sort of heat source surrounding the cell is required. The laser light resonates when its frequency ν equals that of the first absorption line of the alkali atoms. This creates an atomic spin alignment that precesses with a frequency proportional to the modulus of an externally applied magnetic field, $\mathbf{B_E}$. This precession frequency is called the Larmor frequency, given by $\omega_L = \gamma|\mathbf{B_E}|$, where γ is the gyromagnetic constant which has a value of $2\pi \times 3.5$ Hz/nT for cesium. If this precession is coherently driven by an RF magnetic field, B_{rf} oscillating at frequency ω_{rf}, the absorption coefficient of the alkali medium changes, thus modulating the transmitted optical intensity. The oscillating RF magnetic field impinging on the vapor atoms modulates the x component of the magnetization vector inside the vapor cell. The phase difference between the driving RF signal and the probe light transmitted through the vapor cell gives a direct measurement of the Larmor frequency (Tiporlini and Alameh 2013). In weak magnetic fields, such as those produced by bioelectric currents, the mean polarization of the atomic ensemble precesses and the reorientation of the resulting polarization, detected through the interaction with a probe light beam, is a measure of the applied magnetic field strength.

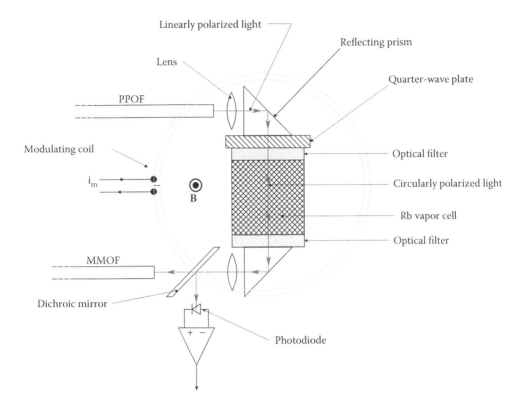

Figure 4.60 Optical magnetometer using Rb vapor.

Kominis et al. (2003) described a prototype SERF atomic magnetometer with a demonstrated sensitivity of 0.54 fT/$\sqrt{\text{Hz}}$, with a measurement volume of only 0.3 cm^3. They used potassium atoms in their device's cell heated to 180°C. (By comparison, typical commercial SQUID magnetometers have a noise of ~5 fT/$\sqrt{\text{Hz}}$, although some SQUID devices have reached sensitivity levels of 0.9 – 1.4 fT/$\sqrt{\text{Hz}}$ with a pickup coil area of ~1 cm^2.) Seltzer and Romalis (2004) designed a three-axis SERF magnetometer with magnetic field feedback used to null the magnetic field in the cell. This magnetometer exhibited ~1 pT/$\sqrt{\text{Hz}}$ sensitivity without magnetic shields.

Figure 4.61 illustrates a simplified schematic of the basic SERF magnetometer of Seltzer and Romalis (2004). As described by Romalis (2008), a high-power, circularly polarized, diode laser beam is directed through the magnetic shields to the glass cell containing vaporized potassium atoms. This beam is absorbed by the potassium electrons, putting them into a spin-polarized state with the electron spins pointing along the direction of circular polarization. A single frequency, diode laser probe beam is used to detect the orientation of the electron spins as they precess in an applied magnetic field. This laser is detuned from the potassium resonance, and as it passes through the polarized vapor, the laser's polarization angle is rotated due to the circular dichroism of the vapor. The degree of rotation is proportional to the degree to which spins are pointing along the probe beam. Two-point measurements or imaging of the magnetic field is done by focusing the probe beam onto an array of photodiodes. In this schematic, the probe laser is imaged onto a linear photodiode array oriented in the y-direction.

4.8.6 Discussion

Biomagnetic recording with SQUID arrays is an active area of research around the world. It is a particularly attractive, NI diagnostic modality because it is, truly, "no-touch." The voxel resolution of present MEG array systems is a few millimeters on a side at the cortex, but decreases to the order of centimeter in deep brain structures such as the thalamus. Loss of resolution with distance is inherent in the mode of measurement, and although deep resolution will no doubt improve with time, the measurement of the MEG with SQUID arrays is ideally suited for the study of brain surface (cortical) (electro-) magnetic activity.

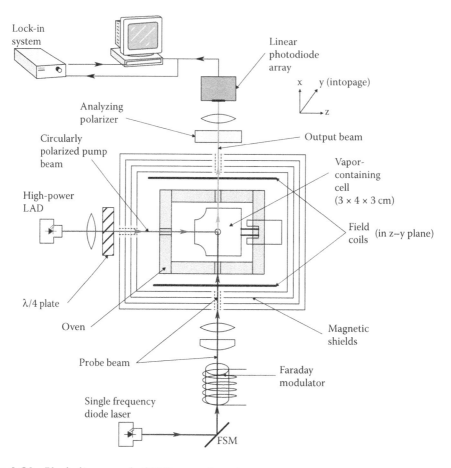

Figure 4.61 Block diagram of a SERF magnetometer.

In the past few years, the physical size of SQUID gradiometers has decreased, and Hi-T_c SQUID arrays have been developed that work at 77°K temperatures, either with LN_2 or special refrigeration units. To eliminate the need for magnetically shielded rooms, researchers have made extensive use of first- and second-order gradiometer SQUIDs in recording MCGs.

Often a low-cost ECG or VCG reveals the nature of a cardiac problem right away. The acquisition cost for a VCG system is probably 1/50th the cost of a SQUID MCG system. The time required for diagnosis is about the same, however. While ventricular ischemia may be simple to spot on a 2-D, color MCG, there are other electrical problems with the heart such as bundle block, or pacemaker dysfunction that can often be resolved with ECG and VCG.

Finally, OM systems have reached a point where they can be miniaturized, and have LOD sensitivities comparable to SQUID MCG and MEG systems. We predict that OMs will replace SQUID systems in the next 10 years because OMs have lower capital cost, do not require liquid helium, and have comparable sensitivity.

4.9 CHAPTER SUMMARY

In this chapter, we have first addressed skin surface electrodes, which are generally of the wet, silver|silver chloride type, giving a C-G-R equivalent circuit model. Amplifiers are described by their terminal properties, that is, their input and output circuits; internal electronic circuit details are avoided. Differential (instrumentation) amplifiers and the CMRR are presented, and the fact that source impedance unbalance can drastically improve or degrade the amplifier's CMRR is described. Also described are sources of noise in amplifiers, and how to calculate amplifier noise figure and output SNR. Low-noise amplifier design is discussed.

Of all the electrical potentials recordable from the body's surface, the ECG is probably the most widely used because of its effectiveness in diagnosing heart pathologies. The ECG is simply obtained at low cost, as is the EEG. We have illustrated how departure from the simple, time-domain, ECG display modality to the VCG in three planes can often aid the diagnostician in locating a specific cardiac pathology.

The SQUID and its uses in measuring the minute magnetic fields produced by nerve action currents in the brain are discussed in Section 4.8. SQUID measurements of the MEG are generally noise-limited, and researchers typically record event-related magnetic field events from the brain by repetitive averaging to improve SNR. Also, the surface of the cerebral cortex is folded in convolutions, hence the neural action currents in the cortex have different directions, causing a complex and often ambiguous vector summation of their B-fields sensed by the SQUIDs. There is probably more information to be realized about the neural activity of the brain from a large EEG electrode array than from a much smaller SQUID array. The MEG, recorded with large arrays of SQUIDs surrounding the head, will probably find little clinical diagnostic application. SQUIDs are expensive to run because of the requirement for liquid helium for their superconductors, magnetic shielding, and the difficulty in interpreting their output signals. A SQUID system, such as the one used for MEF and MCG recording, is truly a no-touch instrumentation modality, however.

5 Noninvasive Measurement of Blood Pressure

5.1 INTRODUCTION

The "gold standard" for blood pressure (BP) measurement is the *invasive measurement* done by inserting a large bore hypodermic needle into the desired artery or vein, and coupling this needle with a saline-filled catheter to a physiological BP sensor, generally of the unbonded strain gauge type. Alternately, in a large blood vessel, a catheter can be inserted with a miniature BP sensor in its tip. In this chapter, unless otherwise noted, BP shall be synonymous with brachial arterial pressure.

During surgery, recovery, intensive care, emergency procedures, pregnancy, childbirth, etc., it is important to know a patient's BP to detect *hypotension* from excessive blood loss, shock, heart failure, etc. or *hypertension* resulting from head trauma, postsurgical release of renin by the kidneys, preeclampsia, etc. BP monitoring under clinical circumstances can either be by catheter/transducer, or be performed noninvasively by a caregiver with a *sphygmomanometer* and stethoscope, or by a calibrated plethysmographic device that sends its output data to a nursing station.

The *brachial artery* in the upper left arm is generally used for NI, sphygmomanometer measurements of BP. The brachial arterial pressure follows the pumping action of the heart, reaching a peak during systole (contraction of the ventricles), and then falling to a minimum, called the *diastolic pressure*, before it begins to rise again during systole. BP is generally given as two numbers, the systolic (peak) pressure "over" the diastolic (minimum) pressure. BP units are generally given in units of mmHg, a holdover from the use of mercury manometers in the nineteenth century to measure physiological pressures (NB: 1 mmHg = 13.60 kg/m^2 = 0.0193 psi). The level of the BP depends on the location of the artery in the body in which it is measured. Generally, the further from the heart, the lower the arterial pressure. Normal BP is also a function of sex and age. In men, the mean brachial artery systolic pressure is ~120 mmHg at 15 years of age, rising to ~140 mmHg at 65; the mean diastolic pressure rises from ~75 mmHg at 15 years to ~85 mmHg at age 65. In women, the mean systolic brachial artery pressure rises from 118 mmHg at 15–143 mmHg at 65 years of age; the mean diastolic pressure is ~72 mmHg at 15 years and increases to ~82 at age 65 (Webster 1992, Section 7.29). A typical brachial BP for a fit, young adult male might be 125/75 mmHg.

BP is sometimes given as mean arterial pressure (MAP), which is simply the time average of BP(t) measured with an invasive sensor. If BP(t) can be approximated by a triangular waveform with peak at P_{syst} and minimum at P_{dias}, then it is easy to show that MAP $\cong (P_{syst} + P_{dias})/2$, that is, the numerical average of systolic and diastolic BPs.

As we are only interested in NI BP measurements, we will not cover catheter sensors here. In the following sections, we describe how the sphygmomanometer works, and how finger plethysmographs can be used to continuously monitor BP.

5.2 CUFF SPHYGMOMANOMETER

Over 120 years ago, in 1896, an Italian pediatrician, Scipione Riva-Rocci, described his invention of the air cuff sphygmomanometer. Figure 5.1 illustrates schematically how the cuff is wrapped around the upper arm just above the elbow. When the rubber bladder inside the cuff is inflated, it exerts pressure inwardly on the soft tissues of the upper arm. The outer surface of the cuff is restrained by a thick, inelastic, fabric cover. The air pressure inside the bladder and cuff is assumed to be the internal pressure of the tissues under the center of the cuff, surrounding the brachial artery. The veins and arteries are the most compressible and elastic of the arm tissues, because blood can be squeezed axially out of them, allowing them to collapse and not conduct blood at high-applied cuff pressure. The cuff's air pressure is measured either with: (1) a mercury manometer; (2) an aneroid pressure gauge; or (3) an electronic pressure sensor. The air is pumped into the cuff by either a rubber bulb pump with a check valve, or in the case of automatic BP measurement, a regulated air supply. To make a BP measurement, the cuff pressure is slowly released by bleeding air out of a needle valve (manual or automatic).

Besides the cuff and pressure gauge, the third essential component of a sphygmomanometer system is a listening device to sense the *Korotkow sounds.* This device can be as simple as a conventional acoustic stethoscope, or a microphone connected to an amplifier, the output of which causes an LED to flash at every Korotkow sound above a fixed threshold. Still another modification of the cuff method is to place two, ultrasound transducers under the cuff, facing the artery: a transmitter and a receiver. The ultrasound system is operated in the CW Doppler mode (see Sections 15.2 and 15.3 of this book). The sudden, pulsatile opening of the artery at systole causes a large,

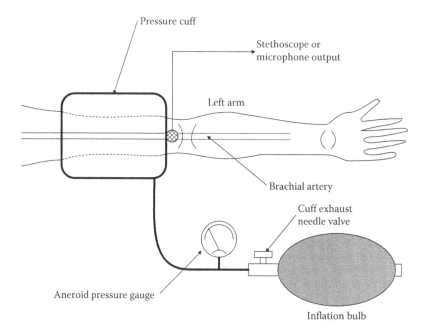

Figure 5.1 Sphygmomanometer cuff and Korotkow sound sensor on a left arm. A simple, vener-able, state-of-the-art, NI instrument. (Not to scale.)

high-velocity transient displacement of the artery's diameter, which is easily sensed as a Doppler frequency shift in the return signal.

The procedure for measuring BP with a sphygmomanometer is to pump up the air pressure to well above that required to collapse the brachial artery under the cuff. The air pressure is then *slowly* reduced at ~2 mmHg/s. When it reaches the systolic BP, the BP in the upper artery forces the artery open momentarily, allowing a bolus of blood to flow. This event is characterized by a thump sound in the stethoscope, the first of the Korotkow sounds. The Korotkow sounds are due to turbulence and the vibration of the elastic artery walls. The thumps occur at successive systolic peaks, gradually becoming softer and more muffled as the cuff pressure falls. Finally, the muffled sounds disappear, marking the transition to normal blood flow in the artery. The cuff pressure that occurs just before this transition is generally taken as the diastolic BP. As the systolic peaks are periodic transient events, and the cuff pressure is released smoothly, it is possible to miss the exact pressures where the first and last Korotkow sounds occur. Thus, the systolic pressure may be underestimated by 5–15 mmHg, and the diastolic pressure overes-timated by 10–20 mmHg. Also, errors can occur if too small a cuff is used on a large arm. The internal pressure in the arm in such a case is not distributed evenly over a significant length of artery; it is concentrated around one spot. The cuff width should be greater than $0.4 \times$ the limb circumference.

Another approach to BP measurement with the pressure cuff that avoids listening for Korotkow sounds is *oscillometry*. In oscillometry, use is made of the small, pulsatile, artery transients super-imposed on the cuff pressure during deflation. These transient increases in cuff pressure come from the volume of each bolus of blood that passes through the brachial artery pushing against the pneumatic compliance of the cuff. The pressure transients are sensed by a piezo-electric pressure transducer attached to the cuff. This type of transducer produces an output voltage proportional to changes in pressure (dp/dt). The overall cuff pressure and the transducer output are shown in Figure 5.2. The transducer output is amplified, low-pass filtered to remove noise, and then rectified to preserve the positive peaks. The average cuff pressure is also sensed by another, dc-reading transducer. Both the average pressure and the positive pulses are sampled and digi-tized by a microcomputer. The computer measures the largest pulse in the record having voltage, V_m. It then finds the first pulse in the sequence with amplitude $V_s \geq 0.85\ V_m$. The pressure when this pulse is found is taken as the systolic pressure. The program then locates the last pulse in the sequence with amplitude $V_d \geq 0.55\ V_m$; the pressure when this pulse occurs is the diastolic BP. In

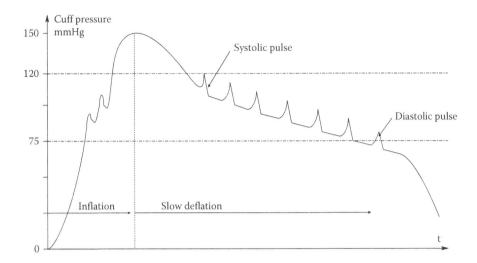

Figure 5.2   Air pressure inside a sphygmomanometer cuff as brachial blood pressure is measured. Note the superimposed air pressure pulses from partially restricted blood flow in the brachial artery. These pulses occur when the Korotkow sounds do, and can be used to detect systolic and diastolic blood pressures. The pulses can be isolated and used to find BP and heart rate.

the opinion of the author, an experienced clinician is probably just as accurate as the computerized oscillometry system described.

5.3 OTHER MEANS OF NONINVASIVELY ESTIMATING BP

A problem with sphygmomanometer measurement is that it does not read the BP in a beat-by-beat manner. It takes a few seconds to inflate the cuff to say 160 mmHg, and then, when in the measuring mode it takes ~50 s to bleed its pressure back to 60 mmHg at 2 mmHg/s. Thus, a complete BP measurement can be made in around 1 min. Continuously using the cuff blocks venous return from the lower arm which will slowly affect the accuracy of succeeding BP measurements made on that arm.

One way to obtain a beat-by-beat estimate of the systolic BP is to use a finger plethysmograph. In one version of this device, a fingertip is inserted into the fingertip of a latex glove. The latex-covered fingertip is inserted into a water-filled chamber with zero compliance. The static water pressure is adjusted to some pressure well below the expected diastolic pressure of the patient. Now, as blood flows into the fingertip at systole, its volume increases. This creates a pressure acting on the compliance of the water pressure sensor. The output of the pressure sensor is a voltage proportional to the static water pressure plus a pulsatile component that follows the peripheral BP forcing blood into the fingertip. The fingertip plethysmograph is thus an inexpensive, NI means of measuring the heart rate and the peripheral BP. Since the peripheral BP in the finger is proportional to the brachial artery BP, a simple one-point calibration with a sphygmomanometer allows the fingertip plethysmograph to yield beat-by-beat, quantitative, BP measurement. Calibration is only valid, however, if the finger position remains fixed in the plethysmograph chamber.

5.4 CHAPTER SUMMARY

Sphygmomanometry, first developed by Riva-Rocci in 1896, is the only effective, accurate, NI means of measuring BP. The only refinement in the procedure is to have a computer automatically control the inflation of the cuff to just above the last known systolic pressure and then release the cuff air pressure at a uniform rate by a servo-controlled valve. The Korotkow sounds are analyzed by a microphone built-in to the cuff. As soon as the last sound occurs, the cuff is rapidly deflated to restore circulation. After a preset pause, the process may be repeated. The pressures are stored with times of measurement.

A continuous, NI estimate of BP can also be obtained with a finger cuff or wrist plethysmometer. Such devices must be individually calibrated, and are not that accurate. They are more useful for measuring heart rate and giving BP estimates for patients in intensive care.

6 Body Temperature Measurements

6.1 INTRODUCTION

The determination of body temperature is generally an NI measurement; a thermometer can be inserted in the rectum, mouth (under the tongue), under the armpit, or in the ear canal. Normal oral (sublingual) body temperature is 98.6°F (37°C), although this value can vary normally over a 24-hour period due to a person's metabolic state, the degree of exercise they may be doing, their food and drink intake, and their environmental temperature. Rectal temperature is about 1°F higher than the orally measured value. Normal rectal temperatures can vary from 97°F due to prolonged cold exposure to 104°F as a result of strenuous exercise under hot environmental conditions.

The body has several adaptive mechanisms (autonomic and behavioral) by which it maintains a relatively constant core temperature. To warm itself and conserve heat, the body may involuntarily shiver, voluntarily engage in aerobic exercise, and control heat loss by autonomically regulating blood flow to the extremities. To bring excess core temperature down, peripheral circulation can be increased to act as a radiator (this is only effective when the body temperature exceeds the air temperature), the body sweats giving evaporative cooling, and behaviorally ceases exercise and seeks shade. If the body cannot compensate for heat loss or heat gain, life is threatened. For example, prolonged immersion in cold water can result in profound hypothermia leading to death. However, the core temperature can drop to less than 75°F and the patient can be revived. Prolonged temperatures over 105°F (40.56°C) can produce heat stroke and brain lesions, and death is almost certain for core temperatures over 110°F (43.3°C) (Guyton 1991).

Elevated body temperature, or fever, is one of the basic diagnostic signs of a severe viral or bacterial infection. A fever normally causes the body temperature to rise between 100°F and 104°F. *Pyrogens* are chemicals that act on thermoregulatory neurons in the hypothalamus to increase the intrinsic, thermoregulatory set point of the body, thereby allowing core temperature to increase. Two strong pyrogens are the cytokine proteins, interleukin-1β (IL-1β), and interleukin-6 (IL-6). IL-1β is released by monocytes/macrophages when they are fighting an infection, notably during antigen presentation to T cells. IL-1β is a *pleiotropic cytokine*, that is, it has many other diverse, stimulatory effects on the immune system besides inducing fever (Northrop 2000). IL-6 is produced by activated macrophages, T and B cells, endo- and epithelial cells, and fibroblasts. It, too, has a pleiotropic role in the inflammation process in infection, and also serves to induce fever. Prostaglandin E_2 (PGE_2) is another pyrogen produced in response to IL1 and IL6 in the hypothalamus. Aspirin and other nonsteroidal, anti-inflammatory drugs (NSAIDs) (e.g., aspirin) inhibit the enzymes that convert arachidonic acid to PGE_2, and thus reduce fever. PGE_2 may be the substance directly responsible for inducing fever.

Probably the most common means of measuring body temperature is the traditional "shake down" mercury-filled, glass fever thermometer. Two versions exist: one for oral (sublingual) use, and the other for rectal use. An oral thermometer generally has an elongated, cylindrical mercury reservoir; a rectal thermometer has short, fatter, Hg reservoir that is mechanically more robust. Both types of thermometers require 1.5–2.5 min to reach thermal equilibrium with their surround. They are easy to read, and hold their reading until their mercury column is shaken down to below the expected body temperature. As their principal disadvantage is their slow response time, many electronic thermometers with faster response times have been developed that have digital readouts. The sale of mercury fever thermometers is being phased out in many states because of the fear of mercury poisoning if they break. The mercury is replaced with colored alcohol.

In the first class of electronic thermometer, temperature is sensed by a change in resistance using a Wheatstone bridge or an active electronic circuit. $\Delta R(T)$ responding devices include both positive- and negative-temperature coefficient thermistors, and platinum resistance elements. Themistors have large, nonlinear resistance tempcos, and must be linearized over the range of interest which is from 92°F to 112°F in most clinical applications. Platinum resistance thermometers have smaller, positive resistance tempcos that are linear enough not to require linearization over the 20°F range in question. Thermistors can be made in small bead configurations, and thus have low-thermal mass and heat quickly to the body temperature being measured. (The tempco of a resistor is defined as $\alpha(T) \equiv (\Delta R/\Delta T)/R_o$. Where $\Delta T \equiv T - T_o$. α of metals such as platinum or nichrome is positive; α itself generally varies with T.)

All electronic IC temperature sensors can also be used to measure body temperature. The Analog Devices, AD590 and AD592 temperature transducers, are two-terminal, current sources that produce 1 μA/K outputs given 4–15 volts across its body. The current is normally converted

119

to voltage proportional to °C or °F by an op-amp transresistor. Although these devices normally come packaged in metal cans or plastic packs, they can be obtained in chip form for custom mounting in a low-heat capacity enclosure. National Semiconductor also makes IC temperature transducers; in the National LM35, the op-amp is on board, and the voltage output is 10 mV/K. Also, the LM135, 235, 335 three-terminal, IC temperature sensors have the same sensitivity as the venerable LM35.

6.2 CONDUCTIVE HEAT TRANSFER AND THERMOMETER RESPONSE TIME

A major problem encountered with the classical glass/mercury fever thermometer is the relatively long time required to obtain a steady-state reading. Ideally, to save clinical staff time, a temperature reading should be stable in not more than 5 s; 2 is preferable. To gain an appreciation of the physical factors that contribute to limiting conductive heat flow from the body (rectum, mouth) to the actual sensing element (Hg expansion, thermistor, IC), we will examine the dynamics of heat flow from an electrical analog circuit viewpoint.

Heat flows from a warmer mass to a cooler mass until the two masses reach thermal equilibrium. In the case of a thermometer, the temperature of the sensor rises until it equals the temperature of the external medium (e.g., body temperature, T_b). It is the time course of the rise of the sensor's temperature that we will examine. Intuitively, we know that if the sensor is covered with a thick layer of thermal insulation, such as plastic or glass, it will take longer for the sensor to reach T_b than if a thin layer of a good heat conductor, such as a metal, covers the sensor. Also, if the sensor has a large mass, it will take longer for its temperature to rise to T_b. It is obviously impractical to directly cover a sensor with metal; if it is an electrical sensor, it will be short-circuited, and if it is an expansion-type liquid such as Hg or colored alcohol, the liquid cannot be seen. An obvious compromise is to cover the sensor with a thin layer of a chemically inert, electrical insulator such as glass or plastic. Thus, the heat from the body must flow through this coating before entering the sensor mass and causing its temperature to rise.

In discussing the physics of heat transfer, we first must examine the units and parameters involved. *Heat* has the units of *energy* or *work*, and can be given in SI Joules, cgs Ergs, gram calories, kilogram calories, British thermal units, etc. Note that 1 gm calorie = 4.186 Joules and 1 kg calorie = 4.186 Joules. The *specific heat capacity* of a material is the quantity of heat that must be supplied to a unit mass of the material to raise its temperature 1°C. The *specific heat capacity* = c = heat capacity/mass has the units of cal./(gm °C). For example, c for Hg is 0.033 cal./(gm °C) and c for glass is 0.199 cal./(gm °C).

If heat is delivered to an object such as a heat sink at a constant rate, P_i (note that Joules/second has the dimensions of *power*), its temperature will rise above the ambient temperature until the combined heat loss rates from the object from conduction, radiation, and convection equal the input rate. This steady-state temperature rise ΔT can be written as

$$\Delta T = P_i \Theta \tag{6.1}$$

In direct analogy to Ohm's law, ΔT is analogous to voltage drop, the heat flow rate, P_i, is analogous to current, and the *thermal resistance*, Θ, is analogous to electrical resistance. The units of Θ are °C/W. The thermal analog to electrical capacitance is *heat capacity*, C_H.

In the electrical case:

$$v = (1/C) \int i \, dt \tag{6.2}$$

In the thermal case:

$$\Delta T = (1/C_H) \int P_i dt \tag{6.3}$$

If we differentiate Equation 6.3, we can write:

$$P_i = C_H \Delta \dot{T} \tag{6.4}$$

C_H has the units of (Joules/s)/(°K/s) = Joules/°K. Note that C_H = mc, where m is the mass of the object, and c is its specific heat capacity. Curiously, there is no thermal analog for electrical inductance, hence thermal systems can be modeled by electrical R–C circuits.

In the case of a glass/mercury fever thermometer, the mercury volume expands with increasing temperature at a greater rate than the glass, forcing it into the capillary tube in the thermometer

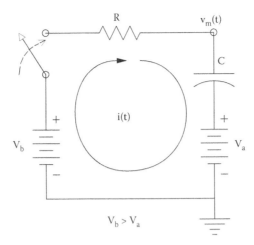

Figure 6.1 Simple R-C analog circuit modeling heat transfer in a glass/mercury fever thermometer. The switch closes when the thermometer is inserted into the body. Voltages are analogous to temperatures, current to heat flow; R is thermal resistance. C is heat capacity.

body. When a thermometer at ambient (room) temperature, T_a, is placed under the tongue in saliva at body temperature, T_b, heat immediately flows into the glass and thence to the mercury, causing its temperature to rise toward T_b. After about 2 min, the mercury in the bulb has reached T_b and the reading is stable. In this case, the glass acts as a thermal resistance, Θ_g °C/W. We assume that the mercury has a negligible heat loss, and that it has a thermal capacitance, C_m Joules/°C. Thus, placing the thermometer in the mouth at constant body temperature is analogous to a step of voltage applied to a resistance in series with the capacitance of the Hg bulb. The equivalent circuit is shown in Figure 6.1. The temperature of the mercury is analogous to the voltage on the capacitance. This simple series, RC circuit, has the well-known step response:

$$v_c(t) = V_a + (V_b - V_a)\left[1 - \exp(-t/RC)\right] \tag{6.5}$$

Note that the voltage source, V_a, in series with C is necessary to model the mercury being initially at ambient temperature. By analogy, the mercury temperature is given by

$$T_m(t) = T_a + (T_b - T_a)\left[1 - \exp(-t/\Theta_g C_m)\right] \tag{6.6}$$

$\Theta_g C_m$ is the thermal time constant of the system. It takes four or five time constants for the mercury to reach $\approx T_b$. Thus, $\Theta_g C_m$ is in the order of 20–25 s for a typical oral glass/mercury fever thermometer. Similar dynamics apply to glass-coated thermistor bead temperature sensors; however, because the bead has a much lower mass than the Hg, and its glass coating is thin, the thermistor thermometer will, in general, respond much faster than the glass/mercury thermometer. Its time constant is on the order of single seconds.

In the case of electronic IC thermosensors, there may be two time constants involved. The heat first must pass through a plastic or epoxy protective coating, and then raise the temperature of the chip substrate, which, in turn, heats the transistors that sense the temperature. Time constants here are typically longer than the thermistor bead but shorter than the glass/mercury thermometer.

In the following section, we examine the theory underlying the operation of no-touch, radiation thermometers that use a pyroelectric sensor to measure surface temperature by using the surface's blackbody (BB) radiation. The generic design of this type of radiation thermometer is also given.

6.3 LIR BB THERMOMETER

6.3.1 Introduction

The long-wave, infrared (LIR) thermometer is a device that comes very close to being an ideal, NI diagnostic medical instrument. It is completely passive, and requires minimum contact with the body surface for a very short time (about 1–2 s) in order to obtain a reading. Its operating principle is based on the same technology used by IR intruder alarms and light switches. That is, when a sensitive, *pyroelectric material* (PYM) is exposed to a surface having a temperature different from its ambient temperature, a minute electric current is generated by the PYM as it absorbs or looses heat to this surface by radiation. The current is converted to a voltage which is a nonlinear function of the temperature difference between the PYM and the surface. In the following sections, we describe the physics of radiation heat transfer, the behavior of PYMs, the electronic circuits required to condition their output signals, and the basic design of the Braun ThermoScan™ 5 LIR ear thermometers.

6.3.2 Physics of BB Radiation

All objects at temperatures above absolute zero radiate heat energy as electromagnetic (EM) radiation. The maximum heat energy that can be radiated from an object is called its *BB radiation*. A BB is a theoretical, ideal, object which is a perfect absorber *and* emitter of EM radiation. When an object is in thermal equilibrium with its environment, the total energy per unit time (power) radiated by it is equal to the power absorbed. This equality is called *Kirchoff's radiation law*. In general, many objects radiate and absorb more poorly than an ideal BB, such objects are characterized by an emissivity constant, ε, and an absorptivity constant, α. In general, both ε and α can be functions of wavelength, λ. Kirchoff's radiation law tells us that $\varepsilon \equiv \alpha$, and $0 < \varepsilon(\lambda) \leq 1$. $\varepsilon = 1$ for an ideal BB; 0.92 for granular pigment (any color); a rough carbon plate = 0.75; oxidized steel = 0.7; polished copper = 0.15. When a beam of EM radiation strikes a transparent object, a fraction is absorbed, a fraction α_t is transmitted, and a fraction α_r is reflected back. For this situation, Kirchoff's radiation law yields (Barnes 1983):

$$\varepsilon + \alpha_t + \alpha_r = 1 \tag{6.7}$$

The distribution of BB radiation as a function of object temperature and wavelength has a well-known form derived from quantum theory. *Planck's radiation law* equation is:

$$W_\lambda = \frac{2\pi hc^2}{\lambda^5 [\exp(hc/\lambda kT) - 1]} (W/m^2)/(\text{meter wavelength}). \tag{6.8}$$

Note that W_λ's units are SI, and it is called a *spectral emittance*. In Equation 6.8, λ is the EM radiation wavelength in meters, c = speed of light (3×10^8 m/s), k = Boltzmann's constant (1.3806×10^{-23} Joule/°K), h = Planck's constant (6.6262×10^{-34} Joule s), T is in °K. W_λ is sometimes put in the form:

$$W_\lambda = \frac{c_1}{\lambda^5 [\exp(c_2/\lambda T) - 1]}, \tag{6.9}$$

where $c_1 = 2\pi hc^2$ and $c_2 = hc/k$. For SI units, $c_1 = 3.742 \times 10^{-16}$ and $c_2 = 1.439 \times 10^{-2}$.

Often workers use "hybrid" or mixed units for W_λ, for example (milliwatts/cm²)/(μm wavelength). The only advantage of using mixed units is that the W_λ scale units at physiological temperatures are simple integers. When these units are used, the constants c_1 and c_2 must be appropriately scaled: sic: $c_1 = 3.742 \times 10^4$ and $c_2 = 1.438 \times 10^4$.

Figure 6.2 illustrates a log-log plot of a family of Planck's distribution curves for ideal BB radiation at different temperatures. Note that as the BB object's temperature increases, the peaks of the W_λ curves shift toward shorter wavelengths. This shift is called the *Wien displacement law*; it can be derived formally by setting $dW_\lambda/d\lambda = 0$. Thus, the W_λ peak occurs at

$$\lambda_{pk} = 2897.1/T°K \, \mu m. \tag{6.10}$$

For a human body at 310°K, the peak W_λ is at 9.35 μm, in the LIR range.

We can find the *total radiant emittance*, W_{bb}, from a BB in W/m² by integrating $W_\nu \, d\nu = W_\lambda \, d\lambda$, where c = $\nu\lambda$. When this is done, we find:

$$W_{bb} = \frac{2\pi^5 k^4}{15 \, c^2 h^3} T^4 = \sigma T^4 \, W/m^2 \tag{6.11}$$

where $\sigma = 5.662 \times 10^{-8}$, the SI Stefan–Boltzmann constant.

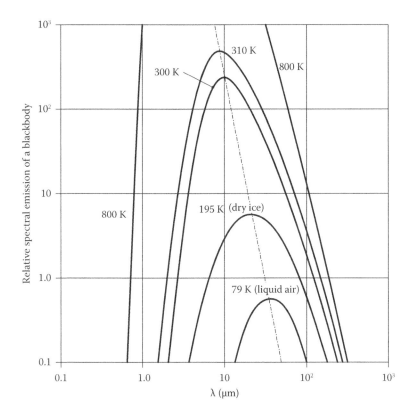

Figure 6.2 Log-log plots of the relative spectral emission of an ideal blackbody at different temperatures.

In the LIR thermometer, heat is transferred by radiation from the object whose temperature is being measured (e.g., an eardrum) to the internal, pyroelectric sensor element at ambient temperature, T_a. The eardrum may be considered to be at constant temperature because it is well supplied with blood at body temperature, and the middle ear behind it is also at T_b. Thus, any heat lost by radiation from the eardrum to the PYM can be assumed to not change the eardrum temperature.

Consider an ideal heat exchange system as shown in Figure 6.3. The surface on the right is the eardrum at temperature T_b. On the left is the PYM at ambient temperature T_a. The conduction lines represent the heat transfer processes taking place at the surfaces and in the space between them. Let H_a be the total *irradiance* from the PYM surface directed at the eardrum. A fraction $a_b H_a$ is absorbed by the eardrum at temperature T_b, and a fraction $(1 - a_b)H_a$ is reflected from the eardrum and returned to the PYM. The *radiant emittance* from the eardrum is $e_b W_b$ so the net irradiance, H_b, to the PYM is (note that $r_b = 1 - e_b$, and $a_b = e_b$, etc.):

$$H_b = (1 - e_b)H_a + e_b W_b. \tag{6.12}$$

Congruent reasoning yields:

$$H_a = (1 - e_a)H_b + e_a W_a. \tag{6.13}$$

Using Cramer's rule, we solve these equations for the irradiances, H_a and H_b:

$$H_a = \frac{W_a/e_b + (1 - e_a)W_b/e_a}{(1/e_a + 1/e_b - 1)} \tag{6.14}$$

$$H_b = \frac{W_b/e_a + (1 - e_b)W_a/e_b}{(1/e_a + 1/e_b - 1)}. \tag{6.15}$$

PYM at T_a Eardrum at T_b

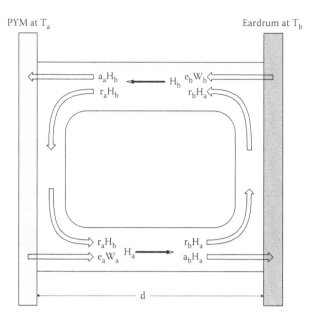

Figure 6.3 Heat flow balance between an eardrum (B-B radiator) and a pyroelectric temperature sensor. Emitted, reflected, and absorbed irradiances are shown.

Thus, the net radiant flux into the PYM can be found from:

$$\Delta H = H_b - H_a = \frac{W_b - W_a}{(1/e_a + 1/e_b - 1)} = \frac{\sigma\left(T_b^4 - T_a^4\right)}{(1/e_a + 1/e_b - 1)} \, W/m^2. \tag{6.16}$$

The net EM power flux into the PYM is simply $P_i = A \, \Delta H$ W. (A is the effective PYM area receiving radiation.) A constant P_i will cause the PYM temperature to rise. However, the BB thermometer is operated with a shutter that only allows P_i to reach the PYM for less than a second, so the PYM returns quickly to its ambient temperature, T_a, and is ready for the next measurement in about 8 s.

6.3.3 Temperature Measurement with PYMs

PYMs are crystalline or polymer substances that generate internal, electrical charge transfer in response to internal *heat flow*. The charge transfer can be sensed as a current or voltage change, depending on the kind of electronic signal conditioning associated with the PYM. In general, PYM materials are also piezoelectric; that is, they also respond to applied mechanical stress by internal charge transfer. PYM sensors include the polymers: *polyvinylidine fluoride* (PVDF) and *polyvinyl fluoride* (PVF), and the crystalline substances: *lithium tantalate* (LiTaO$_3$); *strontium* and *barium niobate; triglycine sulfate* (TGS); *Rochelle salt; KDP* (KH$_2$PO$_4$); *ADP* (NH$_4$H$_2$PO$_4$); *barium titanate* (BaTiO$_3$); *LZT*, etc.

PYM sensors are fabricated by taking a thin rectangle or disc of the material and coating both sides with a very thin layer of vapor-deposited metal such as gold, silver, or aluminum. Electrical contact is made with silver epoxied wires or pressure contacts. The side of the sensor that is to receive radiation is often given an extra, thin, rough, heat-absorbing coating such as gold or platinum black. This coating maximizes the ratio of absorptivity to reflectivity for the PYM sensor. As the original ThermoScan LIR thermometers were designed with PVDF sensors, we will focus our attention on this material in the following developments.

First, it will be seen that PYM sensors respond only to *change* in temperature. In the thermal steady state, there is no net internal charge transfer, and no voltage across their electrodes. Thus, if a constant input radiation power, P_i, is applied, the sensor's temperature rises to an equilibrium value, $T_a' > T_a$, where radiation and conduction heat losses equal the thermal input power. In general, we can write a heat balance differential equation for the PYM sensor:

$$P_i(t) = C_T \frac{d(T_a' - T_a)}{dt} + \frac{(T_a' - T_a)}{\Theta} = C_T \frac{d\Delta T}{dt} + \frac{\Delta T}{\Theta}, \tag{6.17}$$

where C_T is the PYM material's heat capacity in Joules/°K, Θ is its *thermal resistance* in °K/W, and $\Delta T = T_a' - T_a$. T_a is the starting, steady-state, ambient temperature of the PYM and T_a' is the temperature it rises (or falls) to as a result of absorbing (radiating) P_i over some time T_s. Θ depends on the PYM material used, its configuration, and even how it is mounted. (Θ can be reduced by direct thermal conduction (heatsinking) and by air convection.)

C_T is given by

$$C_T = cAh \quad \text{Joules}/°K, \tag{6.18}$$

where **c** is the PYM's *specific heat capacity* in Joules/(cm^3 °K), A is the absorbing surface area in cm^2, and h is the PYM thickness in cm.

If $\Delta T/T$ is small, we can assume that P_i remains constant over T_s. The differential Equation 6.17 can be Laplace transformed and written as a transfer function:

$$\frac{\Delta T}{P_i}(s) = \frac{\Theta}{s\Theta C_T + 1}. \tag{6.19}$$

Now, the short-circuit current from the irradiated PYM is given by

$$i_p(t) = K_p A \dot{\Delta T}. \tag{6.20}$$

Laplace transforming Equation 6.20:

$$I_p(s) = K_p A s \Delta T(s). \tag{6.21}$$

When Equation 6.21 for $I_p(s)$ is substituted into Equation 6.19, we can finally write the transfer function:

$$\frac{I_p}{P_i}(s) = \frac{s K_p A \Theta}{s\Theta C_T + 1}. \tag{6.22}$$

K_p is the PYM's pyroelectric coefficient in Coulombs/(m^2 °K). Table 6.1 gives the important constants of certain common PYMs (note units).

Assume the PYM sensor is at thermal equilibrium at temperature T_a. The radiation-blocking shutter is opened, permitting a *step* of radiation from the warm object at constant temperature T_b to reach the sensor. The short-circuit current is given by Equation 6.22:

$$I_p(s) = \frac{P_{io}}{s} \frac{s K_p A \Theta}{(s\Theta C_T + 1)} = P_{io} \frac{K_p A/C_T}{(s+1)/(\Theta C_T)}. \tag{6.23}$$

In the time domain, this is simply an exponential decay waveform:

$$i_p(t) = (P_{io} K_p A/C_T) \exp[-t/(\Theta C_T)]. \tag{6.24}$$

Table 6.1: Physical Properties of Certain PYMs

Pyroelectric Material	Pyroelectric Coefficient K_p in μCb/(m^2 °K)	Dielectric Constant $\kappa = \varepsilon/\varepsilon_o$	Thermal Resistance Θ °K/W	Specific Heat c in J/(cm^3 °K)
Triglycine sulfate (TGS)	350	3.5	2.5×10^{-3}	2.5
Lithium tantalate (LiTaO$_3$)	200	46	2.38×10^{-4}	3.19
Barium titanate (BaTiO$_3$)	400	500	3.33×10^{-4}	2.34
PVDF film	40	12	7.69×10^{-3}	2.4

Source: Data from Fraden, J. 1993. *Balanced Infrared Thermometer and Method for Measuring Temperature.* US Patent No. 5,178,454. January 12, 1993; Pállas-Areny, R. and J.G. Webster. 1991. *Sensors and Signal Conditioning.* John Wiley & Sons, NY.

ΘC_T is the sensor's *thermal time constant* which is material and dimensionally dependent. P_{io} is assumed constant and is given by

$$P_{io} = A\Delta H = K_s\left(T_b^4 - T_a^4\right) \tag{6.25}$$

$$K_s = A\sigma/(1/e_a + 1/e_b - 1). \tag{6.26}$$

Now examine the circuit in Figure 6.4. The PYM sensor is connected to an op-amp, connected as a transimpedance. Note that the equivalent circuit for the PYM can be configured as an *ideal current source*, $i_p(t)$, in parallel with the sensor's electrical leakage conductance, G_p, and its electrical, self-capacitance, C_p. $i_p(t)$ is given by Equation 6.24 for a step input of IR power. Let us first neglect the op-amp's feedback capacitor, C_F. The output voltage of the op-amp is given by (note the direction of i_p):

$$V_o(t) = R_F i_p(t) = R_F\left(P_{io}K_p A/C_T\right)\exp\left[-t/(\Theta C_T)\right] \geq 0. \tag{6.27}$$

The peak $V_o(t)$ is $V_{opk} = R_F (P_{io}\ K_p\ A/C_T)$ volts; hence, we can calculate the temperature T_b of the warm object from V_{opk} and a knowledge of the system's constants.

$$T_b = \left[T_a^4 + \frac{V_{opk}C_T}{R_F K_p A K_s}\right]^{\frac{1}{4}} = \left[T_a^4 + V_{opk}K_{sys}\right]^{\frac{1}{4}}. \tag{6.28}$$

The problem with this approach is while V_{opk} is measured fairly accurately, the system's constants and T_a are generally not that accurately known; hence a known BB temperature source at T_{cal} can be used to find the lumped constant K_{sys}.

$$K_{sys} = (T_{cal}^4 - T_a^4)/V_{ocal}. \tag{6.29}$$

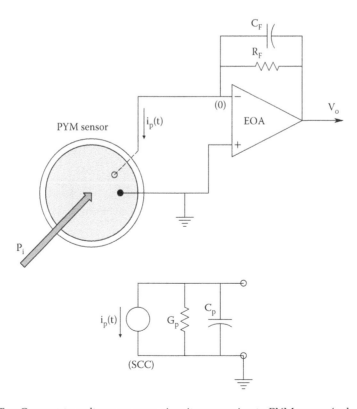

Figure 6.4 *Top*: Current-to-voltage op-amp circuit responsive to PYM sensor's short-circuit current, $i_p(t)$. *Bottom*: Equivalent circuit of PYM sensor alone. See Equations 6.22 and 6.23 for expressions of the sensor's SCC.

Such a BB reference source can be built into the transient radiation thermometer, or be an external BB source, such as the Mikron™ Model M340 BB radiation calibration source, the Omega BB701, BB702, BB703, BB704 Hot/Cold BB calibration sources, or the Isotech 976 Gemini R BB Source IR calibrators.

Another approach to self-calibration is to keep the PYM at a known T_a, then expose it to T_{cal} and measure the peak V_{ocal}, then expose it to T_b and measure V_{opk}. The computer subtracts V_{opk} from V_{ocal} to form ΔV_o:

$$\Delta V_o = \left(1/K_{sys}\right)\left[T_{cal}^4 - T_b^4\right]. \tag{6.30}$$

Solving for T_b:

$$T_b = \left[T_{cal}^4 - K_{sys}\Delta V_o\right]^{1/4}. \tag{6.31}$$

Thus, we see that the calculated T_b of the body relies on measurements of ΔV_o, $K_{sys,}$ and known T_{cal}.

To counteract measurement noise, a low-pass filter was added to the current-to-voltage conversion op-amp in Figure 6.4 by placing capacitor C_F in the feedback path. With C_F in place, the system response to a *step input* of IR radiative power, P_i, is:

$$V_o(s) = P_{io}\frac{K_pA/(C_FC_T)}{[s + 1/(C_FR_F)][s + 1/(C_T\Theta)]}. \tag{6.32}$$

The inverse Laplace transform of Equation 6.32 can be shown to be:

$$v_o(t) = \frac{P_{io}K_pAR_F\Theta}{(C_FR_F - C_T\Theta)}\left\{\exp\left[-t/(C_FR_F)\right] - \exp\left[-t/(C_T\Theta)\right]\right\}\text{volts}. \tag{6.33}$$

This is a positive waveform that rises with an initial time constant $C_T\Theta$, and falls more slowly with time constant, R_FC_F. Its peak is proportional to P_{io}. The measurement noise comes from: (1) Unwanted mechanical vibration of the PYM sensor which is piezoelectric; (2) electronic noise from the op-amp, and (3) thermal (Johnson) noise from the PYM's Norton conductance and from R_F. The $v_o(t)$ transient occurs when the shutter is opened, exposing the T_b BB is sampled and A/D converted. The thermometer's resident microcomputer finds the peak $v_o(t)$ and stores it in memory. Similarly, $v_o(t)$ resulting from the calibration source at T_{cal} is digitized and the peak is found and stored. The microcomputer can then use Equation 6.31 as described above to find T_b.

6.3.4 ThermoScan LIR Thermometers

The original, noncontact, LIR thermometer design using the transient method of exposing the PYM sensor to the BB surface whose temperature is being measured was patented by Fraden (1989a,b, 1993). A full product line of this type of thermometer is currently offered by Braun/ThermoScan, unit of the Gillette Co. of Boston, MA. Figure 6.5 illustrates schematically the basic design of a ThermoScan-type LIR thermometer. The shutter is electromechanical. Accelerating the mass of the shutter vane and stopping it when opening creates mechanical vibrations which are sensed by the piezoelectric PYM, producing an initial, artifact output voltage. However, these initial glitches in $v_o(t)$ are ignored by the resident microcomputer which is programmed to find the peak of the $V_o(t)$ transient, some hundred milliseconds after the shutter opens. The peak $v_o(t)$ is less than but proportional to V_{opk} given by Equation 6.27.

In one version of the thermometer, the shutter has three positions: closed, open to the eardrum at T_b, and open to a calibration source at T_{cal}.

Fraden (1993) showed how the dimensions of the eardrum and LIR thermometer earpiece and PYM sensor affect the BB radiation power from the eardrum absorbed by the PYM. An eardrum is a flat, oval structure with area A_b m^2, maintained at body core temperature, T_b. As a BB, it radiates a total IR power into a solid angle of 4π steradians given by

$$P_e = A_b\varepsilon_b\sigma(T_b^4 - T_a^4)W. \tag{6.34}$$

127

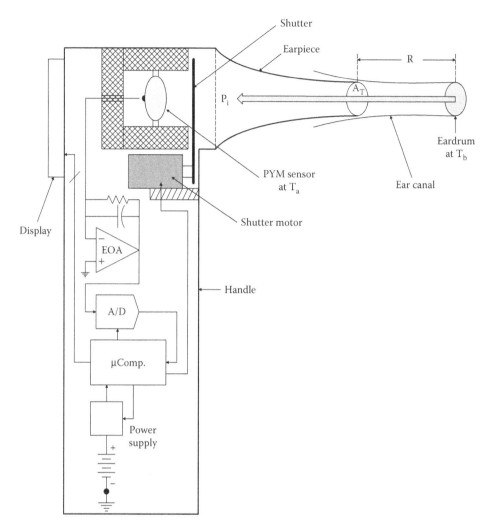

Figure 6.5 Simplified, cutaway schematic of a hand-held, pyroelectric ear thermometer such as that invented by Fraden (1989). See text.

Here, we assume the surrounding space has an absorptivity of 1, and the eardrum an emissivity of ε_b. Assume that the BB radiation from the eardrum is distributed uniformly on the surface of a (hypothetical) hemisphere of radius R. Thus, the irradiance on the surface of the hemisphere is:

$$H = A_b \varepsilon_b \sigma (T_b^4 - T_a^4) / (2\pi R^2) - W/m^2 \tag{6.35}$$

Assume that the end aperture of the otoscope-shaped thermometer probe is R meters from the eardrum. Its opening has an area of A_T m². Thus, the thermal power entering the probe is $P_p = A_T H$ Watts. As the internal surface of the probe is polished and highly reflective to LIR, we can assume that nearly all the LIR power entering the probe impinges on the PYM sensor. Thus, the power absorbed by the sensor is:

$$P_i \cong \varepsilon_s A_T H \ W \tag{6.36}$$

$\varepsilon_s = \alpha_s$ is the emissivity = absorptivity of the PYM sensor. Fraden (1993) made the assumptions that $(1 + T_b/T_a) \cong 2$ and $(1 + T_b^2/T_a^2) \cong 2$ to obtain the final approximation:

$$P_i \cong 2\varepsilon_b \varepsilon_s A_T A_b \sigma T_a^3 \Delta T / \pi R^2 \ W, \tag{6.37}$$

where $\Delta T = (T_b - T_a)$. It takes about 8 s for the PYM sensor in the ThermoScan Model EZ HM3 LIR thermometer to return to T_a and be ready for the next measurement.

Not all of the Braun/ThermoScan LIR thermometers use pyroelectric LIR radiation sensors; however, the Models PRO 3000 and IRT 3520 use *thermopile sensors* (thermopiles are many dc thermocouples in series) that take 8 readings in 1 s and display the highest reading. They are ready for the next reading in 2 s.

The PVDF PYM sensors offer the advantages of being less expensive than thermopiles, they can have large detector areas, are robust mechanically, and are insensitive to moisture. The pyro-electric constant of PVDF is about one-tenth of other crystalline PYMs, but for most applications, this is not a problem, certainly not for ear LIR thermometers. Some ear LIR thermometers use polyethylene Fresnel lenses to concentrate the input LIR radiation on the sensor.

6.3.5 Discussion

We have seen that LIR radiation thermometers are complex devices based on a simple principle, that is, infrared BB radiation from the hotter eardrum causes a net heat flux to the cooler pyroelectric sensor, which warms slightly. When the sensor warms, a current is generated in proportion to the difference of the two surface temperatures raised to the 4th power. The chief advantage of the LIR radiation thermometer is that it is fast, accurate, and has a digital readout. It certainly is more expensive than a simple glass/mercury fever thermometer, but carries no risk to the patient as does a conventional thermometer if it breaks (broken glass and metallic mercury).

6.4 CHAPTER SUMMARY

Body temperature measurements are really concerned with the core temperature. Body temperature is important in diagnosing fever from infection or heatstroke, or hypothermia from immersion in water. It is also useful in predicting the time of ovulation.

Traditionally, core temperature is approximated by use of a glass fever thermometer inserted in the mouth under the tongue, or in the anus. Only in the past 10 years has a no-touch radiation thermometer been developed to the point of clinical acceptance. The ThermoScan series of instruments were described in Section 6.3. They measure the LIR BB radiation from the eardrum, which is richly supplied with arterial blood at core temperature. A ThermoScan instrument's probe (like an otoscope cone) is inserted into the ear canal. Otherwise, there is no contact with the body. Response time of a ThermoScan LIR thermometer is in seconds, versus minutes for a glass/mercury fever thermometer. There is little chance for error in reading an LIR thermometer because of its digital readout, and no hazard from mercury or broken glass if a thermometer's tip breaks.

Thermistors and platinum RTD elements are also used to measure body temperature. These devices require intimate body contact like the glass/mercury thermometers, but are faster than glass thermometers and slower than LIR radiation thermometers in their response. They, too, have digital readouts. Resistance thermometers are generally less expensive than LIR radiation thermometers (simpler electronics).

.

7 Noninvasive Blood Gas Sensing with Electrodes

7.1 INTRODUCTION

The metabolism of all living cells in the body requires oxygen and an energy substrate, generally glucose. As the result of oxidative metabolism, heat and CO_2 are produced as well as regulated molecular by-products, and O_2 in the blood is consumed. The lungs are the organs in which the external atmosphere interfaces with the body's blood supply; O_2 is taken in and CO_2 is exhaled. The partial pressure of oxygen (pO_2) in an alveolus is typically 104 mmHg. Venous blood entering a capillary in the alveolus' wall has a pO_2 of ~40 mmHg. Thus, an initial pressure gradient of $104 - 40 = 64$ mmHg causes O_2 gas to diffuse into the capillary and be combined with hemoglobin in red blood cells (RBCs) and also be dissolved in the water in the blood. The blood exiting the capillary contains ~104 mmHg pO_2. All the oxygenated alveolar blood mixes with venous blood from the nonoxygenating tissues of the lungs, bringing the pO_2 down to about 95 mmHg. This is the pO_2 of arterial blood pumped to the body from the heart's left ventricle.

In the peripheral, systemic capillaries, oxygen diffuses into the interstitial fluid which has a pO_2 of ~40 mmHg. Thus, venous blood returned to the heart and lungs has a pO_2 of ~40 mmHg. The average pO_2 in the systemic capillaries is about 70 mmHg (blood enters with a pO_2 of 95 and exits with 40 mmHg).

Normally, about 97% of the O_2 carried in arterial blood is combined with hemoglobin molecules inside RBCs (erythrocytes), and the remainder of the O_2 is dissolved in the plasma. In terms of partial pressures, ~92.2 mmHg is carried as oxyhemoglobin (HbO), and ~2.8 mmHg O_2 is carried dissolved in arterial blood. The venous blood sent to the lungs under resting (basal metabolic) conditions has about 75% HbO, and a pO_2 of 40 mmHg. Under conditions of intense exercise, the venous HbO can drop to as low as 19% saturation; the interstitial fluid (and venous) pO_2 drops to ~15 mmHg (Guyton 1991, Chapter 40).

Any disease or condition that interferes with the normal exchange of gases in the alveoli, the transport of O_2 to the systemic capillaries, the return of CO_2 to the lungs, and the exchange of O_2 and CO_2 in the systemic microcirculation will give rise to life-threatening hypoxia and/or acidosis. In Section 7.2, we describe NI chemical means of monitoring pO_2 in the body. (Note that in Section 15.8, we cover *Pulse Oximetry*, an NI, optical technique of measuring the percent O_2 saturation (sO_2) of hemoglobin in the peripheral circulation.)

Also considered in this chapter is the NI, transcutaneous measurement of pCO_2 in the peripheral blood, $tcpCO_2$. *High* blood $tcpCO_2$ is a sign of metabolic acidosis, which can have several causes, including damaged alveoli in the lungs. (Damaged alveoli will also give *low* $tcpO_2$ readings.) Normal blood pH is ~7.4. If the pH decreases for any reason, the rate of breathing increases automatically to exhale CO_2 at a greater rate, and the kidneys also compensate for elevated acidity in the extracellular fluid by actively excreting hydrogen ions at an increased rate. Thus another cause of high pCO_2 can be kidney failure, in which the tubular epithelial cells actively transport H^+ ions from their interiors into the collecting tubes for excretion in urine at a reduced rate. Low blood flow to the kidneys, or damaged tubular cells can decrease this normal mechanism for blood pH regulation. High pCO_2 can occur normally in exercise, but it drops in minutes due to increased breathing effort and H^+ elimination by the kidneys. Acidosis can also result from gluconeogenesis in diabetes mellitus. Here, low-intracellular glucose concentration causes liver cells to break down fatty acids to acetoacetic acid and acetyl-Co-A. Acetyl-Co-A is used as an energy source, and acetoacetic acid enters the blood, causing the pH to fall. Even though CO_2 is not involved directly, the lower pH causes the ratio of pCO_2 to $[HCO_3^-]$ to increase. Loss of intestinal bicarbonate in severe diarrhea can also cause acidosis, and an elevated pCO_2 to $[HCO_3^-]$ ratio (Guyton 1991, Chapter 30).

7.2 TRANSCUTANEOUS O_2 SENSING

7.2.1 Introduction: The Clark Electrode

There are several accurate means of measuring the pO_2 of blood, *given direct contact* with a blood sample. For a description of these invasive instrumental methods of measuring pO_2, see Webster (1992). In this text, however, we are devoted to examining NI medical instruments, and there is presently only one, effective means of transcutaneously measuring peripheral tissue blood pO_2. This system is based on the electrochemical *Clark electrode*, first described in 1956 (Tremper 1984, Tremper and Barker 1987, Hahn 1998).

The basic Clark electrode can measure pO_2 in gases or liquids. It is an electrochemical, polarographic system in which a fixed potential is maintained across the electrodes, and a DC current flows which is proportional to the concentration of the rate-limiting reagent, O_2, which participates

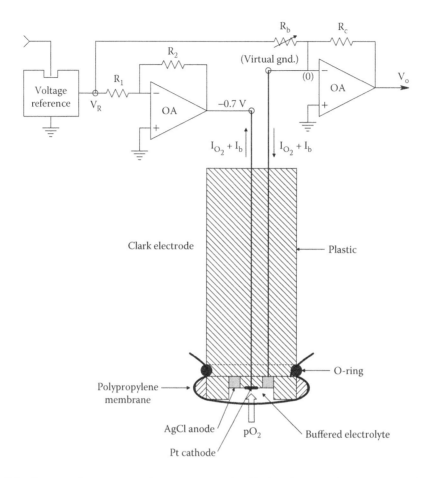

Figure 7.1 Support electronics and cross section of a Clark polarographic O_2 sensor. The left-hand op-amp and DC reference source supply the 0.7 Vdc bias voltage for the cell. The right-hand op-amp acts as a current-to-voltage converter. R_b sets a DC current I_b to cancel out the zero-oxygen current of the Clark cell.

in oxidation/reduction reactions which take place at the electrode surfaces (N.B., oxidation (electron loss) takes place at the anode; reduction (electron gain) occurs at the cathode). A plastic membrane, porous to O_2, separates the *sample compartment* with the *reaction compartment* (around the electrodes). The reaction compartment is filled with an aqueous buffer solution (at about pH 7), containing chloride ions (which can be from KCl). The O_2 that reacts at the electrode surfaces must diffuse in through the membrane from the sample compartment. Figure 7.1 illustrates a cross section through a basic Clark cell. The anode (+ electrode) is an AgCl-coated Ag ring or "washer"; the cathode (− electrode) is the small, exposed tip (12–25 μm diameter) of an insulated platinum wire. The membrane is typically 25 μm polyethylene or polypropylene. The chemical reactions which occur at the Pt cathode are reductions (Hahn 1998):

$$O_2 + H_2O + 2e^- \rightarrow HO_2^- + OH^- \tag{7.1}$$

$$HO_2^- + H_2O + 2e^- \rightarrow 3OH^- \tag{7.2}$$

$$HO_2^- \xrightarrow{\text{catalytic decomposition}} \frac{1}{2}O_2 + OH^-, \tag{7.3}$$

or, as a net reaction:

$$O_2 + 2H_2O + 4e^- \xrightarrow{\text{direct}} 4OH^-. \tag{7.4}$$

The OH$^-$ ions are buffered to maintain neutral pH, and the chloride ions carry charge to the AgCl anode. Four electrons flow for every diatomic oxygen molecule reacted; the Clark cell current at a given temperature is given by

$$I_C = I_b + K_C pO_2. \tag{7.5}$$

By U.S. convention, in metal wires, current flows in the opposite direction to electrons. The Clark cell is generally operated at a fixed potential of 0.7 V; its current is linearly proportional to the pO_2 in the measurement compartment. A small DC, *background current*, I_b, flows at $pO_2 = 0$, this is due to ion drift in the electric field between the electrodes. The current versus pO_2 graph taken with $V_{cell} = 0.70$ V and pH 6.8 is essentially linear, enabling a two-point calibration of a Clark O_2 electrode (at $pO_2 = 0$ and $pO_2 = 160$ mmHg [atmospheric]). The left op-amp in Figure 7.1 acts as a 0.70 V voltage source; the right op-amp is a low-DC drift, FET-input type with very low bias current (I_B) that is used as a current-to-voltage converter (transimpedance). Its output, after subtracting the background current, I_b, is $V_o = K_C pO_2$. The normal temperature coefficient (tempco) of a Clark cell is 2% per °C, and the linearity is better than 1% over the physiological pO_2 range (Hahn 1998).

The response time of a Clark cell to a step change in measured pO_2 is largely governed by the thickness of the membrane, but also depends on O_2 and ion diffusion times in the electrolyte. Typical Clark cell response time (time to reach 1/2 the steady-state value) is on the order of 10 s of seconds. For a theoretical treatment of Clark cell response dynamics, see Hahn (1998). Owing to the low-pass characteristic of the Clark cell's response, it responds to a smoothed, or time-averaged $pO_2(t)$.

7.2.2 Transcutaneous [O_2] (tcpO_2) Sensor

The transcutaneous [O_2] (tcpO_2) sensor uses a Clark cell which is internally heated and temperature-regulated to operate at a temperature of 40–45°C, $\pm$ 0.1° when on the skin. The elevated temperature of the Clark cell membrane is necessary to cause vasodilation and reddening of the skin under the sensor. A thin layer of an aqueous, isotonic contact gel is placed between the skin and the heated sensor's membrane in order to facilitate outward diffusion of O_2 from the skin through the membrane. The sensor has built-in thermistors to monitor the Clark cell's electrolyte temperature and the skin temperature under the membrane. The thermistor outputs are used to control the power supplied to a heater coil surrounding the cell.

Initially, transcutaneous operation of the heated Clark cell was found to be effective in babies and small children because of their thinner skin. Unfortunately, because of the delicate skin of infants, prolonged application of a heated sensor can cause second-degree (blister) burns, unless the sensor is moved every hour or so. There is a time × temperature product which must be observed to avoid skin damage. The heated Clark sensor must be given a two-point calibration at its chosen operating temperature before use.

Heated, transcutaneous pO_2 sensor systems (the TCM instrument series) are made by Radiometer Copenhagen, and sold worldwide. They are used for such applications as monitoring neonatal pO_2 to sense apnea, respiratory distress, etc. They are now also used in adults for applications in hyperbaric medicine, vascular surgery, wound care, and in reconstructive plastic surgery to monitor angiogenesis.

7.3 TRANSCUTANEOUS CO$_2$ SENSING

7.3.1 Introduction: The Stow–Severinghaus Electrode

The basis for transcutaneous pCO_2 sensing is the Stow–Severinghaus (S–S) electrode, developed in 1957–1958 (Hahn 1998). At the heart, literally, of an S–S electrode is the glass pH electrode half-cell, as shown in Figure 7.2. The half-cell EMF of the glass pH electrode is really two half-cell potentials in series: An EMF is developed across the special tip glass envelope that is proportional to the pH, and the EMF of the internal, AgCl coupling electrode immersed in the 0.1 N HCl internal filling solution. In general:

$$E_{GL} = E_{GL}^0 + (2.3026 \, RT/F)[pH], \tag{7.6}$$

where pH is defined as pH $\equiv -\log_{10}(a_{H+}) \cong -\log_{10}([H^+])$, R is the SI gas constant = 8.3147 J/(mole K), T is the kelvin temperature, F is the Faraday number = 96,496, and 2.3026 comes from converting natural logs to $\log_{10}$. At 25°C, (2.3026 RT/F) = 0.059156 V.

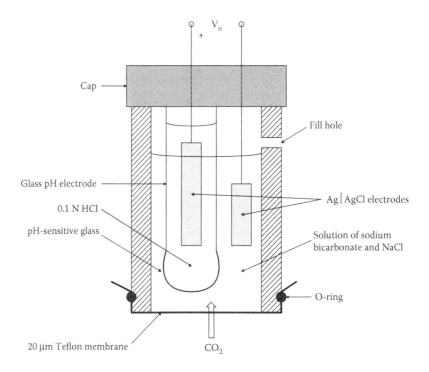

Figure 7.2 Cross section of a Stow–Severinghaus electrode used to sense pCO_2. A glass pH electrode responds to the pH of the inner solution, which is shown to be a function of $\log_{10}(pCO_2)$ in Equation 7.14.

Interestingly, the pH of the 5–20 mM bicarbonate solution surrounding the glass pH electrode is proportional to the negative logarithm of the partial pressure of the CO_2 in the external solution over the range of 10–90 mmHg (Webster 1992, Chapter 10). First, CO_2 must diffuse from the external test solution into the bicarbonate solution through the thin Teflon membrane, where the following equilibria occur:

$$CO_2 + H_2O \Longleftrightarrow H_2CO_3 \Longleftrightarrow H^+ + HCO_3^- \tag{7.7}$$

$$HCO_3^- \Longleftrightarrow H^+ + CO_3^= \tag{7.8}$$

$$NaHCO_3 \Longleftrightarrow Na^+ + HCO_3^-. \tag{7.9}$$

Adding the equations, we find:

$$CO_2 + \overset{XS}{H_2O} + \overset{Solid}{NaHCO_3} \Longleftrightarrow 2H^+ + CO_3^= + HCO_3^- + \overset{Constant}{N_a^+}. \tag{7.10}$$

Note that a constant, a, relating the equivalent concentration of CO_2 gas dissolved in blood to the partial pressure is found from:

$$a = \frac{[CO_2]}{pCO_2}. \tag{7.11}$$

a for blood is $\sim$0.03 (mmol/L)/mmHg pCO_2. At chemical equilibrium, we have:

$$K\{a(pCO_2)\} = [H^+]^2[CO_3^=][HCO_3^-][Na^+]. \tag{7.12}$$

K is the equilibrium constant for reaction 7.10. Also, from Equation 7.8 at equilibrium:

$$K' = \frac{[H^+][CO_3^=]}{[HCO_3^-]} \rightarrow [CO_3^=] = K'\frac{[HCO_3^-]}{[H^+]}. \tag{7.13}$$

Substituting Equation 7.13 into Equation 7.12, we can write:

$$Ka(pCO_2) = [H^+][HCO_3^-]^2[Na^+]K'. \tag{7.14}$$

Taking the logarithm$_{10}$ of terms in Equation 7.14, and noting that pH is defined by pH $\equiv -\log_{10}[H^+]$,

$$\log(Ka) + \log(pCO_2) = -pH + 2\log[HCO_3^-] + \log[Na^+] + \log(K') \tag{7.15}$$

or

$$pH = -\log(pCO_2) - \log(Ka/K') + 2\log[HCO_3^-] + \log[Na^+], \tag{7.16}$$

which is of the form

$$pH = -\log(pCO_2) + A, \tag{7.17}$$

because Ka/K', $[HCO_3^-]$ and $[Na^+]$ are constant. Thus a Stow–Severinghaus pCO$_2$ meter computes the pCO$_2$ by exponentiating (pH − A), sic:

$$pCO_2 = B10^{[-k(pH-A)]}. \tag{7.18}$$

The constants B and k are for display scaling.

Needless to say, the pH electrode and the chemical dissociation reactions involved are all temperature-sensitive. Hence, any application of the Stow–Severinghaus pCO$_2$ sensor *in vivo, in vitro* (with blood), or transcutaneously requires precise temperature regulation in order to maintain calibration.

7.3.2 Transcutaneous tcpCO$_2$ Sensing

The tcpCO$_2$ sensor can be combined with a tcpO$_2$ sensor in the same housing. Such units are described by Hahn (1998) and Webster (1992). Radiometer America (2011, 2012) offers their model TCM™ 4/40, combined tcpCO$_2$- and tcpO$_2$-monitoring systems. The combined sensors can use the same 0.1 N bicarbonate buffer used in the Stow–Severinghaus pCO$_2$ sensor with the addition of NaCl for the Clark cell electrolyte. Figure 7.3 illustrates the author's version of a combined tcpO$_2$ + tcpCO$_2$ sensor. Note that it uses a common electrolyte and membrane. The entire cell is heated and thermostatically regulated (not shown in figure). The elevated (~44°C) temperature causes vasodilation under the sensor and increases upward diffusion of O$_2$ and CO$_2$ through the *stratum corneum* of the skin to the sensor's membrane. The electrometer amplifier used to amplify the pH electrode voltage has an ultralow bias current (in 10 s of fA), and superhigh input resistance (~10^{14} Ω). Thus its bias current will be ~10^{-14} A, which is negligible compared with the 10^{-8} A Clark cell current. OA2 thus can serve as a virtual ground for both the Clark cell and the Severinghaus electrode; its voltage output depends only on the Clark cell current.

7.4 CHAPTER SUMMARY

There are several reliable chemical gas sensors that work well when immersed in blood, *in vitro* or *in vivo*, but only two, as we have seen above, have been adapted to reliable, approved, NI, percutaneous operation.

A wide variety of other sensors work well to sense pO$_2$ and pCO$_2$ in the gas phase. O$_2$ has been sensed by using the fact that it is weakly paramagnetic, that is, O$_2$ gas molecules are attracted by a magnetic field, and thus can be separated from the N$_2$, Ar, and CO$_2$ in air. Oxygen's paramagnetic susceptibility is the basis for several commercial gaseous oxygen meters. Manufacturers and/or vendors of O$_2$ gas sensors include, but are not limited to (Moseley et al. 1991): ABB Measurement & Analytics (EL3000, Magnos 17/106), International Society of Automation (ISA), Rosemount Analytical (X2FD), Siemens Analytical Products and Solutions (the Oxymat 6), Teledyne Instruments (UFO-130-2), Sable Instruments International (PA-10), PASCO (PASPORT PS-2126A O$_2$ gas sensor), Mettler-Toledo (GPro 500), Emerson Process Management (ST3 Series O$_2$ gas sensor), MSA Gas sensors, Servomex paramagnetic O$_2$ analyzers (Model 570A, Pm1111E), and tunable diode laser O$_2$ analyzer.

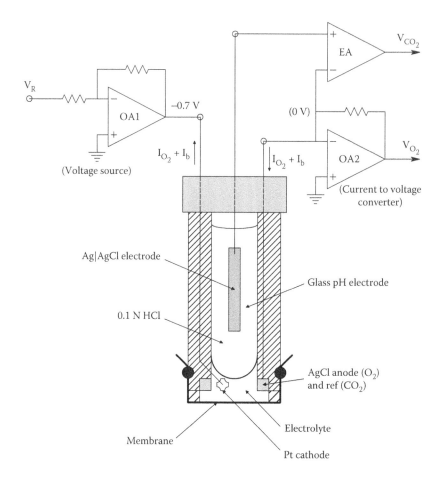

Figure 7.3 Proposed, combined pO_2 and pCO_2 electrode. OA2 outputs a voltage proportional to pO_2, and the electrometer amplifier outputs a voltage $V_{CO_2} \propto -\log_{10}(pCO_2) + A$.

O_2 can also can be used as the rate-limiting reactant in a fuel cell so output voltage is proportional to pO_2, or in a polarographic chemical reaction (e.g., the Clark cell). The speed of sound in O_2 at a given pressure and temperature is different from other gases, and this property has been used to sense the pO_2 in air (Hong and Northrop 1991). The fact that O_2 gas absorbs light at 760 nm is the basis for another, optical, pO_2 sensor using the airpath absorption of light at 760 nm and at another wavelength where O_2 does not absorb, and Beer's law. See the review paper on methods of O_2 sensing by Langridge (2010).

A major means of sensing atmospheric (and respiratory gas) pCO_2 makes use of the IR absorption of the CO_2 gas molecule. Again, two wavelengths are used, one where CO_2 absorbs (e.g., at 4.2 μm) and the other where it does not (e.g., at 3.5 μm). Water vapor interferes in some CO_2 IR absorption bands, so CO_2 sensing in respiratory gases requires the gas input to the IR cell to be dried; the drying can be done chemically, or by heating the gas.

Fiber optic (FO) optical sensors have been used to sense pH through the use of a pH-sensitive indicator dye, such as phenol red bound to the surface of 5–10 μm diameter polyacrylamide microspheres mixed with 1 μm diameter polystyrene microspheres for light scattering. The dye and microspheres are enclosed in a small plastic tube permeable only to H^+ ions. One end of the microtube is sealed; the other is joined to two optical fibers (input and output). Phenol red in aqueous solution has an isobestic wavelength at ~480 nm (the wavelength where reflectance is independent of pH). The wavelength at which maximum change in reflectance versus pH occurs is ~560 nm. By using these two wavelengths to illuminate the indicator dye and computing the difference in reflected intensities over their sum, pH from 6.1 to 7.6 can be measured (Wolfbeis 1991). This type of sensor is called an *optrode*. Note that if this sensor is surrounded by a bicarbonate solution that is separated from the skin by a CO_2-permeable membrane, this pH sensor should be able to be used to measure tcpCO$_2$. Other indicator dyes have also been used in similar pH optrode sensors. These include but are not limited to: sulfo-phenolphthalein, bromothymol blue, and bromophenol blue (Wolfbeis 1991).

Another optrode strategy to measure pH (and possibly pCO$_2$) makes use of light-induced fluorescence which is pH-sensitive. In one system, immobilized *8-hydroxy-1,3,6-pyrenetri-sulfonate* (HPTS) is excited by pulses of 455 nm light. The fluorescence response at 520 nm becomes stronger as the pH goes from 5 to 8. HPTS also has a fluorescence isobestic excitation wavelength at 435 nm. The response here is also at 520 nm, but its intensity does not change with pH. The 99% response time of the HPTS sensor was about 1.7 min (to a step change of pH; $6 \rightarrow 8 \rightarrow 6$, etc.), and its accuracy was ~ $\pm$ 0.1 pH unit. Other fluorescent pH indicators have also been used: *aminofluorescein* and *7-hydroxycoumarin-3-carboxylic acid* (HCC) (Wolfbeis 1991). Again, a H$^+$ permeable membrane serves to isolate the immobilized, fluorescent chemical. This type of sensor, too, has the potential for measuring tcpCO$_2$.

It is possible that certain solid-state pH sensors can be adapted to tcpCO$_2$ operation. It is known that silicon oxynitride is pH-sensitive over a large pH range when used as a coating for the gate of a chemically sensitive field-effect transistor (CHEMFET) (Kelly and Owen 1991). A heated membrane would still be required over the skin, but the analyte gas would diffuse into a low-volume, bicarbonate solution-filled, measurement compartment in which the coated gate of the CHEMFET was in contact.

8 Tests on Naturally Voided Body Fluids

8.1 INTRODUCTION

Naturally voided body fluids obtained noninvasively include urine, saliva, sweat, pus draining from wounds, serum draining from burns, and, for purposes of continuity, feces (arguably not normally a fluid except in the stomach and part of the small intestine). The chemical composition of these substances provides important information which can be used in the diagnosis of infections, cancer, hormonal diseases (e.g., diabetes mellitus, thyroid diseases, diseases of the adrenal glands, gastrointestinal disorders, liver cirrhosis, pathogens, etc.). Much diagnostic information can also be obtained from the blood, but unless it is obtained from a hemorrhaging wound, its collection is certainly invasive or semi-invasive, and therefore its consideration in this chapter is proscribed.

In Section 8.2, we will describe various instrumental means used in laboratory medicine to measure the concentrations of physiologically important ions used in medical diagnosis. These include, but are not limited to: Li^+, Na^+, K^+, Mg^{++}, Zn^{++}, Fe^{++}, Fe^{3+}, Cu^{++}, Hg^{++}, Ca^{++}, Mo^{++}, Cr^{3+}, Mn^{++}, Se^{6+}, $CO_3^=$, HCO_3^-, Cl^-, I^-, $SO_4^=$, phosphates, etc. In addition, in the diagnostic process, it is often required to sense molecules such as glucose, urea, specific antibodies (Abs), certain steroid hormones, various peptide hormones, enzymes, bilirubin, bile, occult blood (from internal bleeding), certain drugs (or their metabolites) used in therapy (e.g., methotrexate, used in cancer chemotherapy, and theophylline used to treat asthma), and drugs used in substance abuse. Specific bacteria can also be sensed by *in vitro* Ab tests, or by surface plasmon resonance (SPR) Ab reactions (Section 8.2.4).

Most tests for disorders of blood electrolytes also have counterparts in the NI measurement of ions in the urine, and urine flow rate. The kidneys, the loops of Henle, and the collecting ducts serve as hormonally controlled regulators for blood volume and blood osmotic pressure (blood sodium ion concentration [Na^+]), blood potassium ion concentration [K^+], blood calcium ion concentration [Ca^{++}], and blood glucose [BG]. Thus, the urine volume and its ionic concentrations reflect the competence of the selective filtering actions of the kidneys. In Section 8.3, we describe necessary (but not sufficient) diagnostic signs based on measurement of urine electrolytes, glucose, proteins, enzymes, etc. Analysis of the feces, described in Section 8.4, aids the diagnosis of GI bleeding, endoparasites, gall stones, etc. Section 8.5 deals with what can be learned from the ionic concentration of saliva, and finally, in Section 8.6, we consider analysis of gases in the breath to detect diseases such as diabetes mellitus, lung infections (lung cancer?), throat infections, sinus infections, gum disease (gingivitis), stomach ulcers, etc. Most breath analysis is still by the physician's nose, but modern analytical techniques such as SPR and gas chromatography (GC) can provide more objective measurements and diagnoses.

8.2 INSTRUMENTAL METHODS

8.2.1 Introduction

In this section, we will describe some of the analytical instruments used in laboratory medicine to measure the concentration of physiologically important ions in body fluids, as well as small and large molecular weight proteins and other molecules (enzymes, hormones, Abs, bilirubin, urobilinogen, stercobilins, etc.), as well as bacteria and viruses. Some of the instruments used are exquisitely sensitive and correspondingly expensive (spectrophotometers, GCs, mass spectrometers [MS]), others are amazingly simple (e.g., specific ion electrodes, flame photometry, SPR) and can be adapted for field use.

We begin the description of instrumental methods used in medical laboratory analysis with consideration of dispersive spectroscopy, in which the substance being measured (the analyte) absorbs, reflects, or transmits light at different wavelengths with a characteristic signature.

8.2.2 Dispersive Spectrophotometry

A *dispersive spectrophotometer* has a *monochromator*, which is an optical system that acts as a narrow-band-pass filter for a broadband, input light source. A monochromator can be made from a prism, or one or two diffraction gratings. The output of a monochromator is a beam of nearly monochromatic light. In an analogy to a tuned, RLC electrical circuit, the "Q" of a monochromator can be defined as the ratio of the wavelength at its peak intensity to the wavelength difference defining the points where its intensity is one-half the peak. For example, a certain grating monochromator may produce an output beam centered at 600 nm, with a 6 nm half-power width, giving it an optical "Q" = 100.

At the heart of *dispersive spectrophotometry* is the interesting property that molecules in solution (or in the solid or gas states) absorb transmitted light more at certain wavelengths than at others. This phenomenon is the basis for spectrographic quantification of many important biological molecules found in blood, serum, urine, saliva, breath, etc. Dispersive spectrophotometry is used to detect the presence of particular molecules and ions, and also to estimate their concentrations. At the heart of spectrophotometry is the fact that molecules have a total energy that is the sum of several components:

$$E_{tot} = E_{translational} + E_{electronic} + E_{rotational} + E_{vibrational} + E_{other}. \tag{8.1}$$

When light at a particular wavelength is passed through a solution of an analyte, the energy from a photon can be absorbed to increase the energy of a molecule in one of its several components. Which component is increased depends on the frequency of the light, ν, in Hz. In general, the energy increase of the molecule is given by

$$\Delta E = h\nu \text{ J}, \tag{8.2}$$

where h is Planck's constant: 6.624×10^{-34} J s.

Note that the light wavelength is $\lambda \equiv c/\nu$ meters. In the visible region, λ is usually given in nanometers (nm), while in the infrared (IR), its dimensions are customarily in micrometers (μm). Often molecular transmittance and absorbance spectra are plotted versus *wave number*, $\xi = \lambda^{-1}$, instead of wavelength. In the IR region, the wave number is related to the wavelength by

$$\text{Wave number in cm}^{-1} = 10^4 / (\lambda \text{ in } \mu\text{m}) = 1 / (\lambda \text{ in cm}). \tag{8.3}$$

Table 8.1 below illustrates the ranges of wavelength over which certain forms of photon absorption occur by molecules, and the energy absorption mechanism.

The energy absorbed from photons by molecules can be reradiated as radio waves, heat (IR), or photons (fluorescence). This reradiation also provides a molecular signature; however, our concern here is in the details of photon absorption.

Most photon absorption by molecules follows the *Beer–Lambert law*, or simply, *Beer's law*. Lambert observed that each unit length of an analyte through which monochromatic light passes absorbs the same fraction of the entering light power (or intensity). Beer extended Lambert's observation to solutions of an analyte at concentration, C. Stated mathematically, this is:

$$dI = -kCI \, dL. \tag{8.4}$$

Rearranging terms, we can write:

$$\frac{dI}{I} = -kC \, dL. \tag{8.5}$$

Integrating, we find:

$$\int_{I_{in}}^{I_{out}} (dI/I) = -kC \int_0^L dL. \tag{8.6}$$

$$\downarrow$$

$$\ln(I_{out}/I_{in}) = -kCL \quad \text{or} \quad \log_{10}(I_{out}/I_{in}) = -(k/2.303)CL. \tag{8.7}$$

In describing spectrophotometric spectra, various measures are used: The *transmittance* is defined as $T \equiv I_{out}/I_{in} = 10^{-kCL/(2.303)} = \exp(-kCL)$. T ranges from 0 to 1. Often the *percent transmittance* is used; $\%T \equiv 100$ T. The *absorbance* is defined as $A \equiv \log_{10}(I_{in}/I_{out}) = -\log_{10}(T) = \varepsilon CL$, where L is the total optical path length through the solution, C is the molar concentration of the analyte, and $\varepsilon = (k/2.303)$ is the *molar extinction coefficient* for the solution. What makes spectrophotometry possible is the fact that ε is a function of λ; it is dependent on atomic bond resonances which are peculiar to the structure of each species of analyte molecule. A is also called the *optical density* (OD); it also can be written as: $A = 2 - \log_{10}(\%T)$.

Table 8.1: Wavelength and Energy Levels in Spectrophotometric Absorption

λ Range	100–10 cm	10–1 cm	1–0.1 cm	100–10 μm	10–1 μm	10^3–100 nm	100–10 nm	10–1 nm	1–0.1 nm	<0.1 nm
Type of radiation	Radio	μ wave	μwv, FIR	Mid-IR	Near-IR	Visible/UV	Vacuum UV	Vac UV/x-rays	X-rays	γ-Rays
Energy transition	Spin orientation	Molec. rotations	Molec. rotations	Molec. vibrations	Molec. vibrations	Valence electron xitions	Valence electron xitions	Inner-shell e^- xitions	Inner-shell e^- xitions	Nuclear xitions
Photon energy range	1.987 E-25–E-24 J	1.987 E-24–E-23 J	1.987 E-23–E-22 J	1.987 E-22–E-21 J	1.987 E-21–E-20 J	1.987 E-20–E-19 J	1.987 E-19–E-18 J	1.987 E-18–E-17 J	1.987 E-17–E-16 J	>1.987 E-16 J
Frequency range	0.3–3 GHz	3–30 GHz	30–300 GHz	3–30×10^{12} Hz	30–300×10^{12} Hz	0.3–3×10^{15} Hz	3–30×10^{15} Hz	30–300×10^{15} Hz	0.3–3×10^{18} Hz	$>3 \times 10^{18}$ Hz

Source: After Reilley, C.N. and D.T. Sawyer. 1961. *Experiments for Instrumental Methods*. McGraw-Hill, NY.

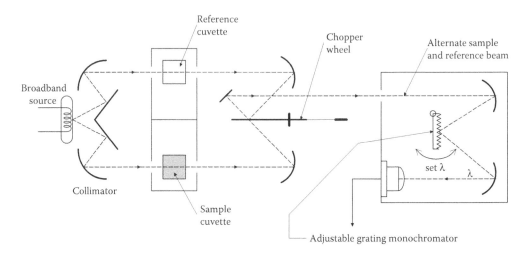

Figure 8.1 Schematic top view of a dual-beam spectrophotometer. In this design, the light first passes through the sample and reference cuvettes, then is chopped and dispersed by a single adjustable grating and passed to a photosensor.

A general purpose spectrophotometer used for chemical analysis uses a monochromator to generate nearly monochromatic light over a wide range of wavelengths. Early monochromators used a glass prism to break white light into its spectral components, and selected the output band with an exit slit. Now one or two *diffraction gratings* are used to disperse the input source light into its spectral components. The desired narrow range of wavelengths is selected by adjusting the grating angle with respect to the input beam of white light, and passing the input and output beams through narrow slits. By adjusting the grating angle and the slits, the spectrum can be scanned from ultraviolet (UV) through the far infrared (FIR). Special gratings, glasses, and mirror surfaces must be used in monochromators used for (FIR), mid-infrared (MIR), and UV (A,B,C). As we have discussed above, the quantum physical mechanisms of photon energy absorption by molecules in the UV, visible, and IR ranges are different. Thus, depending on the application, different types of spectrophotometers are used. These are generally subdivided into instruments that cover the near infrared (NIR) to FIR wavelengths, and instruments that cover the visible spectrum and UV. Figure 8.1 shows the architecture of a dual-beam, IR spectrophotometer. Note that beam forming is done with gold-plated, front-surface mirrors rather than expensive IR lenses. The power from the broadband IR source is divided equally and passed through a reference cuvette, and a sample cuvette containing the analyte(s). Emerging power is next chopped by a chopper wheel having alternate mirror, window, and absorbing segments. The chopped IR is then passed through a monochromator that scans through the desired range of wavelengths. The single photosensor thus receives alternating pulses of light, first from the reference path, then from the sample, and finally a "dark" pulse. The spectrophotometer's electronics stores and averages each like series of pulses and uses this information to compute %T (or A) versus λ (or wave number). An alternate configuration of the dual-beam instrument places the monochromator directly in front of the broadband photon source; two matched photosensors are used. The performance is the same, however. Note that the dual-beam architecture is used for IR, as well as visible/UV applications.

Figure 8.2 illustrates a simple, *single-beam spectrophotometer* designed to be used with visible light/near UV. Often such simple instruments are used to measure a single analyte using only two wavelengths, rather than examine the whole transmission or absorption spectrum. One wavelength, λ_i, is chosen to be at the *isobestic point* where the transmission of the sample is the same regardless of the presence of the analyte, and a second wavelength is chosen where the analyte has a strong absorption peak given by Beer's law.

A third and very important category of spectrophotometer is the *Fourier transform infrared* (FTIR) *System*. As shown in Figure 8.3, a blackbody IR source such as a Globar rod is used to generate a continuous, broadband, IR spectrum given by Planck's radiation law. Collimated radiation from this source is the input to a time-modulated *Michelson interferometer*. The interferometer's mirror is periodically displaced by an amount, δ(t), around a center position, L_2. To understand what

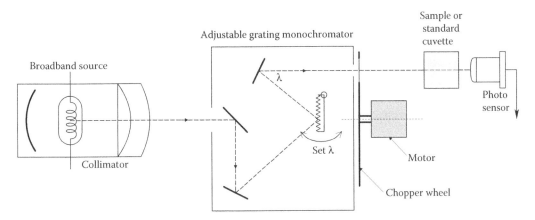

Figure 8.2 Schematic plan view of a single-beam spectrophotometer. In this design, the light is dispersed then chopped before passing alternately through the sample or a reference cuvette.

happens at the interferometer's output, we need to first consider what happens to a *monochromatic input ray* with wavelength λ_1. Assume that the distances L_1 and L_2 are chosen such that there is maximum *constructive interference* at the interferometer output. Thus, neglecting interfacial losses, the output intensity, I_o, equals the input intensity, I_{in}. Now let the mirror move $\delta = \lambda/4$ away from the beam splitter. The light must now travel a total distance of $\lambda/2$ μm more to return to the beam splitter where there is now *destructive interference* and the output intensity has a null. This extra length the light must travel is called the *retardation distance*, ρ. In general, $\rho = 2\delta$. We can write an empirical expression for the output intensity as a function of the wave retardation, ρ, around L_2:

$$I_o(\rho, \lambda_1) = I_{in}\left(\frac{1}{2}\right)\left[1 + \cos\left(2\pi\rho/\lambda_1\right)\right] \text{W}. \tag{8.8}$$

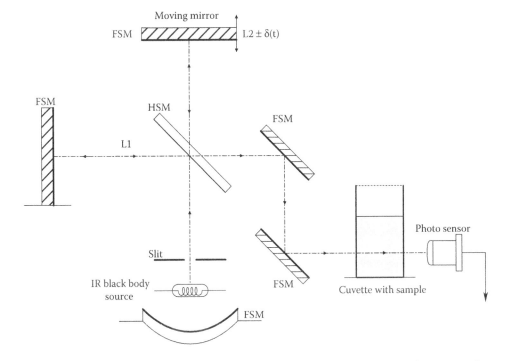

Figure 8.3 Schematic of the optical system of a Fourier transform IR spectrophotometer. A Michelson interferometer is used to modulate the transmitted light.

In terms of wave number, $\xi_1 \equiv \lambda_1^{-1}$, I_o can also be written as

$$I_o(\rho, \xi_1) = I_{in}\left(\frac{1}{2}\right)[1 + \cos(2\pi\xi_1\rho)]\ W. \tag{8.9}$$

Note that $I_o(\rho, \xi_1)$ is an even function in $\rho\xi_1$. When two other beams having wave numbers ξ_2 and ξ_3 are added to the beam of wave number ξ_1, then the output of the time-modulated Michelson interferometer can be written:

$$I_o(\rho) = \sum_{k=1}^{3} I_{ink}\left(\frac{1}{2}\right)[1 + \cos(2\pi\xi_k\rho)]\quad W, \text{ at a given retardation.} \tag{8.10}$$

When this even interferogram function is plotted versus ρ, we see a strong peak at the origin surrounded by ripple, as shown in Figure 8.4. In the more general case, when the source intensity input to the interferometer is described by a *continuous density distribution* in terms of wave number, ξ, the interferogram intensity is given by *the inverse cosine Fourier transform:*

$$I_o(\rho) = \int_{-\infty}^{\infty} W_B(\xi)\left(\frac{1}{2}\right)[1 + \cos(2\pi\xi\rho)]\ d\xi = I_{Wo} + \int_{-\infty}^{\infty} W_B(\xi)\left(\frac{1}{2}\right)\cos(2\pi\xi\rho)\ d\xi, \tag{8.11}$$

where $W_B(\xi)$ is assumed to be even in ξ, so $W_B(\xi) = W_B(-\xi)$. Thus:

$$I_{Wo} = \int_{0}^{\infty} W_B(\xi)d\xi. \tag{8.12}$$

The cosine integral can be considered to be the real, *inverse* Fourier transform of $W_B(\xi)$.

$$\mathbf{I_o}(\rho) = \left(\frac{1}{2}\right)\mathbf{F}^{-1}\{W_B(\xi)\}. \tag{8.13}$$

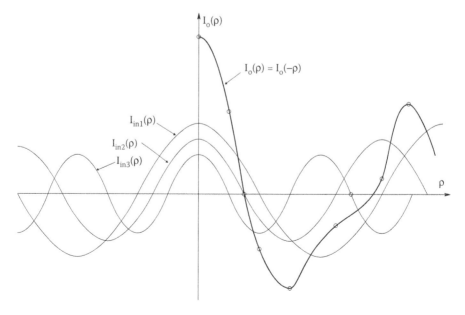

Figure 8.4 Superposition of the output intensity of the interferometer as a function of wave number and retardation distance, ρ, which is time modulated. Note that with just three discrete wave numbers, a peak in the interferogram grows around $\rho = 0$.

Note that by the Euler relation, $e^{-j\omega t} \equiv [\cos(\omega t) - j\sin(\omega t)]$, one definition of the continuous Fourier transform (CFT) is:

$$\mathbf{F}(\omega) = R(\omega) + jX(\omega) \equiv \int_{-\infty}^{\infty} f(t) \, [\cos(\omega t) - j\sin(\omega t)] \, dt. \qquad (8.14)$$

When $f(t)$ is real and even, then

$$F(\omega) \equiv \int_{-\infty}^{\infty} f(t)\cos(\omega t) \, dt \qquad (8.15)$$

and the continuous, inverse, FT is:

$$f(t) \equiv (2\pi)^{-1} \int_{-\infty}^{\infty} F(\omega)\cos(\omega t) \, d\omega, \qquad (8.16)$$

where ω is in radians/s, and $X(\omega) = 0$.

Note that we have defined the blackbody radiation density, $W_B(\xi)$ W/cm^{-1}, as an even function in wave number, ξ. Let ξ be analogous to frequency in Hz, and the retardation distance, ρ, be analogous to time in Equation 8.15, thus $F(\omega/2\pi) \rightarrow W_B(\xi)$. Thus, we see that modulation of the source light's spectral distribution, $W_B(\xi)$, by the Michelson interferometer generates an even, inverse Fourier (intensity) function of $W_B(\xi)$, $I_o(\rho)$, at its output. Sic:

$$I_o(\rho) = \int_{0}^{\infty} W_B(\xi)\cos(2\pi\xi\rho) \, d\xi. \qquad (8.17)$$

Now if we sample the IFT, $I_o(\rho)$, at intervals $\Delta\rho$, and take its DFT, we recover an estimate of the input blackbody intensity distribution, $W_B(\xi)$, as shown in Figure 8.5. This $W_B(\xi)$ estimate is stored in the FTIR system's computer memory. (See Section 7.3.2 for a more thorough discussion of BBR.) Figure 8.6 illustrates a typical interferogram as a function of the retardation distance, ρ.

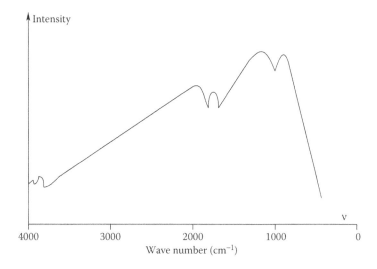

Figure 8.5 Plot of the blackbody source's intensity spectrum versus wave number as determined by taking the Fourier transform of $I_o(\rho)$ given by Equation 8.17.

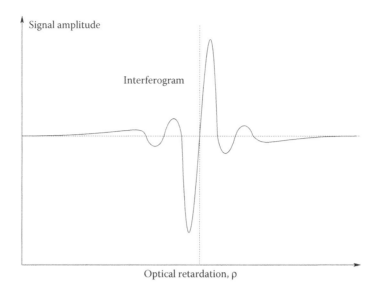

Figure 8.6 Typical, continuous interferogram output of the photosensor.

The next step in the operation of an FTIR spectrometer is to pass the interferometer-modulated IR source radiation through the sample where selective absorption (attenuation) in certain wave number bands occurs. Again, as in Equation 8.9, let us look at one particular wave number, ξ_1. The intensity of the light emerging from the sample, $I_e(\rho, \xi_1)$, is given by

$$I_e(\rho,\xi_1) = I_{in}(\xi_1)T_s(\xi_1)\left(\tfrac{1}{2}\right)[1 + \cos(2\pi\xi_1\rho)], \tag{8.18}$$

where $T_s(\xi_1)$ is the wave number-dependent $(0 \leftrightarrow 1)$ transmittance of the analyte and sample, and $I_{in}(\xi_1)$ is the input intensity at $\xi = \xi_1$.

If the input is replaced by the BB distribution, $W_B(\xi)$, we can write:

$$I_e(\rho) = \left(\tfrac{1}{2}\right)\int_{-\infty}^{\infty} W_B(\xi)T_s(\xi)[1 + \cos(2\pi\xi\rho)]d\xi = I_{ewo} + \left(\tfrac{1}{2}\right)\int_{-\infty}^{\infty} W_B(\xi)T_s(\xi)\cos(2\pi\xi\rho)\,d\xi. \tag{8.19}$$

Clearly, the "DC" term is

$$I_{ewo} = \int_{0}^{\infty} W_B(\xi)T_s(\xi)d\xi, \tag{8.20}$$

and the integral is the *inverse* FT of the frequency-domain product, $W_B(\xi)\,T_s(\xi)$. When the output interferogram, $I_e(\rho)$, is DFTd at intervals, $\Delta\rho$, we obtain an estimate of the output spectrum.

$$S_{Sa}(\xi) = \left(\tfrac{1}{2}\right)W_B(\xi)T_s(\xi). \tag{8.21}$$

Since we already know $W_B(\xi)$, the desired sample transmittance is easily found by the relation:

$$T_s(\xi) = \frac{2S_{Sa}(\xi)}{W_B(\xi)}. \tag{8.22}$$

It goes without saying that a high-speed computer capable of calculating DFTs and generating plots of $T_s(\xi)$ and absorbance $A(\xi)$ is a necessary component of an FTIR spectrometer. We have seen that all spectrophotometers pass light through a cuvette holding the analyte in solution. In some

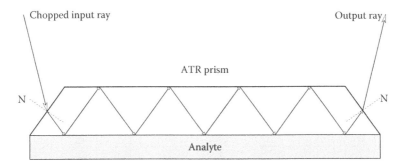

Chopped input ray

Output ray

ATR prism

N

N

Analyte

Figure 8.7 Side view of an ATR prism or plate. Each time the traversing ray reflects off the interface between the ATR plate and the analyte, there is selective absorption by analyte molecules in the interface layer.

designs, the light is broadband (white), and the emergent light from the sample is passed through a monochromator to examine the transmittance or absorbance at particular wavelengths. In other designs, monochromatic light is passed through the sample. In nearly all cases, the light beam is chopped in order that phase-sensitive demodulation can be used (equivalent to a lock-in amplifier) to improve sensitivity and reject noise. In the FTIR spectrophotometer, the modulation is provided by the Michelson interferometer.

Another mode of operation of conventional spectrophotometers is to measure the wavelength-dependent absorption of backscattered light from superficial tissue (skin, dermis, capillaries, etc.). This approach is commonly used to measure the percent oxygen saturation of capillary blood hemoglobin (Hb), and may find application in measuring other blood constituents such as glucose, cholesterol, alcohol, heroin (diacetyl morphine), etc. The measurement of the absorption of backscattered light is greatly facilitated by the use of an *attenuated total reflection* prism (ATRP), as shown in Figure 8.7. The input light enters the ATRP and is directed through its bottom surface into the skin (or absorbing sample). The light that is backscattered from the tissue reenters the ATRP prism, and is totally reflected from its top surface, being directed again into the tissue where it is again backscattered, etc. The repeated re-entry and backscattering of the beam from the tissue increases the sensitivity of the spectrophotometric process by effectively increasing L in Beer's law. Increases in sensitivity by a factor of 20 can sometimes be had.

All sorts of medically important molecules from body fluids can be quantified by spectrophotometry. These include but are not limited to cholesterol, steroid hormones, thyroxine, theophylline, opiates, opioids, tranquilizers, etc. Knowledge of a drug concentration in blood or urine can be used clinically to adjust drug dosage, and also to detect drug abuse.

8.2.3 Nondispersive Spectroscopy

Nondispersive spectroscopy (NDS) is a chemical analytical method that avoids using an expensive monochromator to quantify a specific analyte. Instead of plotting $\%T(\lambda)$ or $A(\lambda)$ versus λ for a sample, and using the resulting peaks and valleys to quantify the analyte, an NDS instrument selects a narrow range of wavelength, $\Delta\lambda$, in which the analyte has a *unique* peak and valley in its $\%T(\lambda)$ curve. The $\Delta\lambda$ band is generated by passing broadband light through a band-pass filter made from one or more *interference filters*. Figure 8.8 illustrates a basic NDS system that uses manual nulling. Light in the band, $\Delta\lambda$, is first chopped, then passed through a half-silvered, beamsplitter mirror. The direct beam passes through the sample cuvette, thence to a photosensor, PS_1. The reference beam passes through an adjustable, calibrated, neutral density wedge (NDW), thence to photosensor, PS_2. The outputs of the photosensors are conditioned to remove DC, then amplified by a difference amplifier (DA). The DA output is a square wave at chopper frequency whose amplitude phase ($0°$ or $180°$) is determined by the relative intensities at PS_1 and PS_2. In calibration, with no analyte present, the NDW is manually adjusted to null the DC signal, V_o, to compensate for reflection and absorption by the sample cuvette. With the analyte present, more light in $\Delta\lambda$ is absorbed and the intensity at PS_1, I_A, is reduced. Now, the NDW must be advanced further to renull V_o. The additional neutral density required to renull the system can be shown to be proportional to the analyte concentration.

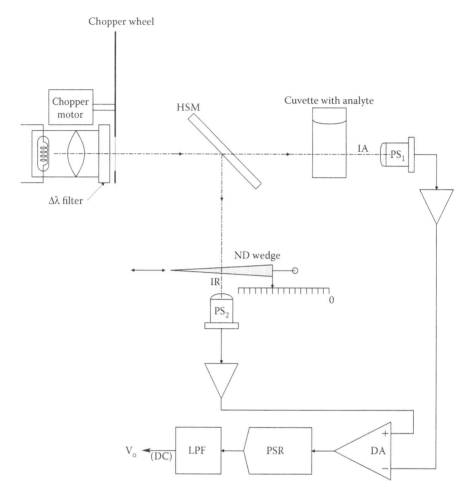

Figure 8.8 Schematic of a manually nulled, single-beam, nondispersive spectrophotometer (NDS). A phase-sensitive rectifier (PSR) and low-pass filter (LPF) are used to change the square wave output of the DA to a DC error signal, V_o. V_o is nulled by adjusting the ND wedge position so that the matched photosensors each have the same total intensity input over the $\Delta\lambda$ filter passband. The passband also contains a wavelength where the analyte absorbs.

A further refinement of an NDS system is to make it self-nulling. Such a design is shown in Figure 8.9. Now, V_o is integrated to make a Type 1 control system with zero steady-state error, and the integrator output, V_o', is conditioned to drive a linear positioning system that moves the NDW. It can be shown that the difference in the voltage V_o' with no analyte, and V_o' with analyte is proportional to the (linear) change in ND, hence in the analyte concentration.

We now demonstrate mathematically how an NDS system works. Assume that the output of the interference filter is a rectangular spectrum of width, $\Delta\lambda$. After being split by the half-silvered mirror (HSM), both source spectrums still have width $\Delta\lambda$, and equal magnitudes, $S_1(\lambda)$ W/nm. The reflected reference spectrum is attenuated by the NDW's transmittance, T_{ND}. In general, $T_{ND} \equiv (I_{out}/I_{in}) \equiv 10^{-\beta x}$, where x is the displacement of the wedge from 0 on the linear x scale, and β is the NDW's attenuation constant, $ND \equiv \beta x$. Note that an ND of 1 means the input light is attenuated by a factor of 0.1, or $I_{out} = I_{in}/10$. Thus, the intensity at the reference photosensor is:

$$I_R = S_1 \Delta\lambda T_{ND} \text{ W.} \tag{8.23}$$

The spectrum that passes through the HSM also passes through the walls of the sample cuvette twice (in and out) and also through the test solution with analyte. The input spectrum

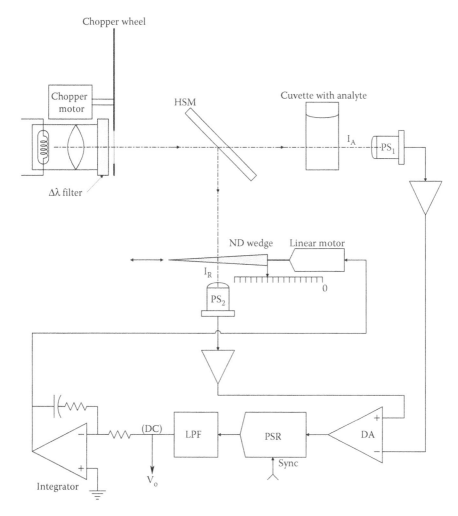

Figure 8.9 Schematic of a servo-nulling, NDS. V_o is integrated and the integrator output drives a linear actuator that moves the ND wedge to automatically null the system. This closed-loop system uses Type I control architecture.

is attenuated by passing through the cuvette by a factor $T_{cuv} < 1$, and also by the test solution independent of the analyte by a factor $T_{sol} < 1$. We assume that in a narrowband, $\delta\lambda$, around λ_o, the analyte has a strong absorption. Hence the spectrum exiting the cuvette, $S_{1A}(\lambda)$, has a reduced total intensity as shown in Figure 8.10. Using Beer's law, the intensity of $S_{1A}(\lambda)$ is simply:

$$I_A = S_1 T_c T_{solv} \Delta\lambda - \delta\lambda S_1 T_c T_{solv}(1 - T_A). \tag{8.24}$$

The transmittance minimum of the analyte is given by Beer's law:

$$T_A = \exp(-kL[A]) \cong 1 - kL[A]. \tag{8.25}$$

Here we have assumed that $kL[A] \ll 1$. $[A]$ is the concentration of the analyte, and the value of k is both wavelength and concentration dependent. Thus after some algebra, we can write the intensity of the light exiting the cuvette as

$$I_A = S_1 T_c T_{solv} \Delta\lambda \left\{ 1 - (\delta\lambda/\Delta\lambda)kL[A] \right\} W. \tag{8.26}$$

If there is no analyte in the cuvette, the V_o null occurs when $I_A = I_R$. That is, when:

$$S_1 \Delta\lambda T_{NDo} = S_1 \Delta\lambda T_c T_{solv}, \tag{8.27}$$

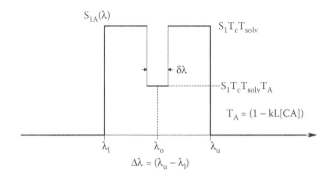

Figure 8.10 Idealized spectral band of width $\Delta\lambda$ after passing through the analyte. The $\delta\lambda$ notch is from the spectral energy in the band that the analyte has absorbed. (See text Equations 8.24–8.30 for analysis.)

or,

$$T_{NDo} = T_c T_{solv} = 10^{-\beta x} \cong (1 - 2.303\beta x_o). \tag{8.28}$$

With analyte present, the wedge is advanced until again, $I_R = I_A$, and $V_o = 0$. Thus at null we have:

$$S_1 \Delta\lambda T_{ND} = S_1 T_c T_{solv} \Delta\lambda \left\{1 - \left(\delta\lambda/\Delta\lambda\right)kL[A]\right\}. \tag{8.29}$$

So,

$$
\begin{aligned}
&T_{ND} = T_c T_{solv}\{1 - (\delta\lambda/\Delta\lambda)kL[A]\} \\
&\downarrow \\
&(1 - 2.3\beta x) \cong (1 - 2.3\beta x_o)\{1 - (\delta\lambda/\Delta\lambda)kL[A]\} \\
&\downarrow \\
&2.3\beta(x - x_o) \cong (T_c T_{solv})(\delta\lambda/\Delta\lambda)kL[A] \\
&\downarrow \\
&\Delta x \cong (T_c T_{solv}/\beta 2.303)(\delta\lambda/\Delta\lambda)kL[A].
\end{aligned}
\tag{8.30}
$$

Thus, the additional displacement of the NDW by Δx to renull the NDS when an analyte is present is simply proportional to the analyte's concentration, [A], assuming Beer's law holds, and the NDW's ND is given by $10^{-\beta x}$, where $\beta x \ll 1$. The 2.3 factor comes from approximating $10^{-\beta x}$ by the use of $e^{-\varepsilon} \cong 1 - \varepsilon$. (Note that $\log_{10}(a) = \ln(a)/2.303$.)

The reader should note that other system configurations for NDS systems have been used, as shown in Figure 8.11. (The choppers for these three systems are not shown.) System A in the figure is basically the one described above, except a blank cuvette filled with solvent is used so that in the absence of analyte in the sample, ND = 0. System B is more sophisticated in that a reference concentration of analyte is used in the input cuvette. System configuration C is an *invalid configuration* in which the sample and the reference cuvettes have been interchanged. Analyses of system B is given below.

In system B, the spectrum $S_2(\lambda)$ exiting the reference cuvette containing a known reference concentration of analyte, $[A_o]$, has intensity I_2, given by

$$I_2 = S_1 T_c T_{solv} \Delta\lambda \left\{1 - \left(\delta\lambda/\Delta\lambda\right)kL[A_o]\right\}. \tag{8.31}$$

This intensity is divided by two at the HSM. The reference beam passes through the NDW thence a blank cuvette. The intensity I_R is thus:

$$I_R = \int_0^\infty S_4(\lambda)d\lambda \tag{8.32}$$

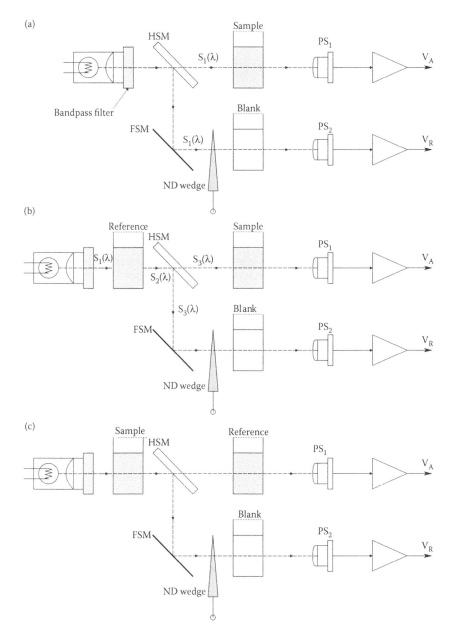

Figure 8.11 Three possible architectures (a, b, and c) for nondispersive spectrophotometers. Choppers are not shown. It can be shown that configuration (c) will not work.

$$I_R = \tfrac{1}{2}\, S_1 T_c^{\;2} T^2{}_{solv} T_{ND} \Delta\lambda - \delta\lambda \left[\tfrac{1}{2}\, S_1 T_c^{\;2} T^2{}_{solv} T_{ND} - \tfrac{1}{2}\, S_1 T_c^{\;2} T^2{}_{solv} T_{ND} T_{A_o} \right]$$
$$\downarrow \tag{8.33}$$
$$I_R = \tfrac{1}{2}\, S_1 T_c^{\;2} T^2{}_{solv} T_{ND} [\Delta\lambda - \delta\lambda + \delta\lambda T_{A_o}].$$

The intensity I_A is given by

$$I_A = \int_0^\infty S_3(\lambda)\,d\lambda \tag{8.34}$$

$$I_A = \frac{1}{2}\, S_1 T_c^{\,2} T^2{}_{solv} \Delta\lambda - \delta\lambda \left[\frac{1}{2}\, S_1 T_c^{\,2} T^2{}_{solv} - \frac{1}{2}\, S_1 T_c^{\,2} T^2{}_{solv} T_{A_o} T_A \right]$$
$$I_A = \frac{1}{2}\, S_1 T_c^{\,2} T^2{}_{solv} [\Delta\lambda - \delta\lambda + \delta\lambda T_{A_o} T_A]. \tag{8.35}$$

Now when the instrument is nulled, $I_A = I_R$, so we can write:

$$T_{ND} = \frac{[1 - (\delta\lambda / \Delta\lambda)(1 - T_{A_o} T_A)]}{[1 - (\delta\lambda / \Delta\lambda)(1 - T_{A_o})]}. \tag{8.36}$$

Recall that the transmittances can be approximated by the relation, $e^{-\varepsilon} \cong 1 - \varepsilon$, $\varepsilon \ll 1$, and also, $1/(1 - \varepsilon) \cong 1 + \varepsilon$, and $\varepsilon^2 \ll \varepsilon \ll 1$. If these relations are substituted into Equation 3.36, we can finally write:

$$T_{ND} \cong 1 - (\delta\lambda / \Delta\lambda) kL[A]. \tag{8.37}$$

Thus, the null setting for the NDW (at low concentrations) is proportional to the concentration of the analyte in the sample solution. It is left as an exercise for the reader to demonstrate why the NDS configuration in Figure 8.11c is a faulty architecture. (Hint: using the approach above, solve for T_{ND} at null.)

To demonstrate the effectiveness of the NDS approach in quantifying an analyte, Fellows (1997) designed, built, and tested an NDS to measure oxyhemoglobin, *in vitro*. Percutaneous measurement of the $\%O_2$ saturation of RBC Hb is an established, NI measurement technique. The pulse oximeter (described in detail in Section 15.8) makes use of the differential absorption of red and NIR light by Hb versus HbO. Pulse oximeters use a red and an NIR light-emitting diode (LED) (not a laser) as a 2-λ source to make the measurement. Fellows' NDS system was developed as a proof-of-concept design, rather than a competing instrument for the very simple pulse oximeter. Fellows' system architecture closely followed the design shown in Figure 8.11b, except instead of a linear, NDW; she used a rotating screen as a variable ND attenuator. Unlike the linear wedge, the screen's transmittance, T_{SC}, is a function of its angle with respect to the beam being attenuated, and is given by

$$T_{SC} = (1 - 2r/d)[1 - (2r/d)\sec(\theta)]. \tag{8.38}$$

Each wire in the screen has radius, r, and d is the center-to-center spacing of the wires; a square mesh is assumed. The ND screen was rotated by a servo galvanometer whose angle, θ, was proportional to its DC input voltage, V_g, that is, $\theta = kV_g$.

Fellows used a filter that passed light in a 650–750 nm band. For the test solution, the standard, and the compensation, 1-cm cuvettes were used. Sigma® freeze-dried human Hb was made up at a concentration of 12 g/L in water buffered to pH 7.4. To make either HbO or Hb, either O_2 gas or CO_2 gas was bubbled through the sample and reference cuvettes, respectively.

Fellows' servo-nulling NDS system was able to measure HbO, but was difficult to calibrate because of the very nonlinear ND relation. A linear wedge or ND disk would have simplified the operation of her system.

A logical application of the NDS system would be to try to noninvasively and percutaneously measure (tissue) blood glucose in the FIR range. Glucose has three absorption peaks in the FIR: One at 10.97 μm, one at 11.98 μm, and one at 12.95 μm. If the LIR bandpass filter passed from 10.5 to 11.5 μm, the peak at 10.97 μm could be used. Figure 8.12 illustrates a basic, FIR, NDS system that might use a finger web or earlobe (always with constant L). The FIR beam is defined by an IR bandpass filter, chopped, and the null is detected using a phase-sensitive rectifier. A light-tight box excludes stray IR from the pyroelectric photosensors (e.g., PVDF). Such a system would be easy to build, but its accurate use would depend on individual calibration with a standard blood glucose test, and the absence of other tissue and blood substances that might overwhelm the glucose absorption peaks.

8.2.4 Chemical Analysis by SPR

SPR sensors are a relatively new and versatile analytical tools. They allow rapid, specific determination of the concentration of a variety of medically and biologically important analytes (Homola 2008).

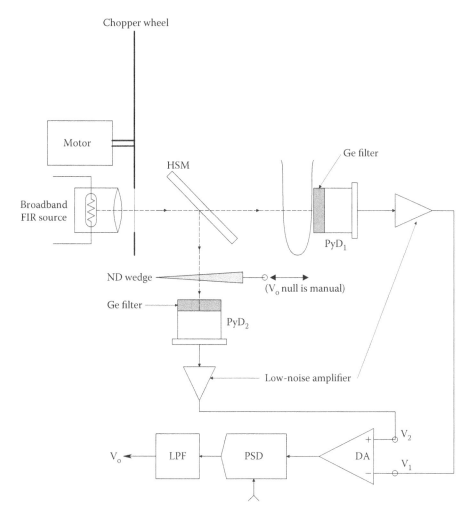

Figure 8.12 Proposed IR NDS applied to measure blood glucose in vascular earlobe tissue. The $\Delta\lambda$ passband might span from 11.5 to 12.5 μm to include the 12 μm glucose absorption peak. A pyroelectric IR sensor could be used in the $\Delta\lambda$ range specified. Such an instrument would have to be individually calibrated against the patient's blood glucose with a fuel cell type blood glucometer. (The Germanium optical filters have an approximate IR passband of 2–20 μm.)

For example, specific bacteria, Abs, theophylline, caffeine, NO_2, pesticides, explosives, controlled substances (opioid drugs), etc. have been sensed with SPR. Threshold sensitivity (limit of detection = LOD) for certain analytes has been reported for a variety of small biomolecules by Mitchell and Wu (2010). For example, an LOD for progesterone of 4.9 pg/mL was reported, and the LOD for a certain Ab was given as 20.1 pg/mL.

SPR technology is relatively simple and inexpensive to implement, compared with analytical systems such as HPLC, mass spectrometry, IR spectrometry, and GC, and it lends itself well to field measurements. Since this text is about NI medical instruments, the analytes are presumably derived from urine or saliva, or smears from mucous membranes, etc. There is no reason, however, why SPR sensors cannot be used on gases, or blood to look for any analyte (chemical, Ab, bacteria, etc.) therein.

SPR is a *quantum* phenomenon which occurs when a beam of monochromatic linearly polarized light (LPL) is reflected off a thin metal film, vapor deposited on one side of a glass prism, or when a beam of LPL is incident at a critical angle on a gold-coated diffraction grating. For illustrative purposes, we will examine in detail the prism SPR system using the so-called *Kretschmann geometry*. This system is shown schematically in Figure 8.13. A thin (~50 nm) film

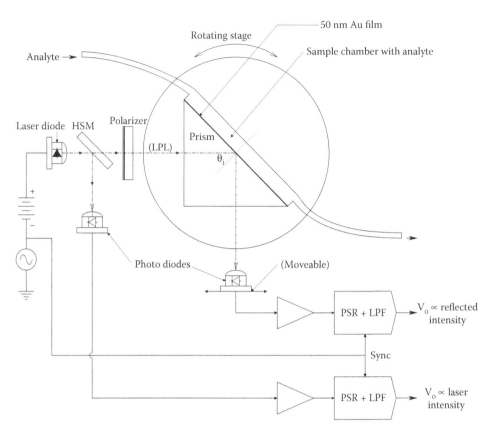

Figure 8.13 Surface plasmon resonance (SPR) analytical system using the Kretschmann geometry. Resonance is reached by varying the angle θ of the monochromatic polarized light incident on the gold film.

of conducting metal such as gold or silver is vapor deposited on one face of a prism, or on the flat face of a half-round rod. A beam of LPL of a known wavelength is directed into the prism or rod so that it strikes the gold film face at an angle of incidence, θ_i. The incident beam's **E** vector must lie in the plane of incidence (be in the TM mode) for SPR to occur. In intimate contact with the other side of the gold film is a thin film of the analyte having a permittivity, ε_a. It has been experimentally observed that when the incoming beam's wavelength and angle of incidence have unique critical values, the intensity of the reflected beam reaches a *minimum*. The depth of the null in the output beam intensity is a function of how much energy from the input LPL beam is coupled into the generation of surface plasmons in the metal film. The degree of coupling is a function of λ, θ_i, and most importantly, the dielectric constant of the analyte material.

Surface plasmons can be thought of as induced, wave-like fluctuations in the density of conduction-band electrons in the thin metal film. These fluctuations exist in both space and time, that is, they can be thought of as traveling waves induced by the incident TM, LPL. The basis for using SPR as an analytical chemical tool is based on the conditions required for resonance. Under conditions of non-SP resonance, the incident beam of LPL reflects off the metallized surface of the prism, and exits the prism to a photosensor. The metal film effectively forms a conducting mirror surface, and conventional refraction and reflection optical laws apply.

The velocity of light *in vacuo* is $c = 2.998 \times 10^8$ m/s. In transparent liquids or glass, light travels more slowly.

The ratio of the speed if light *in vacuo* to the speed of light in the medium is defined as the *refractive index* of that medium, n_m. That is, $n_m \equiv c/v_m$. From electromagnetic (EM) theory, $c \equiv 1/\sqrt{\varepsilon_0 \mu_0}$, and $v_m = 1/\sqrt{\kappa_m \varepsilon_0 \mu_m}$.

However, in nonmagnetic materials, the magnetic permeability $\mu_m \cong \mu_o$. Thus, we can write the refractive index as

$$n_m \cong \sqrt{\kappa_m}. \tag{8.39}$$

v_m and n are generally functions of frequency. An EM wave in a medium or free space such as light, or surface plasmon waves which basically exist in two dimensions can be described by their *wave vector,* **k**. **k** is directed along the direction of wave propagation, and its magnitude *in vacuo* for EM waves is:

$$k_o = \omega/c = 2\pi\nu/c = 2\pi/\lambda. \tag{8.40}$$

The prism has glass with refractive index, n_1, the magnitude of the EM wave vector is (Kraus 1953):

$$k_1 = \omega/v_1 = \omega\sqrt{k_1/c}. \tag{8.41}$$

Surface plasmons are generated on the metal film under the condition that the magnitude of the wave vector in the glass incident on the gold film equals the magnitude of the wave vector at the metal/analyte interface. This can be written as

$$k_i = (2\pi/\lambda)\,\sin(\theta_i)\sqrt{\kappa_1} = (2\pi/\lambda)\sqrt{(\kappa_a\,|\kappa_m|)/(\kappa_a+|\kappa_m|)}, \tag{8.42}$$

where κ_1 is the dielectric constant of the glass prism, κ_a is the dielectric constant of the analyte, and $\kappa_m = \kappa_m' + j\kappa_m''$ is the complex dielectric constant of the gold film. All dielectric constants are generally functions of ν (or λ).

Canceling like terms and solving for the angle of incidence inside the prism, we have the angle criterion for SPR:

$$\theta_{iR} \cong \sin^{-1}\left\{\sqrt{(\kappa_a\kappa_m)/[(\kappa_a + \kappa_m)\kappa_1]}\right\}. \tag{8.43}$$

The resonance condition is due to momentum matching of incident photons with plasmons in the metal. The fact that the permittivity of the analyte layer (typically ~250 nm thick) on the other side of the metal affects SPR may be due to the evanescent field expanding through the metal and coupling into SPs at the analyte surface. The resonance angle, θ_{iR}, is exquisitely sensitive to the dielectric constants of the metal and the analyte in contact with it. Thus, any chemical reaction that takes place at the metal surface, such as binding of Abs to metal-bound antigen, will affect ε_a and the value of θ_{iR}. Thus, surface reactions of analyte can be used to sense Abs, or if the Abs are bound to the metal, it can sense antigen molecules such as those on bacterial and viral surfaces, or analyte molecules in a solution or suspension.

Figure 8.14 illustrates typical SPR curves for a Kretschmann prism system receiving monochromatic light. Note that when the analyte index of refraction increases due to Ab bonding at the metal–analyte surface, κ_a also increases to κ_a', and the SPR curve as a function of incidence angle shifts to the right and broadens. (Note that $n_a \cong \sqrt{\kappa_a}$.) Thus the intensity measured at angle θ_{im} increases, while the intensity minimum moves to θ_{iR}'. Both shifts, either taken together in a formula, or as separate phenomena, can be used to quantify the extent of the binding reaction at the metal surface. The depth of the null at SPR depends in part on the thickness of the metal film.

Another way of using the Kretschmann system is to set the incidence angle at the SPR null for some standard source λ. The source λ is then varied by a monochromator, and the output intensity is plotted as a function of λ as a surface reaction takes place. Typical intensity versus λ curves are illustrated in Figure 8.15. Because the permittivities of the glass, metal film, and analyte are functions of λ, we again see a shifting and broadening of the SPR intensity curves with λ as Ab binding at the metal surface takes place. While varying the source λ can yield good analytical results, it makes the SPR system more expensive because of the need for a precision monochromator.

The reader should be aware that the design of SPR devices for chemical analysis is a rapidly growing field. One alternative configuration of SPR sensor places the analyte solution over the surface of a plastic diffraction grating whose surface has been vapor deposited with gold, silver, or aluminum (gold is generally preferred). The plastic top of the grating acts as an attenuated total reflection (ATR) prism where light reflected from the grating where the beam strikes it initially is reflected back many times to the grating surface. Such a grating SPR design was patented by Simon (1998). Figure 8.16 shows a side-view of Simon's "long range," SPR grating system. SPR

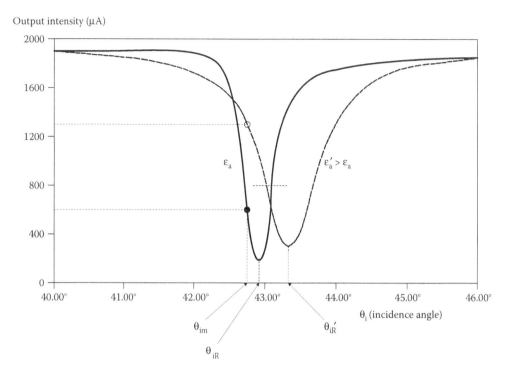

Figure 8.14 Reflected light intensity as a function of incidence angle for the Kretschmann SPR system. The solid curve is the system response in the absence of analyte; the dashed curve is obtained with analyte in intimate contact with the gold film.

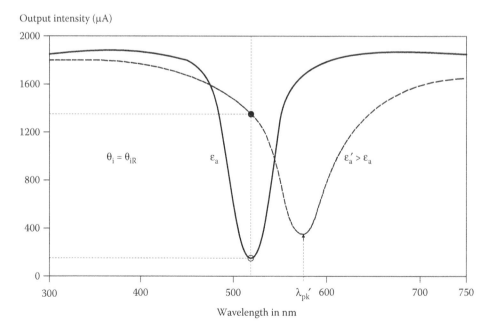

Figure 8.15 Reflected light intensity as a function of the wavelength of the incident polarized beam in a Kretschmann SPR system. The dashed curve is obtained with analyte in intimate contact with gold film.

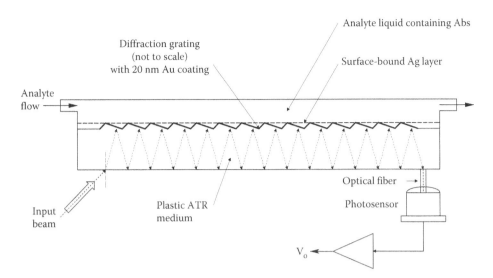

Figure 8.16 SPR system that uses a metal film-covered, plastic diffraction grating. The analyte is in intimate contact with the metal film as in the Kretschmann SPR system. The multiple light reflections in the grating body are reminiscent of the ATR prism. SPR systems have been operated with both liquid and gas phase analytes.

occurs at a critical beam input angle, θ_i, giving a minimum of output light intensity when the coupling component of the monochromatic, TM-polarized input beam wave vector satisfies the relation:

$$(2\pi/\lambda)\sin(\theta_i) + (2\pi/b) = (2\pi/\lambda)\sqrt{(\kappa_a\kappa_m)/(\kappa_a + \kappa_m)}, \qquad (8.44)$$

where b is the grating constant, κ_a is the dielectric constant of the analyte, and κ_m is the magnitude of the complex dielectric constant of the metal film.

A very thin layer of antigen with high affinity to the Ab to be detected is chemically bound to the 20-nm gold film over the grating surface. Abs in the analyte liquid bind the protruding antigen molecules, changing κ_a at the gold-solution interface. This change of dielectric constant changes the interfacial refractive index and "retunes" the SPR to a new input angle, θ_i. Either by changing θ_i to reattain a minimal light output, or by measuring the *increase* in light output due to $\Delta\kappa_a$, the number or density of bound Abs can be quantified. A possible disadvantage of Simon's grating SPR configuration is the formation of bubbles on the grating surface, and the fact that the measurement is a "one-shot" event; a new virgin antigen surface must be reapplied to the gold film, and the output nulled again before another Ab assay can be done. Simon (1998) claimed that the output signal from the ATR layer increases by approximately fivefold when about 2 nm of antigen–Ab complex forms at the gold surface. Also, a refractive index change in the analyte of less than 1% causes a 0.5° shift in θ_i to renull the system.

Other embodiments of the grating SPR system place the analyte over the gold film-covered grating; the monochromatic, TM-polarized light is directed through a thin layer of analyte onto the grating. Jory et al. (1995) reported on an exquisitely sensitive grating SPR system in which an acousto-optical tunable filter (AOTF) element was used to control the wavelength of the incident beam to a precision of 0.0005 nm. They used their system to measure the concentration of NO_2 gas in N_2 (a gas phase analyte). By depositing a thin layer of phthalocynanine over the gold coating, a wavelength shift of only -0.004 nm renulled the system from zero concentration when 0.01 ppm NO_2 in N_2 was applied. They claimed that the sensitivity of their system allowed detection of changes in the refractive index of the gas of 10^{-6}. The fact that very small concentrations of gas are detectable suggests that the grating SPR technology might be developed in the future to detect medical gas concentrations, or even trace gases emanating from controlled drugs and explosives. (At the time of writing this book (2016), trained dogs have the best record for detecting the explosives and controlled drugs.)

The potential application of SPR sensors in medical diagnosis is enormous, and is being actively developed (Homola 2008). As we have seen, both gas and liquid-phase sensing are possible.

Practically any analyte that can react with a reactant bound to the gold film surface on a prism or grating with a strong affinity can be sensed by SPR. The reaction must cause a change in the refractive index or the permittivity at the gold surface in order to affect the SPR conditions (λ and/or θ_i). SPR antigen–Ab reactions can be used to sense specific Abs, bacteria, viruses, proteins, hormones, cytokines, etc. Note that specific, monoclonal Abs can also be bound to the gold film in order to sense any protein or molecule for which they can be made specific.

The problem of quick, efficient, SPR sensor regeneration remains to be solved, however. Once the bound surface reactant has combined with the analyte, the analyte must be totally removed before the next measurement without affecting the bound reactant, or the complex must be removed and the surface reactant layer must be renewed or rejuvenated.

To summarize SPR applications, the technique has been used for food quality and safety analysis, including testing for: pathogens, toxins, veterinary drugs, vitamins, hormones, diagnostic Abs, allergens, proteins, and chemical contaminants. In medical diagnosis, SPR has been used to sense cancer markers, Abs against viral pathogens, drugs and drug-induced Abs, hormones, blood markers for heart attack, and other molecular markers. SPR also has a number of applications in environmental monitoring: pesticides, explosives (e.g., TNT), aromatic hydrocarbons, heavy metals, phenols, polychlorinated biphenyls, and dioxins can be quantified in groundwater and soils. SPR techniques are sensitive; for example, the LOD for DDT in water was 15 pg/mL, the LOD for Cu^{++} was 1×10^{-12} M, the LOD for dioxin was 100 pg/mL (Homola 2008).

8.2.5 Ion-Selective Electrodes

An important analytical tool for measuring the concentrations of electrolyte ions in plasma, urine, saliva, etc. is the *ion-selective electrode* (ISE). ISEs include the well-known, glass, hydrogen ISE used to measure the pH of a solution. All ISEs are used with a *reference electrode* (RE). In electrochemistry, each electrode is known as a *half-cell;* the ISE and the RE together comprise a whole cell, or EMF battery. The half-cell EMF of the RE is generally a constant regardless of the analyte ion's concentration. The half-cell EMF of the ISE is proportional to the logarithm of the analyte ion's *electrochemical activity, a. a* is very nearly equal to the ion's molar concentration at low concentrations.

The EMFs of both the ISE and RE vary with temperature, so all pH and ion measurements have to be done at a constant temperature following the calibration with a standard solution, or an automatic, electronic temperature correction can be made by the instrument by continuously measuring the test solution's temperature.

The net cell potential of the RE and ISE electrodes in the analyte solution is measured under conditions of negligible current flow through the cell. Negligible current flow is required to avoid polarization at the electrodes' surfaces, overvoltages, and ohmic voltage drops (a typical glass pH electrode has an equivalent DC resistance of ~5×10^9 ohms). To meet this condition, the cell's EMF is measured with a direct-coupled, differential, *electrometer amplifier* having bias currents on the order of 10 fA or less and an input resistance on the order of 10^{13} ohms or greater.

As a first example of an ISE application, we consider the glass pH electrode, shown in Figure 8.17. This electrode has a thin glass membrane at its end. It is filled internally with a solution of 0.1 N hydrochloric acid. Internally, a silver|silver chloride electrode makes contact with the HCl. The Ag|AgCl electrode's half-cell potential is a logarithmic function of the Cl^- concentration, which is the same as the HCl's H^+ concentration. The typical reference half-cell for pH measurement is the calomel electrode, also illustrated in Figure 8.17. Thus, the pH measurement system has three half-cells: calomel, glass, and Ag|AgCl. This cell can be written in electrochemical notation: Ag|AgCl(s), 0.1 N HCl|Glass|Solution (pH = x)|Calomel. The definition of pH is: pH $\equiv -\log_{10} a_{H+} \cong -\log_{10}[H^+]$, where a_{H+} is the *activity* of hydrogen ions in the solution under measurement and $[H^+]$ is their concentration. The half-cell EMF of the glass electrode plus the Ag|AgCl(s) electrode is thus:

$$E_G = E_G^0 - (RT/F)\ln(a_{H+}) = E_G^0 + (2.3026\,RT/F)\,pH\,V, \tag{8.45}$$

where R is the SI gas constant [8.31 J/(mol K)], T is the kelvin temperature of the solution, F is the Faraday number (96,500), and 2.3026 comes from converting natural logs to $\log_{10}$.
The half-cell potential of the saturated calomel electrode is then:

$$E_{Cal} = 0.2415 - 7.6 \times 10^{-4}(t - 25°)\,V, \tag{8.46}$$

where t is the Celsius temperature.

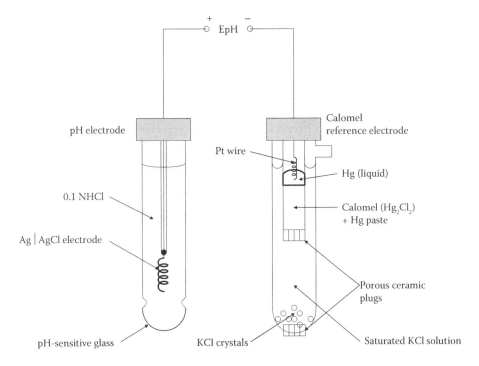

Figure 8.17 Glass pH electrode and calomel reference electrode cell used for measuring pH.

Thus, the net EMF of the pH cell at 25°C is:

$$E_{pH} = E_G^0 + (2.3026 \, RT/F) \, pH - 0.2415 = (E_G^0 - 0.2415) + 0.0591 \, (pH) \, V. \qquad (8.47)$$

Equation 8.47 can be solved for pH:

$$pH = \frac{E_{pH} - (E_G^0 - 0.2415)}{(2.3026 \, RT/F)} = \frac{E_{pH} - \Delta E_G}{0.0591} \text{ at } 25°C. \qquad (8.48)$$

The value of ΔE_G can be determined by calibration with a pH standard solution. ΔE_G is not only a function of temperature but is also different for each glass pH electrode. Commercial pH meters automatically compensate for test solution temperature, and once standardization is done, subtract a DC voltage from ΔE_G so that $E_{pH} = 0.1 \, (pH) \, V$. Thus, a voltmeter with a 0–1400 mV scale can be calibrated in 0–14 pH units. Modern pH meters have a precision of ± 0.01 pH unit, and can be read to ± 1.0 mV on an expanded (2 pH unit or 200 mV) analog scale.

Other ISEs are used in laboratory medicine to measure: NH_4^+, Ca^{++}, Cl^-, CN^-, I^-, Pb^{++}, NO_3^-, NO_2^-, K^+, Na^+, SCN^-, etc. Unless the ISE is combined with the RE in the same housing, each ISR requires a corresponding RE half-cell (usually calomel). *All* ISEs suffer what is known as *interferences* from certain other ions that may be in solution with the analyte. For example, Metrohm® ISEs offer a Cl^--responding electrode with a crystal membrane having a sensitivity range of 5×10^{-5} mol/L to 1 mol/L. This electrode develops erroneous readings in the presence of Hg^{++}, Br^-, I^-, $S^=$, CN^-, NH_3, and $S_2O_3^=$ ions. The Metrohm Na^+ electrode (also known as Ross electrode) has a glass membrane (not unlike a pH electrode) and measures in the range of 1×10^{-5} to 1 mol/L; it is interfered with by $pH > (pNa + 4)$, Ag^+, Li^+, and K^+ ions. pH, silver, and lithium are not normally a problem in biological fluids, but potassium is, and would have to be corrected for. Similarly, the Metrohm K^+ electrode is interfered with by Cs^+, NH_4^+, H^+, and Na^+. The concentrations of cesium and ammonium ions are normally negligible, the pH is relatively constant, and sodium must be compensated for in bio-samples. Some ISEs have polymer membranes, the Na^+ electrode has a glass membrane, and others use a LaF_3 crystal membrane. For example, Pb^{++} and Cl^- electrodes both use crystal membranes, but K^+ and other Cl^- electrodes use plastic membranes. In all ISEs, as in the glass pH electrode, there is an ion-selective barrier (membrane, glass,

159

or crystal), an inner electrolyte, and an inner half-cell. The EMF of an ISE measurement system will generally be of the form:

$$E_i = \Delta E_i - (RT/F)\ln(a_i)\ V, \tag{8.49}$$

where the activity on the ionic analyte is approximated by its molar concentration. If the ion is divalent, such as Ca^{++}, then F is replaced by 2F in Equation 8.49.

Some of the companies that make ISEs are: Beckman Coulter, Inc., Fullerton, OR; Thermo Scientific™, Orion™, ISEs; Hanna Instruments®, Inc., ISEs; Vernier Software & Technology, LLC, Beaverton, OR (www.vernier.com); Metrohm, USA, Inc., Riverview, FL, ISEs; PASCO Scientific, Roseville, CA, ISEs; WTW GmbH, ISEs; METTLER TOLEDO, ISEs; Radiometer Analytical (www. radiometer-analytical.com), ISEs; Cole-Parmer, ISEs.

8.2.6 Flame Photometry

The flame photometer is a relatively inexpensive instrument that is used to determine, *in vitro,* the concentration of physiologically and medically important ions in body fluids such as urine, CSF, and blood plasma. (Of course, invasive procedures are used to collect samples of blood and CSF.) There are two types of flame photometer: The *flame emission spectroscope* (FES), and the *atomic absorption spectroscope* (AAS). Both instruments are described in this section.

FES and AAS are effective in determining the concentrations of the ions of: As, Cd, Ca, Cu, Li, Mg, Hg, K, Rb, Na, etc. in solution. FES is also responsive to the noble gases, the halogens, hydrogen, nitrogen, oxygen, phosphorus, sulfur, Se, and Te (Tel Aviv U. 2015). However, As, Pt, and Zn have relatively high LODs.

As we have seen in Section 8.1, the concentrations of Na^+, K^+, Ca^{++}, Mg^{++} in various body fluids can be used in the diagnosis of many diseases, conditions, and hormonal disorders. Lithium (as carbonate or citrate) is medically important in the treatment of manic-depressive (bipolar) mental illness. The heavy metals, As, Cd, Cu, and Hg, are toxic, and are associated with environmental heavy-metal poisoning.

Figure 8.18 illustrates the architecture of a typical FES instrument. A key component is the burner in which a *fuel* (e.g., H_2, acetylene (C_2H_2), propane, etc.) is mixed with either air or pure O_2. An aerosol of the solution containing the ion to be measured (the analyte) is injected into the base of the flame. All three flows are made constant to insure a stable flame and a stable level of atomic emission. Table 8.2 below gives the approximate flame temperatures for various fuel-oxidizer conditions. Note that the oxyacetylene flame has the highest temperature.

The heat of the flame vaporizes the sample constituents without chemical change. The combination of high temperature and the fuel (reducing gas) decomposes and reduces the analyte ions to *atomic form* in vapor phase. (For example, a Na^+ ion picks up an electron.) The high temperature excites the outer shell electrons of some atoms to higher-energy states. As the excited atoms rise, they cool, and the high-energy state electrons fall back into their normal orbits with the emission of photons of wavelength $\lambda = hc\Delta E$, where $\Delta E \equiv (E_e - E_g)$ in joules, h is Planck's constant (6.624×10^{-34} J s), c is the speed of light *in vacuo* (2.998×10^8 m/s), E_g is the ground state energy of the outer electron, E_e is the excited state energy of that electron, and λ is in meters.

In the gas phase, excited elements such as Li, Na, and K emit multiple, unique, narrow, line spectra. For example, the principle emission lines of Na are at 330.2 nm (600), 330.3 (300), 568.26 (50), 568.82 (300), 589.00 (9000), 589.60 (5000); here wavelengths are in nm, and the numbers in parentheses are relative intensities. Potassium's strongest lines are at 766.50 (9000) and 770.00 (5000) nm. All biological fluids contain both K^+ and Na^+, so either optical interference bandpass filters or a simple grating monochromator can be used to select the unique strong lines for measurement.

The intensity response versus analyte concentration is sigmoid as shown in Figure 8.19. The reasons for this sigmoid curve are easy to understand. It has a low slope at low-analyte concentration (region A) because emission is lower due to reionization of the reduced metal analyte (e.g., $K \rightarrow K^+ + e^-$). At higher concentrations, there is little reionization. The mid-region (B) is linear with intensity proportional to concentration or the number of atoms emitting/s. Finally, at high concentrations, (region C), there is self-absorption of emitted photons by other ground-state atoms in the flame. If a sample is introduced, and the resulting line intensity exceeds I_H, usual practice is to dilute the sample to a known amount to bring the resulting emission intensity back into the linear region where $I(C, \lambda) = b + mC$. If the intensity is below I_L, then vacuum evaporation of the solvent can be used to increase the analyte concentration.

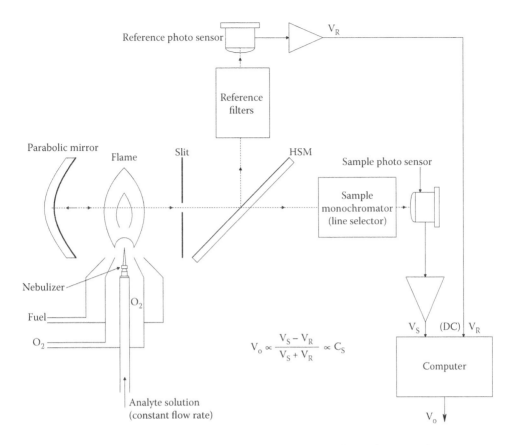

Figure 8.18 Schematic of a flame emission spectroscope. Two channels are used to compensate for intensity noise in the flame.

Other design features of the typical AES instrument include a parabolic mirror to concentrate emission line intensity, a slit to restrict beam width entering the sample monochromator which selects the analyte's principal emission line(s). The HSM splits the beam into the sample beam and a reference beam which is passed through a filter that excludes the analyte's line(s). The reference beam is used to compensate for random fluctuations in flame intensity as shown in Figure 8.18.

The key to flame photometer accuracy is calibration. Two concentrations of standard solutions of an analyte are used to obtain the constants b and m in the $I(C, \lambda)$ relation above. Two-point calibration must also be used with the AAS.

A diagram of a typical AAS instrument is shown in Figure 8.20. This is a more complex instrument than the FES described above. Here the flame is used as a narrowband, Beer's law absorber of light from a special, *hollow-cathode lamp* (HCL). The cathode of the HCL is a hollow cylinder with a cupped end made from or coated with the element whose concentration is to be measured. The anode is generally a tungsten wire. The interior of the HCL is filled with He or Ar at 1–2 mmHg pressure. A high-voltage pulse is used to make a momentary spark which ionizes the gas. Gas ions

Table 8.2: Flame Temperatures for Different Fuel–Oxidizer Mixes

Oxidizer	Fuel	Flame Temp., K
Air	H_2	2000–2100
Air	C_2H_2	2100–2400
O_2	H_2	2600–2700
O_2	C_2H_2	2600–2800

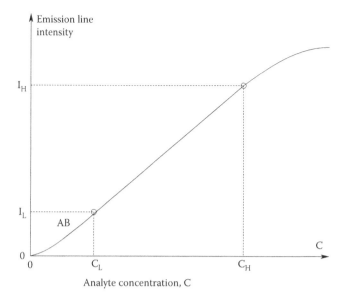

Figure 8.19 Flame emission intensity versus analyte concentration is a sigmoid curve at a selected wavelength with a linear region between C_L and C_H.

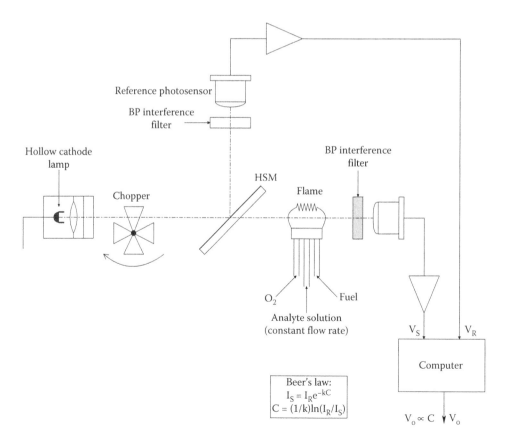

Figure 8.20 Schematic of a flame atomic absorption spectroscope (AAS).

are given velocity by the internal DC **E** field and strike the cathode heating it and forming more gas ions which bombard it. The hot cathode emits the line spectra characteristic of its coating element (the same lines seen from the flame of the FES above). Along with the element's line energy, there is blackbody IR from the hot cathode, and emission lines from the gas. The HCL output beam is chopped before it reaches the flame so that a phase-sensitive detector can discriminate against the flame's intrinsic, DC emission lines. The flame is made long (~10 cm) and narrow; the test solution is atomized into it similar to the FES instrument's flame.

The chopped beam from the HCL passes through the flame and the specific emission line(s) from the HCL interact with the ground state (un-ionized) analyte atoms. The amount emission-line-wavelength light from the chopped HCL beam absorbed is proportional to the density of ground-state analyte atoms in the flame. At the line wavelength, the exiting beam intensity, I_s, is given by the Beer–Lambert law:

$$I_s = I_{in}exp(-kC), \qquad (8.50)$$

where C is the analyte concentration in the sample, and k is a constant proportional to the length the beam travels in the flame.

Note that a reference beam is again used to compensate for fluctuations in the HCL output intensity as it warms up. The analyte aspirated into the flame emits the same line(s) as the HCL. However, the AAS instrument does not respond to it because it is a DC signal. Only the chopper-modulated intensity, I_s, is sensed. The AAS instrument is not as flexible as the FES because a new HCL must be used for each different analyte measured.

The detection limits for the FES and AAS instruments for certain elements are shown in Table 8.3.

While detection sensitivity of an AAS to certain analytes can be very high, overall accuracy of this type of flame spectrophotometer is not high. Qi (1990) reported that the percent standard deviations for the measurement of Cu, Zn, Fe, Ca, Mg, Na, and K in human serum with a Varian "SpectrAA-40" AAS system were 2.2, 2.9, 3.9, 1.3, 1.7, 0.8, and 3.1, respectively. Ten samples of each analyte were measured. The line wavelengths used were: 324.8, 213.9, 248.3, 422.7, 202.5, 330.3, and 404.5 nm, respectively. For each measurement, 10 mL of 1:10 diluted serum were required.

A partial list of manufacturers of commercial AAS flame photometers includes: Sherwood Scientific Ltd.; Labtronics, Haryana, India; Jenway (bibby-scientific.com); Buck Scientific (model PFP-7 and –7C); Spectrolab Systems; PG Instruments (Leicester, UK); Perkin-Elmer; Agilent Technologies (Santa Clara, CA); Shimadzu Corp.; Varian (AA220Z Graphite furnace atomic absorption spectrometer), etc. Many AAS instruments have 8-lamp turrets to permit rapid sequential analysis of eight different analytes. FES instruments include those made by SEAC (FP10 & FP20), and Jenway (PFP7). Precision and reproducibility error for FES instruments are generally about 1%.

It should be noted that a new technique called electrothermal atomic absorption (also known as graphite furnace atomic absorption spectrometry [GFAAS]) has detection limits that are about 1000 times more sensitive (in the ng/mL range) than AAS and FES instruments. Dickson (2010) described the application of a Thermo Scientific iCE 3500 Atomic Absorption (GFAA) Spectrometer to test samples of chocolate for cadmium. The provisional tolerable weekly intake (PTWI) of Cd is currently 7 μg/kg body weight. Typical maximum levels of Cd in foodstuffs are currently between 0.05–0.2 mg/kg wet weight. Excessive ingestion of Cd can cause nausea, gastrointestinal pain, softening of the bones, and kidney damage. Cd accumulates within the kidneys and can eventually

Table 8.3: Detection Limits (LODs) in ng/mL for Selected Elements Using FES and AAS

Element	AAS LOD	FES LOD
Ca	1	0.1
Cu	2	1
Hg	500	4×10^{-4}
Mg	0.01	5
Na	2	0.1
Pb	1	100
Zn	2	5×10^{-4}

cause renal failure (Dickson 2010). The maximum [Cd] in the chocolate samples studied was 40 μg/kg, and the method detection limit (LOD) was reported as 0.029 μg/L (29 pg/L).

8.2.7 Gas Chromatography

GC is an exquisitely sensitive chemical analytical tool that is very competitive with spectrophotometry in terms of the analytes it can quantify in medically derived samples. If an analyte is stable (does not decompose) when in the gas or vapor phase at temperatures up to 400°C, it probably can be identified and quantified by GC. GC works by the simple principle that the volatile components of a sample injected as a bolus travel though the GC's column at different speeds. Each sample component is adsorbed by the column's stationary phase and then released forming a continuous traveling wave of adsorbed component in the carrier gas. The speed of a given traveling wave depends on many physical and chemical factors of the GC system. Of particular importance is the fact that there is very little dispersion (broadening) of an individual analyte's peak as it propagates through the column. Thus, the time that a particular analyte exits the column is peculiar to that analyte, given identical conditions of carrier gas composition, carrier gas flow rate, column temperature, column length and inside diameter, and column stationary phase adsorber. A GC is well-suited to separate mixtures of analytes in samples of complex composition. A GC can be used to identify and quantify such biochemicals as alcohol, acetone, various steroid hormones, drugs such as various tricyclic antidepressants, theophylline, various opioids, etc. The schematic of a typical GC system is shown in Figure 8.21.

A basic GC has seven key components: (1) A source of an *inert carrier gas,* such as dry nitrogen, helium, or argon. The gas literally carries the sample and analyte through the column. (2) A sample injection port. (3) The *capillary column* is a long, thin tube of stainless steel, or fused silica coated on the outside with polyimide resin. Column lengths can range from 10 to 60 m, with 20–30 m being most typical. The *resolution* of a GC (ability to separate two nearly coincident eluent peaks) is proportional to the square root of the column length. Capillary column diameter is typically from 0.32 to 0.25 mm. As column diameter decreases, the retention of a given solute will increase, other factors being constant. This means that a smaller diameter column provides better resolution (wider separation of the eluent peaks). (4) The inside of a GC column is coated with a thin layer of a thermally and chemically stable *stationary phase absorber* (SPA). The thickness of the SPA is another critical parameter affecting GC separation resolution. A thicker SPA will give greater solute retention, hence better resolution of adjacent eluent peaks. SPA thicknesses can range from 0.25 to 1 μm

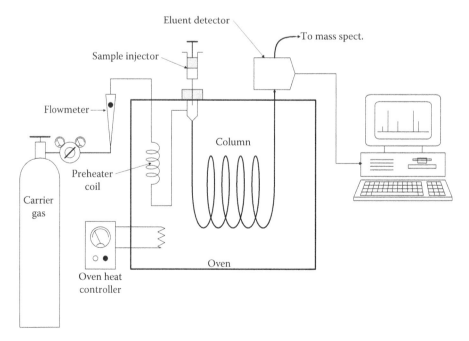

Figure 8.21 Schematic of a modern gas chromatograph. Several different types of eluent detectors can be used. Detector output (exhaust) can be further analyzed using a mass spectrometer.

in capillary columns; the SPA coats the inside walls of the column. The materials used for SPAs are described below. (5) The entire column is placed inside an *oven* that heats the capillary column. The oven temperature can be held constant or programmed to increase (e.g., from 80°C to 280°C at 5°C/min). The temperature limits and rate of increase are set according to the particular analysis. (6) A *detector* senses the changes in eluent gas composition from pure carrier gas when boluses of sample constituents (and the desired analyte) exit the column. There are many kinds of detectors; these are described in detail below. Detector sensitivities allow limits of detection ranging from 100 ppm to 100 ppb (analyte to carrier gas). (7) The detector output consists of voltage peaks of different heights and widths from sample components that exit the column at different times. A complete GC run may take from 5 to 30 min; GCs are not fast instruments. The GC detector output voltage is digitized, and the GC's computer integrates each peak to determine the concentration of each sample component (eluent), including the desired analyte. An analyte sample of known concentration is injected into the column for calibration purposes. The time it exits is peculiar to that analyte, and its area is proportional to the concentration, providing it is in the linear range of the column and detector.

There are many types of GC detectors. Some types of detectors respond to any analyte exiting from the column, others are specific for certain chemical classes of eluents, such as chlorinated hydrocarbon insecticides. As in many branches of measurements, the threshold detection concentration and resolution of a GC system are set primarily by noise arising in the detector and its electronic amplifiers. The *minimum detectable amount* (MDA) of an eluent is defined as the concentration or amount of analyte that will produce a minimum output peak voltage twice the RMS noise voltage. Thus, the practical lower limit of detector operation is set by its MDA. All GC detectors also have a linear dynamic range (LDR) of analyte concentration above their MDAs in which their outputs follow the linear relation: $V_o = b + m[A]$ to within ±5%.

[A] is the analyte concentration in g/mL, or ppm. In Table 8.4 are listed the names and characteristics of some GC detectors.

We shall examine the operating mechanisms of two of these detectors in detail. The thermal conductivity detector (TCD) is one of the simplest, general-purpose GC detectors; it is generally used with helium carrier gas. Figure 8.22 illustrates the circuit of this detector. Note that it is a simple Wheatstone bridge; the resistors of two opposite arms are surrounded with carrier plus eluent gases at temperature T_C, the other two arms are surrounded with pure He at column

Table 8.4: Summary Characteristics of the Major Eluent Detectors Used in Gas Chromatography

Detector Type	MDA (g/mL)	LDR (decades)	Comments
Thermal conductivity detector (TCD)	10^{-7}	≈5	A general detector used with He carrier gas. Temp. differences on Wheatstone bridge resistor arms due to analyte sensed
Flame ionization detector (FID)	10^{-12}	5–7	A mass-sensitive detector for C–H bonds. H_2 is burned, creating ions from analytes
Photoionization detector (PID)	10^{-12}	5–6	Sensitive to aromatics and olefins. Uses 10.2 eV UV lamp to ionize analytes
Electron capture detector (ECD)	10^{-14}	3–4	Uses radioisotopes to ionize halogens, quinones, peroxides, and nitro groups. Used for insecticides and PCBs
Flame photometric detector (FPD)	10^{-11}	3–5	Used for S- or P-containing analytes. H_2 flame causes atomic emission of S at 394 nm and P at 526 nm. A PMT is used
Electrical conductivity detector (ELCD)	5–10 pg (halogens) 10–20 pg (S) 10–20 pg (N)	5–6 4–4 3–4	Eluents react at high T with reaction gas. Products dissolved in solven are passed through electrical conductivity cell
Mass spectrometry (MS)	1–10 pg (selected ion-monitoring mode)	5–6	A mass spectrometer replaces detector. The MS measures the mass/charge ratio of ions fragmented at high T by e^- bombardment
Nitrogen–Phosphorus detector (NPD)	1–10 pg	4–6	Similar to FID except uses *rhubidium bead* to enhance sensitivity to N compounds by X50 and P compounds by X500

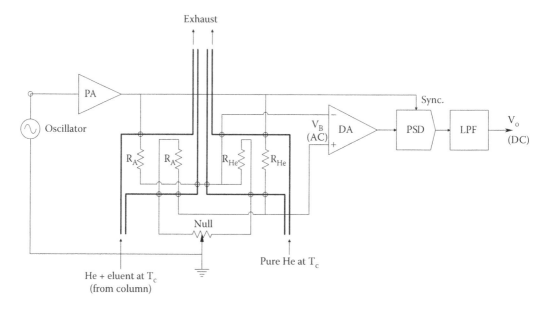

Figure 8.22 Schematic of a Wheatstone bridge, thermal conductivity eluent detector and associated circuitry. See text for analysis.

temperature, T_C, and pressure. The resistors are platinum or nichrome. Current is passed through the bridge arms so that they heat to a temperature, T_B, above T_C. The moving helium gas surrounding the resistors conducts heat away from them lowering their temperature toward T_C. (Helium is unique in that it has a very high heat conductivity.) The drop in resistor temperature is given by the relation:

$$(T_B - T_R) = \Delta T = P_R \Theta_R > 0, \quad T_B < T_R < T_C, \tag{8.51}$$

where T_R is the actual equilibrium resistor temperature in moving He, T_B is the reference temperature, P_R is the electrical power dissipated in each resistor, and Θ_R is the thermal resistance seen by a resistor in moving He. In general, $\Theta_R = \Theta_{Ro} + \beta[A]$. That is, the eluent analyte gas *decreases the ability* of the pure He to conduct heat away from the two R_A resistors. Θ_{Ro} and β are positive constants, and [A] is the eluent analyte concentration in the He carrier gas. A metal resistor has a *positive tempco*, that is, its resistance increases as its temperature increases. This property can be approximated by the relation:

$$R(\Delta T) \cong R_o(1 + \alpha \Delta T), \quad \alpha > 0. \tag{8.52}$$

R_o is the resistance at the reference temperature, T_B. If we combine relations 8.51 and 8.52, we can write:

$$\Delta T = I_B^2 R_o(1 + \alpha \Delta T)\Theta_R. \tag{8.53}$$

Solving for the equilibrium ΔT, we find:

$$\Delta T = \frac{I_B^2 R_o \Theta_R}{\left(1 - \alpha I_B^2 R_o \Theta_R\right)}. \tag{8.54}$$

I_B^2 is the mean-squared AC current through each resistor (assumed constant). $I_B \cong V_s/2R_{He}$. Knowing the temperature drop, we can find the resistance from relation 8.54:

$$R(\Delta T) = \frac{R_o}{\left(1 - \alpha I_B^2 R_o \Theta_R\right)} \tag{8.55}$$

For pure He:

$$R_{He} = \frac{R_o}{\left(1 - \alpha I_B^2 R_o \Theta_{Ro}\right)}.$$ (8.56)

When an eluent analyte ([A]) is present, Equation 8.55 becomes:

$$R_A = \frac{R_o}{[1 - \alpha I_B^2 R_o (\Theta_{R_o} + \beta[A])]} = \frac{R_o}{[1 - \alpha I_B^2 R_o \Theta_{R_o} (1 + \beta[A]/\Theta_{R_o})]}.$$ (8.57)

Now, the general relation for Wheatstone bridge unbalance voltage with two active arms is:

$$V_B = V_1 - V_2 = V_s \frac{R_A}{R_{He} + R_A} - V_s \frac{R_{He}}{R_{He} + R_A}.$$ (8.58)

So

$$\frac{V_B}{V_s} = \frac{R_A - R_{He}}{R_A + R_{He}} = \frac{\dfrac{R_o}{[1 - \alpha I_B{}^2 R_o \Theta_{Ro}(1 + \beta[A]/\Theta_{Ro})]} - \dfrac{R_o}{[1 - \alpha I_B{}^2 R_o \Theta_{Ro}]}}{\dfrac{R_o}{[1 - \alpha I_B{}^2 R_o \Theta_{Ro}(1 + \beta[A]/\Theta_{Ro})]} + \dfrac{R_o}{[1 - \alpha I_B{}^2 R_o \Theta_{Ro}]}}.$$ (8.59)

After some algebra, Equation 8.59 reduces to:

$$\frac{V_B}{V_s} \cong \left(R_{He}/2\right) \alpha I_B^2 \beta[A].$$ (8.60)

That is, the balanced bridge output is zero, and any eluent gas mixed with He will *reduce* the cooling (increase Θ_R), allowing the two R_A resistors to warm slightly, raising their resistance, unbalancing the bridge, and thus producing an output, V_B. An advantage of the TCD is that no chemical change occurs in the eluents. Thus, they can be individually captured by condensation in nearly pure form, or passed on to another type of detector for more detailed analysis such as an MS.

The *electron capture detector* (ECD) is an exquisitely sensitive means of detecting chlorinated pesticide residues and PCBs in and on foods, and in humans and animals. Mass sensitivities to halogenated hydrocarbons from 0.1 to 10 pg are possible with the ECD. Figure 8.23 illustrates a schematic cross-section of an ECD. Ionization is caused by beta particle-emitting isotopes of either tritium (^{3}H) or nickel (^{63}Ni) foil. The electrons are accelerated to and captured by the anode electrode. Chlorinated hydrocarbon molecules in the detector chamber capture some of the radio-electrons and reduce the net anode current signifying the presence of the analyte. The ECD is insensitive to amines, alcohols, and hydrocarbons. The carrier gases used with ECD are N_2 or Ar/CH_4; gas temperature ranges from 300°C to 400°C.

As you can see from Table 8.4, many other application-specific detectors exist. The interested reader should consult Lab Training (2012) for a description of GC detectors and GC technology.

Common stationary phase, GC column coatings (or fillings) range from the mundane zeolite particles (kitty litter), to styrene beads, aluminum oxide particles, to a host of thermally stable liquid polymers, such as the various polysiloxanes and polyethene glycols used with capillary columns. The solid-phase, porous layer open tubular (PLOT) columns are very retentive, and are used to separate analytes whose peaks may be nearly coincident using a conventional capillary column.

In 2001, Yu and Koo of the Lawrence Livermore National Laboratory described a spiral capillary GC column micromachined on a silicon wafer. The object of the instrument development was to create a field-portable GC with rapid response time (~2 min) to sense environmental pollutants. The weight of this GC was ~8 pounds, it measured 8 × 5 × 3″, it consumed ~12 W of electrical power, had a response time on the order of 2 min. It used a glow discharge detector with a sensitivity in the ppb.

Commercial GCs are generally heavy, bench-top instruments because of their ovens, gas supplies, and associated computers. The columns and detectors are relatively compact, however. GC manufacturers and vendors include, but are not limited to: Agilent, APIX Technology, Bruker,

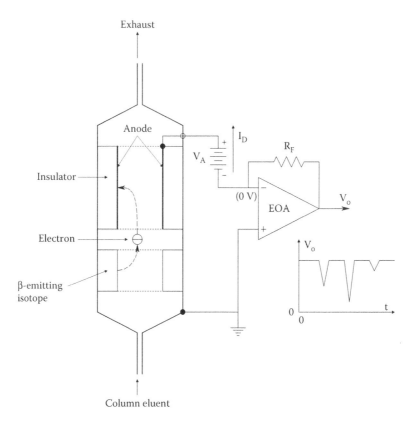

Figure 8.23 Schematic of an electron capture detector used to sense chlorinated hydrocarbon eluents.

Buck Scientific, CDS Analytical, Chemtron Science Laboratory Pvt. Ltd., Defiant Technologies (Frog-4000™ portable GCs), DIAMON Testing Instruments, Falcon Analytical, Gen Tech, GOW-MAC Instrument Co., Inrag, JEOL USA, LECO, Parker-Balston, Perkin-Elmer, Emerson-Daniel (Danalyzer Gas Chromatographs), Quadrex Corp., Shimadzu Corp., Shinbiro, SRI Instruments, Teledyne Tekmar, Thermo-Fisher Scientific, ThermoQuest Corp., Torion, Waters, and Zoex (Lab Manager 2014).

8.2.8 Mass Spectrometry

The MS is another important analytical instrument used in medical diagnosis (Young 1996). While instruments like spectrophotometers and GCs allow investigators to examine intact molecules, the flame photometer and the MS gain their analytical information by breaking molecules apart. In an MS, the sample molecules are bombarded with energetic electrons, moving atoms or photons from a laser beam to break them into component parts; some parts are positively charged (are positive ions or cations), others can be neutral (i.e., have zero charge; they are lost), and negatively charged ions (anions) can also be produced under the right conditions. An MS can perform analysis of elements (isotopes), compounds, and mixtures. It can use gas, liquid, or solid samples, and is fairly rapid yielding results in seconds rather than minutes, as for a GC.

A basic magnetic sector MS design is shown in Figure 8.24. The positive ions are first accelerated in a DC electric field, $E_1 = V_1/d_1$. At the exit slit, S_2, it can be shown that the positive ions having a positive charge magnitude of one electron (q) and a mass m will have a velocity:

$$v = \sqrt{2qV_1/m} \text{ m/s}. \tag{8.61}$$

That is, the velocity is inversely proportional to the square root of the ion's mass. Positive ions with a distribution of velocities determined by their masses next enter a *velocity filter* formed by

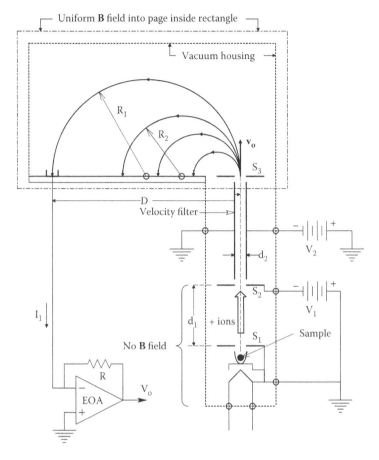

Figure 8.24 Plan view schematic of a conventional magnetic mass spectrometer.

two electrodes parallel to the velocities of the entering ions. The positive ions are attracted to the cathode by a force $\mathbf{F_e} = \mathbf{E_2}q = (V_2/d_2)q\mathbf{i}$. ($\mathbf{i}$ is a unit vector pointing at the cathode.) Because there is a $\mathbf{B}$ field perpendicular to the velocity (into page), the moving ions also experience a magnetic Lorenz force, $\mathbf{F_m} = q(\mathbf{v} \times \mathbf{B})$, the direction of which is given by the *right-hand screw rule*. That is, $\mathbf{F_m}$ points in the direction that a normal right-hand screw would advance if rotated in the direction of rotating vector $\mathbf{v}$ into $\mathbf{B}$. Thus, $\mathbf{F_m}$ is opposite to $\mathbf{F_e}$. Because of the narrow separation (d_2) of the velocity filter's electrodes, only positive ions with velocities such that $F_m \cong F_e$ emerge through slit S_3. This selected velocity can be shown to be:

$$\mathbf{v_o} \cong V_2/(d_2\mathbf{B}) \text{ m/s.} \tag{8.62}$$

Again, the ions with velocity $\mathbf{v_o}$ are acted on by the Lorenz force in the $\mathbf{E}$ field-free chamber of the MS. Because $\mathbf{B}$ is perpendicular to $\mathbf{v_o}$, the ion trajectories are semicircular. The ions strike the detector electrodes at a distance $D = 2R$ from S_3. Basic physics (Sears 1953) tells us that:

$$D = 2R = (2\mathbf{v_o}m)/(q\,\mathbf{B}) = (m/q)\frac{2V_2}{d_2\mathbf{B}^2} \text{ m.} \tag{8.63}$$

Thus, the distance D at which the ion beam strikes the collector is proportional to the ratio of mass to charge (m/q) of the ion exiting the velocity filter. The + ion beam at D can be collected by an electrode (Faraday cup), and the resulting electron current, I_1, converted to a voltage, V_o, by an electrometer op-amp connected as a transresitor.

Compound identification and quantification can also be carried out on analytes with mass ranges less than 10^3 Daltons by *negative ion mass spectroscopy* (NIMS). Negative ions are created in

Table 8.5:   Commonly Lost Mass Fragments

Approximate Mass	Fragment
15	$-CH_3$
17	$-OH$
26	$-CN$
28	$H_2C=CH_2$
29	$-CH_2CH_3$, $-CHO$
31	$-OCH_3$
35	$-Cl$
43	$CH_3C=O$
45	$-OCH_2CH_3$
91	Benzine$-CH_2$

Source: Young, P.R. 1996. *Mass Spectrometry—Background.* Organic Chemistry OnLine. Accessed 1/12/16 at: people.stfx.ca/ tsmithpa/chem361/labs/spec/MS1.htm

a sample by *resonance electron capture,* or direct ionization by low-energy electron bombardment of the sample through a buffer gas such as methane. The methane gas slows down the electrons and stabilizes the resultant *anions.* Now the anions are accelerated through an electric field toward an anode, thence a velocity filter, thence into the magnet chamber. The anions bend to the right, however, because the Lorenz force has the opposite sign.

Unless the investigator has an *a priori* knowledge that a certain compound is present in a sample, identification of a molecular species from its mass fragment peaks can often be challenging. Table 8.5 illustrates commonly lost mass fragments that lack + charges and thus cannot produce peaks (they cannot be accelerated).

Figure 8.25 shows some common stable mass fragment cations (Young 1996). In the analysis of biochemical and drug molecules from respiratory gases, urine, stool, blood, and tissue samples, the investigator often knows the molecules to expect, and thus an MS system can be setup or "tuned" for a specific molecule in terms of the ionization method, and the expected Ds for the expected group of anions. A given analyte molecule can produce as many as 10 or more anions when fragmented and ionized. As in GC, the integral of a peak's area is proportional to the quantity of an ion present.

Approximate mass	Common stable cations
43	$CH_3-\overset{+}{C}\equiv O$
91	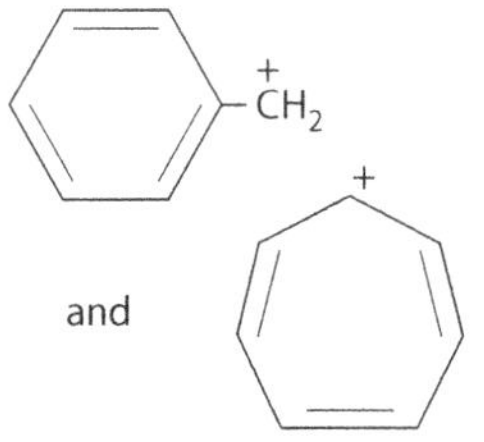 and
$m \rightarrow m^{-1}$	$\overset{O+}{\underset{R\ H}{\overset{\|\|}{C}}} \longrightarrow R\ \overset{+}{C}\equiv O$

Figure 8.25   Some common stable mass fragments encountered in mass spectrometry. (Based on data from Young (1996).)

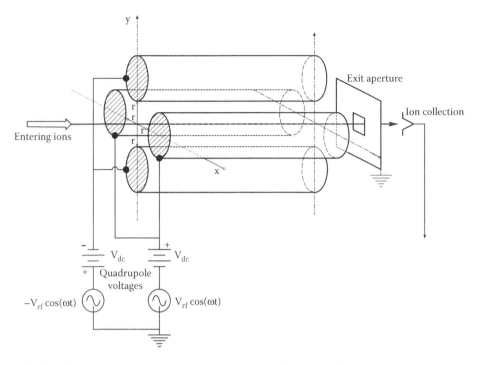

Figure 8.26 View of a quadrupole mass spectrometer. No magnetic field is used.

General-purpose MS instruments with few exceptions are generally large, heavy, and fixed. Smaller, portable MS systems have been designed to measure respiratory gases such as O_2, CO_2, N_2, Halothane, etc. Ion ambiguities exist so that O_2 and CO_2 cannot be measured when ether ($C_4H_{10}O$) or N_2O is present (Webster 1992). N_2 and carbon monoxide also have the same mass number (28).

The *quadrupole MS* (QPMS) was developed in the mid-1950s by Wolfgang Paul and associates at the University of Bonn. The QPMS is a lighter, more portable instrument than conventional magnetic MSs because its ion selectivity does not depend on a magnetic field (or the need for heavy magnets). Instead, ion selectivity depends entirely on the interaction of moving ions with combined AC and DC electric fields maintained between four cylindrical electrodes as shown in Figure 8.26. The voltage applied to the two electrode pairs is the sum of a DC potential and an AC, RF voltage; $V_+ = V_{DC} + V_{rf} \cos(\omega t)$, and $V_- = -[V_{DC} + V_{rf} \cos(\omega t)]$. The QPMS is "tuned" for specific m/q values by linearly increasing the V_{DC} voltage between 0 and 300 V, while simultaneously increasing the peak RF voltage, V_{rf}, from 0 to 1.5 kV. It can be shown that the complex electric field between the tubes causes the entering ions to effectively "run the gauntlet." If an ion has an inappropriate mass/charge ratio, it will collide with an attracting tube and loose its $\oplus$ charge. Such noncharged molecular fragments are pumped out by the vacuum system. An ion with the "tuned" mass/charge will describe a spiral or corkscrew path between the electrodes, emerging through the exit window and striking the ion collector; its charge contributes to the collector current. The voltages on the QPMS's electrodes are increased linearly in time providing a swept tuning of the mass/charge. As the voltages increase, larger and larger mass ions can pass through the quadrupole electrodes without collision. Thus by plotting current peaks from the detector versus the electrode sweep voltage, one can obtain a rapid mass spectrogram. The computer plots relative ion current versus (mass number/charge number) (m/z) (dimensionless). The advantages of QPMSs are that they are relatively inexpensive, smaller, and faster (a scan completed in milliseconds) than conventional electrostatic/magnetic sector MS systems. They also give relative mass readings, have good reproducibility, but do not have the resolution of conventional MSs. Like GCs, QPMS machines must be calibrated with standard samples. Figure 8.27 shows a spectrogram for a methanol sample. Note that the molecular ion has the highest (32) m/z ratio. Relative abundances of the fragments are peculiar to the ionization method used. The very small peaks are due to the natural presence of isotopes of C, H, and O in methanol (Table 8.6). Figure 8.28 illustrates a typical QPMS spectrum of exhaled air.

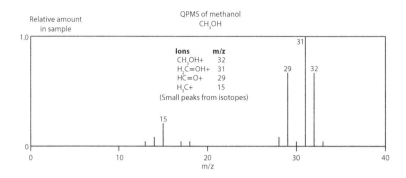

Figure 8.27 Quadrupole mass spectrogram for methanol. Peaks are from various +-charged mass fragments, as well as from the same fragments containing stable element isotopes, giving the fragments slightly different masses. m is the *mass number*, z is the *charge number* (e.g., +1, +2, ...), m/z is *dimensionless*.

Table 8.6: Relative Abundance of Some Naturally Occurring, Nonradioactive Isotopes

Natural Isotope at 100%	Isotope and Rel. Abundance	Isotope and Rel. Abundance
Carbon: ^{12}C	^{13}C: 1.11	
Hydrogen: ^{1}H	^{2}H: 0.16	
Nitrogen: ^{14}N	^{15}N: 0.38	
Oxygen: ^{16}O	^{17}O: 0.04	^{18}O: 0.20
Sulfur: ^{32}S	^{33}S: 0.78	^{34}S: 4.40
Chlorine: ^{35}Cl		^{37}Cl: 32.5
Bromine: ^{79}Br		^{81}Br: 98.0

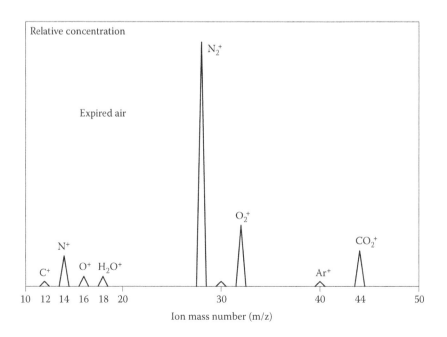

Figure 8.28 Representative quadrupole mass spectrogram of exhaled air.

From the table, for example, we see that for every 100 ^{12}C atoms, we will find 1.11 ^{13}C atoms, while for every 100 ^{79}Br atoms, we find 98 ^{81}Br atoms, a surprisingly large ratio. Thus, a mass spectrogram of a compound containing a bromine atom will exhibit curious double peaks of almost the same size for those ions containing Br.

Several other types of MS exist in addition to the QPMS and magnetic sector MS described above. These include, but are not limited to: the *Time-of Flight MS*, the *Ion Cyclotron Resonance MS*, and the *Fourier Transform Ion Cyclotron Resonance* (FTICR) *MS*.

In summary, we see that compound separation and identification using an MS can be a considerable challenge. An MS gives the total number of each constituent atom in a compound (the empirical formula), but can seldom provide clues about molecular structure that can be given, for example, by an optical spectrophotometer. Often a molecular formula is found by trial and error from the ion mass peaks using information from isotope abundance as well. Because GCs separate pure compounds in time as they traverse the column, feeding the GC column output into an MS simplifies the analysis of an unknown sample under the assumption that the MS will be analyzing one pure eluent compound at a time. Hence, the popularity of GC/QPMS systems.

8.3 WHAT CAN BE LEARNED FROM URINE?

8.3.1 Introduction

Urine is derived from the glomerular filtrate of the kidneys, and is the result of many active and passive exchanges of ions and molecules with the filtrate as it passes through the loops of Henle and the collecting ducts of the kidneys. It is not our purpose here to describe in detail the complex functions of the kidneys in the production of urine, but to describe how substances in the urine can aid in the diagnosis of disease. Urine is either collected noninvasively by a mid-stream catch or clinically by a sterile catheter (a "moderately invasive" procedure).

"Normal" parameters for substances and ions in a healthy person's urine have statistical ranges that can be characterized by means and standard deviations. In Table 8.7, we list the ±1 SD ranges for normal urine contents and parameters:

Table 8.7: Normal Clearance Rates of Ions and Molecules in Urine

Substance	Normal Clearance Range or Concentration
Acetone	0
pH	5.5–7.5
Albumin	0
Ammonia	0.5–1.0 g/24 hour
Amylase	2200–3000 Somogyi units/24 hour
Bilirubin	0
Ca^{++}	100–150 mg/24 hour (4.8 mEq/L)
Cl^-	119 mEq/24 hour (134 mEq/L)
Creatine	<100 mg/24 hour
Creatinine	1.5–2.0 g/24 hour adult males (196 mEq/L) 0.8–1.5 g/24 hour adult females
Erythrocytes	<5.E5 cells/24 hour
Glucose	0.5–0.75 g/24 hour (0)
Leucocytes	1–2.E6/24 hour (1.–4.E3 cells/mL)
K^-	25–100 mEq/24 hour (60 mEq/L)
Na^+	111 mEq/24 hour (128 mEq/L)
Urea nitrogen	20–35 g/24 hour (1820 mEq/L)
Urobilinogen	0–4 mg/24 hour
Mg^{+-}	(15 mEq/L)
$H_2PO_4^- + HPO_4^=$	(50 mEq/L)

Source: Collins, R.D. 1968. *Illustrated Manual of Laboratory Diagnosis: Indications and Interpretations*. J.B. Lippincott Co., Phila; Concentrations in parentheses are from Table 27-1 in Guyton (1991). They are based on a urine production of 1.44 L/24 hour. (Note that these rates and concentrations can vary widely even under normal conditions, and will differ from tabular source to source.) (Note, e.g., E6 = 10^6.)

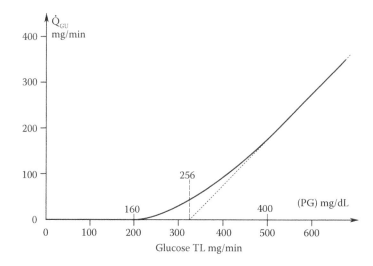

Figure 8.29 Well-known (to physiologists) curve describing glucose loss rate in urine when the plasma glucose concentration exceeds the level at which the kidneys can reabsorb glucose from the glomerular filtrate. Under normoglycemic conditions ~500–750 mg glucose is lost over 24 hours in the urine, or about 0.5 mg/min on the average.

One of the most basic diagnostic tests that can be done on urine is for *glucose*. Normally plasma glucose that is lost from the blood in glomerular filtrate is actively reabsorbed in the tubules and returned to the blood. However, this active reabsorption process can only handle about 320 mg/min (the *transport maximum*). If the blood glucose rises above ~160 mg/dL, then noticeable glucose begins to appear in the urine. When blood glucose exceeds ~260 mg/dL, then the glucose concentration in the urine rises linearly with the blood glucose concentration. This phenomenon is illustrated in Figure 8.29. High blood glucose can be the result of untreated diabetes mellitus. It can also be elevated in renal glycosuria, Cushing's syndrome, pancreatitis, acromegaly, and hyperthyroidism. Urine glucose concentration can be estimated with glucose-sensitive indicator paper, chemical color tests, or quantified with a glucose-specific (fuel-cell) redox electrode.

In cirrhosis of the liver and viral hepatitis, the concentration of urine *urobilinogen* can increase. Carcinoma of the head of the pancreas and gallstones both cause a decrease in urine urobilinogen (Collins 1968).

The urine concentration of Na^+ and K^+, and the pH and volume of urine can be correlated with a number of diseases and physiological conditions. The concentration of Na^+, K^+ can be measured with a flame photometer or specific ion electrodes; pH is measured with a special glass pH electrode. Table 8.8 summarizes some of these correlations.

Tests to determine the concentrations of certain hormones in the urine can also aid in the diagnosis of hormonal regulatory disorders. In Table 8.9, derived from data in Collins (1968), we illustrate the diseases and conditions associated with unbalances of urine *17-hydroxycorticosteroids, 17-ketosteroids, aldosterone,* and *gonadotropins*. At least 13 steroid hormones are made in the adrenal cortex; it is a busy place. The 17-hydroxycorticosteroids are produced from cholesterol in response to ACTH secreted by the anterior pituitary gland; they include the glucocorticoids hormones *progesterone* and *cortisol*. The 17-ketosteroids include the androgenic hormones *dehydroepiandosterone* (DEA), and *testosterone* (made in the testicles). The mineral corticoid, *aldosterone,* is also synthesized in the adrenal cortex (West 1985). Its principle role is in the regulation of plasma potassium ions (Northrop 2000). Human anterior pituitary *gonadotropin hormones* include the glycoproteins, *follicle-stimulating hormone,* and *luteinizing hormone*.

Means of measuring hormones, proteins, and ions in the urine include chemically treated *dipsticks, high-precision liquid chromatography, GC, electrophoresis,* immune methods including *immuno-electrophoresis, radioimmunoassays,* Abs-based *SPR,* and *specific ion electrodes* and *flame photometry* (for Na^+, K^+, Ca^{++}, etc.).

For example, certain urine protein (*proteinuria*) dipsticks respond to as little as 0.5–2.0 mg/mL albumin, the predominant protein found in most renal diseases, but are less sensitive to globulins

Table 8.8:   How Disorders of Blood Electrolytes Affect Na⁺, K⁺, pH, and Volume of Urine

Disease or Condition	Na^+	K^+	pH	Volume
Dehydration	↑	↑	↓	↓
Starvation	N or ↑	N or ↑	↓	↑ with ketones
Malabsorption syndrome (e.g., sprue)	↓	↓	↓	N
Congestive heart failure	↓	N	N	↓
Pyloric obstruction	↓	N	↑	↓
Diarrhea	↓	N or ↓	↓	↓
Diaphoresis with water replacement	↓	N	N	N
Acute renal failure	↓	↓	N or ↑	↓
Pulmonary emphysema	↓	N	↓	N
Salicylate toxicity[a]	↑	N or ↑	↑	N
Adrenal cortical insufficiency	↑	N or ↓	N or ↑	N or ↓
Diabetes insipidus (↓ ADH)	N	N	N	↑↑
Primary aldosteronism	↓	↓	N or ↓	↑
Chlorothiazide diuretics	↑	↑	N or ↑	↑
Hereditary renal tubular acidosis	↑	↑	↑	↑
Chronic renal failure	↑	↑	↑	variable ↑
Diabetic acidosis	↑	↑	↓	↑ with ketones

Source: Collins, R.D. 1968. *Illustrated Manual of Laboratory Diagnosis: Indications and Interpretations.* J.B. Lippincott Co., Phila.
Note: ↑, increase; ↓, decrease; N, no change.
[a] Same symptoms with fever, head trauma, high altitude, and hyperventilation syndrome.

Table 8.9:   Responses of Hormone Levels in Urine to Certain Disorders

Disease or Condition	17-Hydroxy-corticosteroids	17-Keto steroids	Aldosterone	Gonadotropins
Acromegaly	N	N	N	N
Basophilic adenoma of the pituitary	↑	↑	N	N
Panhypopituitarism	↓	↓	N	↓
Pituitary hypogonadism	N	↓	N	↓
Hyperthyroidism	N	N	N	N
Subacute thyroiditis	N	N	N	N
Myxedema	N	N	N	N
Addison's disease	↓	↓	↓	N
Primary aldosteronism	N	N	↑	N
Cushing's syndrome	↑	↑	N	N
Adrenogenital syndrome	N	↑	N	N
Turner's syndrome	N	N	N	↑
Polycystic ovaries	N	↑	N	N
Menopausal syndrome	N	N	N	↑
Pregnancy	↑	N	N	↑
Chorionepithelioma	N	N	N	↑
Seminoma	N	N	N	↑
Klinefelter's syndrome	N	N or ↓	N	↑

and mucoproteins. Albumin in the urine is due to increased permeability of glomerular capillaries, and/or reduced reabsorption of filtered proteins by the tubules. These changes can be due to infection, physical damage (due to injury from jogging, boxing, a fall, etc.), or a neoplasm.

Glucose dipsticks respond with a color change to urine glucose concentrations from about 100 mg/dL to over 1 g/dL. A urine glucose concentration of 100 mg/dL signifies a blood glucose of ~350 mg/dL, well above normal. Glucose in the urine is called *glucosuria.*

Other urine dipsticks are color-sensitive to acetoacetic acid and acetone, both of which are found in the urine of persons with *ketonuria.* Ketonuria is present in uncontrolled diabetes mellitus, starvation, and occasionally in ethanol intoxication. *Hematuria,* or Hb in the urine can also be sensed by a dipstick color test. *Hematuria* is symptomatic of acute renal failure. In *nitrituria,* the dipstick responds to the conversion of nitrate from dietary metabolites to nitrite by certain bacteria in the urine. Normally, no nitrite is present. Thus, a positive *nitrituria* test is seen in about 80% of bladder infections (*bacteriuria*). The urine with nitrate needs to incubate in the bladder in the presence of the bacteria at least 4 hours. Urinary pH is also measured with a color dipstick responsive in the range from 5 to 9. Knowledge of the urine pH helps to identify crystals (e.g., oxalate, phosphate, urate) that may be found on microscopic examination. All dipstick color tests are of low accuracy, 3-bit (1 part in 8) at the most.

Microscopic examination of the urine sediment after centrifuging a specimen allows the clinician to observe the presence of *crystals* (see above), *casts* (cylindrical masses of mucoprotein in which cellular elements, fat droplets, or other proteins may be trapped), *leucocytes* (WBCs), *erythrocytes* (RBCs), and occasional *bacteria.* Over 10 WBCs/μL is diagnostic for urinary tract infection.

GC/mass spectrometry is used to screen urine samples for drugs such as cocaine, marijuana (tetrahydrocannabinol [THC]), amphetamines, and the opiates codeine and morphine. Cocaine use is detected by measuring the concentration of the cocaine metabolite, *benzoylecgonine* (BZG), in urine. BZG concentration in the urine reaches a maximum from 4 to 10 hours after cocaine use, and persists for 2 to 3 days. After the peak, the BZG concentration decays with a $T_{1/2}$ of ~6 hours thereafter. The THC metabolite in urine is *11-nor-9-carboxy-delta-9-THC.* When a marijuana cigarette containing ~33.8 mg of THC was smoked, the peak concentration of 11-nor-9-carboxy-delta-9-THC appeared at a mean time of 13.5 hours. The peak concentrations ranged from 29.9 to 355.2 ng/mL (153.5 ng/mL mean) for six individuals. Many over-the-counter drugs give positive urine tests for amphetamines; these include ephedrine, pseudoephedrine (for sinuses), L-methamphetamine (in Vick's inhaler), and phenylpropanolamine. However, they can be separated from amphetamine and D-methamphetamine by correctly executed GC/MS tests. The opiates codeine and morphine appear in the urine as morphine. Eating foods with poppy seeds can also produce morphine in the urine (they contain morphine). As much as 10 μg/mL morphine has been measured in the urine after a subject ate food with poppy seeds (Thevis et al. 2003).

Also of diagnostic interest is the relatively rare family of diseases called *porphyrias.* Any hereditary deficiency in the biosynthesis of one (or more) of the enzymes involved in heme synthesis causes a porphyria disease in which several metabolic precursors to heme are over-produced (e.g., porphyrins, porphobilinogen [PBG], and δ-aminolevulinic *acid* [ALA]). There are three major categories of porphyria: *acute intermittent porphyria* (AIP), *porphyria cutanea tarda* (PCT), and *erythropoietic protoporphyria* (EPP) (Merk 2000). The latter two porphyrias affect the skin causing rashes, blistering, and lesions. AIP is the result of low levels of the enzyme, *PGB deaminase.* AIP does not affect the skin, but rather the central and peripheral nervous systems, causing acute abdominal and organ pain. Tachycardia, muscle weakness, damage to motor and cranial nerves, tremors, seizures, and psychiatric symptoms can occur in individuals with severe AIP.

A key diagnostic symptom of AIP is that PBG and ALA appear in the urine at high levels (PBG at 50–200 mg/day; ALA at 20–100 mg/day; normal PBG at 0–4 mg/day; normal ALA at 0–7 mg/day). PBG spontaneously forms *uroporphyrin,* and also breaks down into substances called *porphobilins.* The ALA that is oveproduced in the liver may be metabolized to porphyrins in other cells. PBG and ALA are initially colorless, but soon oxidize to a redish purple to brown color (porphyria comes from the Greek word for purple). Uroporphyins fluoresce under UV illumination and all porphyrins have unique IR absorption spectra.

In PCT, the deficient enzyme is *uroporphyrinogen decarboxylase.* In EPP, the deficient enzyme is *ferrochelatase,* which places Fe^{++} in the heme ring. In EPP, there is a build-up of *protoporphyrin IX* in bone marrow and erythrocytes. This excess protoporphyrin enters the plasma, and is excreted by the liver into bile and feces.

Also of diagnostic interest using urine samples is the new development of genetically engineered bacteria that can sense pathological glycosuria resulting from poorly or untreated diabetes (Courbet et al. 2015). Bactosensors made from GE *E. coli* spp. have been imbedded in hydrogel beads; when the beads are placed in a urine sample containing glucose above a designed threshold concentration, the bactosensors turn the urine sample a fluorescent red in almost 89% of cases. They also rarely showed a ~3% false-positive reaction. These measures of sensitivity and specificity make these bactosensors almost as reliable as the urine glucose "dipsticks" currently used in medical practice (Healy 2015). It should be noted that these bactosensors are a qualitative, not a quantitative test for glycosuria. Bactosensors for glycosuria have not yet been approved for clinical use.

8.3.2 Diagnosis of Early-Stage Pancreatic Cancer from Proteins in the Urine

Recently (August 3, 2015), it was reported that a combination of three proteins occurring at high levels in urine can accurately detect early-stage pancreatic cancer (PC) (Radon et al. 2015). This preliminary discovery could lead to a reliable, inexpensive, NI test to screen people who are at high risk for developing this deadly form of cancer.

The researchers screened ~1500 urine proteins; about half were common to both male and female volunteers. In the study, 488 urine samples were examined. Of these, 192 were from patients with PC, 92 were from patients with chronic pancreatitis, 87 were from healthy volunteers, and 117 were from patients with other benign and malignant liver and gall bladder conditions (Radon et al. 2015).

Of the number of proteins in these samples, the concentrations of three specific proteins were found to be statistically significant predictors of Stage I-II PC, namely LYVE-1, REG1A, and TFF1. These urine proteins are described as: LYVE-1 = lymphatic vessel endocytic receptor. It is a homologue of the CD44 glycoprotein, and is a lymph-specific receptor for *hyaluronan* also known as *hyaluronic acid* (HA). REG1A, an *Islet of Langerhans regenerating protein*, also known as *lithostatin-1-α*, or *Islet cell regeneration factor* (ICRF), is a protein encoded by the *REG1A* gene. TFF1 is *Trefoil factor 1*, which has function in maintaining mucosal integrity; its actions are unknown at the molecular level.

Volunteers with PC were found to have increased concentrations of each of the three proteins described above when compared to urine levels from healthy patients. Patients suffering from chronic pancreatitis had significantly lower levels than cancer patients. When combined, the three proteins formed a robust ensemble that can detect patients with Stage I and II PC with better than 90% accuracy.

The 5-year survival rate for PC in the United Kingdom is the lowest of any common cancer, ~3%. This figure has barely improved in 40 years. There is no early diagnostic test available (BioSpace 2015). There is no universal cause of PC; people at higher risk of developing it include those with a family history of PC, heavy smokers, obesity, and persons over 50 years with new-onset diabetes.

The research team headed by Dr. Crnogorac-Jurcevic plans to conduct further tests on urine samples from persons in high-risk groups, also to access urine samples collected from volunteers over an extended period of 5–10 years. By examining samples from donors who went on to develop PC, this "longitudinal information" will allow the researchers to see if the three-biomarker signature persists in the latency period, that is, the time between the genetic changes that will cause the PC to develop, and the clinical presentation.

8.4 WHAT CAN BE LEARNED FROM FECES?

Direct observation of a stool sample under the microscope can lead to the detection of various endoparasites (from their bodies, eggs, or cysts) including *Giardia, tapeworms, round worms (ascarids)*, etc. Infestations of these parasites are often accompanied by cramps, bloating, diarrhea, and bleeding.

Chemical analysis of stool samples can detect whole blood from internal bleeding; this blood can be from stomach ulcers, parasites, colorectal cancer, bacterial toxins, Crohn's disease, etc. The tetramethyl benzidine reagent test and the guaiac test are commonly used to detect occult blood in urine or feces (Collins 1968). They use the principle that heme proteins act as peroxidases, catalyzing the reduction of H_2O_2 to water, giving a color reaction as the indicator substance is oxidized in the reaction. False-positive chemical tests may occur if the patient's diet has recently included foods rich in peroxidases such as brassicas (cauliflower, broccoli, etc.), radishes, and cantaloupe. A false-negative can occur if Vitamin C in excess of 250 mg/day is taken (vitamin C is an antioxidant). A more sensitive and specific test for Fecal occult blood is the FOB Rapydtest® dipstick which uses monoclonal Abs to human Hb. In this test, two colored bands appear on a test strip when a positive result occurs (APACOR 2013). APACOR gives the FOB Rapydtest a sensitivity of 38%, a specificity of 94% and an accuracy of 53% for sensing human haemoglobin.

Bilirubin is a normal by-product of Hb metabolism. Red blood cells, or erythrocytes, have a mean life span of about 120 days. The cell membranes of old erythrocytes rupture, releasing Hb molecules. Special macrophages, the reticuloendothelial cells of the liver, spleen, and bone marrow take up the free Hb and break the protein globin from the heme ring. Normally, 7–8 g of Hb are broken down daily by cells of the reticuloendiothelial system. The heme ring is opened enzymatically and the free Fe^{++} iron is taken up by the enzyme *transferrin* for recycling; the heme is formed into a straight chain of four linked pyrrole nucleii. The tetrapyrrole molecules are first converted to *biliverdin,* then reduced to bilirubin which is released by the reticuloendothelial cells. Once in the blood, the free bilirubin combines strongly with the plasma albumin. It is transported as this stable complex in the blood. The complex is taken up by liver cells (hepatocytes), in which the tetrapyrrole molecule is split from the albumin, and then made water-soluble by conjugation with glucuronic acid to form *bilirubin mono-* and *diglucuronide* (~80%), also, bilirubin sulfate (~10%) and other bilirubin salts (~10%) are formed. It is these water-soluble bilirubin forms that are secreted into the bile, which is injected into the small intestine as part of the process of digestion (Guyton 1991).

The action of certain bacteria in the intestines (in the microbiome) converts the bilirubin salts to the compounds, *urobilinogen* and *stercobilinogen.* In 24 hours, from 50 to 300 mg of bilirubin are secreted as stercobilinogen in a normal adult. This mass is derived from the normal breakdown of from 7 to 8 g of Hb, plus that derived from myoglobins, cytochromes, and catalases. Outside the body, stercobilinogen is further oxidized to *stercobilin.* Some of the intestinal urobilinogen, which is quite soluble, is reabsorbed by the intestinal mucosa, and finds its way back to the liver and the kidneys. Normally, about 4 mg of urobilinogen in 24 hours appears in the urine.

Jaundice is a condition where the skin, mucous membranes, whites of the eye, etc. turn yellow because of an excess of bilirubin in the blood. The presence of jaundice can signal one of two conditions: (1) The rate of red cell destruction is sufficiently above normal (*hemolytic jaundice*) so that the normal hepatocytes cannot keep up with the conversion of the bilirubin–albumin complex in the blood to bilirubin, thence to bile; (2) In *obstructive jaundice,* there may be damage to the hepatocytes from some form of hepatitis (viral, chemical), or the bile ducts may be blocked by bile stones or a cancer. Because of the blockage, bile ducts may rupture and the circulating bilirubin is now of the conjugated form. In the disease malaria, jaundice can be from both damaged hepatocytes and ruptured erythrocytes.

The concentration of urobilinogen in the stool is thus greatly reduced when a gallstone blocks the bile duct (there is also acute pain, which needs no laboratory analysis). Stool urobilinogen is also moderately reduced in viral hepatitis, cancer of the pancreatic head, and in chemical hepatitis.

Celiac disease, or *nontropical sprue* (NTS), is one of several intestinal malabsorption syndromes that can be partially diagnosed from analysis of the stool. Its incidence in the United States is about 1:5000. Celiac disease is a *genetically based autoimmune disease* that destroys the microvilli lining the small intestine preventing the normal absorption of dietary fats, as well as a host of other substances including the fat-soluble vitamins A, D, and K, as well as vitamin B_{12}, and folic acid. In severe NTS, there is malabsorption of calcium, iron, protein, and carbohydrates. Other symptoms presented in NTS include bone demineralization, anemia, failure of blood to clot, and the general symptoms of starvation, although the diet is normal. NTS is caused by the *gliadin* fraction of *gluten protein* in wheat, rye, barley, and oats which are eaten as bread, cereal, etc. Ingested gliadin forms an immune complex in the intestinal mucosa, and the patient's immune system responds with an aggregation of macrophages and killer lymphocytes which generate inflammation and systematically destroy the celiac microvilli through which nutrients are absorbed (Guyton 1991, Merk Manual 2014).

In NTS, the feces contain an abnormally high content of fats (steatorrhea). They are pale, greasy, and float on water. Generally, stool fat over 6 g/24 hour, given a 100 g per day fat in the diet, is diagnostic for NTS. Stool fat can be identified nonquantitatively by staining a smear with the dye, *Sudan III.*

A patient with NTS must be put onto a gluten-free diet. Gluten is also found as a food additive in hot dogs, ice cream, Swiss chocolate, soups, etc., so it can be difficult to eliminate it from the diet. Recovery is accelerated by administering vitamins and minerals to treat the starvation symptoms. Oral corticosteroids (e.g., prednisone) may be given in severe cases to reduce bowel inflammation.

Tropical sprue (TS) is an ideopathic version of NTS. TS may be caused by an unknown parasite, bacteria or virus infection, or a bacterial toxin from spoiled food. It has similar symptoms to NTS, including steatorrhea. The treatment of choice for TS is the antibiotic, tetracycline, which may be given for as long as 6 months. Vitamin B_{12} and folic acid are also given (Merk Manual 2013).

8.5 WHAT CAN BE LEARNED FROM SALIVA?

Saliva is a complex, exocrine secretion of the three pairs of salivary glands: the *parotids,* the *submandib-ulars,* and the *sublinguals.* The parotid salivary glands are the largest. The net output of the salivary glands when a person is chewing is about 2.5 mL/min; however, the secretion rate can vary with the sensed flavor, aroma of the food being eaten, and the individual. Saliva contains two major components, a fluid part containing water, ions, small molecules, and proteins which come from secretory vesicles in the gland cells. Apparently control of the fluid component is by parasympathetic nerve stimulation; sympathetic nerve stimulation causes the release of the proteins. The formation of saliva is a complex, active process; the interested reader should see the book by Edgar et al. (2004).

Some of the proteins and enzymes found in saliva include, but are not limited to, the following: albumin, β-glucuronidase, cystatins, esterases, gustin, abs (IgA, IgG, IgM), lactoferrin, lactic dehydrogenase, mucins, parotid aggregins, phosphatases, ribonucleases, vitamin-binding proteins, α-amylase, epidermal growth factor, fibronectin, histatins, kallikrein, lipase, lysozyme, nerve growth factor, peptidases, salivary peroxidases, etc. Also the low-molecular-weight molecules: glucose, creatinine, lipids, sialic acid, uric acid, urea, etc. The secreted ions include: Na^+ (2–21 mmol/L), K^+ (10–36 mmol/L), Ca^{++} (1.8–2.8 mmol/L), Mg^{++} (0.08–0.5 mmol/L), Cl^- (5–40 mmol/L), I^- (>plasma), F^-, $SO_4^=$, HCO_3^- (25 mmol/L), $PO_4^=$ (1.4–39 mmol/L), also $HPO_4^=$, $H_2PO_4^-$, SCN^-, etc.

Of medical diagnostic significance is the presence in saliva of the bacteria, *Helicobacter pylori* (which normally is not present), signifying possible peptic ulcers, gastritis, or stomach cancer. Saliva has also been used in the detection of all forms of hepatitis. Marijuana (THC), cocaine, codeine, nicotine, and alcohol appear in it and can be detected using the same techniques used with urine. One of the more important, NI diagnostic uses of saliva is in the estimation of blood (plasma) glucose concentration.

Early reports in the literature have made many claims: Ranging from the glucose concentration in saliva is poorly correlated with blood glucose concentration [BG] and cannot be used to manage diabetes (Forbat et al. 1981), to the fact that salivary glucose properly collected is highly correlated with [BG] (with a time delay) and shows promise for an input for a glucoregulation algorithm (Andersson et al. 1998, Yamaguchi et al. 1998). In a pilot study, Yamaguchi et al. gave six healthy young men 75 g oral glucose tolerance tests (OGTTs). They measured salivary glucose [SG] and [BG] with an enzymatic glucose electrode. They observed that individual [BG] responses to the test differed significantly as did the [SG] levels. The averaged regression lines between [BG] and [SG] for the six subjects also varied widely. The correlation coefficients (r^2) for subjects A through F were 0.89, 0.71, 0.65, 0.80, 0.82, and 0.66, respectively. Time lags (t_{bs}) between the first [BG] peak in the OGTT and the first peak in the [SG] curve were highly variable, and in some cases, the means were positive (a phase lead!). For subjects A through F, the lags were: -16 ± 4, -3 ± 4, $+1 \pm 5$, $+6 \pm 11$, -20 ± 7, and $+3 \pm 14$ min, respectively. (I am not sure what a phase lead means in this context; is anticipation a form of noncausality?) In summary, Yamaguchi et al. showed that accounting for time lags, a broad range of the parameters b and a exist in a simple linear model for [BG] = b + a[SG]. Typically, $60 < b < 160$ mg/dL, and $12.5 < a < 63.6$. A typical measured [SG] of 1.5 mg/dL would give a measured [BG] in the range of 110–200 mg/dL.

What the data of Yamaguchi et al. showed is that properly collected saliva samples can indeed be used to estimate [BG]. However, because of *individual variability* in [BG]/[SG], t_{bs}, and r, a salivary [BG] estimator would have to be custom calibrated to an individual using fasting and an OGTT. It remains to be seen whether the NI salivary [BG] estimation method can prove reliable as the finger-prick/blood drop/colorimeter test now most widely used by diabetics.

At present, there is a renewed interest in using measured [SG] to noninvasively estimate [BG] in Type II diabetics. Two types of [SG] nanosensor have been used; a glucose oxidase-based fuel cell (Zhang et al. 2015), and an optical chip based on surface plasmon polaritons (SPP) (Feng et al. 2012). In addition, there has been a recent comprehensive meta-analysis of the dynamics relating [BG] to [SG] in Type II diabetics (Mascarenhas et al. 2014). As described above, saliva is a complex glandular secretion. Measurement of [SG] was made more reliable by the procedure used in gathering samples by Zhang et al. (2015). They first absorbed saliva in the mouth with a sterile dental cotton roll. A syringe was used that had a polyvinylidene fluoride (PVDF) membrane filter fixed to its bottom. The saturated roll was inserted into the syringe and the plunger inserted to exert pressure on the roll, forcing filtered saliva out through the PVDF membrane into a collection tube. The membrane has a protein-binding capacity over 200 $\mu g/cm^2$ and a pore size of 0.2 μm. Thus, it filtered out most of the proteins in saliva rendering glucose measurements by their fuel cell more precise.

The nanoscale plasmonic interferometer developed by Feng et al. (2012) is an optical sensor with wide applications. Their basic plasmonic interferometer consisted of a narrow (0.1 μm), deep slit (etched into a silver metal film on a dielectric substrate) flanked by two, wider (0.2 μm) grooves, all ~10 μm long. The optical tuning of a basic groove-slit-groove plasmonic interferometer is determined by the groove-to-slit distances (p_1 and p_2) and the wavelength λ of the input light. The analyte glucose dissolved in water could be measured with a threshold concentration of ~0.36 mg/dL with the plasmonic interferometer. Details of how SPP optics work can be found in the paper by Zeng et al. (2015).

Measurements of [SG] to estimate [BG] using the new nanosensors still face the problems of individual variability and custom calibration noted by Yamaguchi et al. in 1998, if a reliable, approved NI, salivary [BG] instrument is to be marketed.

8.6 WHAT CAN BE LEARNED FROM BREATH?

From its origin in the lungs, exhaled breath should ideally contain only water vapor, CO_2, O_2, N_2, and traces of CO, H_2, and Ar. Unfortunately, one's breath is not always odorless. *Halitosis* is a term applied to the general phenomenon of unpleasant, malodorous, or bad breath. The offensive odors can be from several sources and in some cases can be of diagnostic value to a physician or dentist.

Other vapor-phase additives to exhaled breath can include volatile substances in the blood such as acetone (present in severe, untreated diabetes mellitus), volatile substances from infections in the nasal passages, sinuses and throat (e.g., from nasal polyps, and/or sinusitis), and substances from the mouth (gum disease, rotting food between the teeth, bacteria on the tongue). Many of the odors of halitosis that come from the bacterial breakdown of food trapped between the teeth (and between the teeth and gums) are due to sulfur compounds. Some of the more obnoxious odorants from the mouth include *hydrogen sulfide, methyl mercaptan, dimethyl sulphide, acetone (from diabetes), dimethylamine, trimethylamine (present in trimethylaminuria* and *uremia, also known as "fish odor"), also putrescene, cadaverine, skatole,* and *indole* (Tangerman and Winkel 2007, 2010).

Other bad breath odors have extra-oral origins. They may be associated with internal organ diseases which may include the lungs, the stomach, pancreas (diabetes), gallbladder dysfunction, and kidney failure. Various carcinomas are reported to cause malodor, as well. Perhaps in the future, an NI screening test for lung cancer can be developed that relies on the enormous sensitivity of FTIR spectroscopy or GC/QPMS to quantify a specific odorant associated with this disease. It is reasonable to expect that if a relatively insensitive human olfactory system can smell an odor, dogs can be trained to identify it, and a modern analytical instrument can also be designed to measure it at far lower concentrations in air.

One of the more successful, NI, diagnostic measurements (rel. sensitivity = 97.6%, rel. specificity = 94.1%) that can be made using exhaled breath is the test for the bacterium that is largely responsible for stomach ulcers, *H. pylori. H. pylori* was discovered by Warren and Marshall in 1982; it is a spiral or corkscrew-shaped bacterium that lives in the stomach in the interface between the mucous gel and the gastric epithelial cells. Topologically, it is outside of the body, and therefore difficult for immune system cells to attack. *H. pylori* is highly correlated with *antral gastritis,* and with duodenal and gastric ulcers. Its presence is also strongly correlated with the incidence of stomach cancer. There is a sixfold increase in the incidence of stomach cancer in patients carrying *H. pylori.*

There are several tests for *H. pylori* (MedlinePlus 2013, Patient 2014). The presence of *H. pylori* in the stomach can definitively be determined invasively by taking a biopsy from a stomach ulcer with a gastroscope. A blood Ab test also is fairly accurate in identifying an *H. pylori* infection. The accurate, NI, "urea breath test" for the bacterium makes use of the fact that *H. pylori* survives on the stomach lining by secreting the enzyme, *urease.* Urease breaks down urea in the stomach contents to ammonia and carbon dioxide. The ammonia forms ammonium hydroxide which neutralizes stomach hydrochloric acid in the vicinity of the bacteria protecting them. The reaction is:

$$2 H_2N(^{13}CO)NH_2 + 2 H_2O \xrightarrow{\text{urease}} 4 NH_3 + 2\ ^{13}CO_2 . \uparrow \tag{8.64}$$

In the ^{13}C test, the patient is asked to swallow 75 mg of urea containing the nonradioactive carbon isotope, ^{13}C. If *H. pylori* are present, they rapidly break down the ^{13}C-urea to NH_3 and $^{13}CO_2$. The $^{13}CO_2$ goes rapidly into the blood, thence to the lungs where most of it is exhaled in the breath, enriching the normal fraction of $^{13}CO_2/^{12}CO_2$ to well above the normal 1.11/100. The ratio of $^{13}CO_2/^{12}CO_2$ is sensed with an MS. Two breath samples are taken at 0 min, and two more at 30 min. A $\geq 4\%$ increase in the $^{13}CO_2/^{12}CO_2$ ratio is considered evidence that *H. pylori* is present in the stomach. The very small amount of ^{13}C-urea ingested is considered innocuous.

An alternate isotope test for *H. pylori* can use ^{14}C-urea. Carbon-14 is a radioisotope that emits 156 keV β particles (electrons) with a half-life of 5730 years. (It is better known for its use in dating organic archeological samples.) One microcurie of ^{14}C-urea is administered to the patient. Again, if *H. pylori* is present, it rapidly breaks down the ^{14}C-urea to ammonia and $^{14}CO_2$. The $^{14}CO_2$ is rapidly passed into the blood and most is exhaled. The β radioactivity of breath samples taken at 0, 6, 12, and 20 min is counted, and these data are used to assess the presence of *H. pylori*. The ^{14}C-urea test is not given to pregnant women. In both tests, some CO_2 becomes bicarbonate and can end up in the bones or other biomolecules. ^{13}C is innocuous, but the long-term presence of even pC amounts of ^{14}C in the body carries some risk of cell damage. That is why the ^{14}C-urea test is not given to pregnant women and the ^{13}C-urea test is favored.

Another breath test that uses an MS or a GC with a molecular sieve is the *hydrogen test* used in the diagnosis of the genetic condition of *lactase deficiency,* otherwise known as *lactose* (milk sugar) *intolerance.* In the normal digestive process, the disaccharide lactose is broken apart to form *galactose* and *glucose* by the enzyme *lactase.* (Lactase is normally found in the brush borders of epithelial cells lining the small intestine. Galactose is also converted to glucose enzymatically.) As a result of this cleavage, the plasma glucose concentration rises. In lactase-deficient individuals, plasma glucose does not significantly rise. The undigested lactose is fermented in the colon by bacteria. Lactose fermentation by-products include hydrogen gas (H_2), which is absorbed into the blood and released through the lungs in exhaled breath. About 21% of H_2 produced in the colon exits the body through the lungs (Simren and Stotzer 2006).

In the hydrogen breath test, 10–50 g of lactose in solution is ingested, followed by periodically monitoring the H_2 gas partial pressure in the exhaled breath by an MS or GC. Normally there is very little H_2 in the exhaled breath; however, it rises in cases of lactase deficiency to over 20 ppm above the baseline pH_2, given a 50 g lactose oral input. Other sugars in the gut (e.g., fructose, D-xylose, sucrose) also can ferment to raise the breath H_2 concentration giving a false-positive reading; so before a patient is given the hydrogen breath test, the preceding day's diet must be low on carbohydrates and free of sweets (especially lactose) and antibiotics (Simrén and Stotzer 2006).

Because CO_2 is another by-product of the metabolic breakdown of sugars, radioactive, ^{14}C-D-xylose and ^{14}C-glycochocolate can also be used in enzyme deficiency breath tests. In this case, $^{14}CO_2$ is assayed in the breath by counting ^{14}C β-emissions with a Geiger counter. There is no reason why safer ^{13}C-sugars could also not be used (as in the case of the *H. pylori* urea test), and the $^{13}CO_2/^{12}CO_2$ ratio can be measured with an MS.

Lee et al. (1991) reported on an exquisitely sensitive tunable IR diode laser spectrometer that could resolve $^{12}C^{16}O$ versus $^{13}C^{16}O$ (isotopic carbon monoxide) in exhaled breath in sub-ppm concentrations. They suggested that their prototype instrument could find application in studies of the catabolism of the heme protein. One molecule of CO is produced along with every bilirubin molecule. Other biochemical applications of their IR diode spectrophotometer could lie in studies of heme formation and its abnormalities such as the porphyrias. They also noted that other molecules with unique IR signatures such as CO_2, NH_3, formaldehyde, H_2O_2, etc., can be quantified in breath by their instrument.

In summary, we see that there are established NI tests using breath gases. At present, the presence of the bacterium, *H. pylori,* associated with ulcers and stomach cancer can be detected, and a variety of digestive enzyme disorders involving sugar metabolism can be verified. GCs, MSs, and Geiger counters are used for these purposes. Other gases in the breath resulting from infections, cancers, etc. will probably be identified, and may eventually be used in diagnostic screening tests. FTIR spectrometers, GCs, MSs, and SPR systems have the requisite sensitivities if correctly applied. These are avenues of research that should be pursued.

8.7 CHAPTER SUMMARY

In this chapter, we have seen that modern analytical instruments can quantify nanomole quantities of analytes in noninvasively obtained body fluids, including saliva, urine, breath, and feces. It appears that certain kinds of bacteria, other pathogens, and cancers emit characteristic molecules into their surrounding milieu. These range from DNA from mitochondria to various metabolites, including hydrogen gas. All of the instrumental methods described in Section 8.2 are well established in laboratory medicine with the exception of SPR. In the future, expect to see SPR used to quantify specific bacterial antigens or Abs in body fluids, as well as to identify other biomolecules. SPR devices will be miniaturized, and perhaps even incorporated into biochips as a readout modality.

Obviously, no one instrumental method is good for all analytical tests. In most cases, at least two modalities can be used on the same analyte. Not every instrumental method was covered in this chapter; for example, liquid and electrophoretic chromatography were not covered; not because I consider them unimportant, but because they have little engineering complexity to justify including them in a text on instrumentation.

Expect photonics in the form of fluorescence, spectrophotometry, SPR, SPP, Raman, etc. to dominate laboratory medicine and NI, nonimaging, diagnostic procedures in the future.

9 Plethysmography

9.1 INTRODUCTION

Plethysmography is a term for a set of NI techniques for measuring volume changes in parts of the body, or even the whole body. The more frequently measured volume changes are those caused by breathing (lung and chest expansion), those due to blood being forced into arteries, veins, and capillaries of the legs, arms, hands, and feet by the pumping of the heart, and the volume change of the heart itself as it pumps. It is also possible to measure local volume changes in arms and legs as muscles contract.

The two main techniques used today for plethysmography are volume displacement using air or water outside the body, and the measurement of the electrical impedance or admittance of the body part being studied. In the latter method, as you will see, volume changes translate into impedance changes. Volume changes can also be estimated by ultrasonic and x-ray imaging. However, introductory imaging is described in Chapter 16 of this book.

9.2 VOLUME DISPLACEMENT PLETHYSMOGRAPHY

Many techniques have been developed to measure volume changes in the body. One of the simplest, used on arms and legs, is the pneumatic sphygmomanometer cuff. The cuff is placed around a limb (e.g., the calf, the upper arm), and is inflated to a pressure, P_o, well below the patient's diastolic blood pressure. Some known air volume, V_o, is required to reach this pressure. The outside of the cuff has little compliance due to the stiff fabric material over the rubber bladder. From elementary physics, we know that $P_o V_o = nRT$, or $P_o = nRT/V_o$. Now, if the limb expands against the compliant bladder by some ΔV, the pressure can be written as

$$P = nRT/(V_o - \Delta V) = \frac{nRT}{V_o(1 - \Delta V/V_o)} \cong \frac{nRT}{V_o}(1 + \Delta V/V_o) = P_o(1 + \Delta V/V_o). \qquad (9.1)$$

By measuring $\Delta P = P_o(\Delta V/V_o)$, we can calculate ΔV of the limb. Constant temperature is assumed.

Another direct means of measuring the ΔV of a limb is to enclose it with a water-filled bladder, the outside of which is noncompliant. (Water displacement is probably the oldest mode of plethysmography.) Because water is not compressible, any positive ΔV of the limb will force water up a capillary tube calibrated in volume. The height of the water in the capillary tube can be converted to an electrical output signal photoelectrically.

A pneumatic, whole-body plethysmograph can be used to estimate the functional residual capacity (FRC) of the lungs (West 1985). The subject sits in a hermetically sealed box of volume V_B. The subject's body volume is V_S, measured by positive water displacement. Thus, the air volume in the box with the patient in it is $V_o = V_B - V_S$. The air in the box is at atmospheric pressure, P_o. The subject is asked to blow into a sealed tube containing a pressure transducer. She creates a pressure, $P_2 > P_o$. This exhalation effort compresses the gas in her lungs so that the lung volume *decreases* slightly by ΔV. Thus the box volume *increases* by ΔV, causing the pressure in the box to drop slightly to $P_3 < P_o$. We apply Boyle's law to both the box and the lungs. For the lungs:

$$P_o V_L = P_2(V_L - \Delta V), \quad \text{so } V_L = P_2 \Delta V / (P_2 - P_o). \qquad (9.2)$$

For the box:

$$P_o V_o = P_3(V_o - \Delta V), \quad \text{so } \Delta V = V_o(P_o / P_3 - 1). \qquad (9.3)$$

ΔV estimates the amount the FRC volume in the lungs is compressed by the exhalation effort against the closed tube. Once found, ΔV can be used in Equation 9.2 to find V_L, the initial lung volume.

9.3 IMPEDANCE PLETHYSMOGRAPHY

9.3.1 Introduction

Yet another way to measure the volume changes in body tissues is by measuring the electrical impedance of the body part being studied. As blood is forced through arteries, veins, and capillaries by the heart, the impedance is modulated. When used in conjunction with an external air pressure cuff that can gradually constrict blood flow, *impedance plethysmography* (IP) can provide NI, diagnostic signs about abnormal venous and arterial blood flow. Also, by measuring the impedance of the chest, the relative depth and rate of a patient's breathing can be monitored noninvasively. As the lungs inflate and the chest expands, the impedance magnitude of the chest increases; air is clearly a poorer conductor than tissues and blood.

IP is often carried out using, for safety's sake, a controlled AC current source of fixed frequency. The peak current is generally kept less than 1 mA, and the frequency used typically is between 30 and 75 kHz. The high frequency is used because the human susceptibility to electroshock, and the physiological effects on nerves and muscles from AC decreases with increasing frequency (Webster 1992). The electrical impedance is measured indirectly by measuring the AC voltage between two skin surface electrodes (generally ECG- or EEG-type, AgCl + conductive gel) placed between the two current electrodes. Thus four electrodes are generally used, although the same two electrodes used for current injection can also be connected to the high-input impedance, AC differential amplifier that measures the vector output voltage, $\mathbf{V_o}$. By Ohm's law, $\mathbf{V_o} = \mathbf{I_s}\mathbf{Z_t} = \mathbf{I_s}[R_t + j\,B_t]$.

At a fixed frequency, the overall (net) tissue impedance can be modeled by a single conductance in parallel with a capacitor. Thus, it is algebraically simpler to consider the *net tissue admittance*, $\mathbf{Y_t} = \mathbf{Z_t}^{-1} = G_t + j\omega C_t$. Both G_t and C_t change as blood periodically flows into the tissue under measurement. The imposed alternating current is carried in the tissues by moving ions, rather than electrons. Ions such as Cl^-, HCO_3^-, K^+, Na^+, Ca^{2+} etc., that drift in the applied electric field (caused by the current-regulated source), have three major pathways: a resistive path in the extracellular fluid electrolyte, a resistive path in blood, and a capacitive path caused by ions that charge the membranes of closely packed body cells. Ions can penetrate cell membranes and move inside cells, but not with the ease that they can travel in extracellular fluid space, and in blood. Of course, there are many, many cells effectively in series and parallel between the current electrodes. C_t represents the net equivalent capacitance of *all* of the cell membranes. Each species of ion in solution has a different *mobility*. The mobility of an ion in solution is $\mu \equiv v/E$, *where* v is the mean drift velocity of the ion in a surrounding, uniform electric field, E. Ionic mobility also depends on the ionic concentration, and the other ions in solution. Ionic mobility has the units of $m^2\,s^{-1}\,V^{-1}$. Returning to Ohm's law, we can write in phasor notation:

$$\mathbf{V_o} = \mathbf{I_s}\,/\,\mathbf{Y_t} = \mathbf{I_s}\frac{G_t - j\omega C_t}{G_t^2 + \omega^2 C_t^2} = \mathbf{I_s}[\mathrm{Re}\{\mathbf{Z_t}\} - j\mathrm{Im}\{\mathbf{Z_t}\}], \tag{9.4}$$

where $\mathrm{Re}\{\mathbf{Z_t}\}$ is the real part of the tissue impedance $= G_t/\left(G_t^2 + \omega^2 C_t^2\right)$, and $\mathrm{Im}\{\mathbf{Z_t}\}$ is the imaginary part of the tissue impedance $= -\omega C_t/\left(G_t^2 + \omega^2 C_t^2\right)$. Note that both $\mathrm{Re}\{\mathbf{Z_t}\}$ and $\mathrm{Im}\{\mathbf{Z_t}\}$ are frequency-dependent. Note that $\mathbf{V_o}$ *lags* $\mathbf{I_s}$.

There are several ways of measuring the tissue $\mathbf{Z_t}$, both magnitude and angle. In the first method, described in detail below, an AC voltage, $\mathbf{V_s}$, is applied to the tissue. The amplitude is adjusted so that the resultant current, $\mathbf{I_o}$, remains less than 1 mA. $\mathbf{I_o}$ is converted to a proportional voltage, $\mathbf{V_o}$, by an op-amp current-to-voltage converter circuit. In general, $\mathbf{V_o}$ and $\mathbf{V_s}$ differ in phase and magnitude. A self-nulling circuit operates on $\mathbf{V_o}$ and $\mathbf{V_s}$. At null, its output voltage, V_z, is proportional to $|\mathbf{Z_t}|$. The second method uses the AC current source excitation, $\mathbf{I_s}$, and the output voltage described above, $\mathbf{V_o}$, is fed into a servo-tracking, two-phase, lock-in amplifier (LIA) which produces an output voltage, $V_z \propto |\mathbf{Z_t}|$, and another voltage, $V_\theta \propto \angle\,\mathbf{Z_t}$.

9.3.2 Self-Balancing, Impedance Plethysmographs

A prototype, self-nulling plethysmograph designed by the author is illustrated in Figure 9.1. A 75 kHz, sinusoidal voltage, $\mathbf{V_s}$, is applied to an opposite pair of chest electrodes. An AC current, $\mathbf{I_o}$, flows through the chest, and is given by Ohm's law:

$$\mathbf{I_o} = \mathbf{V_s}[G_t + j\omega C_t]. \tag{9.5}$$

The current $\mathbf{I_o}$ is converted to an AC voltage, $\mathbf{V_o}$, by the current-to-voltage op-amp:

$$\mathbf{V_o} = -\mathbf{I_o}\frac{G_F - j\omega C_F}{G_F^2 + \omega^2 C_F^2} = -\mathbf{V_s}[G_t + j\omega C_t]\frac{G_F - j\omega C_F}{G_F^2 + \omega^2 C_F^2} \tag{9.6}$$

$$\downarrow$$

$$\mathbf{V_o} = -\mathbf{V_s}\frac{G_t G_F - j\omega C_F G_t + j\omega C_t G_F + \omega^2 C_t C_F}{G_F^2 + \omega^2 C_F^2}. \tag{9.7}$$

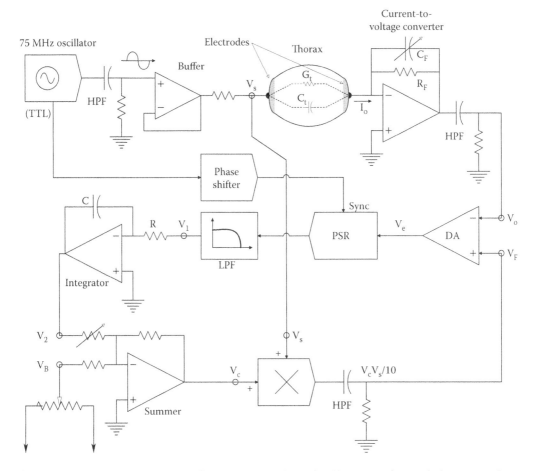

Figure 9.1 Block diagram/simplified schematic of a self-nulling impedance plethysmograph designed by the author. Note the integrator (INT) in the auto-nulling feedback loop.

With the patient exhaled and holding his breath, variable capacitance C_F is adjusted so that $\mathbf{V_o}$ is in phase with $\mathbf{V_s}$. That is, C_F is set so that the imaginary terms in Equation 9.7 $\rightarrow$ 0. That is,

$$C_F = C_{to} / (R_F G_{to}).\tag{9.8}$$

Then, we have

$$\mathbf{V_o} = -\mathbf{V_s} \frac{G_{to}G_F + \omega^2 C_{to}C_F}{G_F^2 + \omega^2 C_F^2} \rightarrow -\mathbf{V_s}R_F G_t.\tag{9.9}$$

Now when the patient inhales, the lungs expand and the air displaces conductive tissue, causing the parallel conductance of the chest, G_t, to *decrease* from G_{to}. Let us substitute $G_t = G_{to} + \delta G_t$ and $C_t = C_{to} + \delta C_t$ into Equation 9.7, and also let $R_F C_F = C_{to}/G_{to}$ from the initial phase nulling. After a considerable amount of algebra, we find:

$$\frac{\mathbf{V_o}}{\mathbf{V_s}}(j\omega) = \frac{-R_F}{[1 + \omega^2(R_F C_F)^2]} \left[G_{to}(1 + \delta G_t/G_{to}) + \omega^2(R_F C_F)^2 G_{to}(1 + \delta C_t/C_{to}) + j\omega C_{to}(\delta C_t/C_{to} - \delta G_t/G_{to}) \right].\tag{9.10}$$

This relation reduces to Equation 9.9 for $\delta C_t - \delta G_t \rightarrow 0$. If we assume that $\delta C_t \rightarrow 0$ only, then Equation 9.10 can be written as

$$\frac{\mathbf{V_o} + \delta\mathbf{V_o}}{\mathbf{V_s}}(j\omega) \cong -R_F G_{to} - \frac{\delta G_t R_F}{[1 + \omega^2(R_F C_F)^2]}.\tag{9.11}$$

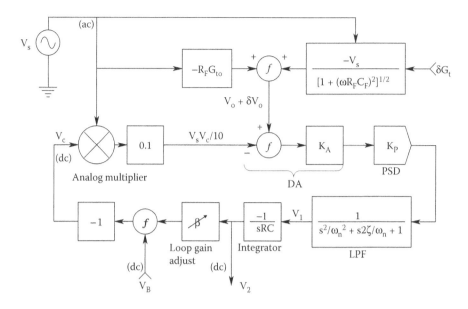

Figure 9.2 Systems block diagram of the self-nulling plethysmograph of Figure 9.1 illustrating system dynamics.

Note that $\delta G_t < 0$ for an inhaled breath.

Figure 9.2 illustrates a systems block diagram for the author's self-balancing plethysmograph, configured for the condition where $\delta C_t \rightarrow 0$. The three, RC high-pass filters are used to block unwanted DC components from $\mathbf{V_s}$, $\mathbf{V_o}$, and $\mathbf{V_F}$. In the first case, we also let $\delta G_t \rightarrow 0$. In the steady state, $\mathbf{V_e} \rightarrow 0$, so:

$$\mathbf{V_s}V_c\,/10 = -\mathbf{V_s}R_FG_{to}. \tag{9.12}$$

Thus,

$$V_c = -10\ R_FG_{to} = -(V_B + \beta V_2), \tag{9.13}$$

and the integrator output is proportional to G_{to}:

$$V_2 = (10\ R_FG_{to} - V_B)/\beta. \tag{9.14}$$

V_B, G_{to}, and $\mathbf{V_s}$ do not change in time, so the steady-state analysis above is valid. Using superposition, we can examine the system's response to a time-varying, δG_t. The transfer function, $\delta V_2/\delta G_t$, can be written as

$$\frac{\delta V_2}{\delta G_t}(s) = \frac{V_sK_AK_p/\{RC[1+(\omega R_FC_F)^2]\}}{s\left(s^2/\omega_n^2 + s2\zeta/\omega_n + 1\right) + V_s\beta K_AK_p/(10RC)}. \tag{9.15}$$

The damping of the cubic closed-loop system is adjusted with the attenuation, β. The steady-state, incremental gain as a function of radian frequency is

$$\frac{\delta V_2}{\delta G_t} = \frac{10}{[(1+(\omega R_FC_F)^2)]\beta}\,\text{v/s}. \tag{9.16}$$

A prototype of this system was run at 75 kHz and tested on the chests of several volunteers after informed consent was obtained. Both $\delta V_2 \propto \delta G_t$ and $V_1 \propto \dot{\delta}\,G_t$ were recorded. System outputs followed the subjects' respiratory volumes, as expected.

A second type of IP made use of a novel, self-balancing, two-phase LIA developed by McDonald (1992) and McDonald and Northrop (1993). An LIA is basically nothing more than a synchronous or phase-controlled, full-wave rectifier followed by a low-pass filter. Its input is generally a noisy,

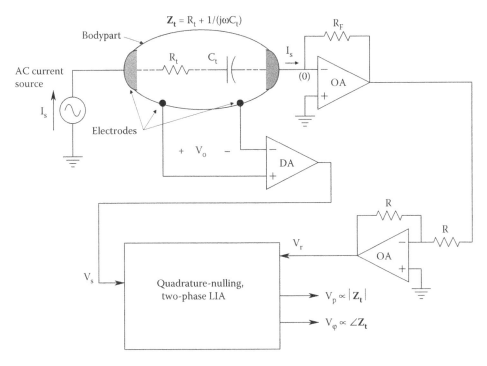

Figure 9.3 Two-phase, self-balancing, lock-in amplifier (SBLIA) developed by McDonald and Northrop (1993) used as an impedance plethysmograph. The SBLIA gives voltage outputs proportional to the body part's admittance vector magnitude and admittance vector angle.

amplitude-modulated, or double-sideband-suppressed carrier AC signal. The LIA output is a DC voltage proportional to the peak height of the input signal; the low-pass filter averages out the noise and any other zero-mean output component of the rectifier. A signal buried in as much as 60 dB of noise can be recovered by an appropriately set-up LIA.

Figure 9.3 illustrates how the LIA is connected to the voltage across the tissue, V_o, where $V_o = I_s (G_t + j\omega C_t)$. Note that if the angle of I_s is taken as zero (reference), then the angle of V_o is $\theta_s = \tan^{-1}(\omega C_t/G_t)$. The AC reference voltage, V_r, in phase with I_s is used to control the LIA's synchronous rectifier. V_r also allows us to monitor I_s since $V_r = I_s R_F$. Figure 9.4 shows a block diagram of McDonald's two-phase, servo LIA.

At the heart of a basic LIA is a synchronous rectifier. One basic form of a synchronous rectifier is a pure analog multiplier (AM), or mixer. Assume one input to the multiplier is a reference signal, $v_r(t) = V_R \cos(\omega_o t + \theta_r)$, the other is a signal whose amplitude we wish to measure: $v_s(t) = V_S \cos(\omega_o t + \theta_s)$. By trig identity,

$$v_p(t) = v_r(t)v_s(t) = (V_R V_S / 2)[\cos(2\omega_o t + \theta_r + \theta_s) + \cos(\theta_r - \theta_s)]. \tag{9.17}$$

When the multiplier output, $v_p(t)$, is run through a low-pass filter, the double frequency term is removed (seriously attenuated), and only the DC component of the product appears at its output:

$$\overline{v_p(t)} = (V_R V_S / 2)\cos(\theta_r - \theta_s). \tag{9.18}$$

If the phase and frequency of the signal and reference are the same, $\overline{v_p(t)} = (V_R V_S/2)$. That is, the output voltage of the LPF is proportional to V_S. (V_R is constant.)

In McDonald's design, the reference signal is phase-shifted by $-90°$ in order to detect any quadrature component of $v_s(t)$. Two analog multipliers are used with two low-pass filters, one for the in-phase component and the other for the quadrature component of V_S. In McDonald's design, a phase-locked loop (PLL) is used as a voltage-controlled phase shifter in a feedback loop that automatically adjusts the reference phase to null the quadrature output, that is, forces $V_q \to 0$. By

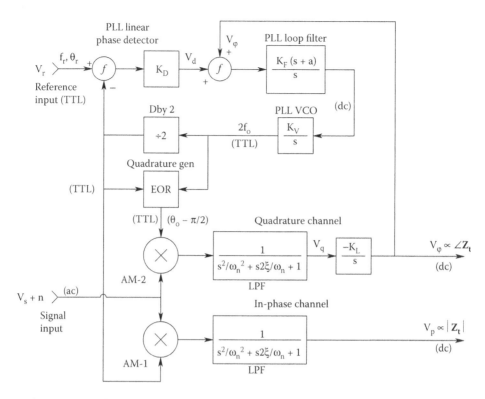

Figure 9.4 Systems block diagram of the self-balancing LIA of McDonald and Northrop (1993).

nulling V_q, we simultaneously maximize V_p, the in-phase output. To see how V_φ can set the phase of the PLL's VCO, we note that the PLL is a Type II feedback system in which in the steady-state, $V_d + V_\varphi = 0$. Note that $V_d = K_D(\theta_r - \theta_o)$. Thus, we can write:

$$\theta_o = \theta_r + V_\varphi / K_D, \tag{9.19}$$

where θ_o is the VCO phase, θ_r is the reference phase, K_D is the phase detector's gain in volts/radian, and V_φ is the DC signal used to adjust θ_o.

In order to generate quadrature phase, the PLL's VCO is forced to run at $2f_r = 2f_o$, and a flip-flop is used to halve its frequency before phase comparison. By inputting $2f_o$ and f_o to an exclusive OR gate, we generate an output TTL signal of frequency f_o and phase $(\theta_o - \pi/2)$. In the steady state, the servo-PLL makes $\theta_o = \theta_s$. $(\theta_r - \pi/2)$ is the quadrature phase reference used in the nulling loop. The reference inputs to the analog multipliers are TTL signals given zero mean by passing through simple RC, high-pass filters (not shown in Figure 9.4). To simplify analysis, we consider the zero mean TTL signals to be represented by their sinusoidal first harmonic components of the Fourier series for the square waves. Thus, the output of the quadrature multiplier channel *before low-pass filtering* is

$$V_q' = V_R \sin(\omega_o t + \theta_r) V_s \cos(\omega_o t + \theta_s) = (V_R V_s / 2)[\sin(2\omega_o t + \theta_r + \theta_s) + \sin(\theta_r - \theta_s)]. \tag{9.20}$$

After low-pass filtering, the double-frequency term drops out and we have the DC voltage:

$$V_q = (V_R V_s / 2)\sin(\theta_r - \theta_s). \tag{9.21}$$

In the steady state, the negative feedback forces $V_q \to 0$, so V_φ assumes a value so that $\theta_r = \theta_s$ and $V_q \to 0$.

Also under this condition, $V_d = V_\varphi$, from which we obtain:

$$V_\varphi = K_D(\theta_s - \theta_r). \tag{9.22}$$

In words, V_ψ is proportional to the phase difference between the I_s reference phase and V_o measured across the tissue under study. As the steady-state θ_o is forced to be θ_s, the output voltage of the in-phase channel is proportional to the $|Y_t|$. Thus the McDonald, self-nulling, quadrature PLL outputs a DC voltage V_ψ proportional to the phase difference between I_s and V_o, and a DC voltage V_p proportional to the magnitude of the admittance of the tissue under study, $|Y_t|$. V_p and V_ψ follow the slow, physiological variations in Y_t caused by blood flow and/or breathing. The modulation of G_t and C_t by pulsatile blood flow or lung inflation can have diagnostic significance.

9.3.3 Applications of Impedance Plethysmography

A major application of IP is in *occlusive impedance phlebography* (OIP). This procedure is used to detect venous blood clots in deep leg veins. IP can also be used to detect blood clots in the lungs. Note that most blood clots in lung vessels are complications of clots in deep leg veins. Also, there are many other signs of clots in the legs and lungs that can be used to verify IP results.

In OIP, an inflatable cuff is placed around the mid-thigh or just below the knee; this is the low-pressure cuff used to block venous return. A high-pressure cuff is placed just above the ankle to occlude both veins and arteries. The IP electrodes are placed high and low on the dorsal (rear) surface of the calf, or on the sides of the calf. When the thigh cuff is inflated, normal venous return is blocked but not arterial blood flow into the lower leg. Restricting venous flow causes blood to pool in the calf veins, and consequently, $|Y_t|$ increases. The thigh cuff pressure is released suddenly, allowing the pooled venous blood to return to the heart. If one or more venous clots are present, it takes longer for $|Y_t|$ to drop to its original value than for normal venous circulation. The OIP test is generally done on both legs for comparison purposes. OIP can also be effectively applied to detect thromboses in proximal (thigh) veins (*femoro-popliteal*). According to one source (Chin and McGrath 1998), OIP is highly sensitive (a 92% detection rate) and specific (95%) when used on patients exhibiting symptomatic, proximal, deep vein thromboses (DVT). The sensitivity of OIP is low in calf vein thromboses (20%) and in screening for DVT in asymptomatic, postoperative, high-risk patients (22%). There are several other NI, diagnostic modalities used in detecting and quantifying DVTs. These include color Doppler ultrasound imaging, magnetic resonance venography, and the iodine-125 fibrinogen scan. Of these NI modalities, OIP is the least expensive.

A multichannel IP investigation of pulsatile blood flow in leg arteries was done by Jossinet et al. (1995). A sinusoidal current of 3 mArms at 64 kHz was injected into the legs through a pair of standard ECG electrodes, one placed on each foot. Sixteen pairs of sensing electrodes were used to record voltages at various sites on the legs. Recording electrode pair spacing was 45 mm on centers. Signal processing of each electrode pair's voltage gave an output voltage proportional to dZ/dt. This information was used to examine the arterial pulse wave velocity in various locations in the legs. This technique may have usefulness in diagnosing asymmetrical problems with arterial circulation in the legs such as might be caused by injury, infection, or embolism.

IP is also used to monitor breathing (and also heart beats) in intensive care and neonatal applications. When used as an impedance pneumograph, electrodes are generally placed on the sides of the chest. Modulations of the peak output voltage are proportional to lung expansion by inhaled air; failure of lung expansion can signify central apnea, and in some cases, extreme obstructive apnea. Since the shape changes of the beating heart are also correlated with expansion and contraction of the aorta, *vena cava*, and pulmonary vessels, the transthoracic Z_t is also modulated at heart rate frequency. In adults, the heart rate is normally higher than the respiration rate, and the two waveforms can be partially separated by band-pass filtering so separate assessments of heart rate and respiration rate and effort can be made. In infants, the respiratory rate can occasionally approach the heart rate, so instead of demodulating the IP voltage for both respiratory and heart rate signals, an ECG amplifier preceded by a pair of low-pass filters can be connected to the IP output electrodes to directly record the ECG signal. The low-pass filters are set to attenuate the $\sim$60 kHz IP modulation signal by at least -120 dB. Often a third modality is used for infant apnea monitoring, for example, a pulse oximeter, to measure the % O_2 saturation of hemoglobin (Section 15.8).

Impedance pneumograph-cardiotachometers used for neonatal and ICU applications have an alarm system that measures a sudden increase in measured impedance such as would be caused by electrodes drying out, coming detached, or falling off the chest. They are also set to alarm for respiration effort or rate, and heart rate under or over preset limits. Many medical instrument manufacturers make ICU and pediatric care monitors that incorporate impedance pneumography functions.

9.3.4 Discussion

IP was seen to have two major applications as an NI, diagnostic method: (1) to measure blood flow (or obstruction) in veins and arteries of the legs, and (2) to measure respiratory effort and rate in ICU and neonatal monitoring applications. The injected AC current is physically and physiologically innocuous because of its low-peak value and high frequency.

9.4 PHOTO-PLETHYSMOGRAPHY

A fingertip photo-plethysmograph can be used to measure heart rate, and to estimate blood pressure when individually calibrated. This device fits over the tip of a finger (or on an earlobe in another incarnation). In one configuration, modulated light from a red or NIR LED is shined into the tissue, and a silicon photodiode senses the back-scattered light. Its signal is demodulated by a phase-sensitive rectifier (PSR) plus low-pass filter. The PSR ensures that only light from the LED is used to derive the pulse rate signal. As blood is forced into the tissue's blood vessels, they expand and the level of back-scattered light changes. This heart-rate change appears as a signal at the output of the LPF.

Once the back-scattered, modulated, NIR light is demodulated, a periodic, analog voltage waveform is available for further processing. This analog waveform is passed through a comparator to derive a heart-rate logic signal. The rising edges of this signal trigger a one-shot multivibrator that makes a train of narrow pulses at the heart rate. The heart rate can be found in analog form by low-pass filtering the one-shot's output pulses and subtracting out the DC offset of the logic LO voltage. To find the heart rate in digital form, the narrow, one-shot output pulses are used to start and stop a fast clock input (e.g., 1 MHz) to a counter. When the leading edge of the second pulse of a pair of output pulses arrives, the counting is stopped and the counter count (total number of microseconds) is downloaded in parallel to an arithmetic unit which takes its reciprocal. The falling edge of the second pulse resets the counter and starts the counting process again. The reciprocal of the count is proportional to the *instantaneous frequency* (IF) of the heart. Several, consecutive instantaneous frequency outputs can be averaged in order to minimize the normal variation in heart rate caused by cardioregulatory action. The appropriately scaled, averaged, IF output drives a digital heart-rate display.

A *pulse oximeter* is a more elaborate incarnation of a fingertip plethysmograph. The oximeter uses two LEDs of different wavelengths in order to measure the percent of blood hemoglobin saturation with oxygen. However, it is also responsive to the blood volume in the tissue on which it is used, and thus can give pulse rate information as well as SpO_2. (Section 15.8 gives a thorough description of pulse oximeters.)

An example of a modern, commercial fingertip pulse oximeter is the Santamedical SM-240 OLED Finger Pulse Oximeter. It displays average pulse rate from 30 to 254 BPM, and SpO_2 from 34% to 99% with ±1% accuracy. It is not intended for medical use, but by mountain climbers, hikers, skiers, aerobic exercisers, etc.

9.5 CHAPTER SUMMARY

We have seen that plethysmography is a relatively simple, NI means of measuring local changes in body volume, generally occurring as the result of respiration, blood flow, or muscle contraction. A device as simple as a blood pressure cuff can be used to measure volume changes in a limb covered by the cuff caused by either blood flow or muscle contraction. Using Equation 9.1, an electronic pressure sensor attached to the cuff can measure $\Delta P = P_o(\Delta V/V_o)$. That is, the change in air pressure, ΔP, is proportional to the increase in limb volume, ΔV. P_o is easily measured, and V_o can be determined by filling the cuff with a known volume of air at P_o.

IP was described, and its applications were discussed. As impedance changes are generally small compared with the overall impedance, it is feasible to use a closed-loop, self-nulling bridge type of circuit to sense the desired $|\Delta Z|$ as a ΔV_o. It appears that many of the applications of plethysmography are in physiological research, rather than in diagnosis.

10 Pulmonary Function Tests

10.1 INTRODUCTION

The principal functions of the vertebrate respiratory system are to keep the arterial blood supplied with oxygen, and to allow the dissipation of a metabolic by-product, carbon dioxide, in the exhaled breath. The biochemistry of the respiratory process is complex, and will not be reviewed here. Rather, we will focus our attention on the physical side of the respiratory process. That is, the mechanics of breathing and the gas exchange processes taking place at alveolar capillaries. Factors that restrict normal breathing and gas exchange are medically important, and have a variety of causes, ranging from heart failure, allergy, infections, cancer, emphysema, COPD, asthma, and hereditary disease. When a patient complains to his or her physician that he or she is "out of breath," the first step in finding out why and how to cure or mitigate this condition is to quantitatively measure the mechanical parameters of his or her respiratory system by *spirometry* and to compare them with those of "normal" persons of similar sex, age, body mass, and height. Deviations from the norm in these tests are only the first step in a complete diagnosis, which can also involve CAT scans, MRI, blood gas tests, etc. The volume-displacement spirometer was invented ca. 1846 by Hutchison, an English anatomist (West 1985).

Spirometers basically measure the respiratory volumes, or in the case of modern units, respiratory volume flow rate which is integrated to determine the volume. Some of the common parameters used in spirometry are:

FVC (forced vital capacity): This is the total volume of air a patient can exhale after a maximum effort inspiration. Patients with *restrictive lung disease* (RLD) have a lower FVC than do patients with *obstructive lung disease* (OLD).

FEV1 (forced expiratory volume in 1 s) (also, FEV1/2): The volume of air expired in the first second following the beginning of maximum expiratory effort. FEV1 is reduced from normal in both OLDs and RLDs, but for different reasons; increased airway resistance in OLD, and decreased vital capacity in RLD.

FEV1/FVC: This ratio is about 0.7 in healthy subjects. It can be as low as 0.2–0.3 in patients with OLD. Patients with RLD have near-normal ratios.

FEF (25%–75%) (forced mid-expiratory flow rate): The average rate of flow during the middle of the FVC maneuver. Reduced in both OLD and RLD.

DLCO (diffusion capacity of the lung for carbon monoxide): The poison gas, CO, can be used to measure the diffusion capacity of the alveoli. The diffusion capacity of the lung is decreased in parenchymal diseases, such as emphysema. It is normal in asthma. (Other gases can be used.)

FRC (functional residual capacity): The volume of air remaining in the lungs and trachea after an exhale in normal breathing.

RV (residual volume): The volume of air left in the lungs after a maximum FVC exhale. It is the "dead space" of the respiratory system; mostly combined trachea and bronchial tube volumes. It cannot be measured directly.

TV (tidal volume): The volume exchanged in normal, relaxed breathing.

AV (alveolar volume): Total volume of all the minute alveoli in the lung parenchyma.

Note that all spirometric tests are NI; however, they require a high degree of patient cooperation. If a patient is unconscious or paralyzed, they cannot be used. The physician must then rely on imaging, or sound transmission tests, as described in Sections 3.4, 15.2, and 15.4 of this book.

Figure 10.1 illustrates the graphical significance of the parameters: FVC, TV, FRC, and RV from a volume spirometer kymograph record. FEV1 is illustrated in Figure 10.2. Computer-generated, flow/volume (F/V) curves are generally made from the outputs of pneumotach (PT) flow meters. Typical F/V curves are shown in Figure 10.3. Note that extensive databases have been compiled to enable the physician or respiratory therapist to compare a patient's volumes and FEV performance to norms for a given age, height, weight, and sex. Such tables can be found at the Australian spirometry web site of Johns and Pierce (2008).

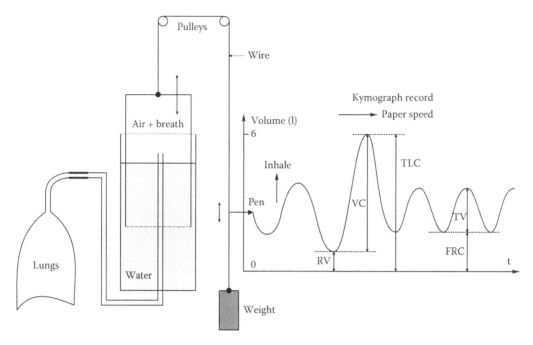

Figure 10.1 Diagram of a basic, water-sealed volume spirometer, showing some critical volumes and capacities on the kymograph readout.

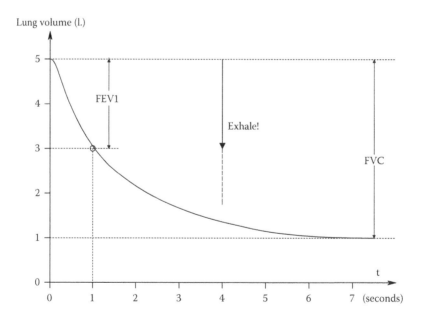

Figure 10.2 Volume of forcibly expired air showing definitions of FEV1 and FVC.

10.2 SPIROMETERS AND RELATED EQUIPMENT

All spirometers can be classified as positive displacement types of instruments using PTs. An example of the positive displacement spirometer is the classic W. E. Collins Model P-600 recording vitalometer (cf. Figure 10.4), which uses a water-sealed, counter-weighted, rigid bell chamber to measure the patient air volumes at near-atmospheric pressure. Other types of positive displacement spirometers use a bellows or a giant piston in a cylinder.

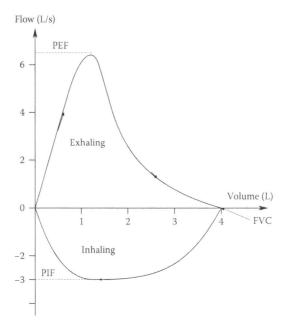

Figure 10.3   Representative computer-generated flow-volume curve; the patient blows into a pneumotach, the output of which is connected to a computer.

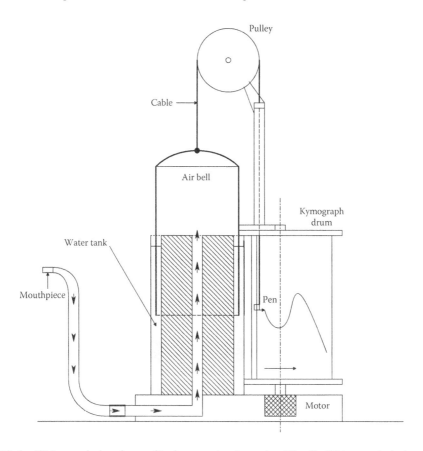

Figure 10.4   Water-sealed, volume-displacement spirometer. The "bell" is counterbalanced so its weight exerts negligible pressure on the trapped gas.

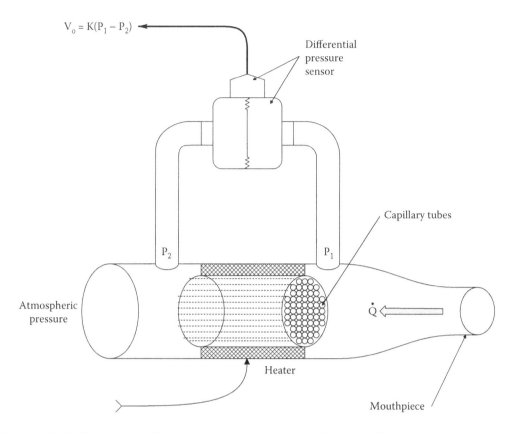

Figure 10.5 Diagram of a Fleisch-type capillary pneumotach. For air flow in the direction shown, $P_1 > P_2$.

The trend now is not to use a bulky volume spirometer that requires sterilization of its connecting tubes for each patient, but rather a small, hand-held *pneumotachometer* (pneumotach). There are three different types of PT. (1) The *flow resistance type* in which a fine screen or a parallel cluster of capillary tubes forms a pneumatic "resistor." The pressure differential across the resistance is proportional to the volume flow in L/s (in analogy to Ohm's law for electric circuits). The resistance made from many parallel capillary tubes is known as the *Fleisch type PT* (Figure 10.5). As condensed water vapor from the breath can clog the tubes or screens and raise the PT resistance causing it to lose calibration, the screens or tubes are often heated to prevent condensation. (2) The second type of PT uses a light, plastic, *turbine fan* mounted in the mouthpiece housing with its axis of rotation in the center of the housing. The fan rotates at an angular velocity proportional to the volume flow rate through the PT. The angular velocity is measured photoelectrically or magnetically without contact with the turbine fan. In both schemes, the pulse frequency is proportional to turbine rpm which is proportional to volume flow rate. (3) A third type of PT uses a *hot-wire anemometer*. This is a nonlinear flow rate sensor in which a fine wire is heated by passing electric current through it. In still air, it reaches a certain temperature $T_o > T_a$ (ambient temperature) and has a certain resistance, $R_o(T_o)$, which is measured. Air flowing past the hot wire cools it, and its temperature drops, lowering its resistance. A feedback circuit senses this lowered resistance and passes more current through the hot wire, reheating it to T_o and R_o. After some nonlinear compensation circuitry, the hot wire anemometer circuit outputs a voltage proportional to the air volume flow rate (cf. Northrop 2014, Section 7.3.2.1). Most modern spirometers use the turbine architecture. The PT's turbine output is connected to a computer's digital interface, and a specialized spirometry software package computes and stores the test parameters described above, and also compares patient performance with the normal entries in its database. Note that the Fleisch PT's output is a voltage proportional to pressure. The pressure is the difference across the pneumatic resistance, which in turn is proportional to flow rate in L/s. Thus, the computer must integrate the differential pressure sensor output signal to determine the lung volumes.

10.3 TESTS WITH SPIROMETERS

In this section, we will describe the uses of gas dilution to measure certain respiratory parameters. For example, Helium dilution can be used to measure RV and FRC. A known concentration of helium in air is put into a positive displacement spirometer. The subject exhales then breathes the mixture in and out several times. Helium is almost insoluble in blood, so that after a few breaths, the helium is diluted by the amount of air in the FRC volume. The initial concentration of helium is C_1 in a total spirometer volume, V_1. So C_1V_1 is the initial amount of He at STP. Since this amount of He does not change because a negligible amount of He is absorbed in the lungs, we can write:

$$C_1V_1 = C_2(V_1 + FRC). \tag{10.1}$$

Solving for FRC:

$$FRC = \frac{V_1(C_1 - C_2)}{C_2}, \tag{10.2}$$

where V_1 is the initial spirometer volume, C_1 is the initial He concentration, and C_2 is the He concentration after several mixing breaths.

C_1 and C_2 can be measured by a mass spectrometer tuned for He, or by measuring the change in sound velocity in the He–air mixture (for details on this latter method, see Section 8.6).

A less accurate means of measuring FRC is by *open-circuit nitrogen washout* (West 1985). In this method, the patient starts in the exhaled condition in which there is 80% N_2 in his or her lungs. He then takes many breaths of pure O_2 from a source, and his exhales are directed into an "empty," large-capacity spirometer. After about 5–7 min, all of the N_2 in the FRC or RV of the lungs has been replaced by pure O_2, and this original N_2 is now in the spirometer along with exhaled O_2, CO_2, and water vapor. (The CO_2 and water vapor can be absorbed if desired.) The concentration of N_2, C_{N_2}, in the final spirometer volume, V_2, is measured. FRC or RV is calculated from:

$$C_{N_1}RV = C_{N_2}V_2. \tag{10.3}$$

This method assumes that all of the N_2 in the lungs is washed out, which may not be the case in certain types of OLD.

Still another, venerable method of estimating FRC and RV makes use of a *whole-body plethysmograph*. The patient sits in a hermetically sealed, coffin-like box. The internal pressure of the box (with patient) can be measured very accurately. Initially, the pressure in the box with the patient is made atmospheric, P_a, before it is sealed. The patient is asked to make a strong respiratory exhale effort, starting at FRC, against a *closed* mouthpiece containing a pressure sensor. As he compresses the gas in his lungs, from P_1 to P_2, the lung (and chest) volume decrease slightly by ΔV, causing the gas volume of the box to increase slightly by the same amount. Since the amount of gas in the box (outside of the patient) has not changed, the gas pressure in the box decreases from P_a to $P_3 < P_a$. Using Boyle's gas law ($P_1V_1 = P_2V_2$ at constant temperature, and amount of gas), we can write for the patient:

$$P_aFRC = P_2(FRC - \Delta V). \tag{10.4}$$

Thus FRC is given by

$$FRC = \frac{P_2 \, \Delta V}{(P_2 - P_a)}L. \tag{10.5}$$

Now ΔV can be found from Boyle's law applied to the box. Initially the box is at P_a, so:

$$P_aV_{BP} = P_3(V_{BP} + \Delta V). \tag{10.6}$$

The increase in box volume caused by the patient's blocked exhalation effort causes the box pressure to fall by $P_3 < P_a$. V_{BP} is the gas volume of the sealed box with patient inside, resting.

$$\Delta V = V_{BP}(P_a / P_3 - 1). \tag{10.7}$$

When this relation for ΔV is substituted into Equation 10.5, we obtain finally:

$$FRC = \frac{P_2 V_{BP}[(P_a/P_3) - 1]}{(P_2 - P_a)} L. \qquad (10.8)$$

P_a, P_2, and P_3 are all directly measured pressures, V_{BP} needs to be determined. One way of measuring V_{BP} with Boyle's law is to include in the box during the above measurements a completely evacuated, thin-walled, gas tank of volume, V_T. With the box sealed, the patient opens the tank's valve and lets it fill with box air. The box pressure drops to a measured P_4. This maneuver effectively increases the box volume by a known V_T. Thus by Boyle's law:

$$P_a V_{BP} = P_4(V_{BP} + V_T)$$
$$\downarrow \qquad \qquad (10.9)$$
$$V_{BP} = V_T P_4 / (P_a - P_4).$$

Equation 10.9 is substituted into Equation 10.8 for a complete solution to FRC from known or measured parameters.

West (1985) observed:

It should be noted that the body plethysmograph and the gas dilution (or washout) method[s] may measure different volumes. The body plethysmograph measures the total volume of gas in the lungs, including any which is trapped behind closed airways and which therefore does not communicate with the mouth. By contrast, the helium dilution and nitrogen washout methods measure only communicating gas, or ventilated lung volume. In young normal subjects these volumes are virtually the same, but in patients with lung disease [OLD] the ventilated volume may be considerably less than the total volume because of gas trapped behind obstructed airways.

Another important respiratory parameter is *alveolar ventilation* (AV). If a person's *tidal volume* (TV) (the volume breathed out in a normal breathing cycle) is 0.6 L, and there are 14 breaths/min, then the total volume leaving the nose each minute is $0.6 \times 14 = 8.4$ L/min. This number is known as the person's *minute volume*. The volume of air entering the nose is slightly greater since more O_2 is taken in than CO_2 is given off. Significantly, not all of the air taken in reaches the alveoli where the actual O_2/CO_2 gas exchange takes place. Of each 0.6 L inhaled, ~180 mL remains behind in the *anatomical dead space* (ADS). Thus, the AV is $(600 - 180) \times 14 = 5880$ mL/min. The AV is an important parameter in evaluating the health of a person's respiratory system. It represents the actual amount of fresh air available for gas exchange.

The calculation of alveolar ventilation depends on measurement of the ADS, which is basically the volume of the gas-conducting airways (the trachea, the bronchial tubes, and various types of bronchioles), and is sex, weight, height and posture dependent. The ADS can be measured by Fowler's method (West 1985). A subject breathes normal air (80% N_2, 20% O_2), then takes a maximum inhale of pure O_2, and then exhales fully into a spirometer that records the exhaled volume. At the same time, a fast mass spectrometer-type N_2 analyzer measures the N_2 in the exhaled breath at the mouth. First, pure O_2 comes out from the upper airways, then as the exhalation continues, the N_2 concentration rises to a plateau whose value is the N_2 concentration in the alveolar gas. Graphs of the typical concentration of N_2 versus time and N_2 versus exhaled volume are shown in Figure 10.6. The ADS is estimated by drawing a vertical line on Figure 10.7 so that the areas A_1 and A_2 are equal (West 1985).

Another means of estimating dead space was described by Bohr (1891) (cited by West 1985). Bohr's technique measures *physiological dead space* (PDS), which is different from ADS. It is obvious that respiratory CO_2 emission comes from the alveoli, and not the PDS. Thus, we can write:

$$TVC_{ECO_2} = AVC_{ACO_2}, \qquad (10.10)$$

where AV is the total alveolar gas volume, C_{ECO_2} is the concentration of CO_2 in the expired breath, and C_{ACO_2} is the concentration of CO_2 in the alveoli just before expiration. It is well known that:

$$TV = AV + PDS. \qquad (10.11)$$

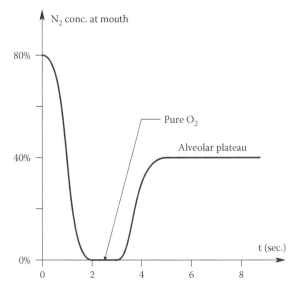

Figure 10.6 Representative graph of exhaled N_2 versus time in the Fowler test to measure anatomical dead space (ADS) in the lungs. The exhaled N_2 concentration is measured with a QPMS.

Hence:

$$AV = TV - PDS. \tag{10.12}$$

Substituting AV from Equation 10.10, we can write:

$$\frac{PDS}{TV} = \frac{C_{ACO_2} - C_{ECO_2}}{C_{ACO_2}}. \tag{10.13}$$

Two more assumptions are made: (1) the partial pressure of a gas is proportional to its concentration, and (2) the P_{CO_2} of alveolar gas is nearly equal to the P_{CO_2} of arterial blood, P_{aCO_2}. Finally, we have *the Bohr equation:*

$$\frac{PDS}{TV} = \frac{P_{aCO_2} - P_{ECO_2}}{P_{aCO_2}}. \tag{10.14}$$

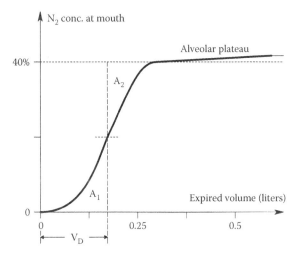

Figure 10.7 Detail of measuring the anatomical dead space.

West (1985) stated:

The normal ratio of dead space to tidal volume is in the range of 0.2 to 0.35 during resting breathing. The ratio decreases on exercise but increases with age.

Bohr's method measures the volume of the lung which does not eliminate CO_2. Because this is a functional measurement, the volume is called the physiological dead space.

Note that in Equation 10.14, TV is directly measured by spirometry, and the partial CO_2 pressures are measured with sensors: in the expired gas by an infrared absorption sensor, and in an arterial blood sample by a Severinghaus P_{CO_2} electrode (Webster 1992). (The Severinghaus P_{CO_2} sensor is described in detail in Section 7.3 of this book.)

It is also of interest in a medical evaluation of the respiratory system to noninvasively measure the alveolar capillary blood flow. One means of measuring the *instantaneous pulmonary blood flow* is to have the subject again sit in the hermetically sealed, full-body, plethysmograph chamber in which there is a collapsible gas bag containing a mixture of 21% O_2 and 79% nitrous oxide (N_2O) at atmospheric pressure. The air inside the chamber is initially at atmospheric pressure, P_o. The subject breathes the gas mixture. N_2O is taken up by the capillary circulation very rapidly; absorption by alveolar capillaries being almost complete in ~100 ms. The transfer of N_2O into the pulmonary capillary blood is said to be *perfusion limited*. As the N_2O volume "disappears" by solution into the pulmonary blood flow, the net gas volume in the chamber *increases* as the N_2O is absorbed.

By Boyle's law,

$$(P_o + \Delta P) = K/(V_o + \Delta V) = (K/V_o)[1 - \Delta V/V_o]. \tag{10.15}$$

The decrement in pressure in the chamber is related to the increase in chamber volume.

$$\Delta P = \frac{K\Delta V}{V_o^2}. \tag{10.16}$$

The chamber pressure thus drops in a slow, stepwise manner, with the steps synchronized with the heartbeat. ΔP is measured, ΔV (of N_2O) is calculated, and from the known solubility of N_2O in blood at atmospheric pressure, it is possible to calculate the blood volume per heartbeat through the alveolar capillaries (West 1985).

10.4 DIFFUSING CAPACITY OF THE LUNGS FOR CARBON MONOXIDE

The DLCO test indirectly measures the extent to which oxygen (or any light-molecular-weight gas) passes from the alveoli into the blood (Hughes and Bates 2003). This test involves measuring the partial pressure difference between inspired and expired carbon monoxide (CO), and thus demonstrates gas uptake by pulmonary capillaries that are less dependent on cardiac output. Note that hemoglobin in RBCs has a very high affinity for CO; a [pCO] of ~0.7 mmHg can be lethal. A [pCO] of only 0.4 mmHg in the alveoli, 1/250 that of the alveolar oxygen, allows the CO to compete equally with the O_2 for combination with hemoglobin; it causes half the blood hemoglobin molecules to become bound with CO instead of O_2 (Guyton 1991, Chapter 40). Naturally, in single-breath DLCO tests, an innocuous [pCO] is used. MacIntyre et al. (2005) stated that the inspired CO should nominally be 0.3% (one breath).

Several factors are found to reduce DLCO; for example:

- Effective thickening of the alveolar wall; from fibrosis, alveolitis, vasculitis

- RLDs and chronic OLDs

- Emphysema

- Pulmonary embolism

- Cardiac insufficiency

- Pulmonary hypertension

- Chronic heart failure

- Anemia (low Hb can cause incomplete absorption of alveolar capillary blood [pCO], leaving residual CO in the exhaled breath)

Factors that can *increase* DLCO include polycythaemia, asthma, and increased pulmonary blood volume flow, left-to-right intracardiac shunting, and alveolar hemorrhage.

More about the physiology and measurement protocol used to calculate the single-breath DLCO can be found in the review paper by Macintyre et al. (2005).

10.5 CHAPTER SUMMARY

Physical pulmonary function tests are an important NI means of diagnosing OLDs. In general, they do require patient cooperation. Modern, turbine-type or Fleisch PTs interfaced with a PC enable clinicians to acquire and store patient data and recall past performance records for clinical comparison. The effectiveness of a bronchodilator can be evaluated in one patient visit. Emphysema only gets worse with time; it is important to be able to quantitatively track the progress of this debilitating condition.

Physiological tests of the ability of the alveolar tissues to exchange gases can also be performed by having the patient breath O_2 plus a tracer gas such as He or N_2O. How readily the tracer gas is taken up, or dissipated (once a steady-state concentration in blood is reached) is an indication of alveolar blood flow and available, gas-exchangeable tissue area.

Asthma and other OLDs are frequent in today's society. The increase of emissions from diesel engines and power plants adds to the bad air quality in urban and industrial regions. Other chemicals, such as gasoline additives, add to the level of air contamination, in spite of sealed gas tanks and catalytic mufflers. (When a car is first started, its catalytic muffler is cold, and ineffective.) Simple, quick, NI pulmonary function testing as a diagnostic tool is becoming more important.

11 Measurement of Basal Metabolism

11.1 INTRODUCTION

Metabolism, in general, is the sum of all of the chemical reactions that occur in the body; both in intracellular and extracellular compartments. Because biochemistry is so complex, we generally focus our attention on certain subsets of metabolic reactions, such as mineral metabolism, further divided into subsets such as calcium, copper, iron, magnesium, potassium and sodium metabolisms, as well as carbohydrate, fat, and protein metabolisms, to cite a few. *Basal metabolism* is defined as the study of *oxidative metabolism* in the mitochondria of cells in a *resting* animal in which certain energy sources such as glucose are oxidized to form molecules of the ubiquitous, energy storage molecule, *adenosine triphosphate* (ATP). The formation of ATP molecules is accompanied by the utilization of respired oxygen, and the production of carbon dioxide, heat, and other "metabolic products." ATP is ubiquitous because the energy stored in two phosphate bonds of the molecule can be released enzymatically to drive many other endothermic biochemical reactions. For example, active ion pumps in cell membranes use ATP as an energy source, including muscle, where it is required to drive the molecular engines that actively take up the calcium ions released in the process of muscle contraction. (Muscle cannot relax unless the Ca^{++} is actively taken up from the actin and myosin and stored in the membrane cells of the sarcoplasmic reticulum.) The structural formula for ATP is shown in Figure 11.1. Each of the two high-energy phosphate bonds contains about 12 calories/mole of ATP (12 Cal = 12,000 calories). Most of intracellular ATP is formed in the mitochondria of cells in which it is used to power various biosynthetic reactions, ion pumps, etc. In the various linked biochemical pathways in which glucose is oxidized to get the energy to form ATP, a net two ATP molecules are formed in the process of *glycolysis* in which one glucose molecule is consumed. Also produced in glycolysis are two *pyruvic acid* molecules per glucose molecule. The two pyruvic acid molecules are enzymatically converted to two molecules of *acetyl CoA,* one of which then enters the *citric acid cycle,* where two more ATP molecules are formed per initial glucose molecule. During glycolysis and the citric acid cycle, 24 hydrogen atoms are released. These hydrogen atoms are further oxidized to give an additional 34 ATP molecules per glucose molecule. Thus, as many as 38 ATP molecules can be synthesized from each glucose molecule. A gram mole of glucose then can produce 456 Cal. stored in the phosphate bonds of the resultant ATP. About 686 Cal. are released during the complete oxidation of a mole of glucose, giving an overall efficiency of 66%. The difference of 686 − 456 = 230 Cal. is released as *waste heat.* This heat acts to raise the temperature of the cells above ambient temperature. In mammals and birds, this temperature average is regulated, and the enzyme systems and metabolic pathways in the body are found to work optimally in the narrow range of normal, regulated body temperature (Guyton 1991).

The processes of ATP synthesis and its utilization in the various intracellular reactions are under closed-loop control by various regulatory hormones. These include thyroid hormone (TH;

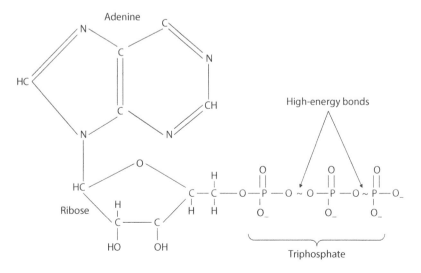

Figure 11.1 Adenosine triphosphate (ATP) molecule.

thyroxine), triiodothyronine, adrenaline, insulin, glucagon, and growth hormone. A disorder or disease affecting the regulation of the concentrations of these hormones affects overall cellular glucose metabolism, including the production of ATP, heat and CO_2, and the consumption of O_2. In order to noninvasively test for problems in the regulation of hormones that modulate metabolism, it is possible to test under standard, resting (basal) conditions, the amount of glucose that is oxidized by the body. One rather elaborate test is to immerse the subject in an insulated tank of water close to, but below normal body temperature. Each calorie released by the body through the skin theoretically will raise each kilogram of water 1°C. In a complex process, the water is chilled by a closed-loop control system that circulates cool water through the tank, keeping its temperature constant. By keeping track of the heat removed from the tank in order to keep it at a constant temperature, and knowing the patient's mass and skin area, it is then possible to obtain a measure of the basal metabolism. The isothermal water tank method may have a sound theoretical basis, but is unwieldy and expensive. Consequently, the measurement of O_2 consumption has proven to provide the same information, is less expensive, and is generally a simpler procedure to perform. The *metabolator* method of measurement of basal metabolism is described in the following section.

11.2 BMR TEST PROCEDURE

Over 95% of the energy expended in the body comes from oxidation reactions with respirated O_2. If 1 L of O_2 at standard temperature and pressure (STP) is used to burn an excess of glucose in a calorimeter, 5.01 calories of energy are released. Excess starches burned with 1 L of O_2 at STP release 5.06 calories; protein releases 4.60 and fat 4.70 calories. It has been found that for the average diet, the adult human metabolism will release 4.825 calories of heat for each liter of

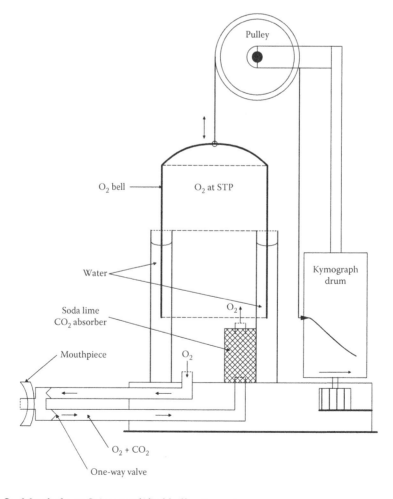

Figure 11.2   Metabolator. It is a modified bell spirometer.

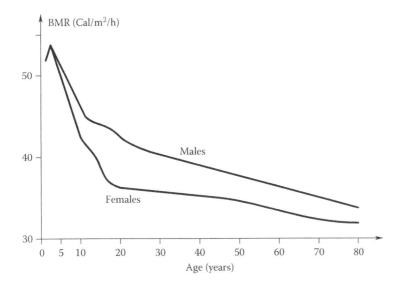

Figure 11.3 Normal basal metabolic rates for men and women according to age. Note the decline of BMR with age.

O_2 "burned" in the body (Guyton 1991). In order to accurately measure the volume of O_2 consumed, a volumetric system called a *metabolator* is used, shown schematically in Figure 11.2. The water-sealed bell is filled with a known volume of O_2 at STP. To measure basal O_2 consumption, the patient must have fasted overnight and be comfortably recumbent in a warm room with no skeletal muscle activity. The patient breathes pure O_2 and exhales a mixture of O_2, CO_2, and water vapor. One-way valves direct the exhaled gases to a canister of soda lime where the CO_2 is totally absorbed, and the exhaled O_2 and some water vapor are returned to the bell. The overnight fast is necessary because as the result of eating a meal, the blood concentration of glucose rises, falls below the resting level, then returns to the resting level. The blood concentration of insulin also rises in response to eating, while the concentration of the pancreatic hormone, glucagon falls during the rise in insulin level. The perturbations in the levels of these glucoregulatory hormones also affect metabolism as do the transients in blood glucose concentration.

The patient breathes the O_2 from the metabolator for about an hour, and the total volume of O_2 consumed is noted. The rate of O_2 consumption under basal conditions depends on the patient's skin surface area, age, and gender. The patient's surface area can be estimated from the formula of DuBois (West 1985):

$$A(cm^2) = (Weight, kg)^{0.425} \times (Height, cm)^{0.725}. \tag{11.1}$$

For example, an 80-kg, 180-cm tall man has $A = 2$ m². Let V be the total liters of O_2 at STP consumed under basal conditions. The total Calories burned are then estimated by

$$H = 2.825 V \, Cal. \tag{11.2}$$

The BMR is found by dividing H by the body area in m² and the time in hours taken to burn V liters of O_2. As a round figure, the BMR of a normal male adult is ~35–40 Cal/m²/h, or in terms of weight, ~1 Cal/kg/h. Figure 11.3 illustrates the age and gender differences in human BMR. (Note the downslope beginning around age 45 for both males and females. If a corresponding decrease in total dietary caloric input does not accompany this reduction in BMR, obesity can result.)

11.3 CHAPTER SUMMARY

BMR is often given as a percent above or below the average BMR for a "standard" person of a given age and gender. If the BMR is abnormally high, it may be indicative of excess circulating thyroxine, which in turn can be symptomatic of a thyroid tumor. Likewise, an abnormally low %BMR can point to a low-TH level. The simple, inexpensive BMR test thus can point to the need for definitive antibody blood tests for TH, as well as other tests such as the uptake of radio-iodine (^{131}I) which is a β and γ ray emitter with a half-life of 8 days. Thyroid cells specifically take up iodine ions, and thus circulating thyroxine and 3-iodotyrosine (3IT) become labeled and can be radioassayed. The thyroid gland itself becomes radioactive and can "take its own picture" on x-ray film, providing an indication of thyroid metabolic activity. There are many other symptoms correlated with high-TH level, so basal metabolism is not necessarily a definitive test for hyperthyroidism.

Other hormones can also produce high %BMR readings. These include adrenaline, anabolic steroids, and growth hormone, all of which stimulate metabolism. Certain neurosecretory endings in the median eminence of the hypothalamus release *thyrotropin-releasing hormone* (TRH), which stimulates the anterior pituitary to release *thyroid-stimulating hormone* (TSH), which in turn causes the thyroid gland cells to increase their output of TH and 3IT. High titers of circulating TH and 3IT inhibit the rate of secretion of TSH, providing feedback regulation of hormone concentration. Brain tumors that interrupt the TRH $\rightarrow$ TSH $\rightarrow$ TH pathway can lead to low TH and %BMR.

In summary, the BMR test is simple, noninvasive, and can point to the need for more detailed tests on the metabolic endocrine system.

12 Ocular Tonometry

12.1 INTRODUCTION

Ocular tonometry is a class of NI measurement that allows an ophthalmologist (and some optometrists) to estimate the internal hydraulic pressure of the eyeballs, called the *intraocular pressure* (IOP). The IOP is the result of the constant production (and outflow) of the liquid *aqueous humor* (AH) into the interior of the eyes. The AH is found around the lens and in the anterior chamber of the eye. It serves as a nutrient solution for the lens, the iris, and the inside of the cornea, and its pressure helps to maintain the proper shape of the eyeball. AH is continuously formed in a normal eye at a rate of about $Q_{AH} = 2$ mm^3/min by the cells of the *ciliary process*, a tissue lying behind the lens having an exposed area of about 6 cm^2 (Guyton 1991). AH is formed by the active, metabolic "pumping" of Na$^+$ ions from inside ciliary process cells to the perilenticular region inside of the eyeball. There is also active transport of ascorbate and certain amino acids into the eyeball. Water, chloride, glucose, and bicarbonate ions follow the ions pumped into the eyeball due to osmotic pressure, and diffusion down concentration gradients. AH contains mainly low-molecular-weight substances, including Na$^+$, K$^+$, HCO$_3^-$, citrate, ascorbate, urea, glucose, etc.

Clearly, in the steady state, the AH must exit the eye at the same volume flow rate that it enters. Outflow of AH is through the *canal of Schlemm*, into the episcleral veins, thence into the main venous circulation, etc. The eyeball is slightly elastic, with most of its compliance coming from the thin, clear cornea. Normal IOP is about 16 mmHg. If there is an increase in the outflow resistance, the normal IOP rises, and if the IOP exceeds its normal high range (about 30 mmHg), the condition known as *glaucoma* can exist. In extreme situations, the IOP can exceed 60–80 mmHg. Such acute glaucoma sharply reduces normal arterial blood flow to the retina, causing poor oxygenation and impaired nutrition of retinal neurons and glial cells. If prolonged, acute glaucoma can lead to the death of retinal neurons, including the loss of retinal ganglion cells, the axons of which comprise the optic nerve. Such neuron loss is irreversible, and it causes loss of visual field, acuity, and even total blindness. Thus, it is medically important as part of every routine eye examination to measure the IOP, especially in the older patients who are more susceptible to glaucoma.

It is important to point out that high IOP is not the only diagnostic sign for glaucoma; it is an important one, however. The retinal nerve damage (cupping) associated with glaucoma has been observed in 50% of the patients with a baseline IOP *less than* 21 mmHg. Also, 50% of the patients with a Goldmann tonometer-measured IOP of over 30 mmHg never developed glaucomatous visual field loss. Less than 10% of the patients with IOP > 21 mmHg have field loss (Spears 1999). Such a loose correlation between elevated IOP and glaucoma indicates that the examining physician should also rely on measurements of losses of the visual field and fundoscopy of the optic nerve head and its blood vessels in the diagnosis of glaucoma.

The simplest, most inaccurate, and subjective means of estimating IOP is by digital (finger, not computer) manipulation of the cornea through the closed eyelid. The examining physician rests his/her hands on the patient's forehead for stability, and presses through the closed eyelid inward and toward the center of the eyeball with his/her index fingers. The perceived ocular compliance is related to extensive personal experience to arrive at an estimate of IOP that may approach 2-bit accuracy (1 part in 4, i.e., low, normal, elevated, and high).

The ideal, *invasive* means of measuring IOP would be to penetrate the eyeball with a saline-filled, hypodermic needle and cannula connected to a pressure sensor. Fortunately, an indirect, NI means of estimating IOP has evolved, called ocular tonometry. There are two major types of tonometer that use the elastic property of the thin cornea: *Applanation tonometers*, such as the Goldmann (1957) type, and various air-puff tonometers (APTs), based on the Forbes APT design, generate a known force that flattens a specified area of the cornea. The IOP is approximately equal to the applied force divided by the flattened area. *Impression tonometers* include the Schiøtz handheld and electronic tonometer and the McLean tonometer, developed in 1919 (Tonometers 2017). Impression tonometers measure the amount of indentation caused by a known force on a small-diameter probe contacting the center of the cornea. All tonometers that directly touch the cornea require its anesthetization and sterile technique.

The simplified mechanics of applanation tonometry are illustrated in Figure 12.1. Here, a force, either from direct mechanical contact with the cornea or from air pressure, causes a small area of the cornea to flatten. In the figure, we assume for simplicity that the entire eyeball is a hollow sphere of radius R, and volume $V_1 = (4/3)\pi R^3$ cm^3. Inside is the intraocular hydraulic pressure which we wish to measure; call it P_1. The external force F_A is increased until a known area A of the cornea is flattened. This area is $A = \pi r^2$ cm^2. As a result of this flattening, it can be shown that

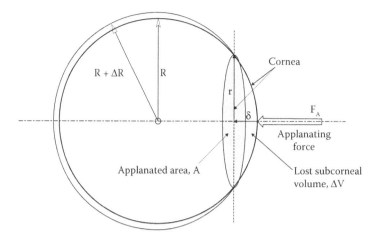

Figure 12.1 Simplified cross section of an eyeball showing corneal applanation. (Internal anatomical features omitted.)

a volume $\Delta V = (1/6)\pi\delta(3r^2 + \delta^2)$ cm^3 is subtracted from the original eye volume, V_1. Assume that the AH is an incompressible liquid, the eyeball is elastic, and no AH leaves the eyeball during the short period of IOP measurement so that applanation causes a small, transient elevation in IOP, ΔP, and an equivalent expansion of the eyeball expressed by a net ΔR. This relation can be summarized by

$$P_1 V_1 \cong (P_1 + \Delta P)(V_1 - \Delta V). \tag{12.1}$$

Furthermore, we assume that the applanating pressure, $F_A/A = (P_1 + \Delta P)$. Thus, we can write:

$$P_1 V_1 = F_A/(\pi r^2)(V_1 - \Delta V). \tag{12.2}$$

This relation reduces to

$$P_1 = (F_A/A)\left[1 - \frac{\Delta V}{V_1}\right]. \tag{12.3}$$

Using Equation 12.3, we can finally write:

$$P_{app} = (F_A/A) \cong IOP\left[1 + \frac{3r^2\delta}{8R^3}\right] \cong IOP. \tag{12.4}$$

F and A are generally known; and from the geometry and real dimensions, $3r^2\delta/(8R^3) \ll 1$, so the approximation is generally valid for the Goldmann and air-puff applanation tonometers. In the sections below, we will first examine the clever APT developed by Forbes et al. (1974), and then describe the classic Schiøtz, McLean, and Goldmann tonometers.

12.2 NONCONTACT, AIR-PUFF APPLANATION TONOMETER

All applanation tonometers are based on the principle that if a sufficient force is applied to the cornea, it will flatten when the (force × flattened area) $\cong$ IOP. This simple assumption neglects the natural stiffness of the cornea. In 1974, Forbes et al. published the design and evaluation of a unique, innovative, no-touch tonometric system consisting of four subsystems. The *first* is a pneumatic system that delivers a short, collimated, air pulse whose force increases linearly in time. The collimated air stream is directed at the center of the cornea. Initially, the force of the air pulse on the cornea increases linearly with time. The *second* is an electro-optical system that detects applanation (flattening) of the cornea due to a critical air pressure with microsecond resolution. The *third* is an electro-optical system that ensures the correct alignment of the first two systems on the patient's cornea. The *fourth* subsystem is a dedicated computer that controls the APT operation, processes sensor output data, and calculates and displays the estimated IOP digitally.

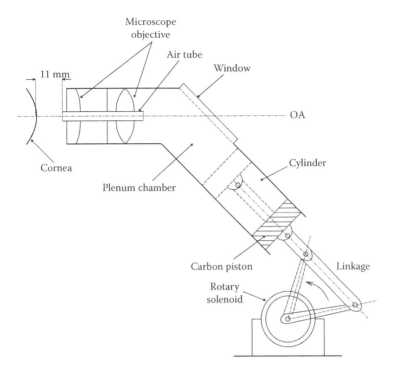

Figure 12.2 Simplified cross section of the mechanism of an air-puff tonometer.

The *first system* is shown schematically in Figure 12.2. A rotary solenoid is coupled by a two-arm crank to a carbon piston sealed in a polished, stainless-steel cylinder. When the solenoid is energized, its rotation forces the piston into the cylinder, compressing the air so that the internal pressure rises as $P = kt^2$ at first. The small tube through the center of the alignment system lens assembly acts as a pneumatic resistance, R_t, so that the volume flow through the tube is given by

$$\dot{Q}_A = P(t)/R_t \text{ cm}^3/\text{s}. \tag{12.5}$$

Hence, the volume flow of air directed at the center of the cornea also increases $\propto t^2$ in time. It takes about 7.5 ms for $\dot{Q}_A$ to reach its maximum square-law value from zero flow, and the entire pulse of air flow is over in about 25–30 ms, before the subject can blink. The force exerted by the air stream on the corneal apex can be given by Newton's second law: $F = ma$. The mass of the air stream (neglecting compression in the short tube) is $m = (AL\rho/g)$ grams, *where* A is the tube's cross-sectional area, L is its length, ρ is the air density, and g is the acceleration of gravity. The acceleration of the gas in the tube can be shown to be:

$$a = \ddot{x} = \ddot{Q}_A/A \text{ cm/s}^2. \tag{12.6}$$

And the rate of change of volume flow can be written as (Northrop 2000):

$$\ddot{Q}_A = \dot{P}\pi r^4/(8L\eta) \text{ cm}^3/\text{s}^2. \tag{12.7}$$

Here, r is the tube's radius in cm and η is the gas viscosity in poise. Thus, the force on the cornea increases approximately linearly in time during the rising phase of the air pulse.

$$F_c = \dot{P}\left(\frac{\rho\pi r^4}{8g\eta}\right) = 2kt\left(\frac{\rho\pi r^4}{8g\eta}\right) \text{dynes}. \tag{12.8}$$

At the critical F_c, the cornea flattens, then becomes concave. As the air flow goes to zero, the cornea again flattens, then becomes normally convex. The orifice of the tube is held about 11 mm from the apex of the cornea.

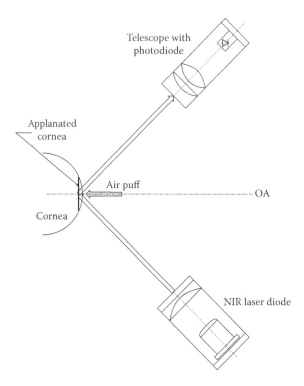

Figure 12.3 Schematic of the applanation-detecting optics used in the air-puff tonometer.

The *second system* that detects the instant of applanation is shown schematically in Figure 12.3. A collimated, low-powered, NIR laser beam is directed at a point at the center of the to-be-applanated cornea. When the cornea is normally convex, the reflected laser beam is dispersed by reflection from the curved corneal surface, and the photodiode receives very low NIR light intensity. When the force of the air puff causes corneal applanation, the collimated laser beam is reflected directly from the flat surface of the cornea into the telescope to the photodiode. A sharp spike of voltage is produced that has two functions: (1) It causes the power to the solenoid to be interrupted, aborting the further increase of air force on the cornea. (2) The pulse signals the tonometer's computer the time at which applanation occurred. Because the air-puff force versus time is the same for every measurement, the applanation time can be related to IOP by previous calibration, and the fact that the force increases linearly with time.

The *third system* is a complex system of lenses and mirrors that allows the operator to align the tonometer's axis perpendicular to a plane tangent to the apex of the cornea and adjust its distance from the corneal apex. In other words, align it along the gaze axis of the eye under measurement when the eye is fixated on an LED fixation target. Alignment is critical because of the air puff is directed off-center from the gaze axis, the measured IOP will be higher than seen for an on-axis measurement. The alignment system uses an LED beam reflection of the normally curved corneal apex to guarantee alignment. Different lenses can be switched into this optical pathway to compensate for near- or far-sighted eyes. If the LED beam is not in registry with its sensor, the system will not generate an air puff, and the operator must realign the tonometer.

For the original calibration of the APT, Goldmann applanation tonometry was done on the same eyes as the air-puff system (Forbes et al. 1974). A total of 570 different eyes were examined, with IOPs ranging from 7 to 60 mmHg. The Goldmann tonometer was considered to be the "gold standard" (true IOP). Linear regression of a scatter diagram of APT versus Goldmann readings showed that:

$$\text{Air-Puff IOP} = 0.953\,(\text{Goldmann IOP}) + 1.01, \quad r = 0.90. \tag{12.9}$$

Thus, the accuracy of the APT was judged acceptable for clinical use. Its advantages are that it is NI, quick, does not require sterile technique, and does not require corneal anesthesia. Because it is computer based, it can store patient data from previous exams, and plot these data so that the treating physician can examine progress in the pharmacological treatment of high IOP. Disadvantages of the APT include the requirements that patients have clear, smooth corneas, and be able to see the fixation target clearly, and fixate.

12.3 CONTACT TONOMETERS

All contact tonometers require sterile technique and anesthetization (e.g., by 0.5% proparacaine) of the corneal surface. They all estimate IOP by exerting an inward force on the corneal surface and either measuring the amount of indentation produced, or the area flattened for some critical force causing flattening. In the latter case, the IOP ≈ applied force/area flattened.

A photograph of a modern *Schiøtz* and an early twentieth-century *McLean indentation tonometer* are shown in Figure 12.4. In both tonometers, a vertical, weighted rod makes contact with the cornea through a hole in the center of a concave cup that rests on the apex of the cornea. In the Schiøtz tonometer, the end of the rod is 3.00 mm diameter, and is slightly concave where it contacts the cornea. The McLean tonometer's rod is 2.50 mm diameter and has a flat face. Both the Schiøtz and the McLean tonometers' cups are about 1.0 cm in diameter. The Schiøtz instrument has a general, 0–20 scale, and can have weights of 5.5, 7.5, and 10.0 g added to the rod. It is used with a lookup table for IOP (the Friedenwald table). The McLean tonometer has a weight built into its rod, and reads IOP directly on its nonlinear scale. Protocol for use of this type of tonometer requires three successive readings; an average is taken.

The *Goldmann applanation tonometer* has been used as a gold standard to evaluate the performance of other types of tonometers (Forbes et al. 1974, Wingert et al. 1995), and is probably the most common tonometer used by modern ophthalmologists and optometrists. A modern Goldmann tonometer is used with the patient's head erect, and the eyes gazing horizontally. The patient rests his head in a three-point headrest (chin and two forehead pads) and looks straight ahead at a fixation point. A drop of saline containing the fluorescent dye, *fluorescein sodium*, is

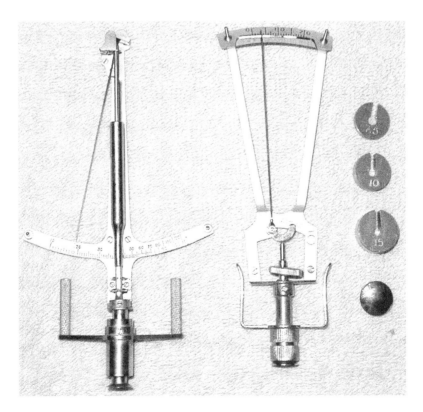

Figure 12.4 Photograph of two hand-held tonometers owned by the author. *Left:* An antique McLean indentation tonometer. *Right:* A modern Schiøtz tonometer with its weights. (Figure from Northrop, R.B. 2002. *Noninvasive Instrumentation and Measurement in Medical Diagnosis*. CRC Press, Boca Raton, FL. ISBN: 0-8493-0961-1.)

placed on the end of the probe. Fluorescein fluoresces yellow-green when irradiated with blue light, which is used in the tonometer. The optical probe of the Goldmann tonometer is slowly advanced until it just touches the apex of the anesthetized cornea. This point is sensed optically. Then the probe is slowly advanced until the operator sees a particular pattern through the optical prism structure built into the probe. The pattern is caused by the probe face flattening a circle on the cornea and forcing a ring of fluorescein to its circumference. The shape of the pattern tells the operator whether the probe is aligned correctly, and also the size of the flattened area. A handheld Goldmann-type tonometer (the *Perkins tonometer*) using a prism probe is also available; it allows IOP to be measured from eyes of supine as well as sitting patients.

There are also electronic tonometers that either measure the indentation displacement with a constant force, or the force required to produce a given flattening area of the cornea. The former is an electronic Schiøtz instrument that uses an LVDT length sensor (linear variable differential transformer) with micron resolution. The latter is called the *MacKay–Marg tonometer.*

12.4 CHAPTER SUMMARY

Tonometry is an important NI diagnostic technique used to detect elevated IOP which may lead to the condition of glaucoma and progressive vision loss. Glaucoma is generally a disease of the elderly. An abnormally high IOP is a necessary, but not sufficient, condition for glaucoma. If high IOP is detected during a routine eye exam, it should be followed up by direct observation of the retina and tests for vision loss.

The APT is a truly no-touch, NI, diagnostic instrument. Most tonometry done during eye exams is done by an electronic, Goldmann-type instrument which makes direct contact with the cornea, and thus requires corneal anesthetization and sterile technique.

13 Noninvasive Tests Involving the Input of Audible Sound Energy

13.1 INTRODUCTION

In this chapter, we will examine how low-intensity, air-coupled, acoustic energy in the range from 0.2 to 5000 Hz can be used to noninvasively characterize the health of the respiratory system (trachea, bronchial tubes, alveoli, and lung tissues), as well as the middle-ear components of the auditory system through the measurement of *acoustic impedance.* The frequency characteristics of sound transmission through the thorax are also considered as candidate NI means of diagnosing obstructive lung diseases.

Acoustic impedance, $\mathbf{Z_A}(j\omega)$, is defined in this chapter as the CGS vector ratio of pressure (in dynes/cm^2) to volume flow (in cm^3/s) caused by that pressure at a given sinusoidal frequency of pressure. It is analogous to electrical impedance in the respect that pressure is analogous to voltage, and volume flow is analogous to electrical current. The units of $\mathbf{Z_A}(j\omega)$ are *CGS acoustic ohms,* and its fundamental dimensions are $ML^{-4}T^{-1}$.

Measurement of a $\mathbf{Z_A}(j\omega)$ can be done with two pressure sensors or two microphones, and a pure acoustic resistance, R_{ac}. This measurement is analogous to measuring electrical impedance (magnitude) with a voltmeter, ammeter, and a resistance. The acoustic circuit generally used is shown in Figure 13.1, drawn as its electrical analog. As you will see below, the only problem with "pure" acoustical resistances is that they develop a phase shift at high frequencies due to acoustic *inertance* (analogous to a series electrical inductance).

It is well known that various anatomical and physical changes happen to the bronchioles and alveoli of the lungs in obstructive lung diseases (e.g., asthma, atelectasis, byssinosis, cystic fibrosis, emphysema, pneumonia, silicosis, asbestosis, tuberculosis, etc.). These changes alter the acoustic impedance of the lungs as measured orally through the tracheal airway. For example, in emphysema, the walls separating adjacent alveoli break down, producing larger alveolar spaces with walls having less elasticity. In cystic fibrosis, the alveoli and bronchioles become clogged with mucus, increasing airway resistance and reducing lung volume, etc. Different physical changes in lung tissues will lead to different $\mathbf{Z_A}(j\omega)$ plots. Hereafter, we will refer to the $\mathbf{Z_A}$ of the respiratory system "seen" through the pharynx and trachea as $\mathbf{Z_{rs}}$.

How these impedance conditions occur may be appreciated by a consideration of the basic components making up a complex acoustical impedance. For example, a cylindrical tube whose diameter is small compared to its length, whose length is small compared to the sound wavelength, and for which $r < 0.2/\sqrt{f}$, has an acoustical impedance given by (Olson 1940):

$$\mathbf{Z_A}(j\omega) = (L/\pi r^2)[8\eta/r^2 + j\omega\, 4\rho/3], \quad \text{CGS ohms.} \tag{13.1}$$

where L is the tube's length, r is its radius, η is the CGS viscosity coefficient of air $= 1.86 \times 10^{-4}$ poise at 20°C, and ρ is the density of air in g/cm^3 $= 1.205 \times 10^{-3}$.

A narrow, *rectangular slit* whose height is small compared to its length, and whose length is small compared to the wavelength has a CGS acoustic impedance given by

$$\mathbf{Z_A}(j\omega) = (6L/wd)[2\eta/d^2 + j\omega\rho/5], \tag{13.2}$$

where L is the length of the slit in the direction of the flow in cm, w = width of slit normal to the direction of flow in cm, and d is the height of the slit in cm. ρ and η are the same as in Equation 13.1.

Note that these impedances are "inertive," characterized by a positive phase angle at high frequencies. The frequency at which the real part of $\mathbf{Z_A}(j\omega)$ equals its imaginary part (ω at which $\angle \mathbf{Z_A}(j\omega_b) = +45°$) is $\omega_b = (6\eta)/(\rho r^2)$ r/s for the tube, and $\omega_b = (10\eta)/(\rho d^2)$ r/s for the slit.

All cavities or chambers of volume V with rigid boundaries have *acoustical capacitance,* C_A. C_A is analogous to electrical capacitance, defined by $i \equiv C_e(dv/dt)$. As we have seen, the current is analogous to volume flow rate, $\dot{Q}$ cm^3/s, and voltage is analogous to acoustic pressure, p. Thus, C_A is defined as the ratio of

$$C_A \equiv \frac{\dot{Q}}{\dot{p}} \tag{13.3}$$

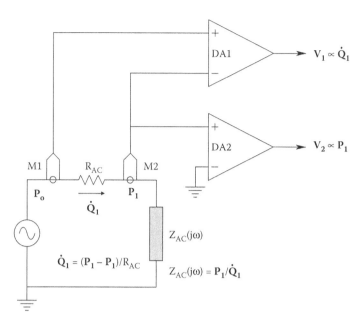

Figure 13.1 Schematic of an analog system modeling the measurement the acoustic impedance of the lungs, eardrum, etc. Acoustic volume flow can be measured, in analogy to Ohm's Law, by using two microphones to measure the sound pressure drop across a pure acoustic resistance. The driving pressure for the impedance being measured comes from microphone M2.

Olson (1940) showed that C_A of a stiff-walled chamber of volume V can be given by (assuming acoustic wavelengths are large compared to the cavity's linear dimensions):

$$C_A = V/(\rho c^2),\tag{13.4}$$

where c is the speed of sound in air (cm/s), and ρ is the mean air mass density in g/cm³.

Another way to realize acoustic capacitance is with a chamber with thin, elastic, low-mass walls, or by a thin, low-mass, elastic diaphragm coupling between two ducts. In these cases, C_A = (mechanical compliance of the diaphragm) × (area squared of the diaphragm). Mechanical compliance is defined as $C_m \equiv X/f_m$, where x is the displacement caused by a mechanical force, f_m. f_m is of course (acoustic pressure) × (diaphragm area). c_m is the reciprocal of stiffness. The fundamental dimensions of acoustical capacitance are $M^{-1}L^4T^2$.

If a tube with Z_A given by Equation 13.1 is terminated in a stiff-walled cavity, the series, driving point Z_A is:

$$\mathbf{Z_A}(j\omega) = (L/\pi r^2)[8\eta/r^2 + 4\rho j\omega/3] + \rho c^2/j\omega V.\tag{13.5}$$

In electrical terms, this impedance is analogous to a series RLC circuit with the capacitor grounded. Thus, it has a resonant frequency, ω_o, at which $\mathbf{Z_A}(j\omega)$ is real and minimum. Elementary complex algebra tells us this is at

$$\omega_o = (cr/2)\sqrt{(3\pi/VL)} \ r/s.\tag{13.6}$$

This type of acoustic circuit is called a *Helmholtz resonator*.

The reactive terms in Equations 13.1 and 13.2 for the $\mathbf{Z_{AC}}$ of a tube are due to the inertance or mass of the air in the tube and slot. In an electrical inductance, we have the well-known relation:

$$v = L(di/dt).\tag{13.7}$$

In acoustic terms, this is analogous to

$$p = M_{AC}(d\dot{Q}/dt).\tag{13.8}$$

M_{AC} is the inertance, analogous to inductance; p is pressure, analogous to voltage; and $\dot{Q}$ is volume flow, analogous to electric current in coulombs/s. Olson (1940) has shown that the inertance of a thin cylindrical tube is simply:

$$M_{AC} = (4L\rho)/(3\pi r^2). \tag{13.9}$$

Inertance has the fundamental dimensions of ML^{-4}.

The acoustic impedance of the ear canal and eardrum at audio frequencies depends on the dimensions of the auditory canal and the mechanical loading of the eardrum at its end. The eardrum drives the three ossicles that couple the sound energy from the outer ear to the cochlea, where acoustic sensory transduction takes place. The "handle" of the *malleus* ossicle is connected to the inside center of the eardrum. At the other end, the malleus is tightly bound by ligaments to the *incus* (anvil). The end of the incus articulates with the *stapes* (stirrup), the base of which moves the membrane of the *oval window*, transmitting sound energy to the fluid in the cochlea. Normally the three ossicles comprise a fairly compliant assembly that is efficient in coupling sound from the eardrum to the cochlea over a wide range of frequencies (20 Hz–15 kHz). If a sudden loud sound occurs, after about 40–80 ms, two small muscles in the inner ear, the *stapedius* and the *tensor tympani*, are caused to contract by the CNS' *auditory attenuation reflex* (AAR). Contraction of the *tensor tympani* pulls the handle of the *malleus* inward, and the *stapedius* forces the stapes outward. These opposing forces cause the ossicles to become very rigid. This rigidity has the effect of attenuating low-frequency sound (below 1 kHz) as much as 30–40 dB. This protects the cochlea from mechanically damaging, low-frequency vibrations and also allows the person to screen out loud, low-frequency sounds while listening to information-carrying sounds above 1 kHz. The AAR causes a change in the acoustic impedance of the eardrum as measured from the ear canal. In normal individuals if $Z_A(j\omega)$ of one ear is measured while the other ear is presented with a sudden, loud, low-frequency sound, the AAR will cause a simultaneous $Z_A(j\omega)$ change in both the ears that can be measured in one ear.

Measurement of the $Z_A(j\omega) = Z_{rs}(j\omega)$ of the lungs or the eardrum can serve as simple NI means of screening outpatients for COLD or hearing problems. In the following sections, we will examine the history of respiratory acoustic impedance measurement systems (RAIMSs), and a RAIMS developed by the author and his graduate students. We will also describe auditory $Z_A(j\omega)$ measurement systems, and a prototype system that measures the acoustic transfer function, $H_{rs}(j\omega)$, of the thorax (including the lungs) using acoustic white noise.

13.2 ACOUSTIC IMPEDANCE MEASUREMENT OF THE RESPIRATORY SYSTEM

Figure 13.2 illustrates the acoustic and electronic components of a general system for measuring the respiratory acoustic impedance. The trachea and lungs constitute a complex, distributed-parameter acoustic impedance, which, at a given frequency, may appear reactive capacitive, reactive inductive, or even real (resistive, a resonance condition).

One of the first efforts to characterize the acoustic impedance of the respiratory system was done by Pimmel et al. (1977). Acoustic pressure was generated by an acoustic suspension loudspeaker (Acoustic Research Corp., AR-3), and volume flow was measured as the pressure drop across a heated Silverman pneumotach (H. Rudolph Co., Model 3700), which served as an acoustic resistance at low frequencies. Two Validyne Model MP-45 pressure sensors were used as low-frequency microphones to measure the sound pressure at the input (loudspeaker) end of the pneumotach, P_1, and P_2 at the mouth end of the pneumotach.

Because of the sinusoidal nature of P_1 and P_2, the phase between these signals (i.e., the phase of $\dot{Q}(t)$ with respect to (P_2)) was measured by passing the conditioned, sinusoidal output voltages from the sensors into zero-crossing comparators to make phase-coherent TTL signals, then passing the TTL signals into a digital phase detector subsystem. The flow was determined by

$$\dot{Q} = [P_1 - P_2]/Z_{pt}(j\omega) = K_m[V_1 - V_2]/Z_{pt}(j\omega), \tag{13.10}$$

where P_1 and P_2 are the actual complex sinusoidal pressures across the pneumotach, K_m is the sensor scaling constant, and $Z_{pt}(j\omega)$ is the complex acoustical impedance of the pneumotach. $Z_{pt}(j\omega)$ is generally of the form:

$$Z_{pt}(j\omega) = R_{pt} + j\omega M_{pt.} \tag{13.11}$$

At low frequencies, $Z_{pt}(j\omega) \cong R_{pt}$ (real), which is what is desired. As the frequency increases, the phase angle of $Z_{pt}(j\omega)$ increases because of the inertance (M_{pt}) inherent in the pneumotach. Pimmel

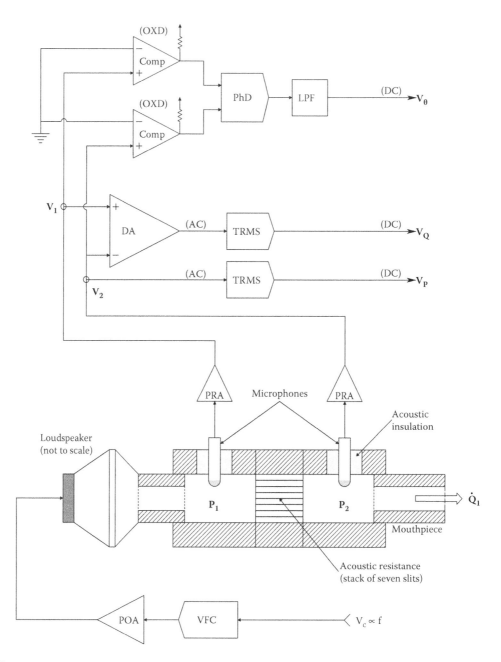

Figure 13.2 Schematic of a system designed by the author to measure the acoustic impedance of the lungs, Z_{rs}. A special low-inertance pneumotach was designed to keep pneumotach impedance resistive to over 300 Hz. DC voltages proportional to volume flow, driving-point pressure, and the angle of Z_{rs} are provided at any frequency from 1 to 200 Hz.

et al. used the frequency where there was a 2° phase in $\mathbf{Z_{pt}}(j\omega)$ as the upper frequency of operation of their instrument. This criterion can be interpreted as

$$\omega_H = (R_{pt}/M_{pt})\tan(2°) = 0.035(R_{pt}/M_{pt})\ r/s \tag{13.12}$$

or

$$f_H = (5.5578 \times 10^{-3})(R_{pt}/M_{pt})\ Hz. \tag{13.13}$$

Pimmel et al. found $f_H = 16$ Hz in their system. They examined the $Z_{rs}(j2\pi f)$ of mongrel dogs over a frequency range of 1–16 Hz. The $Z_{rs}(j2\pi f)$s of normal animals were compared to those given IV physostigmine, a powerful bronchoconstrictor, at a dose of 0.025 mg/kg. The $Z_{rs}(j2\pi f)$ magnitude showed a minimum at about 5 Hz, then increased slowly with frequency. The phase of $Z_{rs}(j2\pi f)$ at 1 Hz was typically about $-70°$, increased smoothly to zero (resonance) at about 5 Hz, then continued to increase, ending at $\sim +70°$ at 16 Hz. The dogs given physostigmine clearly showed a uniform increase in $|Z_{rs}(j2\pi f)|$ at all frequencies, but little change in the phase plot of $Z_{rs}(j2\pi f)$ versus that for normal dogs. Other plots of $|Z_{rs}(j2\pi f)|$ and $\angle Z_{rs}(j2\pi f)$ for a dog who smoked heavily [sic] and a dog with a congenital tracheal hypoplasia showed pronounced increases in $|Z_{rs}(j2\pi f)|$ at all frequencies, and a steeper slope on the phase plots between 5 and 8 Hz. Clearly, the RAIMS of Pimmel et al. could detect respiratory system anomalies. We note that presentation of $Z_{rs}(j2\pi f)$ data as polar plots might have given the investigators a more sensitive tool than separately plotting magnitude and angle. Also, extending the high-frequency range of measurement can provide more useful data, given a pneumotach design with low inertance.

The author realized that the design of a low-inertance pneumotach was essential in developing a prototype RAIMS that could cover at least two decades of frequency (1–>100 Hz). Comparison of the acoustic impedance function for screens, tubes, and slits showed that slits offered an advantage over tubes and screens in terms of their R_{pt}/M_{pt} ratio:

$$[R_{pt}/M_{pt}] = \frac{10\eta}{\rho d^2} \text{(for slits)}. \tag{13.14}$$

Using $\eta = 1.86 \times 10^{-4}$ Poise, $\rho = 1.205 \times 10^{-3}$ g/cm^3, and d = 0.0051 cm (a value we used), the ratio is equal to 5.9345×10^4. Using Equation 13.13 for a 2° phase shift at f_H, we find $f_H = 330$ Hz. Thus, the parallel slit acoustic impedance for the pneumotach appears real until the operating frequency approaches 330 Hz (2° criterion). Putting seven such slits in parallel divides R_{ac} by 7, but does not affect the overall Z_{pt}'s f_H.

Figure 13.2 illustrates the prototype RAIMS developed by the author. In general, $P_1 > P_2$, so $V_1 > V_2$ at any frequency. The sinusoidal signals V_1 and V_2 are converted to DC by true rms converters. Thus, $V_Q = K_D(v_{1rms} - v_{2rms})$ is a DC voltage proportional to the volume flow into the lungs, $\dot{Q}$. The ratio V_P/V_Q is calculated by the system's computer after analog-to-digital conversion; it is proportional to the $|Z_{rs}|$ of the respiratory system. The sinusoidal signals V_1 and V_2 are passed through comparator-zero-crossing detectors to form two TTL signals of the applied acoustic frequency which are shifted in phase relative to the respiratory system input pressure, P_2. A digital phase detector and low-pass filter generate a DC voltage, V_θ, which is proportional to the phase shift. The computer generates the DC voltage input to the voltage-to-frequency converter, V_C, which generates the variable frequency, sinusoidal signal that drives the loudspeaker. The computer makes standard Bode dB amplitude and phase plots versus frequency, polar plots, and $R_e\{Z_{rs}\}$ and $I_m\{Z_{rs}\}$ versus f plots. The system of Figure 13.2 was tested satisfactorily on known acoustic loads and chest phantoms.

In *in vivo* Z_{rs} measurements, the state of expansion of the lungs is an important parameter. Z_{rs} measurements can be made with the airway at ambient atmospheric pressure, or at some mean positive pressure, P_{tr}, to insure complete lung expansion. The applied sound pressure is then a small perturbation on top of P_{tr}. In small-signal, single-frequency Z_{rs} measurements, it was noted generally that both $R_e\{Z_{rs}\}$ and $I_m\{Z_{rs}\}$ are frequency dependent in a complex manner. This is because of the parallel combination of many component Z_{rs}s with different natural frequencies.

If a *large-amplitude, forced oscillation technique* (FOT) is used, three problems can arise: The pneumotach resistance, R_{pt}, used to measure $\dot{Q}$ can become nonlinear due to departure from laminar flow conditions, pneumotach inertance effects can become more pronounced at high-flow rates, limiting the accuracy in the high-frequency range of study, and the elasticity of lung tissues is no longer linear (Hookean).

It should be noted that statistical techniques of estimating Z_{rs} have been used in which the excitation sound pressure, P_1, is pseudorandom binary noise (with zero mean), rather than a sinusoid. Cross-power spectral techniques (Northrop 2000) are then used to extract an estimate of $Z_{rs}(j2\pi f)$. Suki and Lutchen (1992) demonstrated that input signals of the general form of sum of sinusoids, *sic*:

$$p_1(t) = \sum_{k=1}^{N} p_k \cos[2\pi f_\kappa + \varphi_\kappa] \tag{13.15}$$

can also be used to characterize the nonlinear respiratory system's Z_{rs}.

In summary, it appears that the major challenge in making high-frequency measurements of the Z_{AC} (j2πf) of the respiratory system lies in the design of a pneumotach acoustic impedance that remains real over the range of frequencies of interest. Even with this limitation, Z_{rs} measurements have been used in a variety of diagnostic trials. Z_{rs} was measured in horses with heaves (analogous to asthma) using forced oscillations at 1.5, 2, 3, and 5 Hz by Young et al. (1996). They examined $|Z_{rs}$ (f)$|$ and $R_e\{Z_{rs}$ (f)$\}$ and concluded that a significant indicator of heaves was an increase in $R_e\{Z_{rs}\}$ in the 1.5–3 Hz range (no doubt due to bronchiospasm). There was no significant change in the Z_{rs} inertance. Hall et al. (2000) used sinusoidal pressure excitation between 0.5 and 21 Hz to measure Z_{rs} of normal infants under the age of 2 years. The purpose of their study was to study how the different lung tissues (airways and parenchyma) grew in the first 2 years.

Reisch et al. (1999) used the FOT to measure Z_{rs} of persons with *obstructive sleep apnea syndrome* (OSAS). In the OSAS patients, pharyngeal collapses are correlated with a loss of muscle tone in the upper airway, and its consequent partial or total collapse. They concluded that the FOT is a valuable tool for assessing the degree of upper airway obstruction in patients with OSAS.

The broad applications of respiratory FOT were studied and described by Oostveen et al. (2003). These authors commented: "Forced oscillation technique has been shown to be as sensitive as spirometry in detecting impairments of lung function due to smoking or exposure to occupational hazards. Together with the minimal requirement for the subject's cooperation, this makes [FOT] an ideal lung function test for epidemiological and field studies. Novel applications of [FOT] in the clinical setting include the monitoring of respiratory mechanics during mechanical ventilation and sleep."

13.3 ACOUSTIC IMPEDANCE MEASUREMENT OF THE EARDRUM (TYMPANOMETRY)

The auditory canal and eardrum can be modeled by a cylinder closed at its far end by a compliant (elastic) membrane, the eardrum. The degree of eardrum compliance is affected by two significant factors: (1) The difference in mean air pressure between the auditory canal (atmospheric pressure) and the air pressure in the middle ear. (2) The mechanical loading on the eardrum imposed by the ossicles and the oval window (cf. the discussion in Section 13.1). The point of maximum compliance of the eardrum occurs in the absence of loud sound when the air pressure in the auditory canal equals the air pressure in the middle ear. If at the point of maximum eardrum compliance, the contralateral ear is stimulated by a loud, broadband sound, the reflex contraction which occurs in the muscles of the middle ear causes a stiffening of the tympanic membrane and a consequent *increase in the auditory impedance* measured in the ipsilateral ear. Or, in other words, the auditory reflex causes a *decrease in the compliance* of the eardrum and a $\sim$ 30 dB attenuation of sound coupled to the oval window. Measurement of the nonsubjective acoustic reflex by sensing small changes in the acoustic input impedance (or admittance) of the ear canal and eardrum has diagnostic significance in both hearing and neurological problems.

In this section, we will describe two ways that have been devised to quantitatively measure the acoustic attenuation reflex. In measurement of the acoustic impedance of the respiratory system, we saw that it was possible to use an acoustic resistance to measure the volume flow into the oral airway and thus calculate the acoustic impedance as the vector ratio of input pressure to volume flow, given single-frequency, sinusoidal excitation. Because of the much smaller size of the ear canal, the acoustic driving point impedance, Z_A, can be more easily measured by driving the outer ear canal with a sinusoidal volume flow source (analogous in an electrical circuit to an alternating current source) and measuring the resultant pressure across Z_A. Such a scheme was devised by Pinto and Dallos (1968). Figure 13.3 illustrates the Pinto and Dallos system. A volume flow source is approximated by putting the primary, sinusoidal pressure source, P_1, in series with a large acoustic resistance, Z_{LS}(jω). The effective, AC volume flow source is $\dot{Q}_1 \equiv P_1/Z_{LS}$. Z_{LS} couples P_1 to Z_A in parallel with another large Z_m to the microphone. Design makes $|Z_{LS}|$ and $Z_m | \gg Z_A$ at the operating frequency. Thus, $P_A = Q_1 Z_A = P_1 Z_a / Z_{LS}$. (We neglected the volume flow in Z_m as being $\ll$ that in Z_A.) Using superposition, we see that the potentiometer serves as a ratiometric adder to form V_i.

$$V_i = \rho V_m + (1-\rho)V_r, \quad 0 \le \rho \le 1. \tag{13.16}$$

In Figure 13.3, we see how the bridge is nulled. The AC source, V_{in}, is phase shifted by θ, then its amplitude is adjusted by a factor of β in order to make $V_i = 0$ (null). Thus, $V_r = \beta V_{in} \angle θ$ in phasor

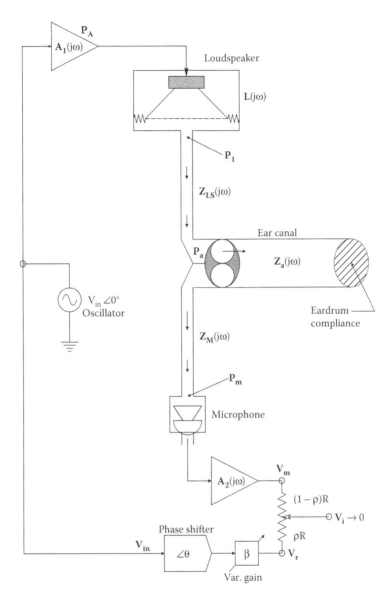

Figure 13.3 Acoustic impedance "bridge" of Pinto and Dallas (1968) used to measure the eardrum acoustic impedance.

notation. $\mathbf{V_r}$ is next attenuated by $(1 - \rho)$ and added to $\rho\mathbf{V_m}$. Note that $0 \leq \rho \leq 1$. $\mathbf{V_m}$ is the conditioned microphone output. $\mathbf{V_m}$ is given by

$$\mathbf{V_m} = \mathbf{V_{in}} \frac{\mathbf{A_1}(j\omega)\mathbf{L}(j\omega)\mathbf{Z_A}(j\omega)}{\mathbf{Z_{LS}}(j\omega)} \mathbf{M}(j\omega)\mathbf{A_2}(j\omega), \qquad (13.17)$$

where $\mathbf{A_1}$ and $\mathbf{A_2}$ are amplifier voltage gains, $\mathbf{L}$ is the loudspeaker transfer function in (dynes/cm²)/ rms volt, $\mathbf{M}$ is the microphone transfer function in rms volts/(dyne/cm²), and $\mathbf{Z_{LS}}$ is the high series CGS acoustic impedance between $\mathbf{P_1}$ and $\mathbf{P_A}$.

Hence, at null:

$$\mathbf{V_i} = 0 = \beta(1 - \rho)\angle\theta + \rho\frac{\mathbf{A_1}(j\omega)\mathbf{L}(j\omega)\mathbf{Z_a}(j\omega)}{\mathbf{Z_{LS}}(j\omega)}\mathbf{M}(j\omega)\mathbf{A_2}(j\omega). \qquad (13.18)$$

Thus, the vector acoustic impedance of the auditory canal and eardrum can be written:

$$\mathbf{Z_A}(j\omega) = \frac{-\beta(1-\rho)\angle\theta}{\rho\mathbf{A_1}(j\omega)\mathbf{A_2}(j\omega)\mathbf{L}(j\omega)\mathbf{M}(j\omega)/\mathbf{Z_{LS}}(j\omega)}, \tag{13.19}$$

where ρ, β, and θ are set to null $\mathbf{V_i}$, and the values of the vectors in the denominator at $\omega = 2\pi f$ are known by prior measurement.

In Figure 13.4, we illustrate a slightly different version of the Pinto and Dallos auditory impedance bridge, modified by the author. The ratiometric voltage divider has been replaced by a difference amplifier with gain K_D. $\mathbf{V_i}$ is now given by

$$\mathbf{V_i}(j\omega) = K_D[\mathbf{V_m} - \mathbf{V_r}] = K_D[V_{in}\mathbf{A_1}(j\omega)\mathbf{A_2}(j\omega)\mathbf{L}(j\omega)\mathbf{M}(j\omega)\mathbf{Y_{LS}}(j\omega)\mathbf{Z_A}(j\omega) - V_{in}\beta\angle\theta]. \tag{13.20}$$

If the complex $\mathbf{V_i}$ is nulled under resting conditions, $\mathbf{Z_A}(j\omega)$ can be calculated from Equation 13.20. When a loud sound is applied to the contralateral ear, the acoustic attenuation reflex causes $\mathbf{Z_A}$ to increase by some $\Delta\mathbf{Z_A}$, unbalancing the null. The unbalanced $\mathbf{V_i}$ can be written:

$$\mathbf{V_i}(j\omega) = K_D[V_{in}\mathbf{A_1}(j\omega)\mathbf{A_2}(j\omega)\mathbf{L}(j\omega)\mathbf{M}(j\omega)\mathbf{Y_{LS}}(j\omega)\{\mathbf{Z_A}(j\omega) + \Delta\mathbf{Z_A}\} - V_{in}\beta\angle\theta]$$

$$= K_D\left[V_{in}\mathbf{A_1}(j\omega)\mathbf{A_2}(j\omega)\mathbf{L}(j\omega)\mathbf{M}(j\omega)\mathbf{Y_{LS}}(j\omega)\right.$$

$$\left.\left\{\frac{\beta\angle\theta}{\mathbf{A_1}(j\omega)\mathbf{A_2}(j\omega)\mathbf{L}(j\omega)\mathbf{M}(j\omega)\mathbf{Y_{LS}}(j\omega)} + \Delta\mathbf{Z_A}\right\} - V_{in}\beta\angle\theta\right] \tag{13.21}$$

$$\downarrow$$

$$\mathbf{V_i}(j\omega) = K_D V_{in}[\mathbf{A_1}(j\omega)\mathbf{A_2}(j\omega)\mathbf{L}(j\omega)\mathbf{M}(j\omega)\mathbf{Y_{LS}}(j\omega)]\Delta\mathbf{Z_A}.$$

Because the magnitude and phase of $\mathbf{V_i}$ are known, as are V_{in}, K_D, and the five vectors, it is possible to calculate the exact $\Delta\mathbf{Z_A}$ elicited by the acoustic reflex. Using two-phase-sensitive demodulators on $\mathbf{V_i}$ with $V_{in}\angle(\phi)$ and $V_{in}\angle(\phi + 90°)$ (quadrature) as references, where ϕ is the net angle of the $\mathbf{A_1}(j\omega)\mathbf{A_2}(j\omega)\mathbf{L}(j\omega)\mathbf{M}(j\omega)\mathbf{Y_{LS}}(j\omega)$ vector at $\omega = 2\pi f$, it is possible to resolve the vector $\Delta\mathbf{Z_A}$ into its real and imaginary values in nearly real time.

Another system for measuring the magnitude of $\mathbf{Y_A} = \mathbf{Z_A}^{-1}$ was described by Ward in the U.S. Patent No. 4,009,707 (1977). Instead of using a constant volume rate flow source, Ward measured $\mathbf{P_A}$ at the entrance to the auditory meatus, and used a type 1 feedback control loop to adjust V_{in} in such a manner to keep $\mathbf{P_A}$ constant as $\mathbf{Z_A}$ changed during the auditory reflex. Although his patent is titled, *Automatic Acoustic Impedance Meter*, Ward's device actually has an output proportional to $\mathbf{Y_A}$: it is not very "automatic," either. Ward's system is illustrated in Figure 13.5. The loudspeaker generates a sound pressure $\mathbf{P_1}$, which creates a volume flow, $\dot{\mathbf{Q}}_1$, in the connecting tube from the loudspeaker to the ear. This tube has impedance $\mathbf{Z_t}(j\omega)$. The acoustic admittance of the auditory canal and eardrum, $\mathbf{Y_A}$, is shunted by the very small admittance of the tube to the microphone.

Thus, practically all of $\dot{\mathbf{Q}}_1$ passes into $\mathbf{Y_A}$. Because of the very small flow in the microphone tube, the pressure at the microphone is essentially the pressure at the auditory meatus, that is, $\mathbf{P_3} \cong \mathbf{P_A}$. These conditions are illustrated in the equivalent electrical analog circuit of Figure 13.6.

To examine how the Ward system operates, we first note that in the steady state, the Type I controller causes $V_e = 0$. Thus, $V_r \equiv V_3 = K_m K_3 p_a$, where K_m is the volts/(dynes/cm^2) conversion gain of the microphone, K_3 is the amplifier gain, and p_a is the rms pressure at the auditory meatus. However, from the analog circuit,

$$\mathbf{P_3} \cong \mathbf{P_A} = \mathbf{P_1}\mathbf{Z_A}/(\mathbf{Z_t} + \mathbf{Z_a}) \tag{13.22}$$

$$\mathbf{P_A}(\mathbf{Z_t} + \mathbf{Z_A}) = \mathbf{P_1}\mathbf{Z_a} = \mathbf{Z_A}[\mathbf{V_s}(1 + \mathbf{V_m})/10]LK_P \tag{13.23}$$

$$\mathbf{P_A}(1 + \mathbf{Y_A}\mathbf{Z_t}) = [\mathbf{V_s}(1 + \mathbf{V_m})/10]LK_P. \tag{13.24}$$

However, the rms $p_a = V_r/[|\mathbf{M}|K_3]$ in the steady state, so we can finally write:

$$\frac{V_r}{|\mathbf{M}|K_3}|(1 + \mathbf{Y_A}\mathbf{Z_t})| = v_s|L|K_P(1 + V_m)/10. \tag{13.25}$$

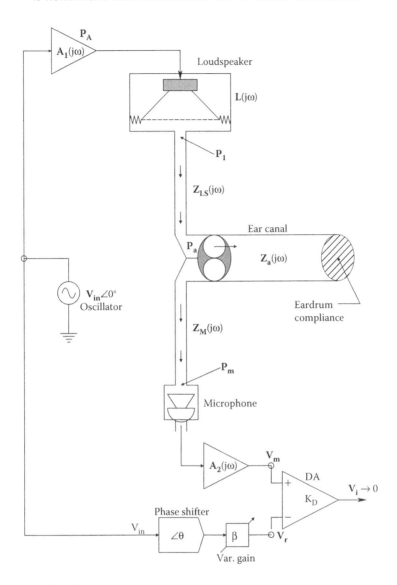

Figure 13.4 Modified Pinto and Dallas bridge.

where v_s is the rms source voltage. The rms input to the loudspeaker is:

$$v_{in} = v_s K_P (1 + V_m)/10. \tag{13.26}$$

Solving for v_s, we can write:

$$v_s = v_{in}/[K_P (1 + V_m)/10]. \tag{13.27}$$

When Equation 13.27 is substituted into Equation 13.25, we find:

$$v_{in} = \frac{V_r}{|M||L||K_3} |(1 + \mathbf{Y_A Z_t})|. \tag{13.28}$$

Now if we make $|\mathbf{Y_A Z_t}| \gg 1$, the final result is that the rms loudspeaker drive voltage is proportional to the admittance looking into the auditory meatus, $\mathbf{Y_A}(j\omega)$:

$$v_{in} \cong \frac{V_r}{|M||L||K_3} |\mathbf{Y_A Z_t}|. \tag{13.29}$$

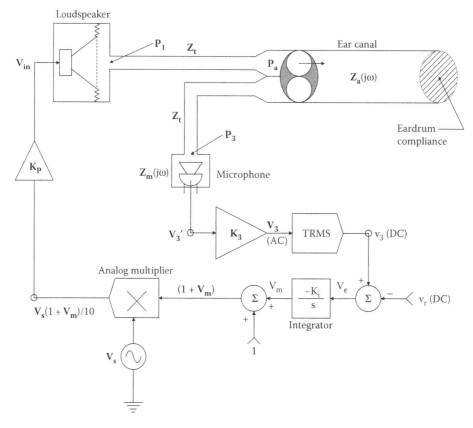

Figure 13.5 Ward's (1977) acoustic admittance measurement system. The source frequency, f_s, is held constant.

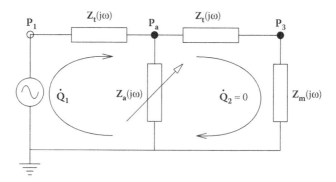

Figure 13.6 Lumped-parameter acoustic circuit relevant to the analysis of Ward's acoustic admittance measurement system.

At a fixed frequency, we can replace $|\mathbf{M}|$ and $|\mathbf{L}|$ with the scalar gains K_m and K_L, respectively. Thus,

$$v_{in} \cong \frac{V_r}{K_m K_L K_3} \, |\, \mathbf{Y_A Z_t}\, |. \tag{13.30}$$

Note that unlike the nulling system of Pinto and Dallos, the Ward system does not give high sensitivity to measure the $\mathbf{\Delta Y_A}$ caused by the auditory reflex. The Ward system does, however, allow the clinician to adjust the air pressure in the ear canal to obtain maximum eardrum compliance under resting conditions. Shown in the original Ward patent is an analog sample-and-hold circuit that allows the user to measure the small, differential output voltage due to $\Delta \mathbf{Y_A}$, that is,

$$\Delta v_{in} \cong \frac{V_r}{K_m K_L K_3} \{ |(\mathbf{Y_A} + \Delta \mathbf{Y_A})\mathbf{Z_t}| - |\mathbf{Y_A Z_t}| \}. \tag{13.31}$$

In general, $|\mathbf{Y_A}/\Delta \mathbf{Y_a}| \ll 1$, so as a final approximation,

$$\Delta v_{in} \cong \frac{V_r}{K_m K_L K_3} |\Delta \mathbf{Y_A Z_t}|. \tag{13.32}$$

In general, the auditory reflex makes $\Delta \mathbf{Y_A}$ negative, so Δv_{in} is negative in response. Ward's system appears useful as a clinical instrument, even though it only measures the *magnitudes* of $\mathbf{Y_A}$ and $\Delta \mathbf{Y_A}$.

Both Ward's and Pinto and Dallos' measurement systems use different approaches to the quantification of the auditory reflex. Both systems also require extensive acoustic and electrical calibration of their components. If Pinto and Dallos' bridge system were made self-nulling, it would be ideal because it could provide vector information on $\Delta \mathbf{Z_A}$ resulting from the auditory reflex.

13.4 TRANSTHORACIC ACOUSTIC TRANSFER FUNCTION AS A POSSIBLE MEASURE OF LUNG CONDITION

13.4.1 Introduction

As we have seen in Section 3.4, a trained clinician, using a stethoscope, can detect pulmonary edema from the lack of intrinsic breath sounds transmitted though the thoracic wall, or internal bubbling and gurgling sounds. Pulmonary edema can be caused by a number of factors, including but not limited to: Congestive heart failure, pneumonia, other infections, allergy, high-altitude syndrome, near drowning, or exposure to toxic chemical fumes or smoke. Pulmonary edema can become life threatening because it decreases active lung volume and decreases O_2/CO_2 exchange, leading to hypoxia and acidosis. X-ray and CAT scan are common NI methods of visualizing pulmonary edema and verifying diagnosis made with a stethoscope.

Another NI approach to detecting and locating volumes of pulmonary edema is to introduce sound into the lungs through the trachea, or by coupling it through the thoracic wall (e.g., on the back), and to use a sensitive microphone on the front of the chest to detect differences in the sound propagation that accompany fluid-filled alveoli. Tissue changes in the lungs that accompany pulmonary emphysema, and the presence of excess mucous in the small airways that occurs with cystic fibrosis, or asthma, can also alter the acoustic transfer function from the source, through the chest walls, through the lung tissues, to the pickup microphone. A medical condition that can affect transthoracic sound propagation is an excess of fluid accumulated in the pleural cavity, between the outside of the lungs and the inside of the chest wall. Factors leading to this *pleural effusion* include blockage of the normal lymphatic drain system of the pleural cavity, heart failure, greatly reduced plasma colloid oncotic pressure, and inflammation of the pleural surfaces caused by infection.

We first consider a model for sound transmission in the lung parenchyma. In a normal lung, the parenchyma can be considered to be a two-phase, elastic continuum in which the alveolar air sacs are embedded in tissue (Rice 1983). In general, the speed of sound in an elastic continuum is given by

$$c = \sqrt{(B/\rho)} \text{ cm/s}, \tag{13.33}$$

where B is the bulk modulus of the medium in dynes/cm² and ρ is its density in grams/cm³.

Let h be the volumetric fraction of the parenchyma that is tissue, and $(1 - h)$ be the fraction that is gas, the composite bulk modulus is:

$$B = [(1-h)B_g^{-1} + hB_t^{-1}]^{-1} \frac{B_g B_t}{(1-h)B_t + hB_g}, \tag{13.34}$$

where the subscripts t and g refer to tissue and gas, respectively. The average density is easily seen to be:

$$\rho = (1-h)\rho_g + h\rho_t. \tag{13.35}$$

ρ of lung tissue is typically from 0.5 to 0.8 g/cm^3. Wodicka et al. (1989) used h = 0.25 for a normal lung, based on an air volume of 2500 cm^3, and an air-free tissue volume of 900 cm^3 in an adult male. They increased h to 0.35 to model edema in the parenchyma.

Sound waves are generally considered to propagate under adiabatic conditions. Thus, $B_g = \gamma\, p_o$, where γ is the ratio of the specific heats = C_p/C_v = 1.4 for air, but in the lung, nearly isothermal conditions occur, so γ = 1.0 is a better value (Wodicka et al. 1989). The mean gas pressure is p_o. When the relations above are substituted into Equation 13.33, we obtain an expression for the net speed of sound in the chest and lungs:

$$c = \left[\left(\frac{1-h}{\gamma p_o} + \frac{h}{B_t} \right) \{(1-h)\rho_g + h\rho_t\} \right]^{-1/2} \text{cm/s}. \tag{13.36}$$

Assuming nearly isolated alveolar gas chambers, the lung may be considered to be like gas bubbles in a fluid. When the bubbles are closely packed, and their radii are $\ll$ a sound wavelength, they do not act as independent scattering centers. For example, at c = 2400 cm/s, and an alveolar radius of 150 μm (0.015 cm), the maximum frequency before the alveoli act as independent scattering centers is $\sim$ 24 kHz. For c = 6000 cm/s, $f_{max} \approx 20$ kHz. Note that in the presence of pulmonary edema, h approaches unity, and c increases.

Wodicka et al. (1989) reported on the results of a computer modeling study of sound propagation from the oral airway, into the trachea and bronchioles, through the parenchyma, thence through the chest wall to an accelerometer or microphone. They used a lumped-parameter, transmission line architecture based on acoustic parameters of the tissue structures, including the chest wall. They concluded that considerable sound energy was coupled into the parenchyma directly from the stiff walls of the large airways. Their model predicted that the decreased transmission of sound to the chest wall at high frequencies was due to thermal (resistive) losses in the parenchyma.

The introduced sound pressure can be sinusoidal, or an input sound pressure of bandwidth-limited, broadband Gaussian noise. Under the assumption that the sound transmission through the lungs and chest is a linear process (i.e., it obeys superposition), linear system theory shows us that the sinusoidal frequency response vector function between the driving point acoustic pressure phasor and the pickup point pressure can be written as

$$\frac{\mathbf{P_o}}{\mathbf{P_i}}(j\omega) = H(j\omega). \tag{13.37}$$

$|\mathbf{H}(j\omega)|$ is generally low pass in nature, and $\ll$ 1.

When the input sound pressure is Gaussian random noise with a two-sided power density spectrum, $\Phi_{ii}(\omega)$, then it is well known that $\mathbf{H}(j\omega)$ can be found from the relation (Northrop 2000):

$$\mathbf{H}(j\omega) = \frac{\Phi_{io}(j\omega)}{\Phi_{ii}(\omega)}, \tag{13.38}$$

providing that the frequency response, $\mathbf{H}(j\omega)$, is from a linear, stationary, and ergodic system. The autopower spectrum, $\Phi_{ii}(\omega)$, is an even, positive-real function. $\Phi_{ii}(\omega)$ is the Fourier transform of the two-sided autocorrelation function, $\varphi_{ii}(\tau)$, of the input pressure given by

$$\varphi_{ii}(\tau) \equiv \lim_{T \to \infty} \frac{1}{2T} \int_{-T}^{T} p_i(t)\, p_o(t+\tau)\, dt. \tag{13.39}$$

The cross-power density spectrum, $\mathbf{\Phi_{io}}(j\omega)$, is a vector function of frequency. It is found by taking the Fourier transform of the cross-correlation function, which is defined by

$$\varphi_{io}(\tau) \equiv \lim_{T \to \infty} \frac{1}{2T} \int_{-T}^{T} p_i(t)\, p_o(t+\tau)\, dt. \tag{13.40}$$

In practice, computation of $\mathbf{H}(j\omega)$ is not as simple as Equation 13.38 would suggest. The signal $p_o(t)$ contains noise from the heartbeating, and other low-frequency noises from digestion and breathing, etc. It also contains electronic noise from amplifiers. Both $v_o(t)$ and $v_i(t)$ must be band-pass filtered to minimize the effect of these noises, and the high cutoff frequency of these filters must be chosen for antialiasing. The filtered $v_o(t)$ and $v_i(t)$ are digitized with a finite number of samples (e.g., 4096) and the windowing, and computation of the auto- and cross-power spectra and the estimate of $\mathbf{H}(j\omega)$ are done by computer using the Fast Fourier transform techniques.

A number of estimates, $\hat{\mathbf{H}}(j\omega)$, of $\mathbf{H}(j\omega)$ are made and then averaged to reduce the noise in the computed frequency response function.

In the sections below, we describe the perthoracic noise method of estimating $\mathbf{H}(j\omega)$ developed by Rader (1998), and the technique of Pohlmann et al. (2001) in which broadband noise sound was introduced into the oral airway.

13.4.2 Transthoracic Propagation of Broadband Acoustic Noise to Evaluate Pulmonary Health

Figure 13.7 illustrates schematically the system used by Rader (1998) to investigate how sound introduced on the back propagates through the chest walls and the lungs. Because her work was the development of a prototype instrument, she used consenting, normal, healthy adult volunteers in her study. The sound input subsystem consisted of a 5″ acoustic suspension loudspeaker mounted in a flexible foam "box," open at the end that made contact with the subject's back. The box was pressed firmly against the subject's back to prevent acoustic leakage into the air. A B&K Model 4117 microphone was mounted through a hole in the foam box to monitor the input sound pressure in the air. Another matched, B&K 4117 microphone was mounted in a 10-cm diameter, soft rubber cup to pick up sound transmitted through the wall of the front of the chest. The cup served to space the microphone about 4 cm from the skin surface, and to exclude other sounds in the air from the microphone.

A *Quan-Tech* Model 420, broadband, analog, Gaussian noise generator (flat from 0 to 100 kHz) was used as a primary noise source. Its output was amplified and band-pass filtered (half-power

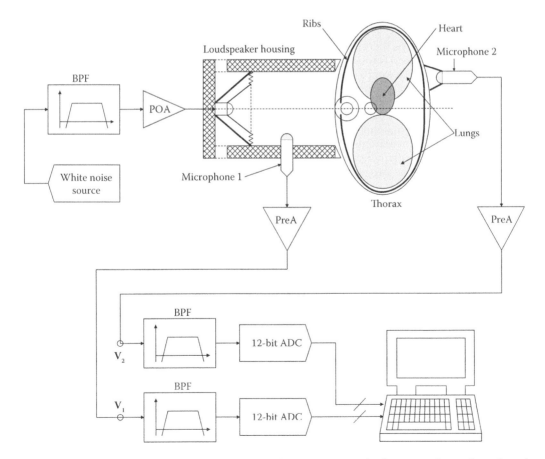

Figure 13.7 Rader's (1998) system to measure the acoustic transfer function of sound conducted through the chest using broadband noise and cross-power spectral techniques.

frequencies of 16 Hz and 1 kHz) to define the input power density spectrum. A total of 4.5 watts noise power was delivered to the 5″ loudspeaker. Both piezo-microphone outputs were conditioned by charge amplifiers to preserve low-frequency signal components, then passed through band-pass filters to exclude heart sounds and their first few harmonics, and sharply attenuate any frequencies above 1000 Hz (for antialiasing filtering). Analog-to-digital conversion of the filtered p_i and p_o microphone signals took place at 5000 samples/s; 12-bit conversion was used. The A/D conversion was under the control of the system computer. In each data epoch, 4096 samples were taken of the p_i and p_o signals, yielding a spectral resolution of 0.8192 Hz in FFT calculations. Rader investigated the suitability of using four different windowing functions on her sampled random data; Rectangular (no window function), Bartlett (triangular), Blackman, and Hanning. In some cases to reduce noise, Rader averaged several like spectra taken by consecutive sampling.

Rader found that the Blackman windowing function gave the best performance in terms of minimizing the noise on the input autopower spectrum and the cross-power spectrums. Figures 13.8a,b and 13.9a,b illustrate representative input-, output-, and cross-power spectrums and coherence for one of Rader's subjects. Note that data acquisition of one epoch (4096 samples at 5 kSa/s) takes 0.8192 s, and five epochs (to average) take a total of 4.1 s. Computation of $\mathbf{H}(j2\pi f)$ using Equation 13.38 takes a few more seconds once data are acquired. Rader only presented the magnitude of $\Phi_{io}(j2\pi f)$ in her dissertation. By inspecting the estimate of $\mathbf{H}(j2\pi f)$ as a polar plot, or as real and imaginary parts versus f, it is expected that more insight into lung condition might be obtained. The technique developed by Rader has the advantage of being totally NI, safe, and rapidly repeatable as an office procedure. Once clinically validated with patients with respiratory problems, it should be able to assess the amount of pulmonary edema in a patient, and track its progress, minimizing the need for more costly CAT scans and x-rays.

13.4.3 Use of White Noise Sound Introduced into the Oral Airway to Assess Lung Condition

Pohlmann et al. (2001) reported on an investigation of acoustic transmission through the respiratory system. In many ways, their study was similar to that of Rader (1998) with the exception that their sound was introduced through the oral airway. Pohlmann et al. used a noise input spectrum with half-power frequencies of 50 and 680 Hz. Sound was recorded with microphones from the left and right, T3 and T6 positions on the posterior chest. A sampling epoch consisted of 2048 samples at a 7.5 kHz sampling frequency. Auto- and cross-power spectra were computed using standard FFT techniques; 12 consecutive epochs were averaged to reduce noise.

Pohlmann et al. found that their acoustic transfer function was both frequency and lung inflation dependent. At the lower frequencies, there was about 20 dB attenuation in $|\mathbf{H}(j2\pi f)|$; attenuation increased steadily with increasing frequency. It also increased with increasing lung inflation. Lung inflation expands the parenchyma by inflating the alveoli, thus decreasing the average

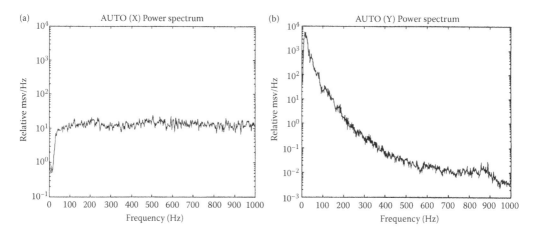

Figure 13.8 Representative power spectra from Rader's study. (a) Input autopower spectrum. (b) Output autopower spectrum. Note attenuation of high frequencies. (Figure from Northrop, R.B. 2002. *Noninvasive Instrumentation and Measurement in Medical Diagnosis.* CRC Press, Boca Raton, FL. ISBN: 0-8493-0961-1.)

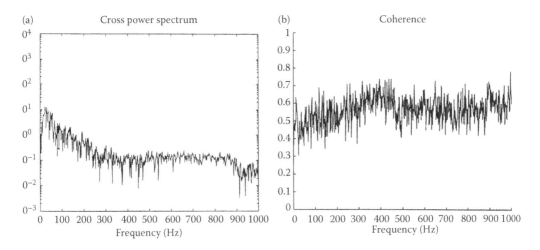

Figure 13.9 (a) Calculated cross-power spectrum magnitude from Rader's study. There are three distinct, spectral regions. (b) System coherence. (Figure from Northrop, R.B. 2002. *Noninvasive Instrumentation and Measurement in Medical Diagnosis*. CRC Press, Boca Raton, FL. ISBN: 0-8493-0961-1.)

density of the parenchyma. Pohlmann et al. commented that the use of vibration sensors (accelerometers) directly on the skin may improve their system's signal-to-noise ratio.

13.4.4 Discussion

The lungs present a complex acoustical impedance to a driving source at the mouth. They also affect the acoustic transfer function between the back and front of the chest. The extent to which obstructive lung disease changes this impedance or transfer function has been the topic of research for a number of years. At present, no clinical application of low-frequency acoustical testing of the respiratory system's acoustical impedance or transfer function has been forthcoming. There must be extensive clinical trials to establish a database for this simple NI testing modality. If the trials are done, will this method be sensitive enough to detect various forms of obstructive lung disease before they become debilitating? Perhaps diagnosis will be more certain using conventional spirometric techniques (cf. Chapter 10). Note that spirometric tests require patient's cooperation, so does lung acoustic impedance measurement, whereas acoustic transfer function measurement does not.

13.5 CHAPTER SUMMARY

In this chapter, we have seen how the transmission of audio-frequency acoustic energy (either as sinusoidal or random pressure waves) through the chest and lungs can be used as an inexpensive, NI diagnostic tool to detect OLD and fluid in the lungs and pleural space. Such systems are at present experimental, as yet they have no clinical application.

Measurement of the acoustic impedance (or admittance) of the ear canal plus tympanic membrane, however, is a widely used clinical test in audiology. The absence of a normal tympanic reflex to sudden, loud sounds is used as a measure of deafness in infants.

14 Noninvasive Tests Using Ultrasound (Excluding Imaging)

14.1 INTRODUCTION

The use of ultrasound (sound with frequencies ranging roughly from 25 kHz to over 30 MHz) in medical diagnosis is best associated with its ability to image internal structures of the body. However, ultrasound, by virtue of its short wavelengths in the body, is also well suited to non-imaging, "A-mode" applications where the phase and frequency of the reflected sound are used to measure the distance to—and velocity of—the reflector or reflecting objects, such as an aortic aneurysm or the fetal heartbeat.

In discussing sound waves, recall that the sound wavelength is given by the simple relation, $\lambda = v/f$, where v is the sound velocity in the medium and f is its Hz frequency. Also in dealing with sinusoidal functions, the sine argument is phase in radians, and frequency in general is the time derivative of phase. That is, if the sound pressure at a point is given by $P_o \sin(2\pi f\, t + \varphi)$, then the phase argument is $(2\pi f\, t + \varphi)$ radians and the frequency is $2\pi f$ r/s.

In this chapter, we first examine the Doppler effect when the source and receiver transducers are collinear and stationary with respect to the moving reflector(s), then consider closed-loop ultrasonic ranging systems that operate under constant-phase conditions with a moving reflector. One such experimental system devised by the author used air-coupled ultrasound to measure the ocular pulse (OP). (The minute, $\pm 10\ \mu m$ expansion of the cornea in response to blood flowing into the eyeball.) The no-touch ocular pulse measurement (NOTOPM) system used a voltage-to-frequency oscillator (VCO) to adjust the transmitted frequency so that the phase difference of the transmitted and received waves remains constant. It is shown in Section 14.4.2 that the sensitivity of the NOTOPM system ($v_o/\Delta x$) is proportional to $1/x_o^2$. The author showed that this nonlinear sensitivity is avoided if a voltage-to-period converter (VPC) oscillator is used instead of a VFC. Use of the VPC permits simultaneous measurement of x and dx/dt in applications such as the NOTOPM system.

In Section 14.6, we describe an experimental system that may have application in the noninvasive measurement blood glucose concentration in a tissue such as an earlobe. This system is based on the closed-loop, constant-phase principle used in the NOTOPM system, except that the ultrasound is transmitted rather than reflected. Small changes in the velocity of sound caused by changes in tissue density, which in turn can be due to changes in glucose concentration in the tissue, will alter the phase lag of the received signal. Other factors, such as the interstitial fluid water concentration, can act as a confounder in this system. The system was tested *in vitro* successfully, followed by tests on the eyes of normal, healthy rabbits, also on consenting, healthy graduate students.

14.2 DOPPLER EFFECT

The Doppler effect can easily be observed with both electromagnetic and sound waves. We are all familiar with the Doppler effect on sound (Magnin 1986). A car moving toward us blows its horn. As it passes, there is a perceptible downward shift in the pitch of the horn. In 1842, Johann Christian Doppler gave a paper, "On the Colored Light of Double Stars and Some Other Heavenly Bodies" before the Royal Bohemian Society of Learning. Doppler was a professor of elementary mathematics and practical geometry at the Prague State Technical Academy. He apparently got little recognition for his work, and died of consumption in 1854 at the age of 49. In 1844, a contemporary of Doppler, Buys Ballot, contested Doppler's theory as an explanation for the color shift of binary stars rotating about an axis perpendicular to a line from the observer to the stars. Ballot actually did an experiment using sound waves, where a trumpet player played a constant note while riding on a flatcar of a train moving at constant velocity. A musician with perfect pitch, standing at trackside, perceived the trumpet tone to be a halftone sharp as the train approached, and a halftone flat as it receded. In spite of this direct evidence of velocity-related frequency shift, Ballot continued to object to Doppler's theory. Ballot's erroneous publications apparently served to discredit Doppler for a number of years. So much for facts.

To derive a mathematical expression of the Doppler effect for sound waves, we will assume a moving, reflecting target and a stationary source/observer, as shown in Figure 14.1. Assume that sinusoidal sound waves leaving the stationary transmitter (TRX) propagate at velocity, c, over a distance, d, to the target, T. The target is moving at velocity, **v**, at an angle θ with the source. Velocity **v** can thus be resolved into a component parallel to the line connecting TRX and the reflecting target, T, and a component perpendicular to the TRX-T line. These components are $|\mathbf{v}|\cos(\theta)$ and $|\mathbf{v}|\sin(\theta)$, respectively. The reflected wave from T propagates back to the

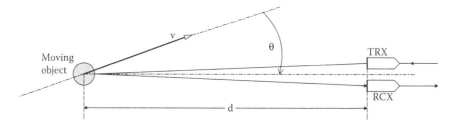

Figure 14.1 Basic Doppler geometry for moving reflector with stationary collinear transmitter and receiver.

stationary receiving transducer, RCX, along path d. The receiving sensor output waveform can be written as

$$V_r = B\sin(\omega_r t + \psi). \tag{14.1}$$

The received radian frequency is ω_r, the transmitted radian frequency is ω_o, and ψ represents the phase lag between the transmitted signal and the received signal. In general, the phase lag, ψ, is given by

$$\psi = 2\pi(2d/\lambda) = 2\pi[2d/(c/f_o)] = \omega_o(2d/c) \text{ radians.} \tag{14.2}$$

However, the distance 2d is changing in time because of the target velocity component along the line from the transducers to the target.

Thus, the frequency of the received signal, ω_r, is the time derivative of its phase:

$$\omega_r = d[\omega_o t + \omega_o(2d/c)]/dt = \omega_o[1 + (2\dot{d}/c)] = \omega_o[1 + (2/c)|\mathbf{v}|\cos(\theta)] \text{ r/s.} \tag{14.3}$$

The Doppler shift frequency, ω_D, is defined by Equation 14.4. It contains the velocity information:

$$\omega_D = (\omega_o 2/c)|\mathbf{v}|\cos(\theta) \text{ r/s.} \tag{14.4}$$

Note that $\omega_r > \omega_o$, because in this example, the target is approaching the source/sensor. The sign of ω_D will be negative for a target moving away from the transducers.

As you will see in Section 14.3, the Doppler effect using ultrasound has many important, noninvasive, diagnostic applications. The Doppler effect is used to measure blood velocity, in veins, arteries, and capillaries. When the diameter of the vessel's lumen is known, true blood flow can be estimated from Doppler measurements. Doppler ultrasound can also detect fetal heartbeats, and the heartbeats of unconscious persons. When the ensonifying beam is perpendicular to the blood vessel and **v**, the radial motion of an aneurysm can be sensed by the Doppler technique. Doppler ultrasound can also measure the heart valve motion.

14.3 DOPPLER ULTRASOUND FOR BLOOD AND TISSUE VELOCITY MEASUREMENTS

14.3.1 Angle-Dependent, CW, Blood Velocity Magnitude Measurement

Doppler velocity measurements of blood suffer from two major problems: One is the angle dependence seen in the equations derived in Section 14.2. The other is noisiness. Practical limitations on noninvasive, Doppler measurement geometry restrict $25° \leq \theta \leq 45°$ with reference to the axis of the blood vessel. Often the angle is not known precisely because of natural anatomical variation, and hand wobble can cause low-frequency noise if the probe is handheld.

The noise associated with Doppler measurements of blood velocity comes from two sources. First, assuming laminar flow, the blood velocity in larger arteries and veins follows an approximately parabolic velocity profile as a function of radial distance from the center of the vessel; the peak velocity is in the center of the vessel, it is zero at the edges. Because the input ultrasound beam has finite width, it simultaneously interacts with a wide range of velocities in the vessel. The ultrasound reflects of red blood cells (RBCs) being carried along in the blood. The RBCs are biconcave disks in shape; they are about 7.5 μm diameter, about 1.9 μm thick at their edges, and are about 1 μm thick at their centers. Typical RBC density is about 5.2×10^6 ($\pm 3 \times 10^5$) cells per cubic mm of plasma for men. Normally, from 40% to 45% of the blood volume is RBCs; this percentage is called the *hematocrit* (Guyton 1991).

The RBCs spin and turn as they flow along in the larger vessels, providing nonstationary targets with varying cross sections for the input ultrasound waves. Thus, instead of a sharp, single Doppler returns frequency, we see a noisy, bell-shaped power spectrum of return frequencies, $S_r(f)$, with its peak at the frequency of the Doppler shift of the maximum RBC velocity in the center of the blood vessel. Any calculation of volume flow necessarily must use the peak velocity, the lumen diameter, and the fact that the laminar flow velocity profile is approximately parabolic.

A simple CW Doppler ultrasound system, such as a Parks Model 811-BTS, typically has an analog (audio) voltage output whose amplitude is proportional to the power in the reflected beam, and whose frequency is proportional to the Doppler frequency shift magnitude, ω_D. Figure 14.2 illustrates the organization of a basic, CW Doppler ultrasound blood velocity system. A sinusoidal oscillator coupled to a power amplifier (POA) drives the transmitting piezoelectric transducer (TRX) at its mechanical resonant frequency. At resonance, the transducer's power output is maximum, and it appears as a nearly real impedance load in the order of hundreds of ohms to the POA. The transmitting transducer may have a concave plastic ultrasound "lens," or a Fresnel-type polystyrene lens (Fjield et al. 2004) that acts to concentrate the transmitted beam at the expected distance where blood vessels are found below the skin. The TRX is placed against the skin with a thin layer of acoustic impedance-matching, ultrasound gel between it and the skin. The receiving transducer (RCX) also has the same resonant frequency as TRX, and is often placed in the same probe housing as TRX. TRX and RCX must be acoustically isolated, so that RCX responds only to the reflected, Doppler-shifted ultrasound. The Doppler-shifted signal from RCX is amplified, and then mixed or detected by effectively multiplying it by the transmitted signal. One easy way to do this is *not* to perfectly isolate TRX and RCX, so that the output of RCX contains the sum of the transmitted signal and the Doppler-shifted return signal. Sic:

$$V_r(t) = A \overset{\text{transmitted}}{\sin(\omega_o t)} + B \overset{\text{received}}{\sin\{\omega_o[1 + (2/c)\,|\mathbf{v}|\cos(\theta)]t + \psi\}}. \tag{14.5}$$

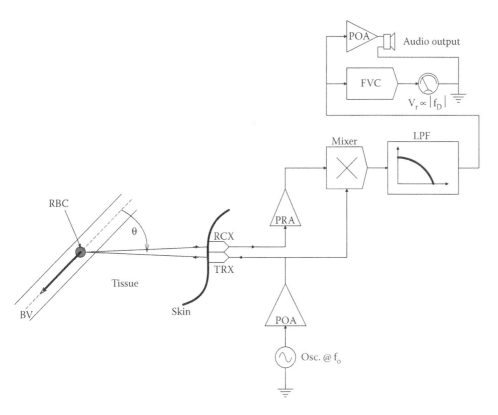

Figure 14.2 Block diagram of a typical CW Doppler blood velocity measurement system. *Key:* RBC = reflecting moving red blood cell; FVC = frequency-to-voltage converter; LPF = low-pass filter; PRA = RF preamplifier; POA = power amplifier; Osc = sinusoidal RF oscillator at frequency f_o; RCX = receiving transducer; TRX = transmitting ultrasound transducer.

Now V_r is conditioned by a square-law transfer nonlinearity, such as a JFET mixer. Squaring V_r, we get:

$$V_r^2(t) = A^2\sin^2(\omega_o t) + 2AB\sin(\omega_o t)\sin\{\omega_o[1+(2/c)|\mathbf{v}|\cos(\theta)]t + \psi\}$$
$$+ B^2\sin^2\{\omega_o[1+(2/c)|\mathbf{v}|\cos(\theta)]t + \psi\}. \tag{14.6}$$

Now by trig identity, the two $\sin^2(*)$ terms give DC + double frequency cosine terms. The middle term above, by the $\sin X \sin Y = \frac{1}{2}[\cos(X-Y)-\cos(X+Y)]$ trig identity, yields the following cosine terms:

$$\cos\{-\omega_o[(2/c)|\mathbf{v}|\cos(\theta)]t - \psi\} \quad \text{and} \quad \cos\{2\omega_o[1+(1/c)|\mathbf{v}|\cos(\theta)]t + \psi\}.$$

By passing $V_r^2(t)$ through an audio-frequency band-pass filter, the frequency of the Doppler shift is actually heard as an audio tone, $V_a(t) = kAB\cos[\omega_o(2/c)|\mathbf{v}|\cos(\theta)t]$. (We do not hear minus signs, constant-phase shifts or DC terms, and ultrasonic terms of frequency ω_o and $2\omega_o$ are not audible.) Thus, the amplitude and frequency of the audio output of the simple CW Doppler ultrasound blood velocity meter are actually the superposition of all the ensonified, low-amplitude, velocity components from the population of RBCs moving at various velocities in the blood vessel under study.

To obtain a DC voltage output proportional to the blood velocity *magnitude* suitable for a strip-chart recorder, the output of the audio band-pass filter, $V_a(t)$, is further amplified and put through a comparator configured as a zero-crossing detector. The TTL logic output of the comparator is HI when $V_a(t) > 0$, and is LO when $V_a(t) < 0$. A one-shot multivibrator is set to trigger on the LO → HI transitions at the comparator's output, generating narrow, positive, TTL pulses of width δT. These pulses are put into a low-pass filter, the DC output of which approximates their average, V_F. It is easy to show that V_F is given by

$$V_F = V_{LO} + \bar{f}_D(V_{HI} - V_{LO})\delta T, \tag{14.7}$$

where V_{LO} and V_{HI} are the TTL low- and high-voltage levels, and $\bar{f}_D$ is the mean, Doppler frequency shift ($\bar{f}_D = \bar{\omega}_D/2\pi$) in Hz, and δT is the pulse width.

Note that the low-pass filter output will be positive for blood velocity toward or away from the transducers; the analog output of this simple Doppler system responds to the velocity magnitude. This simple frequency magnitude discriminator is shown in Figure 14.3.

Webster (1992) gave an expression for the average zero-crossing rate, r_z, of the comparator. It is not a simple function of the Doppler frequency shift, f_D, but instead is given by the relation:

$$r_z = \left[\frac{\int(f_r - f_o)^2 S(f)df}{\int S(f)df}\right]^{1/2}, \tag{14.8}$$

where $(f_r - f_o) = f_D$, the Doppler frequency shift, $S(f)$, is the power density spectrum of $V_r(t)$, in ms volts/Hz, the denominator is P_r, the total ms volts in the return signal, and the numerator can be considered to be the second moment of the Doppler frequency. Note that $S(f)$ is in fact nonstationary because of the pulsatile nature of blood flow. $S(f)$ might be better described by an $S(f, t)$, that is, by joint time–frequency analysis, as described in Section 3.2.3.

The simple, nondirectional, CW Doppler ultrasound system described above provides more qualitative than quantitative information for NI diagnosis. It can provide left/right comparisons of carotid sinus blood velocity and turbulence. A noticeable L/R difference may indicate a unilateral carotid occlusion from cerebrovascular disease (Halberg and Thiele 1986).

More sophisticated Doppler systems exist that: (1) Provide an analog output with the sign of the blood velocity, that is, they are directional. (2) Are angle independent. These systems are described in the following sections.

14.3.2 Directional, CW Doppler System

The organization of a directional, CW Doppler system is shown in block diagram form in Figure 14.4. This system generates a time-varying output voltage whose magnitude is proportional to f_D, and whose sign is + or −, depending whether blood velocity is toward or away from the probe, respectively. To see how this system functions, we will examine its signals and their

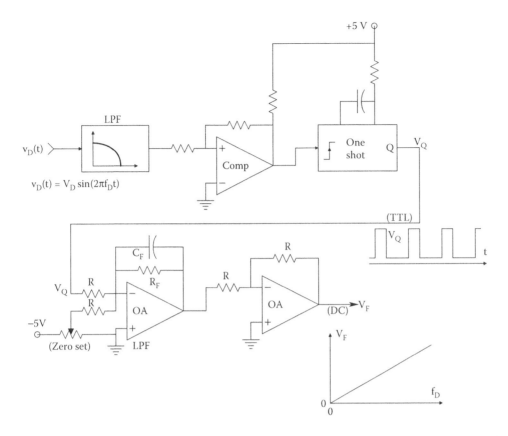

Figure 14.3 Simple VFC circuit that converts an audio-frequency Doppler signal proportional to a DC voltage proportional to f_o by duty-cycle averaging.

functions. Assume the oscillator puts out a voltage, $A \cos(\omega_o t)$. The output of the quadrature phase shifter is $A \sin(\omega_o t)$. The received, Doppler-shifted return signal is:

$$V_r(t) = B \sin\{\omega_o[1 + (2/c)v \cos(\theta)]t + \psi\}. \tag{14.9}$$

$V_r(t)$ is added to $A \cos(\omega_o t)$ and $A \sin(\omega_o t)$ to form the analog sums X and Y, respectively. X and Y are squared by high-frequency analog multipliers. Their respective outputs are:

$$W(t) = K_m(A^2\cos^2(\omega_o t) + 2AB \cos(\omega_o t) \sin\{\omega_o[1 + (2/c)v \cos(\theta)]t + \psi\}$$
$$+ B^2\sin^2\{\omega_o[1 + (2/c)v \cos(\theta)]t + \psi\}) \tag{14.10}$$

$$Z(t) = K_m(A^2\sin^2(\omega_o t) + 2AB \sin(\omega_o t) \sin\{\omega_o[1 + (2/c)v \cos(\theta)]t + \psi\}$$
$$+ B^2\sin^2\{\omega_o[1 + (2/c)v \cos(\theta)]t + \psi\}). \tag{14.11}$$

W and Z are put through audio band-pass filters. The $\sin^2(*)$ and $\cos^2(*)$ terms by trig identity become DC $\pm \cos(2\omega_o t)$ terms, both of which do not appear at the audio BPF outputs. The W(t) middle term can be written by trig identity as

$$K_m 2AB \cos(\omega_o t) \sin\{\omega_o[1 + (2/c)v \cos(\theta)]t + \psi\} = K_m AB\{\sin[2\omega_o t + \omega_o(2/c)v \cos(\theta)t + \psi]$$
$$+ \sin[\omega_o(2/c)v \cos(\theta) t + \psi]\}. \tag{14.12}$$

The $2\omega_o$ term is filtered out, and the analog signal at the output of the "W" BPF is:

$$\overline{W(t)} = K_f K_m 2AB \sin[\omega_o(2/c)v \cos(\theta)t + \psi]. \tag{14.13}$$

231

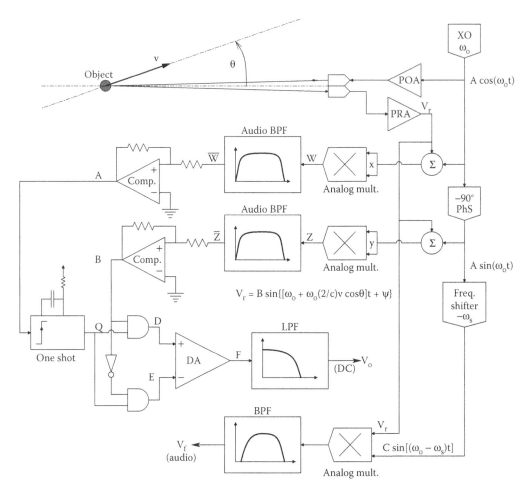

Figure 14.4 Block diagram of a CW directional Doppler system. Quadrature detection allows V_o to have the sign of v. The audio output has a center frequency and is shifted up or down in frequency depending on whether the object is approaching or receding, respectively.

The audible Doppler frequency is $f_D = \omega_o (1/\pi c)\, v \cos(\theta)$ Hz. Similarly, the analog signal at the output of the "Z" BPF is:

$$\overline{Z(t)} = K_f K_m 2AB \cos[\omega_o(2/c)v\cos(\theta)t + \psi]. \tag{14.14}$$

$\overline{W}$ and $\overline{Z}$ are next put through analog comparators configured as zero-crossing detectors (0XDs) with some hysteresis to give them noise immunity. (The hysteresis is the result of the positive feedback around the comparator.) The Doppler signal is demodulated to give an analog V_o, whose magnitude is proportional to ω_D, and whose sign follows **v**. When the reflecting objects are moving toward the probe, the gating (Q) pulse from the one shot is ANDed with the B output from the cosine OXD, producing a pulse of the same width at the D AND gate output. E remains low, so a pulse appears at F at the output of the differential amplifier with amplitude $K_{DA}(V_{HI} - V_{LO})$. The F pulses are periodic at f_D, so the average output voltage, V_o, is:

$$V_o = f_D K_{DA}(V_{HI} - V_{LO}). \tag{14.15}$$

When the objects are moving away from the probe, the sign of the sin(*) term is inverted, and the gating pulse produced by the one shot ANDs with the HI B input to the lower AND gate, producing a pulse at E, while D remains low. Now the peak pulse amplitude at F is $-K_{DA}(V_{HI}-V_{LO})$, and the average output of the low-pass filter is negative:

$$\bar{V}_o = \overline{-f_D} K_{DA}(V_{HI} - V_{LO}). \tag{14.16}$$

The phase shift, Ψ, is common to both sine and cosine channels, $\bar{W}$ and $\bar{Z}$, respectively, so its effect cancels out.

It is also possible to obtain an audio-frequency output from the directional Doppler system that is also responsive to the sign of the object velocity. In this simple system, the return signal, $V_r(t)$, is mixed with a synthesized, constant frequency signal, V_2, that is, $\omega_s = 2\pi 10^3$ r/s *below* the transmitted signal frequency, ω_o. That is, $V_r(t)$ is mixed with $V_2 = C \sin[(\omega_o - \omega_s)t]$. Thus:

$$V_r V_2 = K_m BC \sin\{\omega_o[1 + (2/c)v \cos(\theta)]t + \psi\}\sin[(\omega_o - \omega_s)t]. \tag{14.17}$$

The mixer output is passed through an audio band-pass filter which blocks all DC and high-frequency terms.

Thus, the $\sin(\alpha)\sin(\beta)$ term produces an audio-frequency output given by the $\cos(\alpha - \beta)$ term in the trig identity.

$$V_f = K_F K_m (BC/2)\cos\{[\omega_s + \omega_o(2/c)v \cos(\theta)]t + \psi\}. \tag{14.18}$$

If the object is stationary, V_f has frequency f_s; if the object is approaching the probe, V_f's frequency rises by f_D: if the object is receding, the frequency of V_f is lowered by f_D, just like the trumpet sound on the moving train.

14.3.3 Angle-Independent, CW Doppler Velocimetry

A serious problem in obtaining quantitative Doppler blood velocity measurements is the often imprecise knowledge of the probe angle, θ. Obviously, v is proportional to $f_D/\cos(\theta)$, and an error in θ will give an error in v.

In 1978, Fox derived a closed-form solution to the 2-D Doppler situation, which utilizes the outputs of two independent transmit–receive probes. The probes transmit at two separate frequencies, f_1 and f_2. They are aligned so that their focused beams cross in the volume whose velocity is being measured.

Fox's solution yields the velocity magnitude, $|\mathbf{v}| = \sqrt{v_x^2 + v_y^2}$, and the angle θ_1 between the velocity vector $\mathbf{v}$ and a line from number 1 probe (Figure 14.5). Note that the probes lie in the XY

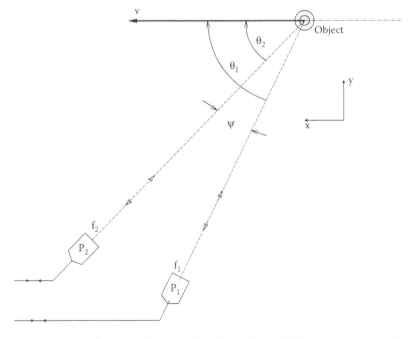

Figure 14.5 Geometry relevant to Fox's angle-independent CW Doppler system. All vectors lie in the plane of the paper.

plane with the velocity vector. The probes are separated by an angle ψ, and their beams converge on the moving, reflecting object. The Doppler frequency shift returned to each probe is given by

$$f_{D1} = f_{o1}(2/c)|\mathbf{v}|\cos(\theta_1) \tag{14.19}$$

$$f_{D2} = f_{o2}(2/c)|\mathbf{v}|\cos(\theta_2) = f_{o2}(2/c)|\mathbf{v}|\cos(\theta_1 - \psi). \tag{14.20}$$

Now we can solve Equations 14.19 and 14.20 for θ_1:

$$|\mathbf{v}| = \frac{f_{D1}c}{f_{o1}2\cos(\theta_1)} = \frac{f_{D2}c}{f_{o2}2\cos(\theta_1 - \psi)}. \tag{14.21}$$

After some algebra and the trig identity for $\cos(x - y)$, we find:

$$\frac{f_{D1}}{f_{o1}} = \frac{f_{D2}}{f_{o2}[\cos(\psi) + \tan(\theta_1)\sin(\psi)]}. \tag{14.22}$$

Fox defined the parameter R as

$$R \equiv \frac{f_{D2}f_{o1}}{f_{D1}f_{o2}} = \frac{1}{[\cos(\psi) + \tan(\theta_1)\sin(\psi)]}. \tag{14.23}$$

From which we find the unknown incidence angle:

$$\theta_1 = \tan^{-1}\left[\frac{R - \cos(\psi)}{\sin(\psi)}\right]. \tag{14.24}$$

The arctangent relation for θ_1 suggests a right triangle with angle θ_1, the adjacent side is length $\sin(\psi)$, the opposite side is $[R - \cos(\psi)]$, and the hypotenuse is $\sqrt{\sin^2(\psi) + [R - \cos(\psi)]^2} = \sqrt{1 + R^2 - 2R\cos(\psi)}$.

Returning to Equation 14.19, and using the trig definition for $\cos(\theta_1)$, we find:

$$|\mathbf{v}| = \frac{f_{D1}c}{f_{o1}2\cos(\theta_1)} = \frac{f_{D1}c\sqrt{1 + R^2 - 2R\cos(\psi)}}{\sin(\psi)}. \tag{14.25}$$

In order to calculate $|\mathbf{v}|$ and θ_1, one must measure f_{D1} and f_{D2}, knowing f_1, f_2, and ψ. The accuracy of the method is limited by the accuracy which one can determine f_{D1} and f_{D2}. Because of the parabolic (laminar) flow profile in blood vessels, the finite size of the ensonified volume (typically 3 mm^3 for a 2.25 MHz carrier (Fox 1978)), and the random scattering nature of moving RBCs, there typically is a bell-shaped distribution of f_Ds, rather than a single, sharp peak. The mode of the distribution is generally taken as the desired f_D. The Fox two-probe method of determining the velocity vector in 2-D is best implemented with a computer system which algorithmically processes the Fourier-transformed Doppler return signals to determine their modes to estimate f_{D1} and f_{D2}, and then calculates $|\mathbf{v}|$ and θ_1 using the relations above and the known parameters, Ψ, f_1, and f_2.

Fox and Gardiner (1988) extended the 2-D closed-form solution for $|\mathbf{v}|$ to 3-D. Their equations are too long to include here, but they have the same general form as the simpler 2-D case described above. Their results showed that the calculated $|\mathbf{v}|$ remained within 5.6% of the theoretical value for Doppler angles up to 50°. Also, their angle estimate agreed with the theoretical values with a correlation coefficient, $r = 0.99937$. The 2- and 3-D Doppler flow velocimetry technique developed by Fox and colleagues is of course not restricted to the ultrasonic measurement of blood velocity. Their technique can be extended to the other Doppler modalities (lasers and microwaves), when a 2- or 3-D estimate of object velocity is required.

14.3.4 Pulsed Doppler Systems

A pulsed Doppler ultrasound system (PDS) emits periodic, sinusoidal pulses of ultrasonic energy. The pulses are characterized by their *repetition rate*, f_r (or period, T_r), their *oscillation frequency*, f_o, and their *pulse envelope*, $e(t)$, which effectively defines the pulse duration and amplitude. A significant advantage of pulsed Doppler ultrasound is that it allows relatively small voxels to be ensonified, giving the ability to describe blood and tissue velocity in detail around structures such as heart valves, aneurisms, atherosclerotic occlusions in major vessels, kidney vessels, and umbilical cord vessels, etc. The output displays on modern pulsed Doppler systems can generally show both velocity versus time plots for a targeted voxel, or be shown as a 2-D image slice of tissues (B-mode display) showing structures as well as velocities in color.

When measuring blood velocity by pulsed Doppler, the return echoes scattered from the moving RBCs are greatly attenuated compared to the echoes from solid tissues of different densities such as bone, muscle, and blood vessel walls. The reflections from blood can be 40 dB less than that from other tissues (Routh 1996). In measuring blood velocity in deep vessels, the pulsed Doppler system (PDS) must wait for the Doppler-shifted echo to return before transmitting the next pulse. If the pulse has a round trip distance of $2L = 0.1$ meters to a fixed reflector, then it will take $T_t = 2L/c = 2 \times 0.1/1540 = 1.2987 \times 10^{-4}$ s to travel 10 cm. Thus, for no-pulse overlap, the maximum rate pulses can be transmitter if $f_r = 1/T_t = 7.7$ kHz at this distance. Shorter distances permit faster pulse repetition rates (PRRs). In summary:

$$PRR_{max} = f_r = c/2L \text{ pps.} \tag{14.26}$$

A major engineering trade-off exists in a PDS between the ability to define a small-sample volume (voxel) in the target, and to simultaneously measure the target velocity. This trade-off is very like the Heisenberg uncertainty principle in quantum physics. The shorter pulse required to define a smaller voxel has a larger transmitted bandwidth and poorer velocity resolution. Another way of stating the trade-off between range and target velocity given by Signal Processing, S.A. (2015), is:

$$L_{max} v_{max} = c^2/[8f_r\cos(\theta)] \text{ m}^2/\text{s.} \tag{14.27}$$

To examine the PDS in the frequency domain, we first consider one pulse alone. In its simplest form, the pulse, $f(t)$, is equal to the time-domain product of a cosine wave at the resonant frequency of the transducer, $\omega_o = 2\pi f_o$ radians/s, and an envelope or gating function, $g(t)$. That is, $f(t) = g(t) \cos(\omega_o t)$. The simplest envelope function is an (even) rectangular pulse: $g(t) = P_r(T_r/2)$. $P_r(T_r/2) = 1$ for $|t| < T_r/2$, and 0 for $|t| \geq T_r/2$. However, the acoustic output of a transducer initially at rest given a narrow, DC excitation pulse rises gradually to a peak amplitude and then dies off to zero. Two simple envelope function models can be used to describe the output tone burst. One is the Gaussian model; $g_g(t) = \exp[-\frac{1}{2}(t/\tau)^2]$, $-\infty \leq t \leq \infty$. Another is the cosine on a pedestal function; $g_c(t) = \frac{1}{2}[1 + \cos(\omega_c t)] P_r(\pi/\omega_c)$. This function is zero for $|t| > \pi/\omega_c$ and has unit value for $t = 0$. Note that $\omega_c = 2\pi/T_c$, so $t = \pi/\omega_c = T_c/2$. Thus, the $g_c(t)$ function makes a tone burst T_c seconds in duration. Typically, $T_c = 8T_o$, where T_o is the period of the transducer's natural frequency (i.e., $T_o = 2\pi/\omega_o$). The Gaussian envelope function, while not finite in length, is mathematically more expedient to use as a model.

Let us examine a single PDS pulse in the frequency domain. We will use the Fourier transform pairs:

$$\cos(\omega_o t) \xleftrightarrow[F^{-1}]{F} \pi[\delta(\omega - \omega_o) + \delta(\omega + \omega_o)] \tag{14.28}$$

$$\exp[-\frac{1}{2}(t/\tau)^2] \xleftrightarrow[F^{-1}]{F} \tau\sqrt{2\pi} \exp[-1/2(\tau\omega)^2]. \tag{14.29}$$

The Gaussian-gated pulse in the time domain is represented by the product:

$$g_o(t) = g_g(t) \cos(\omega_o t). \tag{14.30}$$

Its Fourier transform is given by *complex convolution*:

$$G_o(\omega) = \frac{1}{2\pi} \int_{-\infty}^{\infty} G_g(\omega - u)\pi[\delta(u - \omega_o) + \delta(u + \omega_o)]du$$

$\downarrow$

$$\tag{14.31}$$

$$G_o(\omega) = \frac{\pi\tau}{\sqrt{2\pi}} \{\exp[-\frac{1}{2}\tau^2(\omega - \omega_o)^2] + \exp[-\frac{1}{2}\tau^2(\omega + \omega_o)^2]\}.$$

Thus, the Fourier spectrum of a single-gated pulse has peaks at $\omega = \pm\omega_o$, and at $\omega = 0$, has the value of:

$$G_o(0) = \tau\sqrt{2\pi} \exp[-\frac{1}{2}\tau^2\omega_o^2]. \tag{14.32}$$

Note that the parameter τ is chosen so that a few f_o cycles are included in the pulse envelope before its amplitude becomes negligible.

Next we consider an infinite train of pulses, each pulse of the form of Equation 14.30. These pulses have a repetition rate governed by $f_r = c/2L$, where c is ~1540 m/s, and L is the distance in the tissues (in meters) from the source transducer to the target vessel. In general, $f_r \ll f_o$. Let us represent the infinite pulse train in the time domain by

$$g^*(t) = \sum_{n=-\infty}^{\infty} g_o(t - nT_r). \tag{14.33}$$

Because g*(t) is periodic and meets certain other criteria, it can be represented by a complex Fourier series:

$$g^*(t) \sum_{n=-\infty}^{\infty} C_n \exp[+jn\omega_r t]. \tag{14.34}$$

The complex Fourier coefficient, C_n, is given by (Papoulis 1977):

$$C_n = \int_{-T_r/2}^{T_r/2} g^*(t)\exp[-jn\omega_r t]dt = (1/T_r)G_o(n\omega_r). \tag{14.35}$$

Thus, g*(t) can be written:

$$g^*(t) = (1/T_r) \sum_{n=-\infty}^{\infty} G_o(n\omega_r)\exp[+jn\omega_r t], \tag{14.36}$$

which has the Fourier transform:

$$\begin{aligned}
G^*(\omega) &= (2\pi/T_r) \sum_{n=-\infty}^{\infty} G_o(n\omega_r)\delta(\omega - n\omega_r) \\
&= (2\pi/T_r) \sum_{n=-\infty}^{\infty} \frac{\pi\tau}{\sqrt{2\pi}}\{\exp[-\tfrac{1}{2}\tau^2(n\omega_r - \omega_o)^2] \\
&\quad + \exp[-\tfrac{1}{2}\tau^2(n\omega_r + \omega_o)^2]\}\delta(\omega - n\omega_r).
\end{aligned} \tag{14.37}$$

Thus, the spectrum of the pulse train, g*(t), is a *line spectrum* with lines spaced $\Delta\omega = n2\pi/T_r$ radians/s apart. The exponential terms have maximum amplitude (1) for $|n| = \omega_o/\omega_r$ (nearest integer).

The Doppler return spectrum from a moving object is also a line spectrum. The return signal frequency, f_s, for an approaching, reflecting object is at frequencies:

$$f_s(n) = nf_r[1 + (2v/c)\cos(\theta)] \text{ Hz.} \tag{14.38}$$

Thus, the actual Doppler shift is given by

$$f_d = (nf_r 2v/c)\cos(\theta) \text{ Hz.} \tag{14.39}$$

Note that f_d is not a function of f_o. The Doppler-shifted, return signal's line spectrum is thus:

$$\begin{aligned}
G_{ret}(\omega) &= \beta(2\pi/T_r) \sum_{n=-\infty}^{\infty} \frac{\pi\tau}{\sqrt{2\pi}}\{\exp[-\tfrac{1}{2}\tau^2(n\omega_r\{1 + (2v/c)\cos(\theta)\} - \omega_o)^2] \\
&\quad + \exp[-\tfrac{1}{2}\tau^2(n\omega_r\{1 + (2v/c)\cos(\theta)\} + \omega_o)^2]\} \\
&\quad \times \delta[\omega - n\omega_r\{1 + (2v/c)\cos(\theta)\}].
\end{aligned} \tag{14.40}$$

Note that β is the attenuation of the Doppler signal. The entire return line spectrum is thus seen to be distributed approximately symmetrically around ω_o, the transducer's natural (excitation) frequency.

To gain a heuristic appreciation of how a PDS system works in the time domain, refer to Figure 14.6, where $\cos(\theta) = 1$. Pulses are emitted at a fixed rate, f_r. f_r is set $\leq c/2L$ to prevent aliasing.

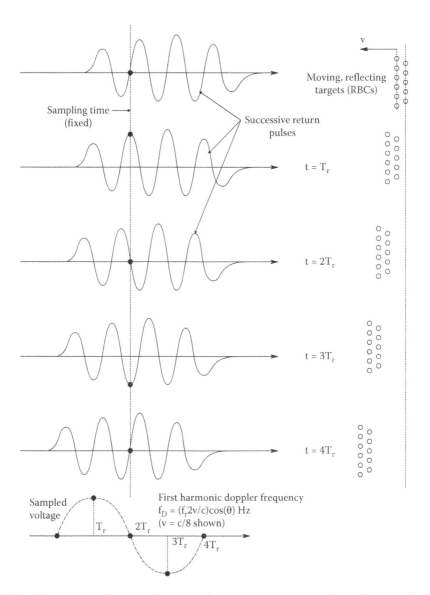

Figure 14.6 Description of how pulsed Doppler velocimetry works. The reflecting objects are approaching the transducer. The Doppler frequency voltage is found by sampling the return pulse at a fixed time relative to the transmission time. The samples are held and used to reconstruct the f_D waveform. T_r is the interval between transmitted pulses.

L is the mean distance to the moving, reflecting target. The returning pulses are amplified and filtered. Each returning pulse is sampled at the same time relative to its emission time; that is, the sampling rate is f_r. If the target is stationary, each sampled return pulse is sampled at the same time and the sampler output is constant (zero Doppler frequency). In the figure, the target is moving toward the transducer at velocity **v**. Thus, each successive return pulse is advanced in phase, creating a periodic, sampled signal, v_s (t). In practice, v_s is noisy and must be averaged over many pulse periods, and then high-pass filtered by a "wall" filter to remove excessive, low-frequency "clutter" noise. The averaged, filtered v_s can be Fourier transformed to form a root power density spectrum, $\sqrt{P_{Vs}}(\omega)$ rms Volts/$\sqrt{Hz}$. The frequency of v_s is the Doppler-shift frequency, which carries the velocity magnitude information. By also sampling the return pulse at a time shift of $1/4f_o$ from the main channel, the quadrature signal obtained can be used to give target velocity sign information, that is, is the target receding or approaching? The electronic analog and digital systems that do this in a PDS are complex. The interested reader should consult the venerable June, 1986 *Hewlett-Packard Journal* for an excellent system's level description of a modern pulsed Doppler system (HPJ 1986).

Modern PDSs can display their data in a time–frequency format in which the Doppler frequency (proportional to velocity) is coded by amplitude. PDSs are also used in an imaging or "B" mode; more will be said of this in Chapter 16 on imaging. The signal-to-noise ratio in PDSs depends in part on the transmitted ultrasonic power.

A fundamental limit to transmitted power is tissue heating; ultrasonic energy absorbed by tissues causes heating due to viscous (lossy) vibration. Only a small portion of the incident ultrasound energy is reflected back at interfaces between structures having different acoustic impedances in tissues. If not dissipated, the heating can cause pain, and excessive heating can denature proteins and destroy cell structures, "cooking" the ensonified tissues. Extreme ultrasound energy density levels can also cause *cavitation* (the formation of gas bubbles), which can rupture cells and otherwise physically destroy tissues. Naturally, ultrasound dosage is rigorously controlled by the FDA and other regulatory agencies, and the dosage from an approved diagnostic PDS does no harm in the applications for which it is designed.

14.3.5 Discussion

In this section, we have described how the Doppler effect used with CW and pulsed ultrasound can measure blood velocity, as well as the velocity of moving tissues in the body, such as aneurisms, fetal heartbeat, cardiac diagnosis (O'Connell 1986), etc. Simple instruments that provide output signals proportional to average blood velocity are not blood flowmeters. To obtain flow, we must multiply blood vessel lumen area by the average blood velocity. Lumen area can be found by ultrasound imaging, or another imaging modality.

The simple, CW ultrasound velocimeter is valuable in screening for obstructive artery disease. When an atherosclerotic plaque forms, partially occluding a blood vessel, Bernoulli's principle dictates that the blood velocity through the restricted area will increase, often causing turbulence. This increase in velocity and the resulting turbulence are easy to spot with a simple Doppler ultrasound system. If the lesion is unilateral, a left–right comparison of velocity at the same anatomical location makes diagnosis easier. The gold standard for verification of arterial obstruction is x-ray angiography.

14.4 NOTOPM SYSTEM

14.4.1 Introduction

The OP is the minute, periodic, radial displacement of the corneal surface caused by arterial pressure pulsations in the intraocular circulation acting through the fluid contents of the eyeball on the compliance of the cornea. Features of the OP waveform have been shown by several workers to be diagnostic indicators of: (1) Cerebrovascular disease (particularly, arteriosclerosis in one or both carotid arteries) (Hørven 1973); (2) Abnormally high-intraocular pressure (IOP), aka glaucoma; (3) Autonomic changes in the cerebral circulatory system in response to changes in blood CO_2 and O_2 levels (Northrop and Decker 1978).

The arterial blood supply for the human eye comes from the *ophthalmic artery* (OA) which branches off the *internal carotid artery* (ICA) below the optic nerve. In addition to the eyes, the OA serves to supply other tissues with blood; notably the extraocular muscles, the sinuses, nasal tissues, etc. Here, we will only consider the OA's role in supplying the internal tissues of the eyeball. The central retinal artery (CRA) branches from the OA and enters the optic nerve and runs inside it. The CRA enters the rear of the eyeball along with the optic nerve fibers. Inside the rear of the eye, the CRA makes numerous fine branches; it also supplies the arterial Circle of Zinn surrounding the optic disc ("blind spot") of the retina. Two, *posterior ciliary arteries* (PCAs) also branch off the OA and divide into some 10–20 branches, which run forward surrounding the optic nerve and pierce the choroid layer of the rear of the eyeball on the medial and lateral sides of the optic nerve. The branches from the *short ciliary artery* enter the sclera on the medial (nasal) side of the optic nerve, while the *long ciliary artery's branches* enter the lateral side of the eyeball and run forward between the sclera and the choroid to supply the ciliary body. They also anastomose with branches from the *anterior ciliary arteries* (ACAs) to form the *circulus arteriosis iridus major* that supplies the iris. The ACAs arise as branches of the muscle branches of the OA. Although the arterial anatomy of the eyeball is complex, the reader should appreciate that it is all derived from the ICA (Kronfeld 1943). Hence, any factor reducing pressure in the ICA will reduce arterial blood flow into the eyeball.

If we take the mean arterial blood pressure (MAP) in the brachial artery to be 100 mmHg, then it can be estimated by *ophthalmodynamometry* that the MAP in the CRA and the PCAs is about 65–70 mmHg (Adler 1933). The static, intraocular pressure (IOP) of a normal eyeball is about 16 mmHg (Guyton 1991). This pressure is due to the constant rate of production of aqueous humor (AH) by the cells of the ciliary process, and the resistance to the outflow of the AH through the trabecular network, the canal of Schlemm and the episcleral veins (Northrop 2000). If the outflow resistance rises, the IOP will rise; a condition known as *glaucoma*. Elevated IOP presses on the arteries within the eyeball which supply the intraocular tissues, restricting the inflow of arterial blood. Prolonged restriction of arterial inflow leads to tissue anoxia which can permanently damage sensitive retinal neurons, leading to visual defects and even blindness.

Under normal IOP, the pulsation of internal arteries creates a periodic pressure variation which is added to the static IOP. This pressure variation causes the elastic cornea to stretch and contract radially in a Hookean manner. It is this displacement of the cornea which can be measured noninvasively as the OP. Because the OP depends on the internal arterial pressure transients, the OP acts, in effect, as a plethysmograph for the ocular circulation. Any factor that alters the pressure as a function of time in the CRA and the ciliary arteries will alter the OP. Such factors can include obstructions in the ICA (or OA), elevated IOP, changes in the hydraulic loading of the ICA beyond where the OA branches off. These latter changes involve arterial perfusion of the brain, which is under tight autonomic control by the CNS. Of course, cardiac output will also affect the OP; the heart stroke volume and rate also being under autonomic nervous control.

Hørven and Nornes (1971), Hørven (1973), and Hørven and Gjønnaess (1974) were among the first researchers to measure the OP and relate it to known circulatory problems and other medical conditions. Hørven and colleagues used an electronic Schiøtz indentation tonometer with a 5.5-g loading weight. The patient lay supine with the tonometer applied vertically to the cornea. The tonometer output was 1 mV per μm of corneal displacement. Thus, the static IOP could be measured along with the OP waveform. Sterile technique was observed and the surface of the cornea was anesthetized. The OP waveforms recorded by Hørven and Nornes on strip-charts were all very smooth; they contained no high-frequency transients or oscillations. They were not quite sinusoidal in form, apparently containing few harmonics beyond the fundamental frequency (heart rate). Hørven and Nornes (1971) examined the OP from six classes of patients: Normal patients, and patients having glaucoma, choroidal melanoma, carotid obstruction, giant cell arteritis, and carotid cavernous sinus fistula. They recorded IOP, pulse rate, peak-to-peak OP amplitude, and the relative crest time (RCT) (the time to an OP peak from the previous OP minimum divided by the period of that OP cycle). Note that the RCT is concerned with the OP wave shape. Another significant OP parameter is the *peak phase delay* (PPD), measured as the time from the ECG R peak to the next OP peak, divided by the period of that cardiac cycle, times 360°. The PPD was not measured by Hørven and Nornes (1971).

In normal subjects, Hørven and Nornes found an average IOP of 16.6 mmHg, and an average peak-to-peak OP amplitude of 30.75 μm (σ = 10.35 μm); the RCT was 41.5% (σ = 2.34%). A significant diagnostic parameter was a significant increase in the RCT. Only in the case of melanoma, there was no significant change in the RCT. The mean RCT *increased* significantly to 43.6%, 45.4%, and 48.6% for glaucoma, carotid obstruction (degree not noted), and giant cell arteritis, respectively. RCT significantly *decreased* to 34.8% for carotid cavernous sinus fistula. Of particular note was that the mean amplitude of the OP increased to 34.4 μm in eyes with glaucoma having a mean IOP of 37.7 mmHg. One might have thought that doubling the normal IOP would *reduce* the OP amplitude and increase the RCT more than it did. (The slight rise in OP amplitude in glaucoma may have its origin in the nonlinear elastic properties of the arteries in the eyeball; a phenomenon similar to that which gives rise to Korotkoff sounds when measuring the brachial blood pressure by sphygmomanometer.)

Another simple contact system for OP measurement was developed by LaCourse and Sekel (1986). A soft ethylene-vinyl acetate (EVM) rubber cup, used to remove contact lenses, made contact with the cornea. The cup was attached to a piezoelectric bender transducer with a short post. An initial cup displacement of 30 μm produced 260 mV across the crystal, and required 2 g force. LaCourse and Sekel examined the OP on New Zealand white rabbits under conditions of normal, carotid flow, and under condition of ipsilateral carotid flow occlusion by an inflatable, hydraulic cuff around the artery. Not surprisingly, a marked attenuation of the OP and change in its waveshape was observed when a carotid occlusion was applied.

Note that a piezoelectric transducer is a band-pass system. That is, it is characterized by a transfer function (relating output voltage to applied displacement) having a *zero at the origin* of the s-plane, a *low-frequency pole* whose value depends on the transducer's electrical loading, and one or more *high-frequency poles* (Northrop 2014, Section 6.2.2.3). Only by connecting a piezoelectric transducer to a *charge amplifier* can one accurately specify the low-frequency pole frequency. LaCourse and Sekel connected their transducer to an isolation amplifier, thus the low-frequency pole of their system depended on this amplifier's input resistance as well as the capacitive load presented to the transducer by amplifier's input capacitance, and the wires connecting the transducer to the amplifier. It is not clear from their paper what the value of their measurement system's low-frequency pole was specified with or without an isolation amplifier. However, there was no evidence of low-frequency OP waveform differentiation in their figures, so the low-frequency pole was probably lower than 1 Hz. It should be noted that Hørven's electronic Schiøtz tonometer output was direct-coupled, hence the OP waveforms he showed in his papers were probably characterized by the frequency response of his strip-chart recorder, typically flat from DC to ~50 Hz. No low-frequency waveform differentiation was possible in his data.

In order to eliminate the need for physical contact with the cornea to measure the OP, and the consequent need for sterile technique and corneal anesthetization, the author and graduate student Shrikant Nilakhe developed an ultrasonic, no-touch means of measuring the corneal displacement. The design and performance of their NOTOPM system are described in the next section.

14.4.2 Closed-Loop, Constant-Phase, No-Touch Means of Measurement of OP

The original NOTOPM system of Northrop and Nilakhe (1977) used continuous-wave, air-coupled ultrasound reflected off the corneal surface to noninvasively measure the OP. The no-touch method obviates the need for sterile technique and corneal anesthesia. Their system is shown schematically in Figure 14.7. A pair of 1/4″ diameter, LTZ-2, air-backed transducers were used as independent, CW ultrasound transmitter and receiver. The transducers were used at frequencies

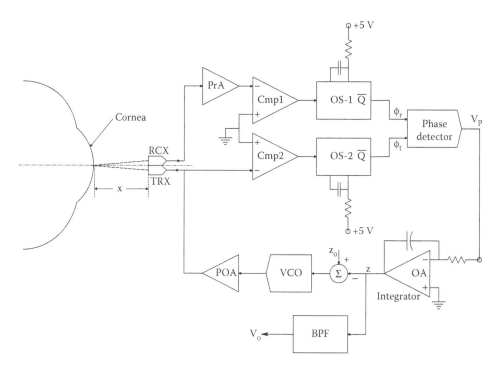

Figure 14.7 Block diagram of the original no-touch ocular pulse measurement system devised by Northrop and Nilakhe (1977). *Key:* RA = receiver RF amplifier; POA = power amplifier; VCO = voltage-controlled oscillator; OS-1, OS-2 = one-shot multivibrators; Cmp1, Cmp-2 = amplitude comparator; TX = transmitting transducer; RX = receiving transducer.

well below their 3-MHz resonant frequency, typically in the range of 850–900 kHz. The system behaved as a constant-phase, Type 1, feedback loop (not a phase-locked loop). Heuristically, the system measures the total airpath distance (transmitter to cornea, cornea to receiver) by adjusting the transmitted frequency so that the same number of ultrasound wavelengths remain in the airpath, regardless of its length. If the cornea expands, the airpath distance is shortened, and the VCO frequency rises; if the cornea contracts, the VCO frequency is lowered to maintain the same number of cycles (phase) in the airpath. Changes in the VCO input voltage are shown to be proportional to the airpath's Δx.

To understand quantitatively how the NOTOPM system works, we first consider it to be in the open-loop, steady state (SS), with no motion of the cornea. The transducers are each at a distance x_o from the cornea, so that the total airpath length is $2x_o$. If the VCO output frequency is f_o, then it is easy to see that the total, SS phase lag between the received ultrasound and the transmitted ultrasound is:

$$\phi_m = 2\pi(2x_o/c)f_o \text{ radians,} \tag{14.41}$$

where c is the velocity of sound in air, nominally 344.0 m/s at 20°C and 40% relative humidity. There can be many wavelengths of ultrasound in the SS airpath at any instant, so the SS ϕ_m can be $\gg 360°$. For example, if the transducer distance is $x_o = 1.5 \times 10^{-2}$ m, and the VCO center frequency is 850,000 Hz, there will be $2x_o\,f/c = 74.128$ cycles or wavelengths of ultrasound in the total airpath.

Changes in airpath length are detected by a digital phase detector (PD). Typical digital PDs have a limited range of operation. For example, the simple R-S flip-flop PD used in the NOTOPM system gives zero output for a 180° phase difference between its input pulses, and has a linear range of 0–360°. If the input phase difference exceeds 360°, its output characteristic is again linear for $360° < \phi_e < 720°$, etc. That is, it has a sawtooth, periodic output characteristic as shown in Figure 14.8. Note that the R-S flip-flop PD has output zeros for input phase differences equal to:

$$\phi_e = 2\pi(k + \tfrac{1}{2}) \text{ radians,} \tag{14.42}$$

where $|k| = 0, 1, 2, 3....$

When the system is initially turned on, the transmitted frequency is $\omega_o = K_v\,V_r$ r/s. A DC voltage V_r is initially applied to the VCO until the return signal is sensed and pulses ϕ_r are available at the PD input. At this time, a PD output voltage, V_p, is presented to the system integrator's input. The integrator's output, V_i, is subtracted from the reference voltage, V_r, changing the input to the VCO from V_r so that its output frequency changes to $\omega = (\omega_o + \Delta\omega) = K_v\,(V_r - V_i)$. In the SS, the Type 1 servo loop forces the integrator *input*, V_p, to be zero. This means that $\phi_e = \phi_m = 2\pi(k + \tfrac{1}{2}) = 2\pi(2x_o\,f/c) = (2x_o/c)\,K_v\,(V_r - V_i)$ radians.

If we assume SS, closed-loop operation, the instantaneous output frequency of the VCO is $\omega_T(t)$. At the Cornea, this instantaneous frequency is $\omega_T(t - \tau)$, where the delay τ is just x_o/c s. If the cornea is moving with velocity $\dot{x}$, the reflected ultrasound is given a *Doppler frequency* shift, so that, at the cornea, the instantaneous reflected frequency is given by

$$\omega_{rc} = \omega_T(t - \tau)[1 + 2\dot{x}(t - \tau)/c] \text{ r/s.} \tag{14.43}$$

At the receiving transducer, we have:

$$\omega_r = \omega_T(t - 2\tau)[1 + 2\dot{x}(t - \tau)/c] \text{ r/s.} \tag{14.44}$$

And the total phase lag between the VCO output and the received signal is:

$$\phi_r = 2\pi \int \omega_r dt = 2\pi \int \omega_T(t - 2\tau)[1 + 2\dot{x}(t - \tau)/c] dt \quad \text{radians.} \tag{14.45}$$

An expression for the total phase error, ϕ_e, must include the periodic, finite range characteristics of the phase detector used. Thus, we can write:

$$\phi_e = -2\pi \int \omega_T(t - 2\tau)[1 + 2\dot{x}(t - \tau)/c] dt - 2\pi(k + \tfrac{1}{2}) + 2\pi \int \omega_T(t) dt \quad \text{degrees.} \tag{14.46}$$

Equation 14.46 can be rearranged to yield:

$$\phi_e = -2\pi \int [\omega_T(t - 2\tau) - \omega_T(t)] dt - 2\pi(k + \tfrac{1}{2}) + 2\pi(2/c) \int \omega_T(t - 2\tau)\dot{x}(t - \tau) dt. \tag{14.47}$$

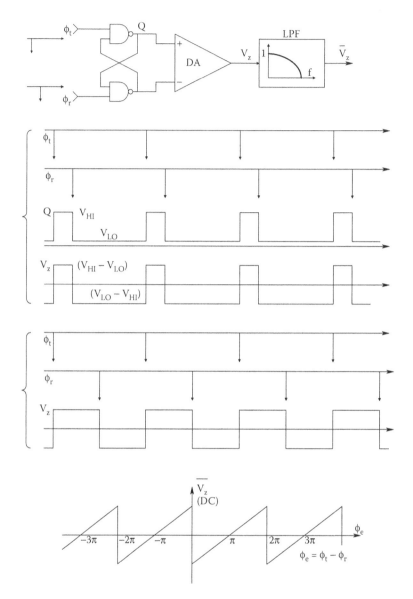

Figure 14.8 *Top:* An RS flip-flop phase detector. *Mid:* Relevant waveforms. *Bottom:* Output DC voltage versus input phase difference characteristic. Note zero output occurs for phase differences which are odd multiples of π.

In normal, closed-loop, small-signal operation, k remains constant, because the peak displacement of the OP is ≪ $\dot{x}_o$. The PD output, V_p, is integrated to form V_i. Thus:

$$V_i = -K_i \int (-K_p) \phi_e dt. \tag{14.48}$$

From Equation 14.48, we obtain:

$$\phi_e = \dot{V}_i / (K_p K_i) \text{ radians}. \tag{14.49}$$

Also, the VCO output instantaneous frequency is given by:

$$\omega_T(t) = K_v (V_r - V_i) \text{ r/s}. \tag{14.50}$$

Substituting Equations 14.49 and 14.50 into Equation 14.47, we obtain

$$\dot{V}_i = -K \int \left[V_i(t) - V_i(1 - 2\tau) \right] dt - 2\pi K/K_v(k + \frac{1}{2}) + K(2/c)V_r x(t - \tau)$$
$$-K(2/c) \int V_i(t - 2\tau)x(t - \tau) \, dt, \tag{14.51}$$

in which $K \equiv K_p \, K_i \, K_v$. Under SS conditions, by definition, $\dot{x} = \dot{V}_i = 0$, $x = x_o$, and $\bar{V}_i = V_i$. Hence, Equation 14.51 can be written as

$$0 = -K\bar{V}_i(2\,x_o/c) - (K2\pi/K_v)(k + \frac{1}{2}) + K(2/c)V_r x_o. \tag{14.52}$$

From which we find that

$$\bar{V}_i = V_r - \frac{2\pi(k + \frac{1}{2})c}{2x_o K_v} \tag{14.53}$$

Thus, we have shown that in the SS, the average value of the integrator output, V_i, is a nonlinear function of the average distance to the cornea, x_o. The corneal Δx from the OP, however, represents a small fraction of x_o, roughly $\pm 15 \, \mu m$ out of $x_o = 15,000 \, \mu m$. Thus, the ΔV_i from the OP can be written:

$$\Delta V_i = \frac{\partial V_i}{\partial x} \Delta x = \frac{2\pi(k + \frac{1}{2})c}{2x_o^2 K_v} \Delta x. \tag{14.54}$$

Thus, in this system, the DC small-signal sensitivity is proportional to x_o^{-2}. This is a drawback to calibration because x_o must be precisely known. Northrop and Nilakhe (1977) showed that loop dynamics also impose a high-frequency real pole at $\omega_b = 2\pi f_b$ on the $\Delta V_i/\Delta x$ transfer function. That is:

$$\frac{\Delta V_i}{\Delta x}(j\omega) = \frac{\left\{ \dfrac{2\pi(k + \frac{1}{2})c}{2x_o^2 K_v} \right\}}{[j\omega/(\omega_b) + 1]}. \tag{14.55}$$

They also showed that $\omega_b = K_p \, K_i \, K_v \, 2x_o/c$ r/s, and the SS value of k is given by the integer value:

$$k = INT[2x_o K_v V_r/(2\pi c)]. \tag{14.56}$$

The SS lock frequency is:

$$\omega_{TL} = \frac{2\pi(k + \frac{1}{2})c}{2x_o} \, r/s. \tag{14.57}$$

Let us evaluate numerically some of the NOTOPM system's key parameters: Take $c = 344$ m/s, $x_o = 15$ mm $= 1.5 \times 10^{-2}$ m, $K_p = 3.1831$ V/radian, $K_i = s^{-1}$, $K_v = 1.06814 \times 10^6$ r/s/V, $k = 74$. From Equation 14.54, The small-signal sensitivity is $S_{Vi}(\Delta x) = 2\pi (k + \frac{1}{2}) \, c/(2 \, x_o^2 \, K_v)$ V/m $= 3.35 \times 10^2$ V/m, or 0.335 mV/μm. The closed-loop system's break frequency is at $f_b = \omega_b/2\pi = K_p \, K_i \, K_v \, 2x_o/2\pi c$ Hz. Numerically, $f_b = 47.2$ Hz for the parameters given. The SS lock frequency is $f_{TL} = c \, (k + \frac{1}{2})/(x_o \, 2) = 850.827$ kHz.

Northrop and Nilakhe (1977) investigated the effectiveness of their ultrasonic NOTOPM system on rabbits and consenting normal human subjects. Adult New Zealand white rabbits were immobilized by IM injection of a mixture of acepromazine maleate 1.5 mg/kg and ketamine HCl 15 mg/kg. The animals were immobile in about 6 min, and stayed that way for about 45 min, unless more drug was given. Recovery was complete in about 2 hours after the last injection. Immobilized rabbits were laid on their sides and their heads were sandbagged. The downward eye was taped shut to prevent drying (the blinking reflex was inhibited by the drugs). The upper eye was held open with tape on the eyelids, and artificial tears were used to prevent corneal drying. The ultrasound transducers were positioned at $x_o = 15$ mm from the cornea, and ECG electrodes were attached to shaved spots on the forelimbs.

Examples of rabbit OP waveforms are shown in Figures 14.9 and 14.10. The peak outward corneal deflection occurs at approximately a 175° phase lag following the ECG R spike. Corneal expansion generally proceeds without inflection, that is, the OP's first derivative does not go to zero once expansion starts until the peak is reached; similarly, the contraction phase has no inflection until minimum corneal radius is reached. Peak-to-peak OP was about 13 μm. The effects of (external, bilateral) carotid compression on rabbit OP were shown to be a reduction in its amplitude. In addition, CNS autonomic changes in cerebral circulation induced by breathing different gas mixtures

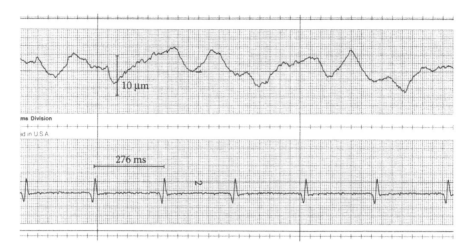

Figure 14.9 A strip chart recording of the ocular pulse waveform recorded from an anesthetized New Zealand white rabbit along with its ECG QRS complex for reference. Note the noise on the OP waveform. (Figure from Northrop, R.B. 2002. *Noninvasive Instrumentation and Measurement in Medical Diagnosis*. CRC Press, Boca Raton, FL. ISBN: 0-8493-0961-1.)

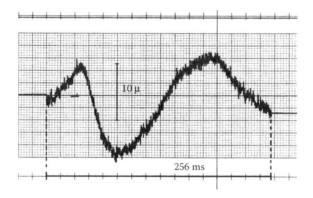

Figure 14.10 The same rabbit's OP averaged over 128 cardiac cycles. (Figure from Northrop, R.B. 2002. *Noninvasive Instrumentation and Measurement in Medical Diagnosis*. CRC Press, Boca Raton, FL. ISBN: 0-8493-0961-1.)

(pure O_2, air, and air + 5% CO_2) produced OP amplitude changes. In some cases, there was as much as a 50% reduction in OP amplitude when breathing pure O_2. On the other hand, air with 5% CO_2 caused the OP amplitude to increase, sometimes as much as 75% above the air value. The waveshape of the OP remained substantially invariant, however, regardless of the gas breathed. Rabbit heart rate also changed less than ±10% with different gases (Northrop and Decker 1978).

The protocol for measuring human OP used the same transducers and 1.5 cm x_o distance used with the rabbits. x_o was set by a calibrated pulse echo delay. No drugs were used. Monocular OP was measured; the subject rested his/her forehead on an optometrist's head rest. Instead of a chin rest, extra head stability was achieved by using a bite bar. In later measurements, we adapted a pair of optometrist's trial frames worn by the subject to carry transducers for the left and right eyes, permitting simultaneous, binocular OP recordings.

One salient feature of all OP recordings done on human subjects was their noisiness. The sources of noise were found to be eyelash tremor, micronystagmus of the eyeball, air currents, weak return signal due to misalignment of the transducers, electronic noise from the phase-tracking loop's amplifiers, etc. Some of the noise could be minimized by instructing the subjects to open their eyes wide and fixate on an LED fixation spot on the centerline of the transducers. Band-pass filtering was also used to restrict the noise to the OP bandwidth. It was generally necessary to average 32 OP waveforms synchronized by the ECG R spike to reduce the noise to an acceptable

(a)   (b)

(c)   (d)

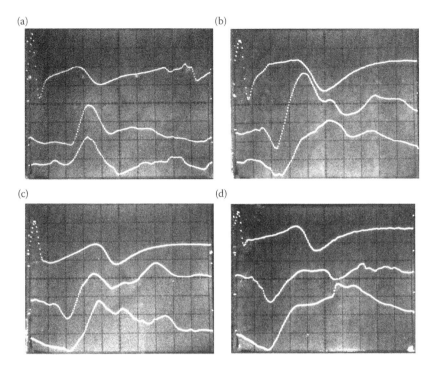

Figure 14.11   Averaged, representative, normal human, bilateral OP waveforms with ECG. In all four plates, the top trace is the ECG, middle trace is left eye's OP, bottom trace is right eye's OP. All OPs are averaged 64 times in sync with the ECG QRS spike. *Plates:* (a) Male age 31; normal vision. (b) Male age 23; normal vision. (c) Male age 24; farsighted. (d) Male age 24; normal vision. We noted that no subjects' eyes had identical OP waveforms. Vertical scale in all figures given by the 12 μm initial peak height in the bottom trace of plate (A). (Figure from Northrop, R.B. 2002. *Noninvasive Instrumentation and Measurement in Medical Diagnosis.* CRC Press, Boca Raton, FL. ISBN: 0-8493-0961-1.)

level. Figure 14.11 illustrates some of the variability in normal, averaged, human OP waveforms. Note variability between averaged OPs of OS and OD.

Northrop and Nilakhe's (1977) research on normal human OP, and Northrop and Decker's (1978) study of the effect of respiratory gases on the OP led to some surprising observations and conclusions about using the OP as a noninvasive, diagnostic screening tool for the detection of cerebrovascular disease. First, human OP was found to have a more complex shape than that of rabbits; there were generally more inflections, and often two positive peaks during a cardiac cycle. There were also differences between individuals, and often significant left/right OP differences in the same subject. As a further complication, we discovered that when subjects held their breath in the process of concentrating on holding their eyes wide open and fixating their gaze, their OP waveforms increased in amplitude. This increase was probably due to an increase in blood pCO_2, and an autonomic compensatory increase in flow in the ICA to the brain.

While their OP was being measured, human subjects were asked to breath either USP oxygen, air, or air + 5% CO_2. There was a consistent and significant OP amplitude *decrease* with O_2 with reference to air, and a consistent and significant OP amplitude *increase* when breathing air with 5% CO_2. Clearly, there was an autonomic compensation for both high O_2 and high CO_2 partial pressures. The stroke/volume of the heart and the hydraulic admittance of the ICA may have been increased by the high pCO_2, and decreased by pure O_2.

14.4.3 Discussion

Besides the labile nature of the human NOTOP waveform and its relative noisiness, another drawback to the NOTOPM system is that it requires patient cooperation (and some practice) in keeping the eyes open wide and fixated over a 30-s or so interval required to average 32 pulse cycles. The NOTOPM system is not suitable for use on persons who are unable to cooperate in this manner. These problems mean that it cannot be used as an absolute indicator of reduced carotid blood flow. It must be used under controlled conditions, generally on the same individual. The NI contact methods of OP measurement used by Hørven and Nornes (1971), and by LaCourse and Sekel (1986) are far less noisy than the NOTOPM system. They do require sterile technique and corneal anesthesia, however.

It is clear that more work needs to be done in establishing the OP diagnostic parameters for cerebrovascular disease that are transferable among individuals. No one appears to have examined the OP in the frequency domain, either as an impulse response (to the ECG R wave) or to display the OP's Fourier series harmonics under various conditions.

14.5 CLOSED-LOOP, TYPE 1, CONSTANT-PHASE DIFFERENCE RANGING SYSTEM

14.5.1 Introduction

The author has described a means of linearizing a CW, constant-phase difference, closed-loop, ultrasonic distance measuring systems such as the NOTOPM system described in Section 14.4. This innovation was also extended to laser and microwave distance measurement systems (Nelson 1999, Northrop 2014). At the heart of the constant-phase difference ranging system (CPDRS) is the use of a VPC instead of a voltage-to-frequency converter (VFC). The VPC is a type of voltage-controlled oscillator (VCO) in which the *period* T of the output waveform is directly proportional to the input (control) voltage, that is,

$$T = 1/f = b + K_p V_c \, s. \tag{14.58}$$

(In a VFC, $f = 1/T = a + K_v V_c$ Hz). Thus, the output radian frequency of a VPC is given by

$$\omega_o = 2\pi/(b + K_p V_c) \, r/s. \tag{14.59}$$

For small changes in V_c, we can write:

$$\Delta\omega = \left(\frac{\partial \omega_o}{\partial V_c}\right)\Delta V_c = \frac{-2\pi}{(b + K_p V_{co})^2}\Delta V_c. \tag{14.60}$$

The closed-loop CPRS system is made a Type I feedback system by the inclusion of an electronic integrator in the feedback path; it is easy to show that the input to the integrator is proportional to the target (reflecting object) velocity, and the integrator output is linearly proportional to target range ($2x_o$). Unlike the NOTOPM system described above, there is no distance dependence in the velocity and range sensitivity expressions; they remain constant over the system's target operating range. Examples of an analog and a digital VPC are shown in Figures 14.12 and 14.13,

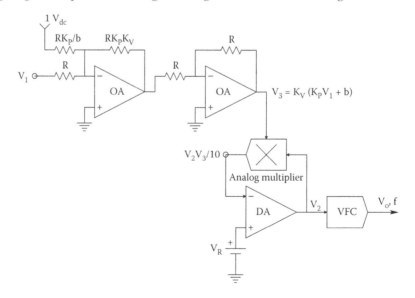

Figure 14.12 All-analog voltage-to-period converter (VPC). A conventional voltage-to-frequency converter (VFC) is driven by a voltage V_2. It is easy to show that $V_2 = 10V_R/V_3$, ($V_3 > 0$). V_R is made 0.1 V so $V_2 = 1/V_3$. Now, as shown in the figure, $V_3 = K_V(K_P V_1 + b)$. The VCO generates $f_o = K_V V_2$ Hz $= K_V/K_V(K_P V_1 + b)$, hence the output period is $T_o = 1/f_o = K_P V_1 + b$, which is the desired characteristic of a VPC given input V_1.

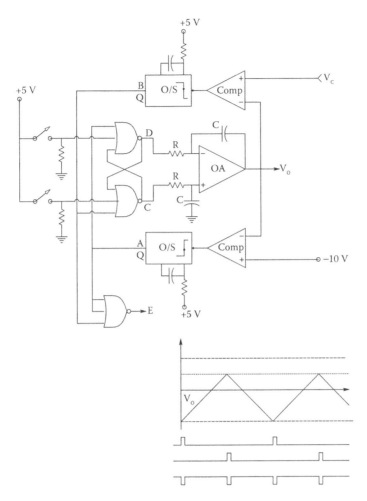

Figure 14.13 Digital/hybrid VPC. The AD840 high-speed op-amp integrates the complimentary TTL outputs, D and C, of the RS flip-flop. We assume initially D is HI and C is LO. V_o ramps negative. When V_o reaches −10 V, the lower AD790 comparator's threshold, this comparator goes HI, producing a narrow positive TTL pulse at A that resets the flip-flop so D = LO and C = HI. The integrator output now ramps positive until V_o reaches threshold V_C. Now the upper AD790 comparator output goes LO, triggering a narrow positive pulse at the upper one-shot's output, B. This B pulse again resets the FF so D is HI and C is LO, and again V_o ramps negative. You can see intuitively that the lower the V_C, the higher will be f_o and the smaller the period. It can be shown that the pulses at E have a period given by: T = KPVC + b, as in Equation 14.55.

respectively. Note that the analog VPC uses a standard VFC but takes the reciprocal of the input analog control voltage. As in the case of VFCs, there are practical limits to the range of the output frequency in VPCs.

We now examine how the use of a VPC linearizes the distance and velocity sensitivities of the NOTOPM system.

14.5.2 Analysis of a Linear NOTOPM System Using a VPC

Figure 14.14 shows the organization of a NOTOPM system using a VPC. Its system block diagram is shown in Figure 14.15. In addition to the VPC, this system uses a compensating zero in its integrator to ensure closed-loop stability. The transfer function of this integrator is:

$$\frac{V_o}{V_p}(s) = \frac{-K_i(\tau s + 1)}{s}. \tag{14.61}$$

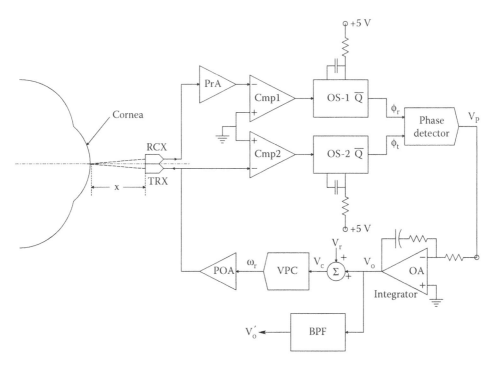

Figure 14.14 Block diagram of an improved, no-touch ocular pulse measuring system using a VPC instead of a VFC.

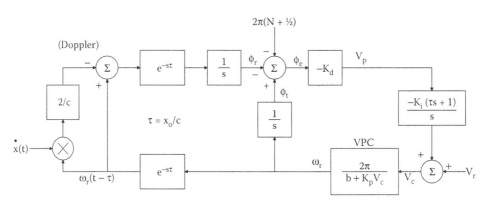

Figure 14.15 Systems block diagram of the NOTOPM system of Figure 14.14.

From Equation 14.61, we can write the ODE:

$$\dot{V}_o = -K_i(\tau \dot{V}_p + V_p).$$ (14.62)

The phase error is given by the expression:

$$\phi_e = -\int \omega_T(t - 2\tau)[1 - 2\,\dot{x}(t - \tau)/c]\,dt - 2\pi(N + \tfrac{1}{2}) + \int \omega_T(t)\,dt.$$ (14.63)

Rearranging terms in the integral equation above, we have:

$$\phi_e = -\int [\omega_T(t - 2\tau) - \omega_T(t)]\,dt - 2\pi(N + \tfrac{1}{2}) + (2/c)\int \omega_T(t - 2\tau)\dot{x}(t - \tau)\,dt.$$ (14.64)

From the VPC:

$$\omega_T(t - 2\tau) = \frac{2\pi}{b + K_p\left[V_r + V_o(t - 2\tau)\right]}.$$ (14.65)

We now note that $V_p = -K_d\dot\phi_e$ can be substituted into Equation 14.62, giving:

$$\dot V_o = K_i[\tau(-K_d\dot\phi_e) - (K_d\dot\phi_e)], \tag{14.66}$$

which is solved for ϕ_e:

$$\dot\phi_e = -[\tau\dot\phi_e + \dot V_o/(K_iK_d)]. \tag{14.67}$$

Thus, we can write:

$$-[\tau\dot\phi_e + \dot V_o/(K_iK_d)] = -2\pi K_p \int \frac{[V_o(t) - V_o(t-2\tau)]}{[b^2 + \cdots]} dt - 2\pi(N + \tfrac{1}{2})$$
$$+ (4\pi/c) \int \frac{\dot x(t-\tau)}{b + K_p[V_r + V_o(t-2\tau)]} dt. \tag{14.68}$$

In the SS: $\dot V_o = \dot\phi_e = 0$, $V_o = \bar V_o$, and $\bar x = x = x_o$. Thus, Equation 14.68 becomes:

$$0 = 0 - 2\pi(N + \tfrac{1}{2}) + \frac{4\pi\bar x}{c[b + K_p(V_r + V_o)]}. \tag{14.69}$$

Let $V_r \equiv -b/K_p$. Rearranging Equation 14.69, we find:

$$V_o = x_o \left[\frac{2}{K_p c(N + \tfrac{1}{2})} \right]. \tag{14.70}$$

The small-signal range sensitivity is obviously $[2/(K_p c(N + \tfrac{1}{2})]$ at frequencies $\ll$ the closed-loop system's ω_n. From algebraic manipulation of the equations above, it also can be shown that the system's transfer function in response to *target velocity* is:

$$\frac{V_P}{\dot X}(s) = \frac{\dfrac{-2}{K_i K_p c(N + \tfrac{1}{2})}}{(\tau s + 1)}. \tag{14.71}$$

The real pole at $s = -1/\tau$ is inherent in the compensation filter.

We now examine the dynamics of the closed-loop system. Figure 14.16 illustrates the negative feedback loop that determines the closed-loop system's ω_n and damping. The system's loop gain is:

$$A_L(s) = \frac{-(\tau s + 1)}{s^2} \frac{K_d K_i 2\pi c^2 (N + \tfrac{1}{2})^2}{4x_o^2} \tag{14.72}$$

The closed-loop system's transfer function's denominator (DEN) is the numerator of $F(s) = 1 - A_L(s)$. Thus:

$$DEN = s^2 + s2\xi\omega_n + \omega_n^2 = s^2 + s\tau \frac{K_i 2\pi c^2(N + \tfrac{1}{2})^2}{4x_o^2} + \frac{K_d K_i 2\pi c^2(N + \tfrac{1}{2})^2}{4x_o^2}. \tag{14.73}$$

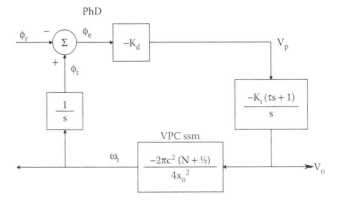

Figure 14.16 Linearized systems block diagram of the system of Figure 14.14. From the single-loop system, we can find the closed-loop system's poles.

The right-hand term in Equation 14.73 is ω_n^2. The damping factor can be shown to be equal to:

$$\xi = \tau\sqrt{2\pi K_d K_i}\,\frac{c(N+\frac{1}{2})}{2x_o}. \tag{14.74}$$

It is now useful to define and to calculate some of the system parameters. The mean distance to the moving object (e.g., cornea) is taken as $x_o = 1.5 \times 10^{-2}$ m = 15 mm, the speed of sound in air is c = 344 m/s, and the closed-loop, center frequency of the system is $f_o = 850$ kHz. Thus, in the airpath under SS conditions, there are $(2x_o/\lambda_o) = (2x_o f_o/c) = 74.128$ cycles. Hence, we take N = 74. Take $K_i = 0.01$ and $K_d = 0.1$ V/radian. The VPC was designed so that with b = 0, $V_c = 5$ V will produce $f_o = 850$ kHz. That is, $8.5 \times 10^5 = 1/(K_p\, 5\,V)$, so $K_p = 2.353 \times 10^{-7}$ s/volt. Hence, the range sensitivity is $2/[c\, K_p\, (N + \frac{1}{2})] = 3.317 \times 10^2$ V/m, or 3.317×10^{-1} mV/μm. The velocity sensitivity is $-2/[K_i\, K_p\, c(N + \frac{1}{2})] = -3.317 \times 10^4$ V/m/s. The undamped natural frequency, ω_n, of the system is 6.77×10^4 r/s, or $f_n = 1.078 \times 10^4$ Hz. In order for the damping factor to be 1 (critically damped), the compensation zero's time constant must be $\tau = 1.478 \times 10^{-5}$ s (15.8 μs). These parameter values are entirely reasonable for the redesigned NOTPM system.

14.5.3 Other Applications of the CPDRS Architecture Using Ultrasound

In the sections above, we have considered the use of air-coupled ultrasound to noninvasively measure the periodic, corneal displacements caused by the ocular arterial blood supply. This OP was shown to have some diagnostic value in screening for severe cerebrovascular disease. In this section, we will examine the possible use of a CPDRS ultrasound system to detect aneurisms of the aorta and common carotid arteries. Because the CPDRS system architecture provides simultaneous outputs proportional to both target velocity and position that are range independent, it has the potential to provide useful data on aneurysm size and type, without the risk of dye-injection angiography. Its use would be similar to conventional, directional Doppler ultrasound except the CPDRS method will give an exact displacement measurement of the aneurysm surface [$\Delta x(t)$] as it pulsates, as well as a quantitative record of its velocity. It will allow quantification of the mechanical properties of an aneurysm which might have been first seen on a static x-ray image. Needless to say, An NI CPDRS system would be far less expensive than a real-time ultrasound imaging system, and would carry negligible risk.

The CPDRS system design for aneurysm-sensing system can use a CW ultrasound frequency of about 1 MHz, and an acoustic lens to concentrate the sound energy at the expected depth of the aneurysm (Macovski 1983). Sufficient acoustic energy would be reflected from the interface between the aneurysm and surrounding soft tissue to enable phase lock. An alternate mode of operation would be to use pulsed ultrasound. For example, taking c = 1540 m/s as the mean velocity of sound in tissue, a 2-cm distance to the aneurysm would cause a $\delta T = 25.97$ μs delay in the return echo. In order for δT to represent a 45° phase lag at the phase detector (PD), the transmitted average pulse rate, f_o, would have to be 4.81 kHz. The CPRS system keeps this 45° phase lag constant as the target distance, x, varies around x_o by adjusting the pulse rate with the VPC. If the aneurysm is aortic, say at $x_o = 10$ cm, then the average pulse rep rate would be 962.5 pps for a 45° phase shift. Even at this slower f_o, the system bandwidth would be high enough to characterize an aneurysm moving with a period of about 1 s.

Besides aneurisms, the pulsed, ultrasonic CPDRS system could be used to measure the distance to, and motion of such organs as the heart, the uterus, and the bladder. The CPDRS system is not intended to replace conventional, real-time, x-ray tomographic systems which can image the heart in 3-D. However, it could find application in emergency medicine to see quickly whether or not a patient's heart is beating, or a uterus is contracting in an unconscious patient.

14.5.4 Discussion

The CPDRS makes use of the voltage-to-period oscillator rather than the conventional VFC/ VCO. By doing so, its simultaneous range and velocity output gains are independent of range, that is, are properly constants, unlike the same system using a VFC/VCO. Nelson (1999) successfully designed and built and tested a pulsed laser range finder (for use in air or space) using the CPDRS architecture. The CPDRS system architecture can easily be adapted to CW or pulsed ultrasound. It does not appear that CPDRS is suitable to measure blood velocity; it requires a coherent, relatively noise-free return signal for closed-loop, constant-phase operation.

14.6 MEASUREMENT OF TISSUE GLUCOSE CONCENTRATION BY CLOSED-LOOP, CONSTANT-PHASE, CW ULTRASOUND: A PROTOTYPE SYSTEM

14.6.1 Introduction

The design of an instrument to make rapid, accurate, *noninvasive* measurements of blood glucose in diabetic patients has been an elusive technical objective for biomedical engineers for over 36 years. One physical means proposed by the author would make use of the fact that excess dissolved glucose solute in extracellular body fluids slightly raises the density of those fluids, hence slightly reducing the speed of sound, c, in tissues containing those fluids. If it was possible to accurately and consistently measure the speed of sound, or a quantity dependent on it such as phase, one could estimate the glucose concentration, *providing no* other confounding physiological factor alters tissue density, hence c.

The system described below is a prototype, constant-phase, self-nulling, Type I, control loop that maintains a constant-phase lag in the transmitted, CW ultrasound wave path by automatically adjusting the frequency of a VCO. The system's block diagram is shown in Figure 14.17. The small changes in tissue density due to changes in blood glucose concentration produce changes in the velocity of sound in the tissue, leading to small changes in the VCO input voltage, hence its frequency. Theoretically, the system is linear in that Δf and ΔV_o are linearly proportional to ΔG, the change in glucose concentration.

14.6.2 Approximate Model of How c Varies with Density, ρ

For a homogeneous, liquid medium, such as seawater at 12.5°C, the speed of sound is given by

$$c = \sqrt{(B/\rho)} = \sqrt{(3.31 \times 10^9 \, \text{N/m}^2 / 1025 \, \text{kg/m}^3)} = 1501.2 \, \text{m/s},$$

where B is the liquid's bulk modulus, ρ is its density. We assume that soft, vascular tissue such as an earlobe, or the web between the thumb and forefinger can be treated in the same manner as seawater as far as sound velocity is concerned. (Obviously, soft tissues contain inhomogeneities, including skin, fat, muscle, cartilage, blood vessels, etc., that complicate the picture.) The vascular tissue is assumed to be uniformly perfused with glucose at a concentration equal to the plasma glucose concentration, [pG]. Normally, the tissue density includes the normal [pG] = 100 mg/dl = 1 g/l = 1 kg/m³. A frequent condition in untreated or poorly treated diabetes is an elevated [pG], which can rise to 4 or 5 g/l above the normal level. A concentration rise above the normal glucose concentration of 1 g/l is defined as ΔG. Thus, we can write:

$$c(\Delta G) \cong \sqrt{B/(\rho_o + \Delta G)} = \sqrt{B/[\rho_o(1 + \Delta G/\rho_o)]} \cong c_o/(1 + \Delta G/2\rho_o) \cong c_o(1 - \Delta G/2\rho_o). \quad (14.75)$$

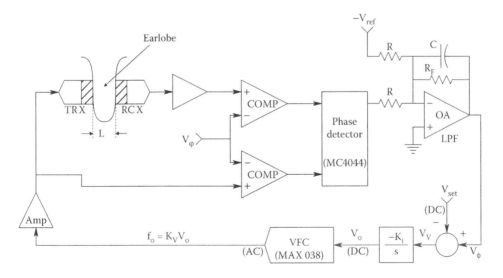

Figure 14.17 Block diagram of a proposed system to estimate blood glucose concentration by nulling the difference between the transmitted and received ultrasound phase through the earlobe. It is shown that the fractional change in VCO frequency required to null the system's phase detector output is proportional to the change in the glucose concentration in the earlobe.

Here we have assumed that $1 \gg \Delta G/\rho_o$, so $\sqrt{(1+\varepsilon)} \cong (1+\varepsilon/2)$, and $1/(1+\varepsilon/2) \cong 1-\varepsilon/2$.

Thus, a small increase in the density of the sound-conducting medium from elevated plasma glucose concentration results in a small decrease in the speed of sound in the medium.

14.6.3 Phase Lag between the Transmitted and Received CW Ultrasound Waves

It is easy to show that the received wave's phase lags the transmitted wave's phase by φ_r.

$$\varphi_r = 360° \, Lf_o/c(\Delta G) \cong \frac{360° \, Lf_o(1+\Delta G/2\rho_o)}{c_o} \text{ degrees,} \quad (14.76)$$

where L = sound transmission path length in tissue in m, f_o = VCO output frequency in Hz.

14.6.4 System Block Diagram for the Constant-Phase Glucose Sensor System

Figure 14.18 illustrates the closed-loop system that adjusts the VCO output frequency so that the SS phase difference remains fixed, regardless of the small changes in the speed of sound in the transmission medium (vascular tissue). The sound transmission path length, L, is assumed to be constant. Because the system is a type 1 control system, there will be zero SS error in φ_r. Thus, in the SS, $V_V = 0$, hence $V_{set} = V_\varphi$, and we can write:

$$V_{set} = \frac{K_\varphi 360L \, K_V V_o}{c_o}[1+\Delta G/(2\rho_o)]. \quad (14.77)$$

From this equation, we find that:

$$V_{oSS} = \frac{V_{set}c_o}{K_\varphi 360L \, K_V}[1-\Delta G/(2\rho_o)]. \quad (14.78)$$

Also, the VCO output frequency is:

$$f_o = \frac{c_o V_{set}}{K_\varphi 360L}[1-\Delta G/(2\rho_o)] \text{ Hz.} \quad (14.79)$$

The change in frequency due to an incremental increase in glucose concentration is simply:

$$\Delta f = \frac{-c_o V_{set}}{K_\varphi 360L2\,\rho_o}\Delta G \text{ Hz.} \quad (14.80)$$

Also in the SS, it is obvious that $\varphi_r = V_{set}/K_\varphi$.

The dynamics of the system can be estimated from consideration of the system's loop gain, $A_L(s)$. Input ΔG and DC quantities are $\rightarrow 0$.

$$A_L(s) = -\frac{360L \, K_\varphi K_i K_V}{sc_o}. \quad (14.81)$$

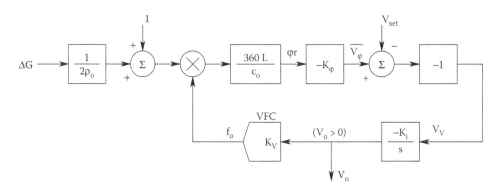

Figure 14.18 Block diagram for the system of Figure 14.17. Note that the system is nonlinear because of the multiplier in the loop.

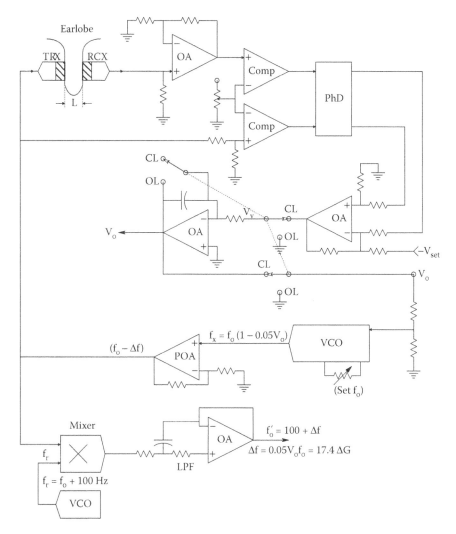

Figure 14.19 Simplified schematic diagram of an ultrasonic tissue glucose sensor built by the author and tested *in vitro*. Operating frequency range was around 35.7 kHz. See text.

The denominator of the linearized closed-loop transfer function is the so-called return difference, $F(s) \equiv 1 - A_L(s)$. The zeros of the return difference are the poles of the closed-loop system transfer function. In this case, the closed-loop system has one real pole.

$$F(s) = 1 + \frac{360L \, K_\varphi K_i K_V}{s c_o} = \left[s + \frac{360L \, K_\varphi K_i K_V}{c_o} \right] / s. \tag{14.82}$$

Thus, we see that the closed-loop system's real pole has a break frequency, ω_b:

$$\omega_b = \frac{360L \, K_\varphi K_i K_V}{c_o} \text{ radians/s.} \tag{14.83}$$

Substituting system design parameters: $K_i = 1$, $c_o = 1501$ m/s, $K_V = 10^5$ Hz/V, $V_{set} = 6$ V, $K_\varphi = 0.2$ V/degree, $L = 0.0035$ m, $c_o = 1501$ m/s, we find $\omega_b = 16.79$ r/s, $f_b = 2.67$ Hz. This small bandwidth describes the speed with which the system will come to the SS lock with $\varphi_r = 30°$. The low closed-loop bandwidth is beneficial in that it limits output noise arising within the system. The same parameters yield $V_{oSS} = 0.35738$ V, $f_o = 35.738$ kHz, and $\Delta f = -17.433 \, \Delta$GHz. ΔG is in g/L or kg/m³ of glucose.

14.6.5 Discussion

Even though tissue density changes due to $\Delta G = 1$ g/L are on the order of 0.1%, the absolute frequency changes are of the order of 17.4 Hz, and are easily detectable. If the VCO output frequency is mixed with a fixed frequency f_r, and the lower sideband extracted by an LPF, the resultant mixed frequency will be:

$$f_m = f_r - [f_o - \Delta f] = 35.838 \times 10^3 - [35.738 \times 10^3 - (-17.433 \, \Delta G)] = 100 - 17.4 \, \Delta G \text{ Hz.} \quad (14.84)$$

Thus, the percentage change of $\Delta f / f_o{}'$ can be made much larger after mixing. Note that f_r must be from a very stable frequency source.

The path length L can be held constant by mechanical means. The tissue temperature is relatively constant if the patient is indoors at room temperature. One possible confounding factor which must be explored in the future development of this instrument is how much the effective tissue density changes with normal water intake (drinking) in normal and diabetic subjects.

It is anticipated that because of anatomical differences between individuals, the ultrasonic glucose estimator will have to be calibrated for every patient by direct blood glucose measurement.

Figure 14.19 illustrates the circuit of a prototype ultrasonic, glucose sensor built by the author. It was tested on a 1 cm, *in vitro* chamber containing glucose in normal saline rather than an earlobe, however. Linear regression fits of output voltage to chamber glucose concentration were not as tight as might have been expected, probably because of standing waves in the test chamber. Typical fit correlation values ranged from 0.987 to 0.993.

14.7 CHAPTER SUMMARY

We have seen in this chapter that there are many important, nonimaging uses for ultrasound in noninvasive medical diagnosis. The Doppler blood velocimeter is an accepted clinical instrument. In its simplest form, it has about 3-bit resolution because of noise and uncertainty of the incidence angle, θ. The uncertainty comes from estimation of the external probe angle as well as a poor knowledge of the internal path of the ensonified vessel.

I have also included descriptions of three prototype, NI instruments using ultrasound. All three instruments use a closed-loop architecture in which the period of an oscillator is adjusted to maintain a constant-phase difference between the transmitted and reflected ultrasound waves. The NOTOPM system was used to experimentally study the minute pulsations of the cornea of the eye (the OP) in response to blood flow into the eye. The CPRS system used a systems improvement in which the VCO was replaced by a VPC/VFO. This replacement was shown to allow range-independent measurement of the corneal velocity and its displacement.

The third prototype system used the small changes in the velocity of sound in a chamber of known width and temperature to estimate its glucose concentration. The principle of this system should be tested on a tissue such as an earlobe to try to estimate the blood glucose. Not known are to what extent other physiological factors will change c in the tissue. Such a system would have to be calibrated for each individual.

15 Noninvasive Applications of Photon Radiation (Excluding Imaging)

15.1 INTRODUCTION

Photon radiation is also electromagnetic radiation (EMR), a wave phenomenon traditionally described by Maxwell's equations. At very low-power levels and at high frequencies, the quantum photon description of EMR is used. For example, we count "single photons" at ultra-low light levels with photomultiplier tubes (PMTs), not single waves, yet most of optical phenomena such as reflection, refraction, interference, polarization, and imaging are described by the use of the mathematics of waves and EMR.

Wavelength bands used in nonimaging, diagnostic applications range from x-ray and gamma radiation (0.2 pm–50 nm), ultraviolet (50–400 nm), visible (400–700 nm), and infrared (0.7–1000 μm). Little diagnostic use is made of radio-frequency EMR, including microwaves. The energy in a photon is given by the simple relation, $E = h\nu$, where E is the energy (joules), h is Planck's constant (6.624×10^{-34} J s), and ν is the frequency of the EMR in Hz. Note also that $\nu\lambda = c$, where λ is the EMR wavelength (meters) and c is the speed of light in the medium in which the photons are traveling ($c = 3 \times 10^8$ m/s *in vacuo*). Often x- and gamma "rays" are described by the energy of their photons in electron volts (eV) (1 eV = 1.603×10^{-19} J). For example, an x-ray with a wavelength of 50 pm has a frequency of $\nu = 3 \times 10^8/(5 \times 10^{-11}) = 6 \times 10^{18}$ Hz (6 Exahertz). Thus, a 50-pm photon has an energy of $E = h\nu = 3.974 \times 10^{-15}$ J, or $3.974 \times 10^{-15}/1.603 \times 10^{-19} = 24.8$ keV. In general, the wavelength in picometers (pm) of an x- or gamma ray is related to its energy in eV by

$$\lambda = \frac{1.2397 \times 10^{-6}}{W(\text{in eV})} \text{ pm}. \tag{15.1}$$

When directed at the body, the EMR used for medical diagnosis interacts with the biomolecules of the body in several interesting ways. Incident photon energy is reflected or backscattered, absorbed in tissues, and transmitted through the tissues to emerge attenuated. The energy spectrum of emergent and backscattered radiation can show peaks, and valleys at wavelengths where certain biomolecules have absorbed more energy than at others. This selective absorption is the basis for several interesting kinds of *absorption spectroscopy*; it is due to "tuned" energy absorption by different classes of interatomic bonds. Energy absorption at selected frequencies by interatomic bonds is also the basis for *Raman spectroscopy*, where scattered light from an incident monochromatic beam exhibits spectral peaks and valleys. Incident photons with sufficient energy (e.g., blue light) can also produce *fluorescence* in biological molecules. Fluorescence is where an incident photon strikes a particular molecule where it is absorbed and causes secondary photon(s) to immediately be generated having longer wavelength(s) (lower energy). The spectrum of the emitted fluorescent light is unique for each species of fluorescing molecule, and thus can be used for detection and measurement of an analyte's concentration.

Very high-energy photons (e.g., from UV light, x- and gamma rays) can create free radicals having unpaired electrons (peroxides, leading to hydroxyl radicals); they can actually break molecular bonds and damage parts of critical biomolecules such as DNA and RNA, causing genetic damage, apoptosis, mutations, cancer, and leukemia. These high-energy photons are called *ionizing radiations,* and as you might expect, their use in diagnosis is not without statistical risk to the patient for diseases such as cancer and leukemia. The reason they are classified as ionizing radiation is that when these photons interact with certain molecules or atoms they can cause the net loss (or gain) of one or more electrons creating an ion. UV generally has little penetration and generally affects surface (e.g., skin tissue) molecules. Long-term UV exposure is associated with skin cancers (e.g., melanomas), corneal damage, and cataracts. High-energy x- and gamma rays penetrate the entire body, and can cause radiation damage to biomolecules anywhere in the body. Particularly sensitive are tissues in which cell division is continuously underway to replace cells lost by natural turnover *(apoptosis)*. These cells include *blood stem cells* in bone marrow, *intestinal epithelial cells,* and skin cells. A 1 meV gamma ray has ~2×10^6 times the energy of visible light and can generate tens of thousands of ions as it passes through the body. It also can break DNA and RNA strands, which, if not repaired by natural intranuclear enzymes, can lead to cell mutation and/or premature cell death. The reader interested in probing the effects of ionizing radiation in greater depth can begin by visiting the ACHRE (1994) website which contains an excellent primer on the basics of radiation science.

The following sections of this chapter treat the use of photon radiation: bone density analysis by x-rays (15.2); the use of tissue fluorescence to detect cancers (15.3); the use of interferometry to measure the nanometer displacements of body surfaces (15.5); the use of laser Doppler velocimetry (LDV) to measure capillary blood flow (15.7); the use of transcutaneous IR (TIR) spectroscopy to measure blood analytes (15.9); the use of Gilham polarimetry to measure the glucose on the aqueous humor (AH) of the eyes (15.10); the use of pulse oximetry to measure the percent of oxyhemoglobin in capillary blood (15.11); and applications of Raman spectroscopy in NI medical diagnosis (15.12).

15.2 BONE DENSITOMETRY

15.2.1 Introduction

The disease of *osteoporosis* is a slow, progressive loss of bone calcium (and bone strength) which, in 2014, affected ~8 million women and ~1–2 million men in the United States, and in 2013, an estimated 22 million women and 5.5 million men in the European Union. Osteoporosis leads to ~1.5 million fractures each year in the United States, having an estimated treatment cost, including physical therapy, of $16 billion in 2002, rising to $22 billion in 2008 (Blume and Curtis 2011). Most of the persons at risk from osteoporosis are postmenopausal women who are not on estrogen therapy. A comprehensive, current paper on Osteoporosis facts and statistics is available from the International Osteoporosis Foundation (IOF 2015).

In osteoporosis, there is a decrease in the activity of *osteoblasts* (cells that build the bone matrix) and in the rate of production of bone growth factors. Also, estrogen deficiency causes the rise of the concentrations of the following cytokines: Interleukin-1, tumor necrosis factor-α, granulocyte-macrophage colony-stimulating factor, and interleukin-6. These cytokines enhance bone resorption through the stimulation of *osteoclasts,* the cells which break down bone and bone matrix. There are many external factors that increase the rate of osteoporosis in both men and women. These include malnutrition, prolonged physical inactivity, a prolonged zero-G environment (space travel), lack of dietary calcium, lack of exposure to sunlight (to generate endogenous vitamin D), excessive dietary protein consumption, smoking, alcoholism, rheumatoid arthritis, excessive caffeine consumption, and taking corticosteroids (NOF 2015).

The natural decline in bone density and consequent decrease in bone strength following menopause can eventually lead to debilitating and sometimes fatal bone fractures. Falls can lead to broken wrists, fractures to the head of the femur, the pelvis, the spine, and other bones. The rate of osteoporosis in postmenopausal women can be slowed by avoiding some of the aggravating factors listed above. A good diet, moderate exercise, and moderation in caffeine and alcohol consumption are indicated.

To assess the degree of osteoporosis in a patient, there are several invasive tests (bone biopsy, certain chemicals in blood) which we will not consider here, and some fairly definitive, NI tests. Bone density can be measured by quantitative CAT scan techniques, and less expensively by dual-energy x-ray absorption (DXA or DEXA) scans of bones (described in the following section), and tests of urine of a fasting patient for excess Ca^{++}, *hydroxyproline-containing peptides,* and *pyridinium peptide* (from the breakdown of bone matrix) (Merk Manual 2015). The purpose of these NI tests is to assess the degree of risk a person may be at for broken bones and other orthopedic complications of osteoporosis.

15.2.2 DXA Method

The DXA (originally DEXA) method is an inexpensive and accurate means of measuring bone mineral density primarily from the calcium content in bone salts (Bonnick 1998). DXA is typically used on bones in the heel, wrist/forearm, femoral neck, lumbar spine, or whole body. A typical DXA system is shown schematically in Figure 15.1.

X-rays are characterized by their photon energy, hν, in thousands of electron volts (keV) (or alternately, by their wavelengths, λ, in picometers, pm), and their intensity in W/m^2. X-rays can be formed into fairly collimated pencil beams or floodlight-like fan beams. Both types of beams are used in various DXA systems. The operation of a DXA system is reminiscent of spectrophotometry at two wavelengths (see Section 15.8 on pulse oximetry). To obtain a heuristic appreciation of how a DXA system works, consider x-ray transmission through a homogeneous, dense material (e.g., bone) of thickness, L. Some of the x-rays entering the material are absorbed and do not exit. Most of these absorbed x-rays are ultimately converted to heat, and some cause chemical bonds to rupture, creating ions and free radicals that can lead to genetic damage, even cancer. The x-rays that emerge are "counted" by an x-ray sensor. Some x-ray sensors are of the ionization type (acting like Geiger counters), producing a current pulse for every x-ray photon that creates an ion pair. Another type of x-ray sensor uses a scintillation crystal that emits secondary,

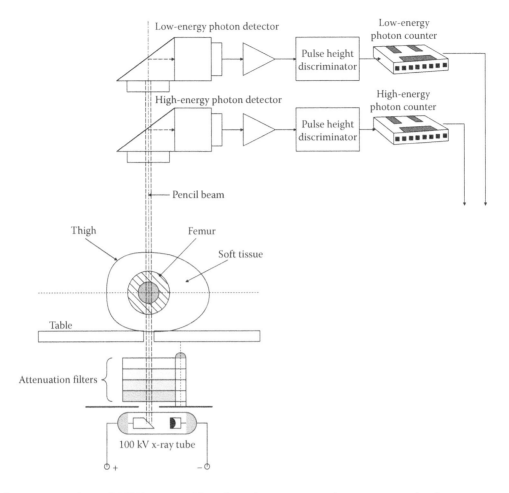

Figure 15.1 Typical DEXA system. Note that it has two x-ray photon counters for the two energy levels are used.

visible photons when struck by an x-ray photon; the visible photons are in turn sensed by a PMT. The law that governs x-ray absorption (or transmission) in bone is very like Beer's law in spectrophotometry:

$$\frac{I_{out}}{I_{in}} = \exp[-\mu_\lambda \rho L], \qquad (15.2)$$

where I_{out} is the intensity of the transmitted x-rays, I_{in} is the intensity of the input x-rays, μ_λ is the wavelength-dependent *mass attenuation coefficient* (MACs; also known as x-ray cross section) in cm²/g, ρ is the volume density of the absorbing medium in g/cm³, and L is the length of the path the x-rays travel in the medium. μ_λ is a function of the absorbing element (in the case of bone it is significantly calcium) as well as the x-ray's wavelength, λ.

Note that x-ray photon energy is $h\nu$, and $\nu = c/\lambda$. "Soft" x-rays have energies in the range of 1–20 keV. Intermediate energies range from 20 keV to 0.1 MeV. Hard x-ray energies are above 0.1 MeV. Figure 15.2 illustrates the relative intensity/$h\nu$ versus x-ray photon energy $h\nu$ in keV for various conditions in a DEXA x-ray system. The top curve is the intensity spectrum of x-ray photons leaving the x-ray tube. The second curve is the intensity spectrum of attenuated photons entering the tissue and bone, and the bottom curve is the intensity spectrum of photons exiting the bone. In this example, the x-ray tube's tungsten anode is bombarded with 100 keV electrons. Note the presence of line spectra added to the smooth *bremsstrahlung* spectrum. Tungsten has line spectra at 57.9, 59.3, 67.4, and 69.3 keV photon energies. The total energy in these spikes amounts to ~10% of the total emitted energy. The spikes are generated by the bombarding

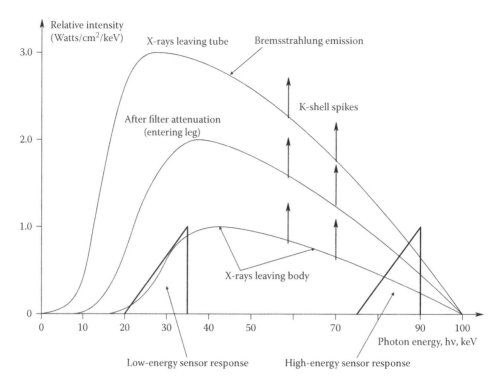

Figure 15.2 X-ray energy spectra in a DEXA system.

electrons in the x-ray tube interacting with K-shell electrons in the tungsten anode atoms (Jacobson and Webster 1977). The two triangular graphs on the spectrum plots represent the spectral sensitivities of low- and high-energy x-ray detectors that respond to the photon intensities in the exiting x-ray beam.

The general x-ray absorption equation (15.2) can be modified to find the effective density of calcium in a bone of thickness L. One approach to this problem is to consider the incident x-ray spectrum to be absorbed by calcium in the bone, and "other tissue" including soft tissue surrounding the bone, and the collagen in the bone matrix. As the x-ray photon detectors select low- and high-energy photons, and two absorbers have been defined (Ca and "other"), there are four MACs associated with the DEXA system: μ_{Hc}, μ_{Lc}, μ_{Ho}, and μ_{Lo}. They are, respectively, the mean MAC for Ca at high $h\nu$, the mean MAC for Ca at low $h\nu$, the mean MAC for other tissue at high $h\nu$, and the mean MAC for other tissue at low $h\nu$. For example, the MAC for Ca at $h\nu = 30$ keV is 3.97 cm^2/g; the MAC for Ca at $h\nu = 62$ keV is 0.63 cm^2/g, a ratio of 6.3:1. All four MACs are assumed to be known from prior measurements. Thus, the detected x-ray intensities can be written as

$$I_L = I_{inL}\exp[-\mu_{Lc}\rho_cL]\exp[-\mu_{Lo}\rho_oL] \tag{15.3}$$

$$I_H = I_{inH}\exp[-\mu_{Hc}\rho_cL]\exp[-\mu_{Ho}\rho_oL]. \tag{15.4}$$

where I_{inL} is the total input intensity of x-rays to the tissue defined by the low-energy detector's acceptance spectrum, I_{inH} is the total input intensity of x-rays to the tissue defined by the high-energy detector's acceptance spectrum. I_L is the transmitted intensity of the low-energy x-rays, I_H is the transmitted intensity of the high-energy x-rays, L is the x-ray path length through the sample, ρ_c is the unknown density of Ca in the bone, and ρ_o is the mean mass density of other tissues in the sample.

The equations above can be rewritten as

$$I_L = I_{inL}\exp[-\mu_{Lc}\rho_cL - \mu_{Lo}\rho_oL] \tag{15.5}$$

$$I_H = I_{inH}\exp[-\mu_{Hc}\rho_cL - \mu_{Ho}\rho_oL]. \tag{15.6}$$

When we take the natural logarithm of both sides of each equation above, we have the simultaneous equations:

$$\ln(I_{inL}/I_L) = + \rho_c \mu_{Lc} L + \rho_o \mu_{Lo} L \tag{15.7}$$

$$\ln(I_{inH}/I_H) = + \rho_c \mu_{Hc} L + \rho_o \mu_{Ho} L. \tag{15.8}$$

These equations are solved for the calcium density, ρ_c, g/cm^3 by the DXA system computer which has values for the μ matrix, L, I_{inL}, and I_{inH} stored in memory.

$$\rho_c = \frac{\mu_{Ho}\ln(I_{inL}/I_L) - \mu_{Lo}\ln(I_{inH}/I_H)}{L\,[\mu_{Lc}\mu_{Ho} - \mu_{Hc}\mu_{Lo}]}. \tag{15.9}$$

Once measured on a patient, ρ_c and ρ_o are compared to the data base value for the same bone in a healthy 30-year-old woman or man (peak calcium density). A measured bone density (ρ_c) of less than 1 standard deviation from the peak bone mass mean is considered to be a normal or safe bone mass loss in aging. The condition of *osteopenia* is considered to exist when the measured ρ_c is between −1 and −2.5 SD down from the peak mean. When ρ_c is <−2.5 SD from the peak mean bone mass, the patient is considered to have severe osteoporosis and be at risk for stress fractures, falls, etc. These classifications with respect to peak bone mass are called a T-score. Another type of scoring (the Z-score) for bone mass loss compares the measured ρ_c with that for age- and sex-matched controls. The Z-score can be misleading, however, because of its relative nature.

If a CT scanner is used to measure the bone density, it must be calibrated with a standard of reference to give quantitative output. Such physical bone density standards (phantoms) are made by CIRS (Computerized Imaging Reference Systems, Inc.) of Norfolk, VA (CIRS 2015). Physical standards are also used to field-calibrate DXA systems.

15.2.3 Discussion

Modern DXA (also known as DEXA) systems use pencil beams, fan beams, narrow-angle fan beams, or cone beams, depending on the application. Pencil beam DXA systems, such as the GE Lunar DPX Duo and the GE Lunar DPX Bravo, minimize patient exposure to x-rays but have a longer scan time than a fan-beam instrument. The Hologic QDR series DXA systems utilize fan-beam technology. Fan-beam densitometers have not only the advantage of improved geometrical resolution but also the disadvantage of errors induced by magnification effects caused by beam geometry. In addition to the DXA systems mentioned above, there are the Hologic Discovery Series, and the Norland XR series (Brownbill and Ilich 2005).

A typical DXA system uses a 100-kV x-ray source which is attenuated by a bank of 8 samarium metal filters, giving 256 possible intensity levels. Hence, the system can be adjusted to minimize the patient exposure and at the same time to optimize the dynamic range of the low- and high-energy x-ray photon counting sensors over a range of tissue thickness from 12 to 22 cm.

The DXA method is definitely the "gold standard" of bone densitometry. It is an accurate, NI procedure that can be done in a doctor's office or clinic at low-patient cost. (Use of a quantitative CT scanned for the same purpose costs about 10 times the DXA procedure's cost.)

15.3 NI DIAGNOSIS BY TISSUE FLUORESCENCE

15.3.1 Introduction

Fluorescence occurs when a molecule absorbs one or more high-energy photons (generally from blue or UV light depending on the molecule), and immediately reradiates a low-energy photon, generally in the visible range of wavelengths. Many naturally occurring molecules in cells exhibit fluorescence, and specially engineered, fluorescing, *fluorophore molecules* can be attached to probe molecules that have affinities for various natural cellular components. Thus, *fluorophore tags* can be used to identify specific cellular components (surface proteins and receptors). Fluorophore taggants are now generally used in *in vitro* studies and are becoming more common for *in vivo* applications as their safety is established. One reason for the intense interest in fluorescence in NI medical diagnosis is the incredible analytical sensitivity of the method. Conventional spectrophotometric absorbance methods can reliably detect a molecular species at concentrations of 10ths of a μmole/L; fluorescent techniques can accurately measure concentrations 1 million times smaller in the range of pm/L. For example, the PTI Quantamaster 400® steady-state spectrofluorometer has an LOD for fluorescein in 0.1 M NaOH of 400 attomoles. It has an SNR of 20,000:1 or better, given

Table 15.1: Naturally Occurring Biomolecules That Fluoresce

Molecule	Excitation Peak, nm	Emission Peak, nm	Comment
Tryptophan	285 (290)	340 (330)	Amino acid emits; in UV
Tyrosine	274	303	"
Phenylalanine	257	282	"
GFP	490	509	Green fluorescent protein from jellyfish
NADH	350	450	Nicotinamide adenine dinucleotide. Found in mitochondria
FAD	450	525	Flavin adenine dinucleotide concentrated in mitochondria, also found in cytoplasm
Flavins	445–470	500–700	"
Protoporphyrin IX	375–440	520, 635, and 704 (3 peaks; 635 largest)	In erythroid cells and Ca cells treated with 5-ALA

350 nm excitation, 5 nm spectral band-pass, and 1 s integration time (PTI 2014). As techniques improve, quantities less than an attomole ($<10^{-18}$ mole) may be detected.

The short wavelength light required to excite fluorescence is rapidly attenuated in the skin and other tissues, so NI, *in vivo* studies of cell fluorescence are limited to the first few mm of tissue depth. Two major sources of excitation light exist: *Lasers*, including the 337 nm nitrogen laser, the argon ion laser with 7 emission lines between 457 and 529 nm, and various solid-state diode lasers, and *Xenon tubes* coupled to grating monochromators are used. The latter source is commonly used in research spectrofluorometers and can produce wavelengths from 200 to 700 nm. Quartz lenses and optical fibers are used for wavelengths <400 nm. UV light is classified as UVA (320–400 nm), UVB (280–320 nm), and UVC (100–280 nm).

15.3.2 Properties of Fluorescent Molecules

Fluorescent molecules used in diagnosis include intrinsically fluorescent substances as well as the fluorophore tags mentioned above. Table 15.1 lists some of the major intrinsic fluorescent molecules, their optimum excitation wavelength, their peak emission wavelength, and where they are found. It should be stressed that all fluorescent molecules have a broad excitation action spectrum, sometimes with two peaks. Their emission spectra are also broad and can have more than one peak; often the long wavelength tail of the excitation spectrum overlaps the short wavelength tail of the emission spectrum. Also, conditions of pH, ionic environment, and the proximity (<6 nm) of other nonfluorescing molecules can shift or attenuate the excitation and emission spectra. The intensity of the induced, fluorescent irradiance is thousands of times lower than the irradiance of the excitation source. In cancerous lung tissue, the ratio of blue laser light irradiance to fluorescent emission irradiance is about $64 \times 10^6 : 1$ (Turner Designs 1998).

Table 15.2 lists some common fluorophore molecules used for marking specific cellular molecules and structures. The marking can be due to one of the following mechanisms: The fluorophore is bound to another molecule (e.g., an antibody) that has a high-selective affinity to a molecular species within (or without) a cell. The fluorophore can also be bound to the active site of an antigen, and thus be used to detect specific, circulating antibodies. The fluorophore may fluoresce when in the presence of a high-ionic concentration of calcium or some other molecule or ion that activates it.

Note that each fluorophore molecule has a finite working lifetime. Typically, $<10^5$ photons can be emitted before the molecule is damaged and undergoes a structural change that makes it nonfluorescent. Thus fluorophore-tagged cells cannot be illuminated by CW UV excitation without gradual loss of fluorescence or "bleaching." Often short nanosecond-length pulses are used having a very low-duty cycle. The use of excitation pulses allows the dynamics of the fluorescence to be studied at a given wavelength including the latency, the time to peak, the emitted pulse shape, and the decay time. *Phase fluorometry* looks specifically at the dynamics of pulse-excited fluorescence.

15.3.3 Fluorescence in NI Cancer Diagnosis

A recent, important trend in medical diagnosis is the use of fluorescent molecules to screen for superficial cancers, that is, cancers that lie on or near the skin surface, or on or near the surface of the

Table 15.2: **Partial List of Synthetic Fluorophore Molecules, Their Emission Spectral Peaks, Their Excitation Peaks (Where Available), and Their Applications**

Fluorophore	Excitation Peak, nm	Emission Peak, nm	Specificity
Bisbenzimide Hoechst 33342	UV	390–440	Binds to DNA
Rhodamine 123	545, (485)	Red (green)	Binds to mitochondria
Wheat germ agglutinin + fluorescein isothiocyanate	488 (Ar laser)	520	Plasma membrane and endosomes, but not mitochondria
Texas Red coupled to streptavidine	595 (dye laser)	620	Binds to biotin
FURA-2	340	515	Fluorescence depends on [Ca^{++}]. Chelates Ca^{++}
Alexa	?	603 or 617	These fluorophores attach to taggants
Phenol red	?	575	
Resorufin	?	587	"
Red phycoerythrin (R-PE)	488 (Ar laser)	576	"
Allophycocyanin (APC)	595 (dye laser)	660	"
Cy-3 (cyanine dye)	?	565	"
Cy-5	488 (Ar laser)	667	"
Cy-Chrome tandan Conj. of R-PE and cyanine	?	670	"
Cascade blue	406 krypton	430	"
EDANS aminonaphthalene-1-sulfonic acid	336	490	"

tissues that are accessible to endoscopes such as the lungs, bladder, and cervix. At the present time, cancer diagnosis by fluorescence is generally done as an imaging process. The examining physician illuminates the tissue being evaluated with monochromatic light ranging from 330 nm wavelength (UVA) to green light, depending on the optimum excitation range of the fluorescing molecules. UV light with wavelengths shorter than 330 nm is known to damage cellular DNA by inducing thymine dimers (Heintzelman et al. 2000), and so is avoided when examining tissues *in vivo*.

In 1990, Xillix®, a Canadian medical imaging company, developed a fiber optic, *LIFE-Lung Fluorescence Endoscopy System*™ used to detect lung cancer (Takehana et al. 1999). ("LIFE" stands for "Light-Induced Fluorescent Endoscopy.") It is used as an adjunct to white-light endoscopy. A HeCd laser produces deep blue light at 442 nm with an irradiance of ~64 mW/mm² that is shined on lung tissues from a bronchoscope probe inserted into the bronchi. Both normal and precancerous lung tissues emit similar quantities of red light, but normal cells also emit about eight times the intensity of green light. The fluorescence is picked up by over 10⁴ optical fibers in a coherent (imaging) bundle. The emitted light is split into green and red color bands by a dichroic mirror and further refined in bandwidth by interference filters. The intensity of the faint red and green spectral images is then amplified by two image intensifiers up to ×10⁴. The images are captured on two, 512 × 512 pixel CCD cameras and encoded as digital video signals. To compensate for the $1/r^4$ law of *in vivo* fluorescence attenuation with distance, the red emission, which is the same for both healthy and cancerous cells, is used to normalize the green channel signals. Lung tissues fluorescing proportionally less green light than red then can be marked as suspect regardless of their distance from the endoscope tip. The Xillix system was approved to be used with the Olympus type BF20D bronchoscope.

Xillix claims that after a large, multicenter clinical study of their LIFE system versus white-light endoscopy done on suspected lung cancer patients, detection improved from 37% to 75% on a per-patient basis and on a per-lesion basis, detection improved from 25% to 67%.

In summary, the Xillix LIFE-Lung system is a mildly invasive diagnostic system that uses computer-enhanced spectral imaging of lung tissues to detect precancerous cells by fluorescence. The blue light used does not damage tissues like UVA and B wavelengths. No special systemic drugs are required for the Xillix diagnostic system; it works with endogenous fluorescent molecules.

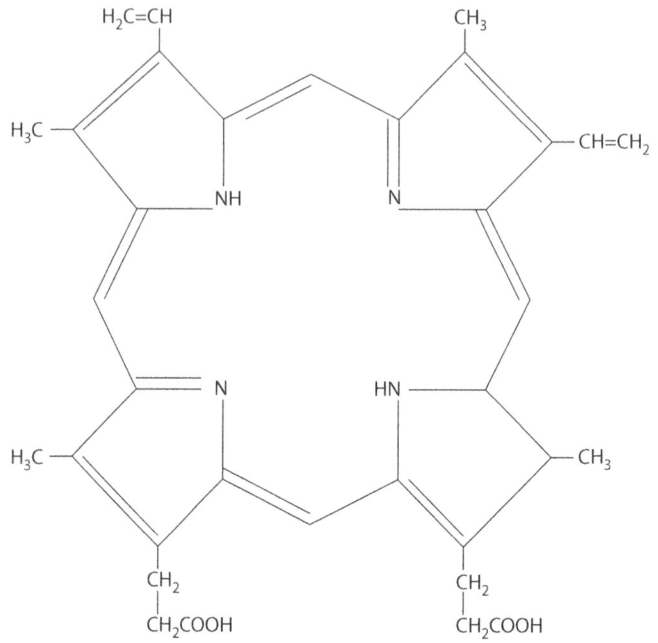

Figure 15.3 Fluorescing Protoporphyrin IX molecule.

The cytochrome proteins found in the mitochondrial oxidative phosphorylation process are *heme proteins,* that is, they contain one or two heme residues in one polypeptide chain. *Cytochrome c* contains a modified iron protoporphyrin called *heme c.* All three forms of heme found in cytochromes are derived biochemically from *iron protoporphyrin IX* (PpIX), also called *heme b.* The 2-D molecular schematic of PpIX is shown in Figure 15.3. PpIX has emission peaks at 520, 635, and 704 nm.

The red (635 nm) major fluorescent emission peak from PpIX has been investigated as a marker for oral carcinoma. In one study, 410-nm excitation elicited PpIX-like fluorescence spectra from 85% of oral carcinomas irradiated. Analysis of the emissions was by spectrofluorometer (Inaguma and Hashimoto 1999). In another study, topical application of *5-aminolevulinic acid* (5-ALA) was found to enhance the PpIX fluorescent emission from neoplastic tissue in the oral cavity. There was a maximum fluorescent contrast of 10:1 between cancers and normal tissues at about 1–2 hours after the 5-ALA treatment, allowing a demarcation of tumors even to the naked eye (Leunig et al. 1996). In a similar study, 5-ALA (a 0.4% solution) used as a topical rinse was used to enhance PpIX red fluorescence of oral leukoplakias (also known as squamous cell carcinomas). The identified lesions were treated with *retinyl palmitate* (vitamin A) which caused complete remissions in 15 out of 20 cases. The cured cancers lost their PpIX fluorescence (Leunig et al. 2000). In another study of basal cell (skin) carcinoma, varied doses of orally administered 5-ALA were given to determine optimum fluorescence response of PpIX in the cancers versus side effects. *In vivo* spectrofluorometry was used (Tope et al. 1998).

NADH stands for (reduced) *nicotinamide adenine dinucleotide.* NADH plays an important biochemical role in Complex 1 of the mitochondrial oxidative phosphorylation process. As noted above, NADH has an intrinsic blue fluorescence emission with a peak at 450 nm which can be excited by 337-nm UV pulses from a nitrogen laser. NADH fluorescence of bladder cancer cells was observed using a quartz fiber to deliver the short laser pulses, and another fiber to collect the fluorescence radiation. The optical fibers and a conventional, white light, FO cystoscope are inserted up the urethra, a process that is arguably as about as invasive as a semi-invasive procedure can be (König et al. 1994).

In an *in vitro* fluorescence study, cervical epithelial cancer cells were shown to have high levels of tryptophan offering the possibility that they can be discriminated from inflammatory immune system cells (leucocytes) and normal cervical cells (Heintzelman et al. 2000). Unfortunately, the wavelength required to excite tryptophan fluorescence is 290 nm (UVB), which can cause DNA damage in normal cells *in vivo*. Clearly, what is needed is a fluorescent taggant with a high affinity to a surface protein unique to cervical cancer cells, and which has an excitation wavelength longer than 330 nm. Direct, *in vivo* excitation of tryptophan fluorescence appears to carry an unacceptable risk.

15.3.4 Discussion

The use of NI and semi-invasive fluorescent imaging methods to detect surface cancers on the skin, oral mucosa, lung tissues, cervix, and bladder is an area of medical diagnosis being rapidly developed. As most intrinsic, fluorescent biomolecules generally require potentially tissue-damaging short wavelengths for excitation, the use of fluorophore taggants excitable at wavelengths longer than 330 nm is expected to grow.

The most satisfactory approach for fluorescent diagnosis appears to be digitally enhanced endoscopic imaging using appropriate interference filters to contrast the cancerous cells with the normal surround. A more complex approach is to use quantitative spectrofluorometry to map the lesion, and to use pulsed excitation so the dynamics of the fluorescence can be studied (e.g., rise and fall times). The behavior of fluorescent molecules changes with their chemical environment; this fact offers another tool to differentiate what molecules are fluorescing and how much of each is there.

15.4 OPTICAL INTERFEROMETRIC MEASUREMENT OF NANOMETER DISPLACEMENTS OF BIOLOGICAL SURFACES

15.4.1 Introduction

There have been several areas of NI diagnosis in which information is gained by the no-touch optical interferometric measurement of extremely small (e.g., on the order of nanometers) mechanical displacements of external surfaces. One such displacement is the extremely small vibration of the eardrum in response to incident sound pressure. Such measurement can be useful in the study of the mechanics of hearing, including the tympanal reflex in response to sudden loud sounds. Another physical displacement is the movement of a tooth *in situ* in response to a lateral force. Such measurement of the mechanical compliance of teeth can be useful in orthodontic research and in the study of dental health. Still another application of optical interferometry lies in the measurement of very small displacements of the skin caused by blood flow in capillary beds. Microplethysmography of the skin surface can have application in studies of the control of peripheral circulation and in assessing microcirculation following vascular surgery. Quantitative measurement (amplitude and frequencies) of skin displacement caused by fine tremors in underlying muscles can have application in studies of neurological disorders, such as Parkinson's disease.

There are many types of optical interferometers which can be used to make the measurements described above; most use one coherent light source (i.e., a laser) and split the coherent beam into two optical paths, R and M, then combine the beams in such a manner that there is a linear summation of the output beam **E** vectors (E_M and E_R) at a common output plane or photosensor. At the output plane, there is alternate constructive and destructive interference. There are bright rings or lines where there is constructive addition; dark rings or lines appear where there is destructive interference. In order to measure a physical quantity such as surface displacement, it must change the phase between E_M and E_R by changing the M beam's path length. As you will see, a convenient way of doing this is to stick a mirror on the moving surface and use the phase change in the reflected light in the M path. (Other physical quantities can be measured by interferometry when they cause a phase change between the M and R beams.) For an elementary discussion of the use of interferometry in length or displacement measurement, see Chapter 4 and others in the text by Sirohi and Kothiyal (1991). A detailed mathematical analysis of several major types of interferometer can be found in Chapter 9 in the *Optics* text by Hecht (1987).

Direct measurement of an object's displacement with an interferometer is generally limited to motions of less than $\pm \lambda/4$. Greater motion will result in a periodic output of the interferometer, and some means must be used to count interference "fringes" during the motion of the object to keep track of the total object displacement.

Before describing specific types of interferometers, let us examine a general, heuristic treatment of optical interference. For interference to occur, the electromagnetic light wave must be temporally and spatially *coherent*. That is, the frequency and phase of the E-vectors of the interfering waves must remain constant in time and space for interference to occur. A stable, monochromatic source such as a laser is ideal for interferometry. The optical intensity changes associated with interference occur as the result of the superposition of the $\mathbf{E}$ vectors at a point on the detector. The intensity at the detector is proportional to the net $\mathbf{E}$ vector squared. That is:

$$I_d \propto (e_r + e_m)^2 \, W/m^2, \tag{15.10}$$

where:

$$e_r = e_r(t) = E_{Ro}\cos[(2\pi c/\lambda)t] \tag{15.11}$$

$$e_m = e_m(t) = E_{Mo}\cos\left[(2\pi c/\lambda)t + 2\phi_m + (2d/\lambda)2\pi\right], \tag{15.12}$$

where e_m and e_r are the time-varying $\mathbf{E}$ vector magnitudes of EM plane waves at a point at the detector surface.

The fixed phase of e_r is taken as zero; the phase of the measurement wave, e_m, has a fixed component, $2\phi_m$, due to the out and back propagation delay, and a variable component, $(4\pi d/\lambda)$ radians, due to the small, relative displacement of the reflecting surface, d. Note that the frequency of both waves is $\nu = c/\lambda$ Hz. Substituting Equations 15.11 and 15.12 into Equation 15.10, we find:

$$I_d = \left(E_{Ro}^2/2\right)[1 + \cos(4\pi\nu t)] + \left(E_{Mo}^2/2\right)\left\{1 + \cos\left[4\pi\nu t + 4\phi_m + (4d/\lambda)2\pi\right]\right\}$$
$$+ E_{Ro}E_{Mo}\left\{\cos\left[4\pi\nu t + 2\phi_m + (2d/\lambda)2\pi\right] + \cos[2\phi_m + (2d/\lambda)2\pi]\right\} W/cm^2. \tag{15.13}$$

Of course, the photodetector does not respond to terms at frequency 2ν Hz. Thus, the detector output is given by

$$V_o = -K_d\overline{I}_d = -K_d\left\{\left(E_{Ro}^2/2\right) + \left(E_{Ro}^2/2\right) + E_{Ro}E_{Mo}\cos\left[2\phi_m + (2d/\lambda)2\pi\right]\right\} V. \tag{15.14}$$

We use the trig identity, $\cos(A + B) \equiv [\cos(A)\cos(B) - \sin(A)\sin(B)]$. If d is slowly varying (i.e., is a DC quantity), we can make $2\phi_m = q\pi/2$, (q 1, 5, 9, 13, ...) so that $\cos(2\phi_m) = 0$ and $\sin(2\phi_m) = +1$. Thus, the detector output is given by

$$V_o = -K_d\left\{\left(E_{Ro}^2/2\right) + \left(E_{Mo}^2/2\right) - E_{Ro}E_{Mo}\sin\left[(2d/\lambda)2\pi\right]\right\}. \tag{15.15}$$

If d is moving at an audio frequency so that $d = d_o\sin(\omega_m t)$, the DC terms are filtered out by high-pass filtering and again $2\phi_m$ is made equal to $q\pi/2$, $q = 1, 5, 9, 13, ...,$ so

$$v_o(t) = K_d E_{Ro} E_{Mo}\sin\left[(4\pi/\lambda)d_o\sin(\omega_m t)\right]. \tag{15.16}$$

To keep the system in its linear output range, the argument of the $\sin[.]$ term must not exceed $\pm\lambda/4$. That is, d_o must be $< \lambda/4$. If $d_o > \lambda/4$, periodicity in the output versus d_o is observed, and unless one counts output maxima and minima, there will be ambiguity in the true value of d_o. Equation 15.16 can be expanded by the Bessel–Jacoby identity (Stark, Tuteur and Anderson 1988) to

$$v_o(t) = K_d E_{Ro} E_{Mo}\sum_{n=-\infty}^{\infty} J_n(\xi)\sin(n\omega_m t), \tag{15.17}$$

where obviously, $\xi \equiv (4\pi/\lambda)d_o$, and $J_n(\xi)$ is a *Bessel function of the first kind*. It can be shown that $J_n(\xi)$ can be approximated by the series (Stark et al. 1988):

$$J_n(\xi) = \sum_{k=0}^{\infty} \frac{(\xi/2)^{(n+2k)}(-1)^k}{(n+k)!k!} \tag{15.18}$$

If $\xi \ll 1$, Equation 15.18 can be approximated by

$$J_n(\xi) \cong (\xi/2)^n/n! \quad n > 0, \text{integer} \tag{15.19}$$

and in general (Dwight 1969, #807.4),

$$J_{-n}(\xi) \equiv (-1)^{|n|} J_n(\xi). \tag{15.20}$$

Thus, the first few terms of Equation 15.17 can be written, assuming $\xi \ll 1$:

$$v_o(t) \cong \overset{n=0}{0} + K_d E_{Ro} \overset{n=\pm1}{E_{Mo}}$$

$$\left\{ \xi \sin(\omega_m t) + \overset{n=\pm2}{0} + \left(\xi^3/24\right) \overset{n=\pm3}{\sin}(3\omega_m t) + \overset{n=\pm4}{0} + \left(\xi^5/1920\right) \overset{n=\pm5}{\sin}(5\omega_m t) + \ldots \right\}. \tag{15.21}$$

As even, high-order harmonic terms are zero, and $\xi \ll 1$, the fundamental frequency term dominates the series of Equation 15.17. d_o, the quantity under measurement, can be found by phase-sensitive rectification of $v_o(t)$ using a ω_m-frequency reference signal, followed by low-pass filtering. If the low-pass filter has gain K_F, then its DC output, V_o', will be:

$$V_o' = K_F K_d E_{Ro} E_{Mo} \left(4\pi/\lambda\right) d_o \text{ DC V}. \tag{15.22}$$

We next examine some examples of optical interferometers that have been used in biomedical applications.

The first is the fiber-optic Fizeau interferometer developed by Drake and Leiner (1984).

15.4.2 Measurement of Tympanal Membrane Displacement By Fizeau Interferometer

This prototype instrument, shown in Figure 15.4, was used to sense the minute displacement of the tympanal membrane of a common cricket subject to external audible sound. Drake and Leiner used a 15 mW HeNe (633 nm) laser as their source. The half-wave plate was rotated to minimize the observed intensity, indicating that all of the linearly polarized light (LPL) from the laser was going into the 10×0.255 NA microscope objective used to direct all of the incident light into the proximal end of the polarization-preserving glass optical fiber (PPOF). The PPOF was of two-step design; it had a 5 μm core diameter and a 125 μm cladding diameter. By experimentally adjusting the PPOF loop diameter, D, and twisting it some small angle, θ, around the axis from the objective to the object, the PPOF loop could be made to act as a quarter-wave plate. Thus, the light returning to the proximal end of the PPOF was rotated 90° with respect to the entering light. Drake and Leiner stated:

> All of the interfering light is then reflected toward the detector by the polarizing beamsplitter, while light reflected from the back side of the beamsplitter, from the elements of the microscope objective, and from the proximal end of the fiber, all pass straight back through the polarizing beam splitter and does not contribute unwanted radiation at the detector.

As the Fizeau interferometer gives an output signal proportional to *relative object displacement,* Drake and Leiner mounted their object (a cricket tympanum) on a piezoelectric crystal that could be displaced toward or away from the PPOF's distal end by $> \pm \lambda/2$ by applying a 10 Hz, triangular, voltage waveform and observing the magnitude of the AC signal output at the acoustic stimulus frequency, f_m. The AC output was maximum when the distance, a, was some multiple of $\lambda/4$. This particular DC voltage was applied to the crystal for subsequent tests of tympanal membrane response, d. Calibration of the Fizeau interferometer was accomplished by applying a 1 kHz triangular wave around the DC bias voltage to the piezo crystal. The triangle wave amplitude was adjusted until the output peaks just began to fold over as seen on an oscilloscope display. The target was then known to be undergoing a $\pm \lambda/4$ displacement. Thus, an output calibration factor was determined in V/nm displacement ($\lambda/4 = 158.2$ nm).

Drake and Leiner displayed their output signal on an oscilloscope and on a spectrum analyzer. The typical ratio of fundamental frequency to second harmonic amplitude was 0.16. They found that their instrument could resolve 0.01 nm $< d_o < 30$ nm linearly. This is an amazing sensitivity considering that a lock-in amplifier was not used. They commented that the working distance, a, from the distal end of the fiber to the moving object can be increased to over a few mm by adding a SELFOC® lens to the tip of the PPOF cable.

Drake and Leiner mentioned that future applications of their Fizeau interferometer could include studies of human eardrum displacement, measurement of the ocular pulse (a typical

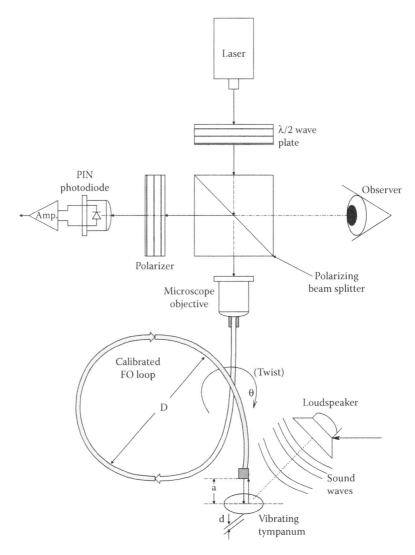

Figure 15.4 Schematic of the fiber optic Fizeau interferometer used by Drake and Leiner to measure very small deflections of an insect tympanal membrane. The linear range measured was from 0.01 to 30 nm.

human ocular pulse is $\sim \pm 8\ \mu$m, beyond the described range of their instrument), basilar membrane deflection in the cochlea (presumably done *in vitro*), measurement of nerve axon displacement during an action potential, and dental strain measurements.

15.4.3 Measurement of Skin Vibration By Optical Interferometry

The Michelson interferometer was used to measure skin surface microvibrations (Hong and Fox 1993, Hong 1994). A true Michelson interferometer is illustrated in Figure 15.5 (Hecht 1987). Note that it uses a compensating plate in optical path L_1 so that each beam travels the same distance through glass. The compensating plate is identical to the half-silvered mirror beam splitter, except that it does not have silvering. Use of the compensation plate corrects for refractive index dispersion with λ, and lets the Michelson interferometer be used with broadband (semicoherent) light sources. If a monochromatic laser source is used, the compensation plate is not necessary. A Michelson interferometer without the compensation plate is often called a *Twyman–Green interferometer* (Sirohi and Kothiyal 1991). As we showed above with the Fizeau interferometer, the optical

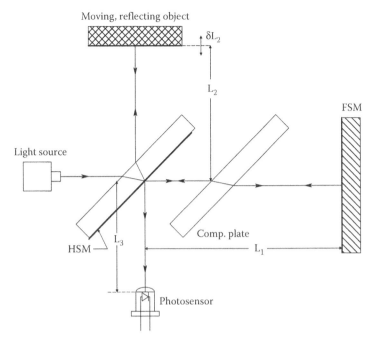

Figure 15.5 Schematic of a Michelson interferometer.

intensity at the photodetector is proportional to the square of the sum of the two **E** vectors imping-ing on the detector. Let us take point **O** on the half-silvered mirror as the phase origin. Neglecting the half silvered mirror thickness, we can write for the Twyman–Green/Michelson interferometer:

$$e_r(t) = E_{Ro}\sin[2\pi\nu t + 2\pi(2L_1 + L_3)/\lambda] \tag{15.23}$$

$$e_m(t) = \eta E_{Ro}\sin[2\pi\nu t + 2\pi(2L_2 + L_3)/\lambda], \tag{15.24}$$

where the lightwave frequency $\nu = c/\lambda$ Hz, the distances are defined in Figure 15.5 and $\eta < 1$ represents the fraction of incident light reflected back to the detector. The intensity at the detector is proportional to $[e_r(t) + e_m(t)]^2$. That is,

$$I_d \propto (E_{Ro}^2/2)\{1 - \cos[4\pi(\nu t + 2L_1 + L_3)/\lambda]\} + \eta^2(E_{Ro}^2/2)\{1 - \cos[4\pi(\nu t + 2L_2 + L_3/\lambda)]\}$$
$$+ 2E_{Ro}\eta E_{Ro}\sin[2\pi\nu t + 2\pi(2L_1 + L_3)/\lambda]\sin[2\pi\nu t + 2\pi(2L_2 + L_3)/\lambda]. \tag{15.25}$$

As the detector does not respond to the double light frequency terms, Equation 15.25 reduces to

$$I_d \propto (E_{Ro}^2/2)(1 + \eta^2) + \eta E_{Ro}^2\{\cos[4\pi(L_1 - L_2)/\lambda] - \cos[4\pi\nu t + 4\pi(L_1 + L_2 + L_3)/\lambda]\}. \tag{15.26}$$

Again, the double light-frequency term drops out and we have:

$$I_d \propto (E_{Ro}^2/2)(1 + \eta^2) + \eta E_{Ro}^2\cos[4\pi(L_1 - L_2)/\lambda]. \tag{15.27}$$

Using the $\cos(A - B) = [\cos(A)\cos(B) + \sin(A)\sin(B)]$ identity, we can write:

$$I_d \propto (E_{Ro}^2/2)(1 + \eta^2) + \eta E_{Ro}^2\{\cos(4\pi L_1/\lambda)\cos(4\pi L_2/\lambda) + \sin(4\pi L_1/\lambda)\sin(4\pi L_2/\lambda)\}. \tag{15.28}$$

Now, we adjust L_1 so that $\cos(4\pi L_1/\lambda) \to 0$ and $\sin(4\pi L_1/\lambda) = 1$. We can now consider a small sinusoidal skin vibration at frequency f_s and peak amplitude, $\delta_{L2o} < \lambda/4$:

$$L_2(t) = L_{2o} + \delta_{L2o}\sin(2\pi f_s t). \tag{15.29}$$

Thus:

$$I_d \propto \left(E_{Ro}^2/2\right)(1+\eta^2) + \eta E_{Ro}^2 \sin\{(4\pi/\lambda)[L_{2o} + \delta_{L2o}\sin(2\pi f_s t)]\}. \tag{15.30}$$

Using the $\sin(A + B) = [\sin(A)\cos(B) + \cos(A)\sin(B)]$ trig identity, we can finally write:

$$I_d \propto \left(E_{Ro}^2/2\right) + \eta^2\left(E_{Ro}^2/2\right) + \eta E_{Ro}^2 \left\{\sin\left(4\pi L_{2o}/\lambda\right)\cos\left[\left(4\pi\delta_{L2o}/\lambda\right)\sin(2\pi f_s t)\right]\right.$$
$$\left. + \cos\left(4\pi L_{2o}/\lambda\right)\sin\left[\left(4\pi\delta_{L2o}/\lambda\right)\sin(2\pi f_s t)\right]\right\}. \tag{15.31}$$

The $\cos[\xi \sin(2\pi f_s t)]$ and $\sin[\xi \sin(2\pi f_s t)]$ terms can be represented as Bessel functions (Stark, Tuteur and Anderson 1988), sic:

$$\cos[\xi\sin(2\pi f_s t)] = \sum_{n=-\infty}^{\infty} J_n(\xi)\cos(n2\pi f_s t) \tag{15.32}$$

and

$$\sin[\xi\sin(2\pi f_s t)] = \sum_{n=-\infty}^{\infty} J_n(\xi)\sin(n2\pi f_s t), \tag{15.33}$$

where $\xi \equiv (4\pi\delta_{L2o}/\lambda)$. Thus, the voltage output of the detector contains DC terms, a fundamental frequency term (at f_s) and harmonics (at nf_s, $n \geq 2$). The DC terms can be eliminated by a high-pass filter, but there is no way to eliminate the harmonics; however, they will be small for small ξ. Thus, the output of the Michelson interferometer is nonlinear even with a reflecting object's small motion.

If the object motion is fast enough, there will also be a significant *Doppler frequency shift* associated with the lightwave frequency of $e_m(t)$. This shift can be expressed as a change in frequency of the e_m **E** vector:

$$e_m(t) = \eta E_{Ro}\sin\left[\left(2\pi\nu_m/c\right)t + \left(2\pi\nu/c\right)(2L_2 + L_3)\right] \tag{15.34}$$

and

$$e_r(t) = E_{Ro}\sin\left[2\pi\nu t + \left(2\pi\nu/c\right)(2L_1 + L_3)\right], \tag{15.35}$$

where $\nu_m \equiv \nu + \Delta\nu$. The *Doppler shift* is $\Delta\nu \equiv \nu(2\,\dot{L}_2/c)$ Hz. Now, ignoring light-frequency terms, the intensity is of the form:

$$I_d \propto \left(E_{Ro}^2/2\right)(1+\eta^2) + 2\eta E_{Ro}^2\cos(A)\cos(B), \tag{15.36}$$

where $A \equiv [2\pi\nu t + (2\pi\nu/c)(2L_1 + L_3)]$ and $B \equiv [2\pi\nu(1 + 2\,\dot{L}_2/c)t + (2\pi\nu/c)(2L_2 + L_3)]$. Using the identity, $\cos(A)\cos(B) \equiv (\frac{1}{2})[\cos(A - B) + \cos(A + B)]$, we have:

$$I_d \propto \left(E_{Ro}^2/2\right)(1+\eta^2) + \eta E_{Ro}^2 \left\{\cos\left[\left(2\pi\nu 2\dot{L}_2/c\right)t + (4\pi\nu/c)(L_2 - L_1)\right]\right.$$
$$\left. + \cos\left[4\pi\nu t + \left(2\pi\nu 2\dot{L}_2/c\right)t + (4\pi\nu/c)(L_1 + L_2 + L_3)\right]\right\}. \tag{15.37}$$

The second term in the $\{.\}$ is dropped because it is twice lightwave frequency. The first term is at the Doppler shift frequency, $\Delta\nu$ Hz, which is generally in the audio range and resolvable by the photosensor. We can now use the trig identity, $\cos(C + D) \equiv [\cos(C)\cos(D) - \sin(C)\sin(D)]$, to find:

$$I_d \propto \left(E_{Ro}^2/2\right)(1+\eta^2) + \eta E_{Ro}^2 \left\{\cos\left[\left(2\pi\nu 2\dot{L}_2/c\right)t\right]\cos\left[\left(4\pi\nu/c\right)(L_2 - L_1)\right]\right.$$
$$\left. - \sin\left[\left(2\pi\nu 2\dot{L}_2/c\right)t\right]\sin\left[\left(4\pi\nu/c\right)(L_2 - L_1)\right]\right\}. \tag{15.38}$$

If the skin motion is sinusoidal so that

$$L_2 = L_{2o} + \delta_2\sin(\omega_s t). \tag{15.39}$$

Then

$$\dot{L}_2 = \omega_m \delta_2 \cos(\omega_s t). \tag{15.40}$$

We set $L_1 = L_{2o}$, and after some mild algebra we get the messy result:

$$1_d \propto \left(\frac{E_{Ro}^2}{2}\right)(1 + \eta^2) + \eta E_{Ro}^2 \left\{\cos\left[\left(\frac{4\pi\delta_2}{\lambda}\right)(\omega_s \cos(\omega_s t))t\right]\cos\left[\left(\frac{4\pi\delta_2}{\lambda}\right)\sin(\omega_s t)\right]\right.$$

$$\left. -\sin\left[\left(\frac{4\pi\delta_2}{\lambda}\right)(\omega_s \cos(\omega_s t))t\right]\sin\left[\left(\frac{4\pi\delta_2}{\lambda}\right)\sin(\omega_s t)\right]\right\}. \tag{15.41}$$

The $\cos[\xi\sin(\omega_s t)]$ and $\sin[\xi\sin(\omega_s t)]$ terms in Equation 15.41 give rise to the motion-frequency Bessel function series of Equations 15.32 and 15.33. It is not known what sort of temporal modulation of the Bessel series the Doppler $\cos[\xi\omega_s t \cos(\omega_s t)]$ and $\sin[\xi\omega_s t \cos(\omega_s t)]$ terms will provide. For example, let us calculate the maximum Doppler shift for a peak sinusoidal skin deflection of 120 nm at 1 Hz, using a HeNe laser with $\lambda = 633$ nm. From above, $\Delta\nu_{max} = 2_{max}/\lambda$ Hz. So:

$$\Delta\nu_{max} = \left[2 \times 2\pi(1) \times 1.2 \times 10^{-7}/(633 \times 10^{-9})\right] = 2.38 \text{ Hz}. \tag{15.42}$$

Thus, the peak Doppler shift is about three times the 1 Hz displacement frequency.

Hong and Fox (1993) reported on an "optical stethoscope" that used a 670-nm laser diode as a coherent light source with a Michelson (actually, a Twyman–Green) interferometer to sense skin vibrations. Their interferometer was housed in a metal box about $5'' \times 3.5'' \times 3.5''$; its AC-coupled photodiode output was observed in real time on a digital oscilloscope with FFT spectrum analysis capability. A more refined version of this instrument was described by Hong (1994), in which he used a HeNe laser source and a fiber-optic cable to impinge the light on the skin. In most of the phantoms and human subjects studied by Hong, object displacements were periodic at the heart rate, but displacements were in hundreds of μm rather than hundreds of nm. Thus, the Twyman–Green interferometer was well out of its $\pm\lambda/4$ linear range, and the apparatus served only as a *mixer* to extract the lightwave Doppler shift frequency in the measurement beam. The Doppler frequency shifts extracted followed the shape of the *magnitude* of the time derivative of the pressure waveform in the phantom studies, as evidenced by the output of a frequency-to-voltage converter (FVC). (Apparently, the "skin" surface displacement of the phantom was proportional to the vessel pressure.) In human studies, Hong cited the peak displacement of the skin over the common-carotid artery to be 510 μm over 86 ms. This is a velocity of 5.93×10^{-3} m/s, and the peak Doppler lightwave frequency is $\Delta\nu = 2 \times 5.93 \times 10^{-3}/633 \times 10^{-9} = 18.74$ kHz. Obviously, this output frequency will vary over the cardiac cycle. Because there is no way to sense the sign of $\Delta\nu$, the voltage-to-frequency converter (VFC) V_o was determined by

$$V_o \propto \Delta\nu \propto |\dot{L}_2| \propto |\dot{p}|. \tag{15.43}$$

Thus in summary, Hong's interferometer was apparently used as a Doppler mixer, not an nm distance measuring system.

15.4.4 Discussion

Interferometers are generally suited for precise displacement measurements of body surfaces when the range of deflection is $<\lambda/4$. When the surface is moving at a high frequency, the interferometer output contains many harmonics due to the $\cos[\xi\sin(\omega_s t)]$ terms and lightwave Doppler shift terms. They are better-suited to measuring small, slow displacements, such as tooth drift in orthodontic research.

15.5 LASER DOPPLER VELOCIMETRY

15.5.1 Principles of LDV

LDV provides a "no-touch" means of measuring the linear velocity of fluids, including air, water, hydraulic fluid, and, for our purposes, blood. The Doppler effect is observed as a frequency shift in coherent, monochromatic light waves reflected or scattered from particles moving in the

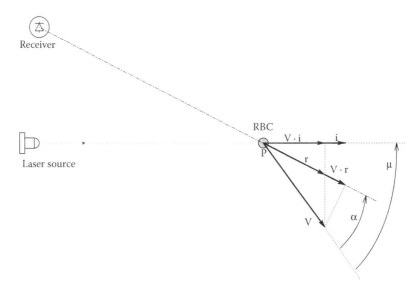

Figure 15.6 Vectors required to describe laser Doppler velocimetry (LDV). All vectors lie in the x–y plane (plane of the paper).

fluid whose velocity is to be measured. As in the case of Doppler ultrasound used to measure blood velocity, the reflecting particles are the erythrocytes (red blood cells [RBCs]) in the blood. However, unlike Doppler ultrasound, the return wave path is seldom colinear with the path from the laser source to the reflecting particle, P.

To understand how LDV works, let P move with a velocity **V**, which is to be measured. Refer to Figure 15.6 in which all vectors lie in the x–y plane. Let us define a *unit vector,* **i**, directed from the source S to P. Assume that $|\mathbf{V}|/c \ll 1$, so that relativistic effects are negligible. When $\mathbf{V} = 0$, the number of wave fronts striking the object per unit time is

$$f_s = c/\lambda_s \text{ Hz}, \tag{15.44}$$

where c is the velocity of light in the medium in which V is being measured, and λ_s is the wavelength of the source laser. (f_s for a HeNe laser in plasma striking an RBC is $(3 \times 10^8/1.336)/(632.8 \times 10^{-9}) = 3.5348 \times 10^{14}$ Hz. $n_p = 1.336$ is taken as the refractive index of plasma.)

It is easy to show that the number of wavefronts hitting a moving RBC/s is:

$$f_p = [(c/n_p) - \mathbf{V} \cdot \mathbf{i}]/\lambda_s \text{ Hz}. \tag{15.45}$$

The *vector dot product* gives the RBC velocity component parallel to the *unit vector,* **i**. **i** points in a line from the source to the moving RBC. Thus, the wavelength apparent to the RBC is:

$$\lambda_p = c'/f_p = (\lambda_s c')/[c' - \mathbf{V} \cdot \mathbf{i}] = (\lambda_s c')/[c' - V\cos(\mu)], \tag{15.46}$$

where $c' = c/n_p$ = the velocity of light in the medium (plasma) in which the RBC is moving.

Now the *unit vector,* **r**, points from the instantaneous position of the moving RBC, P, to the stationary receiver, R. An observer at R sees a scattered wavelength, λ_r, emanating from P. This is:

$$\lambda_r = (c' - \mathbf{V} \cdot \mathbf{r})/f_p = (c' - V\cos(\alpha))/f_p. \tag{15.47}$$

The dot product, $\mathbf{V} \cdot \mathbf{r}$, gives the velocity component of the RBC in the **r** direction. Thus, the frequency of the received, scattered, Doppler-shifted radiation is:

$$f_r = c'/\lambda_r \text{ Hz}. \tag{15.48}$$

Substituting from Equations 15.47 and 15.48, we find:

$$f_r = c'(c' - \mathbf{V} \cdot \mathbf{i})/[\lambda_s(c' - \mathbf{V} \cdot \mathbf{r})] = f_s \frac{(c' - \mathbf{V} \cdot \mathbf{i})}{(c' - \mathbf{V} \cdot \mathbf{r})} \text{ Hz}. \tag{15.49}$$

Now, if the f_s and f_r signals are mixed, and the difference term is examined, the Doppler shift is:

$$f_D \equiv (f_s - f_r) = (c'/\lambda_s) = \left[1 - \frac{(c' - \mathbf{V} \cdot \mathbf{i})}{(c' - \mathbf{V} \cdot \mathbf{r})}\right] \text{Hz.} \tag{15.50}$$

Now, since $V \ll c'$, Equation 15.50 reduces to

$$f_D \cong \frac{V[\cos(\mu) - \cos(\alpha)]}{\lambda_s} \text{ Hz.} \tag{15.51}$$

For example, if $V = 0.1$ m/s, $\lambda_s = 632.8 \times 10^{-9}$ m, $\mu = 50°$, and $\alpha = 30°$, fD is equal to -35.278 kHz. fD is negative because the object is receding. There is no simple way to extract the sign of $\mathbf{V}$.

The *mixing* of the input and return (Doppler-shifted) signals can be thought of as occurring on the photocathode (PC) of the receiver PMT. The transmitted and received light sinusoidal $\mathbf{E}$ vectors add linearly and vectorially at the PMT PC surface. However, the PMT responds to the net *intensity* of light at its PC surface. The intensity is proportional to the net, instantaneous, $\mathbf{E}(t)$ vector magnitude *squared*. Thus, the PMT photocurrent can be written as

$$i_P(t) = K_p \int |\mathbf{E_s}(t) + \mathbf{E_r}(t)|^2 dt, \tag{15.52}$$

where $\mathbf{E_s}(t)$ is the electric field vector of non-Doppler-shifted laser source light of frequency c'/λ_s, and $\mathbf{E_r}(t)$ is the sum total of Doppler-shifted, backscattered light electric field vectors.

Thus, when the resultant $\mathbf{E}(t)$ vector magnitude at the PC surface is squared, it gives terms with frequencies of $2f_s$, $2f_r$, $(f_s + f_r)$, $(f_s - f_r)$, and 0 (DC). Of course, the $f_D = (f_s - f_r)$ term is of primary interest. Normally, the PMT responds to the 0 frequency terms, but in this case they are filtered out by a band-pass filter to select the distribution of f_D frequencies in $i_P(t)$.

15.5.2 LDV Applied to Retinal Blood Vessels

Figure 15.7 illustrates a simple geometry for sensing RBC velocity in the large blood vessels surrounding the head of the optic nerve (macula) at the rear of the eyeball. Measurement of the flow in these vessels is important in diagnosing glaucoma. The system is responsive to velocity vectors lying in a plane defined by the $\mathbf{i}$ and $\mathbf{r}$ unit vectors. The Doppler frequency shift from the component of RBC velocity lying in the $\mathbf{i}$–$\mathbf{r}$ plane can be shown to be equal to that derived in the section above. That is:

$$f_D \cong \frac{V[\cos(\mu) - \cos(\alpha)]}{\lambda_s} \text{ Hz.} \tag{15.53}$$

Note that both angles, μ and α, must be known to obtain accurate velocity estimates. These angles are very difficult to estimate, so simple ocular blood vessel LDV lacks accuracy.

To overcome the uncertain angle problem, a system was designed by Feke et al. (1987) that used two PMT receivers with their optical axes separated by a small, fixed angle, γ. Figure 15.8 illustrates the vector geometry of their system in three dimensions. The RBC velocity vector $\mathbf{V}$ is described in a spherical coordinate system by its length, V, angle ϕ with the z-axis (vertical), and angle θ with the x-axis (horizontal). We assume that the input laser beam and the two receiver axes all lie in the x–y (horizontal) plane. It is the vector component of $\mathbf{V}$ in the x–y plane that is relevant in finding the system output. The magnitude of this projection is $V_{xy} = |\mathbf{V}|\sin(\phi)$. For simplification, Figure 15.9 shows the relevant vectors in the x–y plane. As in the previous developments, the moving RBC at P "sees" an illuminating frequency, f_p:

$$f_p = \frac{c' + \mathbf{V_{xy}} \cdot \mathbf{i}}{\lambda_s} = \frac{c' + V_{xy}\cos(\pi - \mu)}{\lambda_s} = \frac{c' - V_{xy}\cos(\mu)}{\lambda_s} \text{ Hz.} \tag{15.54}$$

A "+" sign is used in the numerator of Equation 15.54 because the object has a velocity component parallel with the $\mathbf{i}$ vector adding to the apparent light speed from the source. Thus, the wavelength of the laser light seen by the RBC is given by

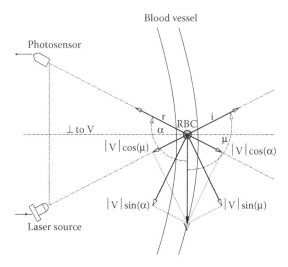

Figure 15.7 Vectors used to describe the application of LDV to retinal blood vessels. The unit vectors i and r define the plane in which the vectors lie.

$$\lambda_p = \frac{c'}{f_p} = \frac{c'\lambda_s}{c' - V_{xy}\cos(\mu)} = \frac{\lambda_s}{1 - (V_{xy}/c')\cos(\mu)} \cong \lambda_s\left[1 + \left(V_{xy}/c'\right)\cos(\mu)\right]. \tag{15.55}$$

Note that there is a "red shift" (stretching of the perceived source wavelength) at a receding RBC. Now an observer at R_1 sees a scattered wavelength, λ_{r1}, emanating from the RBC.

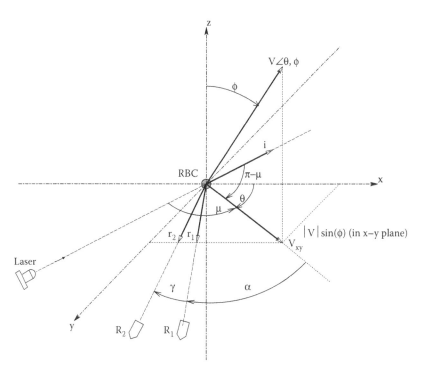

Figure 15.8 LDV vectors in 3-D space, following the system of Feke et al. (1987). The projection of the object velocity V into the x–y plane is V_{xy}.

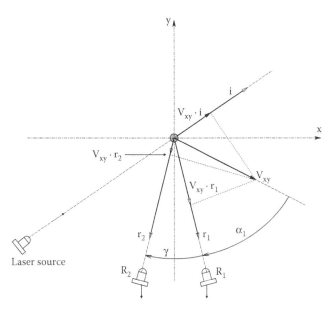

Figure 15.9 LDV vectors projected into the x–y plane. The laser and two detectors lie in the x–y plane.

$$\lambda_{r1} = \frac{[c' + V_{xy} \cdot r_1]}{f_p} = \frac{[c' + V_{xy}\cos(\alpha_1)]}{f_p} = \frac{\lambda_s[c' + V_{xy}\cos(\alpha_1)]}{c' - V_{xy}\cos(\mu)} \tag{15.56}$$

$f_{r1} = c'/\lambda_{r1}$, so:

$$f_{r1} = (c'/\lambda_s)\frac{[1 - (V_{xy}/c')\cos(\mu)]}{[1 + (V_{xy}/c')\cos(\alpha_1)]} \text{ Hz.} \tag{15.57}$$

The Doppler frequency of the RBC at R_1 is found by mixing f_s and f_{r1} at the R_1 PC:

$$f_{D1} = (f_s - f_{r1}) = (c'/\lambda_s)\left[1 - \frac{1 - (V_{xy}/c')\cos(\mu)}{1 + (V_{xy}/c')\cos(\alpha_1)}\right] \text{ Hz.} \tag{15.58}$$

If we assume that $(V_{xy}/c') \ll 1$, then Equation 15.58 reduces to

$$f_{D1} \cong (V_{xy}/\lambda_s)\,[\cos(\alpha_1) + \cos(\mu)] \text{ Hz.} \tag{15.59}$$

By the same development, we can show that

$$f_{D2} = (V_{xy}/\lambda_s)\,[\cos(\alpha_1 + \gamma) + \cos(\mu)] \text{ Hz.} \tag{15.60}$$

The output of the system is the *difference* of the two Doppler frequencies, obtained by mixing and filtering f_{D1} and f_{D2}.

$$\Delta f_D = (f_{D1} - f_{D2}) = (V_{xy}/\lambda_s)[\cos(\alpha_1) + \cos(\mu) - \cos(\alpha_1 + \gamma) - \cos(\mu)] \text{ Hz.} \tag{15.61}$$

Note that the $\cos(\mu)$ terms cancel. The $\cos(\alpha_1 + \gamma)$ can be expanded by trig identity:

$$\Delta f_D = (V_{xy}/\lambda_s)\,[\cos(\alpha_1) - \cos(\alpha_1)\cos(\gamma) + \sin(\alpha_1)\sin(\gamma)] \text{ Hz.} \tag{15.62}$$

Because system design made $\gamma < 10°$, we can let $\sin(\gamma) \rightarrow \gamma$ in radians and $\cos(\gamma) \rightarrow 1$. Thus, Δf_D simplifies to

$$\Delta f_D \cong (V_{xy}/\lambda_s)\gamma\sin(\alpha_1) \text{ Hz} \tag{15.63}$$

or:

$$V_{xy} \cong 2\pi\Delta f_D \lambda_s / [\gamma \sin(\alpha_1)], \tag{15.64}$$

where Δf_D is measured, λ_s and γ are known, and now only α_1 needs to be estimated.

Figure 15.10 shows a very simplified schematic of the optical setup used by Feke et al. (1987). A flat, front-surface contact lens (a Goldmann-type fundus lens) was fitted to the eye to permit precise optical alignment. After attenuation to 18 μW, a collimated HeNe laser beam was directed at the large blood vessels surrounding the head of the optic nerve. The area illuminated was about 3.14×10^4 μm². The backscattered, Doppler-shifted light rays were directed through two apertures to a pair of matched photomultiplier light sensors. The vergence angle on the sensor optics was 11.5°, which translates to an internal γ angle of 8.3° in an eye with normal vision (an emmetropic eye). The Doppler frequency signals from the PMTs were processed by VFC (e.g., comparators, one-shots, and low-pass filters), and their difference was used to estimate the $|V_{xy}|$ of RBCs in retinal veins and arteries using Equation 15.64.

Figure 15.11 was redrawn from Figure 8 in Feke et al. (1987). It shows a plot of Δf_{Dmax} versus time (one cardiac cycle) for a superior temporal retinal artery in the right eye of a normal subject without the noise. Peak (systolic) velocity was 2.7 cm/s; minimum (diastolic) velocity was 1.0 cm/s. Corresponding Δf_Ds are shown on the vertical axis. Feke et al. calculated the mean blood flow rate in these retinal arteries from the formula:

$$\dot{Q}_s = \overline{V}_{xy} S / 2 \text{ cm}^3/\text{s}, \tag{15.65}$$

where S is the cross-sectional area of the artery in cm², estimated from fundoscopy, and V_{xy} is the mean blood velocity in the vessel in cm/s.

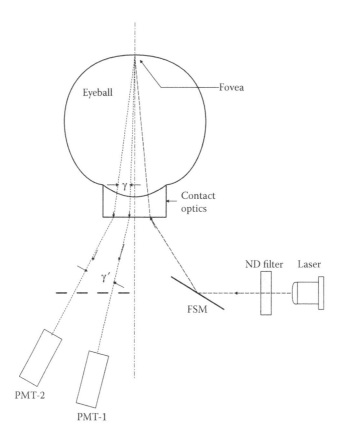

Figure 15.10 The Feke LDV system applied to an eye to measure the retinal blood flow. A contact lens is required to match the refractive index of the cornea.

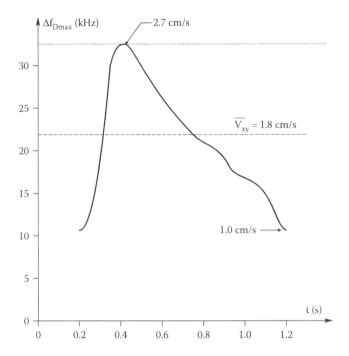

Figure 15.11 Representative plot of Δf_{Dmax} versus time over one cardiac cycle for a retinal artery. (Based on data from Feke, G.T. et al. 1987. *IEEE Trans. Biomed. Eng.* 34(9): 673–680.)

15.5.3 LDV Applied to Skin and Other Tissues

At the time of this writing (2016), several manufacturers make percutaneous LDV systems for experimental and diagnostic study of the microcirculation in the surface of various tissues. These instruments are generally called laser Doppler blood flowmeters, even though they respond to the velocity of erythrocytes in subdermal blood vessels. The NI use of LDV systems includes measuring RBC velocities in blood vessels under the skin, in teeth, in the retina, and in internal sites still considered to be NI, including the inner surface of the trachea, the colon, nose, rectum, esophagus, etc. Some of the companies that make LDV blood velocity systems include but are not limited to: Advance Co, Ltd. (Japan), ADINSTRUMENTS, Transonic Systems, Inc., Abb Automation, Inc. (Instrument Division), Moor Instruments, Inc., TSI, Inc., and Wallach Surgical Devices.

Most of these LDV systems use diode lasers, and couple the laser light to the tissue, and the Doppler-shifted backscattered light back to the photomultiplier with optical fibers. Both source and output fibers are terminated in a small probe, not unlike that used in Doppler ultrasound applications. LDV probes have various sizes and shapes depending on the application. Here, we will focus out attention on dermal circulation. Figure 15.12 illustrates some of the circulatory features of the skin. In the deep layers (4000 μm below the surface), we find *horizontal* networks of arterioles and venules. Closer to the surface (1000–4000 μm) are arteriovenous shunts under autonomic control and *vertical branches* of arterioles and venules. Just below the epidermis (150 μm) are extensive capillary beds running *parallel* to the skin's surface. The effective penetration of the input laser light depends on its wavelength, with red HeNe light (633 nm) penetrating between 0.6 and 1.5 mm. The HeNe beam allows the observance of blood Doppler signals from throughout the dermis, while blue argon (458 nm) laser light penetrates ~250 μm, and so is responsive to the blood velocity in the upper subpapillary capillary plexus beneath the epidermis (Duteil et al. 1985).

The laser illumination of many subepidermal capillaries, the paths of which are generally horizontal, but nevertheless torturous, means that the RBCs in them are moving with a broad range of angles {μ} and speeds with respect to the **i** vectors of the divergent rays from the optical input fiber. There is also a broad spectrum of **r** vectors that can pass into the acceptance cone of the pickup optical fiber. Thus, there is a broad, low-frequency spectrum of Doppler frequencies generated by the skin's microcirculation.

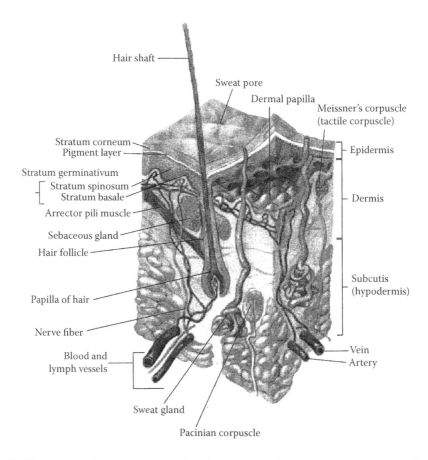

Figure 15.12 A section through human skin. Many anatomical features are shown; of principal interest are the blood vessels. Note that blood flow in larger vessels is parallel to the skin surface, while the smaller capillary loops carry vertical flow. (Public domain figure at: https://commons. wikimedia.org/wiki/File:Skin.png)

As the PMT photocurrent, $i_P(t)$, is a random signal derived from the random distribution of **i** and **r** vectors with respect to many RBCs moving in many different directions, it can be characterized by its two-sided *autocorrelation function*, $R_{ii}(\tau)$, and its *power density spectrum*, Φ_{ii} (f). (Φ_{ii} (f) is simply the Fourier transform of $R_{ii}(\tau)$; it shows how the power in the frequency spectrum of Doppler signals is distributed). Duteil et al. (1985) described and discussed mathematical models that describe the observed Φ_{ii} (f)'s seen in percutaneous LDV. They chose an exponential model to fit the measured autocorrelation functions:

$$R_{ii}(\tau) = \sigma_i^2 \exp(-|\tau|/\tau_D). \tag{15.66}$$

The two-sided power density spectrum thus has the Lorentzian form:

$$\Phi_{ii}(\omega) = \frac{2\sigma_i^2(1/\tau_D)}{\omega^2 + 1/\tau_D^2}, \tag{15.67}$$

where $(1/\tau_D)$ is the half-power frequency in r/s and:

$$\tau_D = \frac{1}{(2\pi f_D)} \text{ s.} \tag{15.68}$$

Many of the LDV skin blood flow power spectra given by Duteil et al. (1985) do appear to be fit by Equation 15.67; however, others drop off more sharply at low frequencies and might be better modeled by exponential functions or simple rectangular hyperbolas (saturating, first-order Hill functions) of the form:

$$\Phi_{ii}(f) = \Phi_{max} \left\{ \varepsilon^1 / (\varepsilon^1 + f) \right\}. \tag{15.69}$$

In addition to parameters of the power spectrum of Doppler return signals such as the half-power frequency and the peak power (modal) frequency, a parameter known as the "flux" is also used:

$$\text{flux} = k_1 \int_{f_L}^{f_H} \frac{f\Phi_{ii}(f)}{I^n} df = k_2(\text{Ave. speed of RBCs}) \times (\text{Number concentration of RBCs}). \tag{15.70}$$

The integral computes the normalized first moment of the PDS over the bandwidth, $\{f_H - f_L\}$. I is the mean light intensity on the PMT, and n is an exponent, generally 2.

If instead of illuminating a small, fixed, subcutaneous voxel with a fiber-optic probe, a laser beam in air is scanned over an area of skin with moving mirrors, and a 2-D, LDV plot of the subcutaneous blood flow can be constructed. The Doppler-shifted backscattered light propagates back through the same mirror assembly that scans the laser, through telescope lenses to the detector PMT. This type of LD imaging (LDI) system can be used on a whole torso or smaller skin surfaces such as a breast or a face. Here, left/right differences in velocity signature or local changes may signal asymmetrical cerebrovascular disease, or a tumor. LDI applications on the skin surface also include the assessment of wound and burn healing, and studies of angiogenesis in plastic surgery, and success in reattaching accidentally amputated limbs and appendages. Although accurate measurement of subcutaneous blood flow is impossible with LDV and LDI, these techniques do allow precise comparisons between normal and abnormal skin circulation on a given individual, and allow quantitative measurement of how vasoactive drugs affect skin perfusion.

15.5.4 Discussion

LDV has the advantage over ultrasound velocimetry of being able to measure the blood velocity in extremely small vessels, such as capillaries in the skin and in mucous membranes, and also in larger vessels in the retina. The laser beam can be focused down to illuminate an area of only a few μm^2. The probe beam will only penetrate a few mm in the skin, so is suited to measure average blood velocity in the subdermal capillaries. Thus, LDV can be used to assess the angiogenesis that accompanies wound, burn, and skin graft healing. LDV signals from the skin are very noisy not because of laminar velocity in capillaries but because the capillaries run in different directions and twist and turn. In an effort to treat LDV output signals quantitatively, autocorrelation and autopower spectra are sometimes used.

Laser Doppler uses and limitations are described in an online paper by Transonic (2012).

15.6 TIR SPECTROSCOPY

15.6.1 Introduction

Infrared light is EMR whose wavelengths (λ) are too long for human eyes to perceive. IR light wavelengths cover from 750 nm to over 1000 μm; the IR spectrum is subdivided somewhat arbitrarily into near-infrared (NIR) (IR-A) (750–1500 nm), intermediate (IIR) or mid-range (MIR) (IR-B) (1500 nm–7 μm), and far-infrared (FIR) (IR-C) (7–1000 μm) (Barnes 1983). (Different references differ slightly on their three IR band definitions.) Spectral bands are often described in terms of wave number (WN), ν. WN is defined as $\nu \equiv k/\lambda$ cm^{-1}, where λ is in nm, and k = 10^7 (the ratio of cm to nm).

Many biological molecules absorb IR energy in narrow bands of wavelength due to the transfer of energy from photons to the molecular bonds binding various molecular subgroups together, exciting the vibration and stretching of bonds connecting, for example, hydroxyl, methyl, and amino radicals in various modes. Figure 15.13 illustrates the approximate wavelengths at which certain types of chemical bonds absorb photon energy (Wordpress 2008). These narrow absorption bands provide unique signatures that make *in vitro*, IR spectrographic analysis effective, and offer many possibilities for identifying biomolecules, *in vivo*, through the skin, either by transmitted- or backscattered IR light.

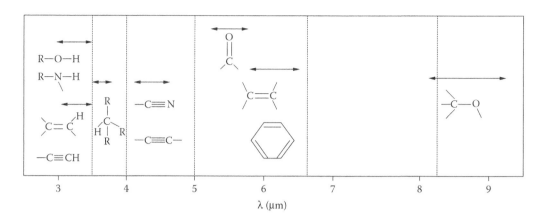

Figure 15.13 IR wavelength bands where certain molecular groups selectively absorb IR photon energy. Absorption bandwidth depends in part on the presence of other nearby groups and the solvent.

Often IR *absorbance* or *percent transmittance* spectra are plotted versus WN in cm^{-1}. WN in cm^{-1} is related to wavelength in μm by: WN $= 10^4/\lambda$. When monochromatic light passes through a cuvette containing the analyte in solution, the intensity is attenuated exponentially. That is, by Beer's law model,

$$I_{out} = I_{in} 10^{-\alpha(\lambda)L[C]}. \qquad (15.71)$$

If the input intensity is I_{in}, and the output intensity is I_{out}, the $\% T \equiv 100(I_{out}/I_{in})$, and the *absorbance, A*, is defined as

$$A \equiv \log_{10}\left(\frac{I_{in}}{I_{out}}\right) = 2 - \log_{10}(\%T) = \alpha(\lambda)L[C]. \qquad (15.72)$$

A depends on the wavelength-dependent *molar absorptivity (molar extinction coefficient)*, $\alpha(\lambda)$, the concentration of the analyte, [C], as well as the optical path length, L. The absorbance is also called the *optical density* (OD).

One of the better-known NI medical uses of NIR light is in the two-wavelength fingertip pulse oximeter used to measure the oxygen saturation of hemoglobin (Hb) in the capillaries. (Pulse oximetry is described in detail in Section 15.8.) A general problem in applying IR spectroscopy to percutaneous measurements is the absorption and attenuation of IR intensity by skin (*stratum corneum* and other layers), skin pigment, fat cells, and water in extracellular tissues, all of which can overwhelm the absorption by the targeted analyte. Water absorbs IR strongly between 5.5 and 7 μm and also around 2.7 μm, and beyond 25 μm (Barnes 1983).

A very active area of research at present is the development of an NI, TIR, blood glucose sensor. The perfection and FDA approval of such an NI device will revolutionize the management and care of persons with diabetes mellitus and other glucoregulatory dysfunctions. By analyzing the intensity of backscattered IR light at two or more wavelengths, it is theoretically possible to estimate blood glucose concentration from the glucose absorption signature. Such a device would need to have a two-point calibration based on actual blood samples from the individual using it. The IR photons can come from LEDs, tunable IR diode lasers, from a *globar* blackbody IR source passed through a grating monochromator, or even the black-body radiation from deep body tissues (at ~310°). (Recall that Section 8.2.2 described *dispersive spectroscopy* and *Beer's law*.) When nondispersive, IR spectrophotometry is used, an interference-type optical band-pass filter selects the input band from a broadband IR source such as an incandescent filament lamp. For reasons of noise reduction, all radiation sources are chopped to permit synchronous detection (e.g., with a lock-in amplifier). Transduction of the backscattered light can be done with one sensor which covers the IR wavelengths used. This can be an InGaAs photodiode (covers 0.9–2.6 μm), a HgCdTe photodiode (covers 2–11 μm), or a pyroelectric IR sensor (covers 2–25 μm). Pyroelectric sensors have lower temporal signal bandwidths compared to photodiodes. IR sensors are often thermoelectrically or cryogenically cooled to reduce noise and improve IR photon detection efficiency.

There are many medically important molecules that theoretically can be measured by TIR spectroscopy. These include but are not limited to: *cholesterol, cocaine, codeine, diacetyl morphine (heroin), ethanol, glucose, morphine, Δ^9-tetrahydrocannabinol,* and other *opioids.* Many of these molecules have unique absorption peaks in the range from 6.5 to 14 μm.

Complications arise in TIR measurements because everyone's anatomy is different in terms of skin thickness, pigment, vascularization, fat deposits, etc. To make TIR spectrophotometric measurements, we need body parts with high vascularization, thin skin, low pigment, and low fat. For transmission TIR measurements, the webs between the fingers or the earlobes are suitable. For backscattered light, the tissues under the finger nails, the thin skin on the medial surface of the forearms, the tongue, and the lips offer possible sites.

15.6.2 Direct Measurement of Blood Glucose with IR Spectrosopy

At present, the FDA-approved, practical, semi-invasive means to measure blood glucose is the finger prick, blood drop on chemical strip, colorimetric analysis (FPCA) method, or the use of miniaturized amperometric sensor strips using a catalyst. As obtaining a blood sample requires breaking the skin, the FPCA method is semi-invasive, causes discomfort, and the risk of possible infection. Couple these "cons" with the fact that Type II diabetics generally have to test their blood four or more times a day in order to adjust their diet, insulin dose, and exercise to try to achieve normoglycemia. Clearly, an accurate, glucose-measuring system is needed that is truly NI, and which can be used as many times as needed without pain or risk. In Section 15.7, we describe one possible NI means of estimating blood glucose using the natural optical rotation (OR) of LPL by glucose molecules in the AH of the eye. In this section, we consider the use of IR absorption by glucose molecules in tissues under the skin. For reference, Figure 15.14 illustrates an IR percent transmittance spectrogram of pure *anhydrous* glucose (dextrose). The glucose powder was suspended in nujol liquid. Note the three, evenly spaced absorption peaks at ~11.0, 12.0, and 13.0 μm; also, there are smaller peaks at ~8.7, 9.0, and 9.6 μm (not shown). In the body, in blood, cells, and interstitial fluid, glucose is dissolved in water, and surrounded with proteins, lipids, etc. which significantly change the character of its percent transmittance spectrum.

Between the strong IR absorbance regions for water, there are three "windows" that permit *in vivo,* NIR absorption spectroscopy to proceed with minimum interference from water absorption: (1) The *combination region* from 2.0 to 2.5 μm (5000–4000 cm⁻¹). (2) The *first overtone region* from 1.54 to 1.82 μm (6500–5500 cm⁻¹). (3) The *short wavelength NIR region* from 0.7 to 1.33 μm (14,286–7500 cm⁻¹). Glucose also has measurable NIR absorbance peaks at 1.61, 1.69, 1.73, 2.10, 2.27, and 2.32 μm (Burmeister et al. 1998).

One of the first *in vitro* studies of IR spectroscopy of whole blood using an *attenuated total reflection* (ATR) prism was reported by Kaiser (1979). Kaiser first made a percent transmittance spectrogram of distilled water over 2.5–20 μm. Then citrate-buffered blood was scanned with a

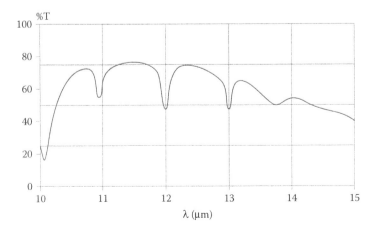

Figure 15.14 Percent transmittance of anhydrous glucose in the range from 10 to 15 μm.

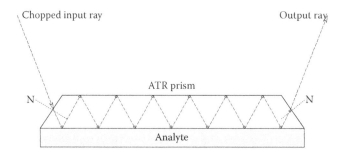

Figure 15.15 Vertical section through an ATR prism.

conventional spectrometer using a 25 μ cell and again using the ATR prism in direct contact with the blood. Finally, a tunable CO_2 laser IR source was used in a two-beam ATR spectrometer to resolve ethanol from glucose in the 1060–1030 cm^{-1} range. Measurement sensitivity for glucose and ethanol was ~3.5 mg/dL, or 35 ppm. (Normal fasting blood glucose concentration is ~90 mg/dL.)

Another, *in vitro* study that demonstrated that the concentration of glucose in whole blood could be measured accurately by IR absorption was reported by Mendelson et al. (1990). They first made an IR percent transmittance spectrogram of distilled water over a WN range of 1900–800 cm^{-1} (5.26–12.5 μm wavelength) using an ATR prism. An ATR prism (or plate) is an optical, surface-effect device used to couple the source IR energy to the sample where absorption occurs. An entering beam of IR energy reflects back and forth between the ATR plate's inner surfaces. Mendelson et al. used a ZnSe, IR-transmitting ATR plate that was 20 mm × 50 mm × 3 mm thick. There were 17 internal reflections of the IR beam before it exited (Figure 15.15). The refractive index, n_1, of the ZnSe is ~2.42 for 9.66 μm light; n_2 of water is 1.33. (n is the ratio of the speed of light *in vacuo* to the speed of light in the medium at a given wavelength.) With water as the absorbing medium, Mendelson et al. calculated that the penetration depth of the light at the interface was only 1.3 μm at λ = 9.6 μm. They passed the sample (water or blood) over both flat surfaces of the ATR plate. When Mendelson et al. used whole human blood as the sample with glucose added to give 10 g/L (10 × higher than normal blood glucose), definite absorption "wiggles" were seen in the spectrogram between 1000 and 1200 cm^{-1}. By subtracting the percent transmittance spectrum for distilled water, and expanding the WN scale, a very sharp absorption peak was observed (percent T went from ~90 down to 66.5) at 1035 cm^{-1} (9.663 μm). This wavelength was also available from an 8 W tunable CO_2 laser. Mendelson et al. built a single wavelength, ATR-based blood glucose-measuring system around their CO_2 laser source; they chopped the beam at 193 Hz and used a broadband pyroelectric IR detector to sense the emergent beam. A reference channel was used to compensate for laser intensity fluctuations. As the output power of the CO_2 laser was 3 W (~10^3–10^5 times the power from a standard IR spectrophotometer), and the CO_2 laser has a spectral line width which is between 10^{-3} and 10^{-6} cm^{-1} (vs 1–10 cm^{-1} for a grating monochromator), the *in vitro* measurement of blood glucose with the ATR plate was quite accurate. Mendelson et al. (1990) used pig blood samples doped with glucose between 90 and 270 mg/dL and plotted relative absorption versus glucose concentration [G] in mg/dL (measured with a YSI Model 23A, electrochemical glucose analyzer "gold standard"). The regression line was RA = 0.64 + 1.37 × 10^{-3} [G]. The correlation coefficient was r = 0.98 and the standard error of the estimate (SEE) was 0.001. Mendelson et al. pointed out that the nonzero intercept (0.64) is due to the other absorbing substances in the blood; whole blood is a biochemically complex substance.

15.6.3 Transcutaneous Measurement of Glucose with IR

To achieve a truly NI means of estimating the blood glucose concentration, the measurement must be made through the skin without direct contact with blood, fluids, or internal tissues. From the success described above with ATR plates in direct contact with blood, it was suggested by Kaiser (1979) that an ATR plate could be placed over lip tissue to measure the glucose absorption in the underlying vascular tissue. Heise et al. (1999) attempted to measure the tissue glucose by its absorbance spectrum using an ATR prism pressed against the tissues of the inner lip. IR from 1750 to 750 cm^{-1} (5.71–13.3 μm) was used. Heise et al. found that there was *no good correlation* between the spectral features measured and the subjects' measured blood glucose concentration. This is probably because the evanescent IR light from the ATR prism scarcely penetrates the skin's *stratum corneum* into the underlying vascular tissue layers. The ATR method works with direct blood contact because glucose molecules are on the prism's surface.

Blank et al. (1999) made a study of diffuse reflectance from tissue in the forearm using NIR light in the range from 1.05 to 2.45 μm. A custom-built, scanning, NIR spectrophotometer was used with a sampling interval of 1 nm. Indium gallium arsenide detectors were used. These authors claimed an SNR of 90 dB at the peak (reflectance intensity); they concluded:

> The results reported here lead to a cautious optimism that non-invasive glucose measurement using NIR spectroscopy in the 1050–2450 nm range is possible … Many factors, including variations in skin surface roughness, variations in measurement location, skin hydration on the surface and [in] underlying tissue, the effect of tissue displacement (contact pressure) by the [fiber optic] probe interface, and variations in skin temperature can contribute to significant changes in the sampling of the tissue volume elements. Parameters that are internal to the tissue sample may not be controllable but their impact on the measurement must be compensated.

The big problems with the glucose measurements of Blank et al. (1999) were consistency, repeatability, and the maintenance of calibration. In fact, many workers who have tried the transcutaneous, NIR spectrophotometric approach using either transmitted or reflected light conditioned by passing through vascular tissue have encountered these same problems.

Burmeister et al. (1998) claimed that an effective human tissue phantom for the finger web can be made from a water layer of 5.0–6.3 mm, and a fat layer of 1.4–4.2 mm thick. The water in such a phantom can contain dissolved glucose and the phantom can be "tuned" as a reference for a given subject. Burmeister et al. concluded:

> Successful noninvasive clinical measurements [of glucose] require the ability to collect reproducible noninvasive spectra from human subjects. Between run variations must be avoided in the thickness, composition, and temperature of the sampling site. This demand for spectral reproducibility makes the human-to-spectrometer interface critical. The temperature of the interface must be controlled to minimize thermal induced spectral shifts. The compressibility of human tissue further complicates the interface which must fix the amount and thickness of the tissue being sampled while avoiding excess pressure which can degrade tissue integrity.

Thus, we see that to obtain consistent, accurate readings, the interface-to-tissue geometry must be preserved from measurement to measurement, and the optical path length in the tissue must also be long as possible, and remain constant during a measurement, and from measurement to measurement. The tissue chosen to measure and the optical and mechanical details of the spectrophotometer/tissue interface appear to be critical.

The idea of using vascular body tissues in place of a cuvette in a dispersive, NIR spectrophotometer was patented by Dähne and Gross (1987). Their system used the earlobe. A patent is not a research paper, so the performance of the instrument described was not evaluated. In 1989, Schlager patented a nondispersive, correlation, NIR spectrophotometer (see Section 8.2.3 of this book) designed to measure the tissue glucose, again in the earlobe. By placing an IR mirror at the back of the earlobe, glucose absorption resulting from two passes through the lobe was obtained. The principal advantage of this instrument's architecture is that it does not require an expensive, NIR monochromator. After passing the broadband light from the source through the tissue, the beam is imaged on a slit, then the slit (as a source) is refocused onto a beamsplitter. Half the beam energy is passed through a *negative correlation filter* (NCF), that is, a cuvette, containing a glucose solution that absorbs strongly at the glucose absorption wavelengths. Light emerging from the NCF is sensed by a lead sulfide IR sensor. The other half beam from the tissue sample is passed through a neutral density filter (NDF), thence to a (matched) lead sulfide sensor. Figure 15.16 illustrates a nondispersive IR spectrophotometer based on the Schlager system, and shows the necessary chopper. Note that this is a *proposed,* NI, glucose sensor architecture which needs clinical evaluation.

A relatively new spectrophotometric approach to the measurement of blood glucose uses the *Kromoscopy*™ system architecture (Sodickson and Block 1994, 1995). *Kromoscopy* is simply a nondispersive technique in which broadband IR is passed through the sample (*in vitro* or *in vivo*). The emergent beam is split into four equal intensity beams using three half-silvered mirrors, or beamsplitters; each separate beam is then passed through a particular, broadband, optical band-pass filter, thence to an InGaAs IR photodiode. The transmittance curves of the four filters overlap at their edges. There is nothing sacred about four detection channels; more channels

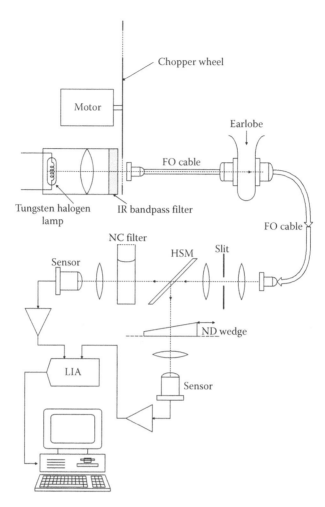

Figure 15.16 Schematic of a proposed nondispersive IR spectrophotometer used to measure the glucose concentration in earlobe tissue. (Based on a system patented by Schlager, K.J. 1989. *Non-Invasive Near Infrared Measurement of Blood Analyte Concentrations.* US Patent No. 4,882,492. (Transcutaneous non-dispersive spectrophotometry used to sense blood glucose using 900–1800 nm light.))

could theoretically lead to more robust measurements. A given, absorbing, chemical species in the sample is said to have a unique *Kolor* [sic] *vector* as the result of processing the four element vector made from the sensor signals.

In other aspects of the Kromoscopic system, one or more of the filters can be made narrow band-pass, band-reject, or a comb filter with multiple narrow passbands. Such complex filters can aid in the discrimination of the desired analyte from other, interfering, analytes. A detailed description of the basic theory underlying the Kromoscopic system, with examples, can be found in the *Detailed Description of the Invention* of Sodickson and Block (1995). The algorithms for processing the detector outputs appear to be proprietary.

It should be remarked that a similar, multidimensional, Kolor-type vector can be generated with a system using N, IR laser diodes, each emitting at a different wavelength. (The wavelengths are chosen to coincide with several of the absorption peaks and valleys of the analyte being measured.) After normalizing for the intensity of each laser, the transmitted or reflected output from the sample can be sensed by one photodiode assuming sequential chopping is used. No fil-ters are required. Such a laser diode-based system would be more expensive than the Kromoscopy system with its simple incandescent source and four filters; however, it may be more accurate and robust because of the narrow emission bandwidths of the lasers.

Finally, it is worthwhile to describe the MIR spectroscopic measurement blood glucose using the 310° blackbody radiation of the body as the IR source. First, the tissue containing the glucose to be

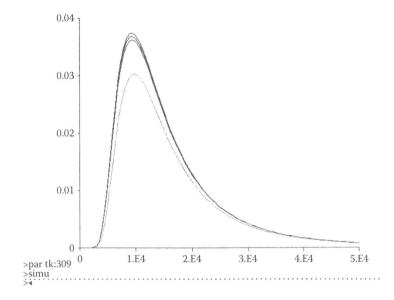

```
>par tk:309
>simu
>◄
```

Figure 15.17 Theoretical energy spectrum of an ideal blackbody at 25°C, 36°C, 37°C, and 38°C. The top curve is for 38°C. W_λ units are (W/m²)/nm. Note linear scales.

measured must itself be at a temperature less than the 310° source, or else no absorption spectrum will be seen. At 310°, the sample will only radiate as a blackbody (Klonoff et al. 1998). Figure 15.17 shows the spectral emission of an ideal blackbody calculated using Planck's radiation equation, at 25°C, 36°C, 37°C, and 38°C. Note that the peaks are at about $\lambda = 10\,\mu$m and W_o is down to 10% of the peak at ~4 μm.

Braig et al. (1997) described a means to measure the absorption of certain blood analytes in U.S. Patent # 5,615,672, using the body's own 310° blackbody radiation as a source. The medial surface of the forearm was illustrated as the source/analyte for the system. The system did not use a monochromator, but like the Kromoscopy approach, a filter wheel was used containing various IR band-pass filters; a single, cryo-cooled HgCdTe detector was used. The IR radiation from the object (forearm) was first chopped and then filtered before impinging on the detector. A microcomputer was programmed to calculate the estimated analyte concentration from the detector outputs for the various filters. It should be pointed out that this system only works because there is a temperature gradient from the 310° core of the forearm to the skin (298°). The IR absorption from the analyte in capillaries immediately underlying the skin would provide the system's signal.

Klonoff et al. (1998) tested the invention of Braig et al. on human subjects. The system, built by Optiscan Biomedical Corp., was reported to estimate blood glucose (verified by the YSI blood glucometer) with an $r^2 = 0.94$ and an overall standard error of 24.7 mg/dL. (The relative glucose absorption around 9.8 μm was examined.) This performance needs improvement before clinical application of the instrument. This type of instrument will always be bothered with sequential nonrepeatability and the need for calibration when used on different individuals and on the same individual at different times; the exact site on the skin, the skin temperature, the optical distance, etc., all need to be controlled.

M. J. Block was awarded U.S. patent # 6,002,953, 1999, for *Non-invasive IR Transmission Measurement of Analyte in the Tympanic Membrane*. In Block's system, the 310° blackbody IR from the *inner ear* acts as the radiation source for a cooler eardrum (tympanic membrane). (The tympanic membrane is oval in shape, contains many fine blood vessels, and is about 100 μm thick with an area of ~40 mm². It consists of three anatomical layers: (1) On the outside, a thin skin layer without papillae. (2) On the inside, a thin layer of simple, cuboidal ciliated epithelium. (3) In the center, a layer of radial fibers of connective tissue and a layer of circularly ordered connective tissue fibers. It is the connective tissue layers that give the eardrum its stiffness. The tympanum is also supplied with pain-sensing nerve endings. Block cooled the eardrum by exposing it to a heatsink consisting of a thermoelectrically cooled element inserted into the ear canal. Eardrum temperature reduction is by radiation from the eardrum to the chilled element and by conduction to air molecules in the ear canal. The sensing elements can be a cluster of four, miniature, MIR-sensing photodiodes covered with appropriate, miniature, optical band-pass filters, forming a Kromoscopy-type system. IR radiation from the inner ear passes through the cooler, vascular, tympanic membrane where absorption of photon energy occurs at certain wavelengths depending on the concentration of analytes in the blood including glucose. The emergent radiation from the tympanic membrane can be analyzed by a four-channel Kromoscopy system, as described above, or can be passed to another dispersive or nondispersive spectrophotometer outside the ear canal by direct focused radiation or by an MIR-conducting optical fiber. A problem with the use of the tympanic membrane to measure blood glucose is that it is thin, and from Beers' law, the resultant short optical path length produces a poor signal-to-noise ratio. Also, it is a mechanical challenge to chop the output radiation in the ear canal. As the peak of the natural 310° blackbody radiation is from 7 to 13 μm, the complex absorption peaks of glucose from 7 to 10 μm can be used, as well as its three, single peaks at 11, 12, and 13 μm. When working in the MIR, one needs special optics: gold-plated mirrors, IR-transmitting lenses such as Ge, Irtran, or plastic Fresnel lenses, special MIR-conducting optical fibers, and detectors such as pyroelectric or cryo-cooled HgCdTe sensors.

Kottmann et al. (2012) described a prototype system using photoacoustic (PA) signal generation from pulsed MIR photons of a set WN selectively absorbed by glucose in skin capillaries. As the name suggests, the photon-evoked PA signal is an acoustic pressure wave sensed by a microphone. PA signal amplitude is proportional to [bG]. The pulsed laser's output WN was tuned from 1010 to 1095 cm^{-1} to select maximum PA response. Kottmann et al. reported that their detection limit for epidermal glucose was 100 mg/dL (SNR = 1). They stated:

> Although this lies within the human physiological range (30–500 mg/dL), further improvements are necessary to noninvasively monitor glucose levels of diabetes patients. Furthermore, [PA] spectra of epidermal tissue with and without glucose content have been recorded with the tunable quantum-cascade laser, indicating that epidermal constituents do not impair glucose detection.

> One cause for their lack of detection sensitivity may be that the PA studies were carried out *in vitro* using fresh tissue samples (foreskins). There was no constant perfusion of blood.

An *in vivo* study by Hewlett-Packard using IR spectroscopy was reported by Hopkins (2006). They used the 1–2.5 μm spectral range because glucose has measurable absorption in this range and test beam photons penetrate into tissue sufficiently to sample glucose in capillary blood and interstitial fluid. Sadly, they concluded: "We were not successful at measuring blood glucose concentration accurately enough for home monitoring." Their accuracy was *approximately* three times poorer than required for a home-monitoring instrument.

An accurate, prototype, NI, *in vivo* glucose-sensing system using reflected IR light between 8 and 10 μm wavelength was described by Liakat et al. (2014). They used a quantum cascade laser source coupled to the skin by a hollow core fiber 500 μm diameter. The target skin was the web between the thumb and forefinger. The incident laser light was chopped at 55 kHz with a 1% duty cycle; it had peak powers of 50–125 mW (depending on wavelength), which yielded average powers that were on the order of solar radiation, and met limits set by ANSI for acceptable skin IR radiation intensity. Backscattered IR light from the skin was collected by a bundle of six fibers identical to the input fiber. The six fibers were arranged in a circular bundle around the input fiber and directly coupled to a commercial liquid nitrogen-cooled mercury cadmium telluride (MCT) detector. The conditioned detector output was input to a lock-in amplifier whose output was digitized and underwent DSP. The laser was scanned from 1040 to 1140 cm^{-1} (9.62–9.77 μm) in ~20 s; up to 10 scans were taken for each glucose concentration number. In addition, scans from 1075 to 1085 cm^{-1} (9.30–9.22 μm) were done around a prominent glucose absorption feature which gave very promising results.

A commercial electrochemical blood glucose meter "gold standard" was used at the beginning and end of each scan set. Liakat et al. (2014) concluded:

> In summary, we show that mid-IR spectra obtained *in vivo* from human skin yield clinically accurate predictions for blood glucose levels for concentrations between 75 and 160 mg/dL using both PLSR and derivative spectroscopy techniques. … Based on these results, we conclude that this application of mid-IR light to noninvasive *in vivo* glucose sensing yields a robust and clinically accurate system that transcends boundaries set in the past which limited the scope of mid-IR *in vivo* applications.

It will be interesting to see how the promising mid-IR spectroscopy system of Liakat et al. (2014) succeeds in its formal clinical trials. Note that any NI, transcutaneous, IR spectroscopic glucometer must rely on at least one calibration point from an electrochemical, blood drop glucose sensor. Skin colors, vasculature, and fat layers which all absorb, scatter, and reflect IR vary among individuals.

15.6.4 Discussion

All of the systems described above are ingenious, and their development into FDA-approved versions all face problems cited above. At best, such systems might be adjusted to work with a given individual after a two-point calibration using drawn blood and a "gold standard," such as the Yellow Spring Instruments Model 2300 STAT Plus™ glucometer. Repeatability will always be a problem because of anatomical differences over a given body region, and changes in instrument placement geometry. At this writing, there are only two, fairly reliable means for personal monitoring of blood glucose: the much-maligned, fingerprick-chemical-strip-colorimetric and amperometric methods which use a drop of blood.

While this section has focused on the measurement of glucose using TIR light, the reader will recall that there are other *intrinsic* analytes in blood that IR absorption/transmittance/reflection techniques may be able to measure including cholesterol. *Extrinsic* drug molecules that show promise for NI, transcutaneous, IR spectroscopic measurement include ethanol, cocaine, THC, etc. However, because of the problems of individual anatomical differences in skin and underlying tissues (fat, pigmentation, blood vessels), calibration and repeatability remain constant obstacles.

15.7 ESTIMATION OF BLOOD GLUCOSE FROM NI MEASUREMENT OF OPTICAL ROTATION OF THE AQUEOUS HUMOR OF THE EYE (A PROTOTYPE SYSTEM)

15.7.1 Introduction

Over the past three decades and more, a number of workers have tried to develop effective, accurate sensors for blood glucose measurement to aid in the management of diabetes mellitus. Most of these sensors require samples of a body fluid such as blood or interstitial fluid, and are by nature invasive or semi-invasive. More recently, attention has been given to the development of truly NI blood glucose measurement means. One such approach has attempted to use the wavelength-selective absorption or transmission of NIR light by glucose in vascular tissues. Another approach, which was followed by the author and his graduate students, was first described by March (1977, 1984), March et al. (1982), and Rabinovitch et al. (1982). March and Rabinovitch realized that the AH in the anterior chamber of the eye could be used to estimate blood glucose (BG) concentration. The glucose concentration of AH follows that of the BG with a few minutes time lag, and at about an 80% level. They proposed to measure the OR of a beam LPL directed through the anterior chamber of the eye. This OR is mostly due to the glucose dissolved in the AH. Hence, measurement of the OR should enable an estimate the blood glucose concentration to be made. The approach of March and Rabinovitch made use of the fact that aqueous solutions of glucose are *optically active*, that is, they rotate the vibration axis of the E vector of transmitted LPL by an angle given by the simple relation:

$$\phi = [\alpha]_{\lambda}^{T} LC, \tag{15.73}$$

where L is the optical path length through the solution, C is the concentration of the optically active solute (i.e., glucose), T is the Kelvin temperature, λ is the wavelength of the light, and $[\alpha]_{\lambda}^{T}$ is the specific rotation constant in degrees/(cm path length × concentration unit); α is both temperature and wavelength dependent. In general, the magnitude of $[\alpha]_{\lambda}^{T}$ increases as the wavelength gets shorter. $[\alpha]_{\lambda}^{T}$ can have either sign (L or D OR) depending on the solute.

If more than one optically active solute is in solution together, the net rotation is given by the relation below, which implies linear superposition of optical activities:

$$\phi = \sum_{k=1}^{N} [\alpha]_{\lambda k}^{T} C_{k} L. \tag{15.74}$$

Finding the concentration of the desired substance under this condition can be as simple as assuming the other optically active constituents are at negligible or constant concentrations, or it may require N measurements of ϕ at N different λs. From the N simultaneous equations, $C_{1} \ldots C_{N}$ can be solved for using Cramer's rule, the N measured ϕ's, and the N^2 known $[\alpha]_{\lambda k}^{T}$.

The author and certain of his graduate students developed a prototype NI instrument to measure the OR of glucose in the AH. The small rotation caused by the glucose in the AH was

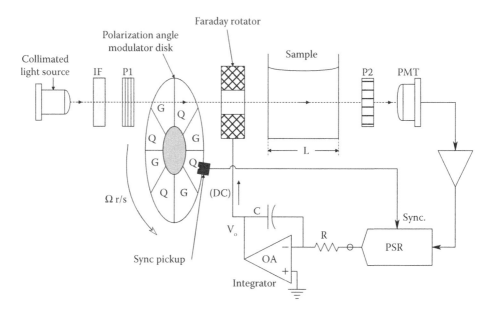

Figure 15.18 Schematic of Gilham's original closed-loop microdegree resolution polarimeter. PSR = phase-sensitive rectifier. Square-wave polarization angle modulation was done by the rotating disk that had alternating windows of glass and polarizing quartz.

accurately measured in the presence of "confounders," that is, other optically active substances in the AH and the birefringence of the cornea in an optical model eye.

A.F. Browne (1998) designed, built, and tested a proof-of-concept, optical model system that demonstrated the validity of our instrument design. This prototype NI electro-optical instrument hopefully will lead to the development of an inexpensive, approved, medical instrument that will allow diabetics to quickly, accurately, and painlessly estimate their blood glucose concentrations. The chemical composition of AH has been well-described (de Berardinis et al. 1965). D-glucose is known to be the principal optically active substance in the AH that rotates LPL (Rabinovitch et al. 1982). Thus, a means of measuring the OR of the AH can be used to estimate the blood glucose concentration.

Our prototype system used an improved microdegree ocular polarimeter based on the original design by Gilham (1957). (Gilham's original system is shown in Figure 15.18.) We developed our microdegree polarimeter as part of a Phase I SBIR research project in 1995; it was applied to the NI measurement of the OR caused by D-glucose in the AH. In our configuration of the instrument, a beam of monochromatic LPL of innocuous intensity was polarization angle modulated by a Faraday rotator (FR), then directed through the cornea, the pupil, the AH, and was reflected off the front surface of the lens. The reflected beam emerged from the eye with a greatly reduced intensity, and an additional, small OR due to other optically active substances in the AH, and the birefringence of the cornea. The emergent beam was directed to a polarizer/analyzer, P2, and thence to a photomultiplier light sensor. Details of the operation of the modified, closed-loop, Gilham-type polarimeter are given below. A schematic of the proposed system is shown in Figure 15.19. Browne (1998) demonstrated theoretically, and physically with a model system, that there is a restricted range of polarized light entry angle relative to the gaze vector over which the system will work.

15.7.2 Open-Loop Gilham Microdegree Polarimeter

The heart of the ocular polarimeter for blood glucose estimation is the modified Gilham polarimeter developed by the author and graduate students, Aidan Browne and Todd Nelson. Before describing the operation of the modified, closed-loop Gilham polarimeter, it is important to understand how an *open-loop* Gilham polarimeter works. Figure 15.20 illustrates the open-loop system. Linearly polarized monochromatic light is derived by passing collimated, monochromatic, polarized light from a source through a high-quality Glan calcite polarizer, P1. Polarizers P1 and P2 have extinction ratios of $>5 \times 10^4$:1. P1 and the laser source are aligned so that the linearly

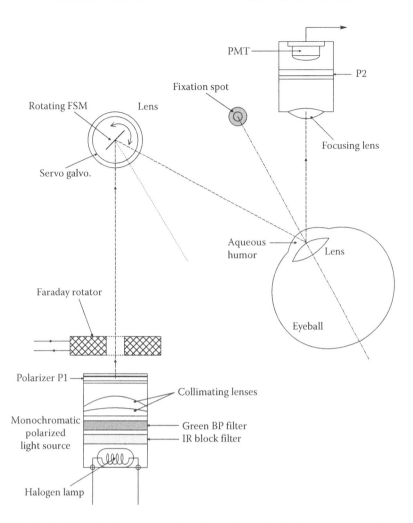

Figure 15.19 Optical layout of a proposed ocular polarimeter that can measure the optical rotation of the aqueous humor (AH) in the eye which is largely due to glucose. The measurement of glucose in the AH can be used to estimate the blood glucose concentration. The sinusoidal polarization angle modulation of the incident beam is done with a Faraday rotator. The moving mirror is used to align the beam; it is stationary during a measurement. P1 and P2 are linear polarizers, PMT = photomultiplier tube.

polarized electromagnetic **E** vector vibrates in the X–Z plane at a frequency $\nu = c/\lambda$ Hz as it propagates with velocity c. This LPL is next passed through an FR. The FR consists of a dense glass rod with optically polished and antireflection (AR)-coated flat ends. An axially directed magnetic **B** field passes through the axis of the rod. The linearly polarized electromagnetic light waves interact with the material of the rod and the axial B field ($\mathbf{B}_z$) to cause a total OR, θ_{mo}, as they exit the rod (Hecht 1987). The total **E** vector axis rotation is given by the relation:

$$\theta_{mo} = VB_zL, \tag{15.75}$$

where V is the rotator material's *Verdet constant*, which is material, temperature, and wavelength dependent.

In general, V increases with decreasing wavelength. $\mathbf{B}_z$ is the mean Z axis component of the magnetic field (parallel to the *Poynting vector*), and L is the length that the light travels in the Faraday rod and B field.

Practically all transparent liquids (e.g., water) and solids (e.g., glass) exhibit the Faraday magneto-optic effect. That is, they can rotate the axis of the **E** vector of LPL when subjected to an axial magnetic field.

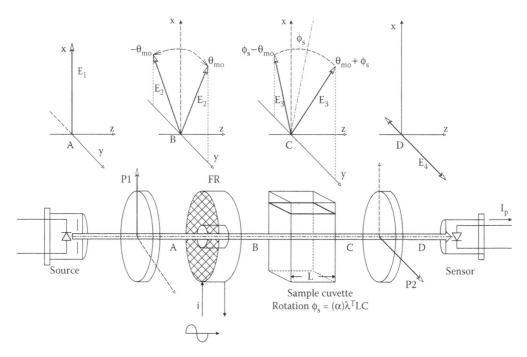

Figure 15.20 Schematic of an *open-loop* Gilham polarimeter. The Faraday rotator sinusoidally modulates the polarization angle of the input beam. Mathematical analysis of this system is in the text.

In the open-loop Gilham polarimeter, the FR is used to sinusoidally modulate the axis angle θ_m of the emergent **E** vector. This modulation is accomplished by passing an audio-frequency AC current through a solenoidal coil wound around the FR glass rod. This current causes the axial B field to vary as $B_z(t) = B_{zo} \sin(2\pi f_m t)$. Thus from Equation 15.75, the polarization angle of the emergent **E** vector varies as

$$\theta_m(t) = (VLB_{zo})\sin(2\pi f_m t) = \theta_{mo}\sin(2\pi f_m t). \tag{15.76}$$

System parameters are chosen so θ_{mo} typically ranges from $1°$ to $3°$. The modulation frequency, f_m, can range from 20 Hz to 2 kHz depending on coil design.

After modulating the angle of the **E** vector of the LP light emerging from the FR, the light is passed through an optically active (e.g., glucose) solution, where the **E** vector picks up a fixed clockwise rotation, ϕ_s, from the D-glucose in solution following Equation 15.74. From Figure 15.20, we see that the **E** vector of the polarized light emerging from the sample cuvette swings sinusoidally from $(\phi_s - \theta_{mo})$ to $+(\phi_s + \theta_{mo})$ in the X–Y plane at the FR modulation frequency. The next critical optical element in the open-loop Gilham polarimeter is the calcite analyzer polarizer, P2. The pass axis of polarizer P2 is adjusted to be exactly $90°$ from the input beam **E** vector axis, along the y-axis. If we assume P2 is an "ideal" polarizer, then only the y-component of the **E** vector at point C emerges from P2 at D. The peak amplitude of $\mathbf{E_x}$ at D is $\mathbf{E_4}$. By *Malus' law*, the peak $\mathbf{E_4}$ is given by

$$E_4(t) = E_{4o}\sin[\phi_s + \theta_{mo}\sin(2\pi f_m t)]. \tag{15.77}$$

The *irradiance* of this beam, i_4, is proportional to E_4^2 (Hecht 1987). Thus:

$$i_4(t) = E_{4o}^2\left(c\varepsilon_o/2\right)\sin^2[\phi_s + \theta_{mo}\sin(2\pi f_m t)] \; W/m^2. \tag{15.78}$$

Now by trig identity, $\sin^2(x) = [1 - \cos(2x)]/2$, so

$$i_4(t) = E_{4o}^2(c\varepsilon_o/2)[1 - \cos\{2\phi_s + 2\theta_{mo}\sin(2\pi f_m t)\}]/2. \tag{15.79}$$

The photosensor output is proportional to the irradiance; sic:

$$V_D(t) = K_P i_4(t) = K_P E_{4o}^2(c\varepsilon_o/2)[1 - \cos\{2\phi_s + 2\theta_{mo}\sin(2\pi f_m t)\}] / 2. \tag{15.80}$$

Since the cos{*} angle argument is small, that is, $|2(\phi_s + \theta_{mo})| < 3°$, we can use the approximation, $\cos(x) \cong (1 - x^2/2)$ in Equation 15.80. Thus, the photosensor output can be written as

$$V_D(t) = K_P I_{4o}[\phi_s^2 + 2\phi_s\theta_{mo}\sin(2\pi f_m t) + \theta_{mo}^2\{1 - \cos(4\pi f_m t)\}]. \quad (15.81)$$

Thus in the photosensor output voltage, we see 2 DC (average) terms, a sinusoidal term at the modulation frequency, f_m, whose amplitude is proportional to the unknown ϕ_s, and a double frequency cosine term. The phase-sensitive rectifier (PSR) (or lock-in amplifier) responds only to the fundamental frequency term. The DC photosensor output to the PSR is blocked by a simple RC high-pass filter. After suitable low-pass filtering, the PSR's DC output can be written as

$$V_L = K_L K_P I_{4o} 2\phi_s\theta_{mo} \text{ DC V}. \quad (15.82)$$

V_L is seen to depend not only on the unknown ϕ_s but also on the beam intensity, I_{4o}, and on the depth of modulation, θ_{mo}. While θ_{mo} can be held constant, I_{4o} can be subject to considerable variation especially from a nonstabilized laser source. It is this dependence on the constancy of I_{4o} that can be troublesome in open-loop operation. We show below that the Type 1 closed-loop operation of the Gilham polarimeter yields robust results, including independence from certain system parameters, including I_{4o}.

15.7.3 Dynamics and Sensitivity of the Closed-Loop Polarimeter

In the author's version of the closed-loop Gilham polarimeter, a DC current proportional to the DC error angle, ϕ_E, is fed-back to the solenoid coil of the FR to produce a DC component of the magnetic field that causes a counter rotation of the optical **E** vector axis, ϕ_F, that exactly cancels the rotation, ϕ_s, caused by the sample. Thus at any instant, the DC error angle is:

$$\phi_E = \phi_s - \phi_F. \quad (15.83)$$

Figure 15.21 illustrates the modified, closed-loop Gilham system as developed by Browne (1988). It is shown measuring the OR of a sample in a 1 cm cuvette. The average (DC) output of the PSR is now proportional to the error angle in OR, ϕ_E. Nulling of the system occurs when $\phi_s = \phi_F$. The effective gain of the PSR is $2K_L K_P I_{4o}\theta_{mo}$. (The intensity I_{4o} is proportional to the source laser's beam

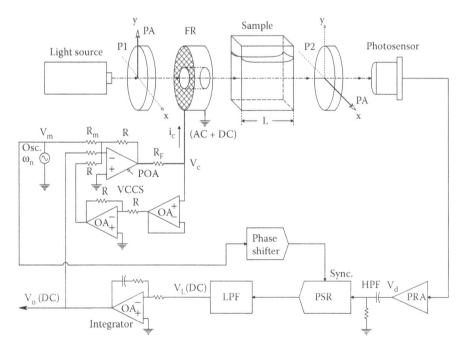

Figure 15.21 Schematic of the improved, closed-loop Gilham polarimeter developed by the author. The same Faraday rotator is used for polarization angle modulation and for DC feedback to automatically null the system.

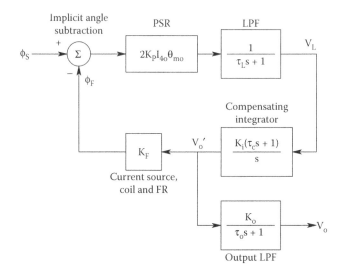

Figure 15.22 Block diagram describing the linearized dynamics of the polarimeter of Figure 15.21.

intensity.) A first-order low-pass filter with DC gain $=1$ and time constant, τ_L, follows the PSR to extract its average output voltage, V_L. V_L is then input to a proportional + integral (PI) controller element to make the closed-loop system Type 1 with zero steady-state error. The DC output of the PI element drives a voltage-controlled current source (VCCS) that sets the DC nulling current through the FR solenoid coil. A high-voltage power op-amp is used as the actual FR coil driver supplying both the DC nulling current and the AC polarization modulation current.

The block diagram of the system is shown in Figure 15.22. If we examine the closed-loop transfer function relating V_o' to ϕ_s, we find that it has a quadratic denominator. This transfer function can be used to describe the system turn-on transient or the transient response of the system to transient changes in ϕ_s. It is:

$$\frac{V_o'}{\phi_s} = \frac{2K_P I_{4o}\theta_{mo} G_M K_i(\tau_c s+1)/\tau_L}{s^2 + s(1 + 2K_P I_{4o}\theta_{mo} G_M K_i \tau_c K_F)/\tau_L + 2K_P I_{4o}\theta_{mo} G_M K_i K_F/\tau_L}. \tag{15.84}$$

From the transfer function above, we see that the closed-loop system has an undamped natural frequency of

$$\omega_n = \sqrt{2K_P I_{4o}\theta_{mo} G_M K_i K_F/\tau_L} \ \ \text{r/s}. \tag{15.85}$$

And a damping factor of

$$\zeta = 1/(2\omega_n) + \tau_c/2. \tag{15.86}$$

In the steady state, the system's DC gain is simply:

$$\frac{V_o'}{\phi_s} = \frac{1}{K_F}. \tag{15.87}$$

Equation 15.87 is a rather profound result because it tells us that determination of the steady-state ϕ_s *does not* depend on the laser beam intensity or the peak modulation angle, θ_{mo}, or certain other system constants. To be sure, the beam intensity and θ_{mo}, etc. must have values chosen for practical reasons for satisfactory robust system operation. Thus, only the physical factors affecting K_F affect system accuracy. By using a VCCS to drive the FR coil, the effect of coil resistance changing with temperature is eliminated. However, the Verdet constant of the FR glass rod is a function of temperature; the rod will be heated by the power dissipation of the coil. Unfortunately, there is no easy way to keep the FR glass rod temperature constant. If we measure the rod's Verdet constant's tempco and put a temperature sensor in intimate contact with the rod, we can then compensate for temperature-caused changes in the Verdet constant. The system's steady-state sensitivity is dependent of source intensity fluctuations, and modulation depth, θ_{mo}, contributing to its robustness. However, electronic noise arising within the loop can degrade system resolution and accuracy.

A significant source of broadband noise injected into the loop is from the photosensor and its signal conditioning amplifier. A wise choice of components, PSR filtering time constant, and further low-pass filtering of V_o' will help maximize the system signal-to-noise ratio. The closed-loop system should be designed to have a low ω_n (~12 r/s) and a damping factor lying between 0.5 and 0.707.

In bench tests of the self-nulling polarimeter, we found that its resolution (LOD) was better than 150 microdegrees of OR. The polarimeter was able to measure the OR of aqueous D-glucose solutions in the physiological range of concentrations in a 1 cm cuvette with an LMS linear data fit having an $r^2 = 0.9986$. (The average rotation of a 100 mg/dL dextrose solution in a 1 cm path at 633 nm wavelength was 4.53 millidegrees.)

15.7.4 Application of the Modified Gilham Polarimeter to the Measurement of the Optical Rotation of Aqueous Humor in a Model system

Figure 15.23 illustrates the modified Gilham system's components in the horizontal plane, illustrating how a monochromatic beam of LPL is directed into the eye, reflected off the front surface of the lens, and passed out through the cornea to the analyzer and photomultiplier. The input beam intensity is adjusted to be at an eye-safe level; bright, but not harmful.

Browne (1998) mathematically analyzed the optics of polarized light reflection at a dielectric reflecting surface with particular attention to the AH of the eye and the front surface of the lens. In discussing the optics of the reflection of LPL off the plane surfaces, we first define the *plane of incidence*. The plane of incidence holds the incoming and reflected rays and the normal vector to the reflecting surface. In general, it is always perpendicular to the plane reflecting surface. For our purposes, we will define it as the X–Z plane. A ray always propagates in the direction of its Poynting vector, here defined as the local y-axis. In general, the unit vectors are related by the vector cross product: $\mathbf{x} \times \mathbf{y} = \mathbf{z}$. A simple planar surface diagram of the boundary and reflection is shown in Figure 15.24.

The reflecting surface is transparent and has an index of refraction, $n_2 = c/v_2$ (c is the velocity of light in free space, and v_2 is the velocity of light in the reflecting medium). Reflection occurs at the interface of AH with index of refraction, n_1, and the reflecting front surface of the lens having index,

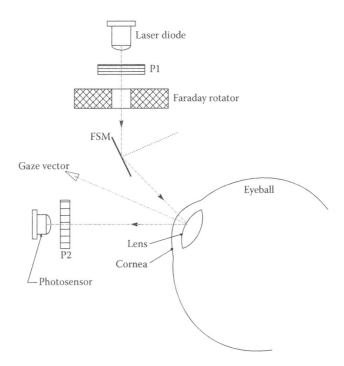

Figure 15.23 Simple optical architecture of the polarimeter applied to the measurement of the glucose concentration in the AH. (See Figure 15.19.)

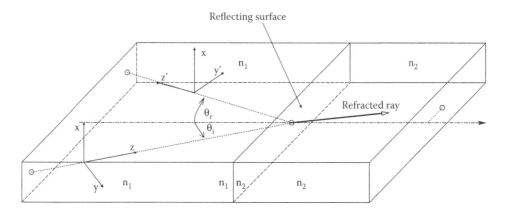

Figure 15.24 Relevant vectors describing how TEM linearly polarized light acts at a plane boundary between two transparent media having different refractive indices.

n_2 $(n_2 > n_1)$. The incident ray's **z** vector can be normal to the reflecting surface, but more generally it is at some angle β to the unit vector, **n**, which is normal to the reflecting surface at the point where the ray strikes it.

The incident **E** vector of the LPL can have a component in the y direction, which lies in the plane of incidence; this is called the *TM component* of **E**. The **E** component parallel with the x-axis (and thus normal to the plane if incidence) is called the *TE component*.

We are interested in what happens to the intensity of the reflected ray at the n_1/n_2 interface, and what happens to its **E** vector when it reaches the corneal boundary. The n_1 medium (AH) is optically active because it contains glucose; hence, the axis of the **E** vector of the incoming ray is rotated by a small clockwise angle, α. What happens to the reflected **E** vector depends on the incidence angle, θ_i, the initial angle of **E**, the OR, α, and n_1 and n_2. In his analysis, Browne (1998) considered three input angle conditions: $\theta_i < \theta_B$, $\theta_i = \theta_B$, and $\theta_i > \theta_B$. θ_B is the Brewster angle, defined by

$$\theta_B \equiv \tan^{-1}\left(\frac{n_2}{n_1}\right). \tag{15.88}$$

When the **E** vector of LPL of the input beam is all in the TM mode (**E** lies in the plane of incidence), there will be *zero* light intensity reflected when $\theta_i = \theta_B$. Browne assumed an arbitrary polarization angle with respect to the x-axis; that is, the polarization angle of the input beam of LPL is ϕ just as it enters the n_1 medium. As it propagates to the n_1/n_2 boundary, the optical activity of the n_1 medium causes **E** to rotate an additional α degrees. Thus, just before the reflection boundary, the incoming beam has a TM component (in the plane of incidence) of $E_o \sin(\phi + \alpha)$, and the TE component of **E** (in the x-direction) is $E_o \cos(\phi + \alpha)$ as the input wave strikes the n_1/n_2 boundary. In the reflected wave, the TE component of **E** undergoes an 180° phase change for all input angles. The TM component behaves differently depending on θ_i: for $\theta_i < \theta_B$, there is no phase change. For $\theta_i = \theta_B$, the reflected TM component = 0. For $\theta_i > \theta_B$, there is an 180° phase change in the reflected TM component of **E**. The bottom line of Browne's analysis was that when $\theta_i > \theta_B$, the polarization angle of the ray emerging from the n_1 medium into air was shown to be $\beta = \phi + 2\alpha$. When $\theta_i < \theta_B$, $\beta = \phi$, that is, there is no sensitivity to OR; the outward rotation cancels the inward rotation. For a real eye, $\theta_B \cong 46.9°$.

Browne concluded:

A reflection angle relative to gaze normal [the gaze vector] anywhere in the range of fifty to fifty-five degrees is achievable for all cases. Over this range, the incident beam input angle can be any value in the range of fifty-five to sixty degrees, relative to gaze normal; this range is well within the limits of the Brewster angle on the low end and the maximum angle due to physical limitations on the high end.

"These results clearly show that the geometry of the eye is very tolerant of parameter changes in regard to light pathway through the anterior chamber."

Browne also considered the light intensity budget of the eye and the safe exposure energy for the retina. Calculable losses due to reflections occur at every boundary between two media with different refractive indices. At the lens, most of the light is refracted and sent to the retina, only a small fraction is reflected. Assuming 5 mW of 512 nm laser light enters the eye, about 6.1 μW exits the cornea as a result of reflection off the front surface of the lens. This amounts to an attenuation factor of 9.37×10^{-4}.

Safety standards for laser light shined into the eye are quite strict (OSHA 1999, FDA 2015a,b). The maximum power density that is considered eye safe at 512 nm is 2.5 mW/cm² for 0.25 s. This is the same as 25 μW/mm² over 0.25 s. Thus, if the laser beam has a diameter of 2 mm on the retina, its area is 3.14 mm², and the maximum beam power cannot exceed 78.5 μW for 0.25 s. This power translates to an *output beam power* from the eye of 95.8 nW for 0.25 s. This is adequate power for a PMT to sense. If the modulation frequency, f_m, is 2 kHz, the PSR has a total of 500 modulation cycles to average to find $V_o' \propto \alpha$. If the SNR is poor, this may not be enough time to average out the noise.

To avoid the government safety restrictions on laser input power to the eye, the polarized light can be derived from a conventional tungsten (quartz-halogen) lamp. The light is filtered to exclude IR, band-pass filtered with an interference filter to define a narrow bandwidth and then collimated. It is then linearly polarized and sent to the FR, thence to the eye. Optometrists' and ophthalmologists' ophthalmoscopes and slit lamps use high-intensity quartz-halogen lamps, and are considered safe for prolonged use in eye exams. Tungsten lamps are considerably less expensive than stable diode lasers and are a viable alternative in configuring this type of instrument.

Browne (1998) evaluated the modified Gilham ocular polarimeter with an *analog model eye*. This eye was built with a glass meniscus lens "cornea" having a refractive index of 1.439. It was 0.8 mm thick at the center; 11.78 mm diameter; front radius of curvature 7.7 mm; rear radius of curvature 6.8 mm. The inside apex of the meniscus lens was mounted about 3 mm from the outer apex of the inner lens. The plano-convex inner lens was made from SF5 glass; its front radius of curvature was 10.09 mm. Artificial AH containing various glucose concentrations could be introduced into the "anterior chamber" of the model eye. In one plot of V_o versus glucose concentration over a range of 0–3 g/L, The LMS linear fit to data had an $r^2 = 0.9989$, quite a good, linear fit. These measurement were made using the full 6 mW output of the 512 nm diode laser.

In adapting this system to take accurate measurements from human eyes, the input light power will have to be seriously reduced, as discussed above. Also, the system must be calibrated for each user by taking several conventional finger-prick blood samples at different, steady-state blood glucose levels along with V_o measurements. It will be a considerable challenge to develop a clinical and home version of this instrument.

15.7.5 Discussion

In the preceding sections, we have described the prototype of an NI, electro-optical system designed to enable diabetics to quickly, painlessly, and frequently monitor their blood glucose concentration, and so adjust their intake of insulin, food, and exercise to better achieve normoglycemia.

The present state of the art for home blood glucose monitoring requires taking a blood sample; not more than one or two drops of venous blood using a small lancet or needle. Usually one of the fingertips or an earlobe is pierced. The blood drops are smeared on a chemically treated plastic strip, which after about a 60 second reaction time is read in a two-wavelength colorimeter, the output of which is an estimate of the blood glucose concentration. This method strongly discourages frequent use by the patient, especially children, and has the following *disadvantages*:

1. The procedure is *semi-invasive*. It provides an opportunity for infection in a population already predisposed to infections of the extremities.

2. The procedure is *painful*, especially when 5 or 6 pricks a day are required.

3. The procedure is *not accurate*. Accuracy can be off by as much as ±20% due to age and lot variations in the chemical strips, as well as changes in ambient temperature and nonadherence to a uniform testing procedure.

4. The procedure is *expensive*. While the monitors are generally inexpensive as medical devices go, the manufacturers' profit is assured through the sale of the strips. The average cost of an electrochemical test strip is $0.98.

The overall mean utilization for pharmacy-based, self-monitoring, blood glucose test strips is 764.3 strips/year. This amounts to an average yearly cost of $749 (Yeaw et al. 2012).

The overall objective of the research described was to develop a prototype of an accurate, NI, ocular polarimeter to estimate blood glucose concentration that will successfully replace the present finger prick-test strip-colorimeter technology at a cost comparable to 1 year's supply of test strips. Any prototype instrument developed would have to undergo FDA approval before it could be marketed to help diabetics. To be marketable, it must have a reasonable cost, be easy to use, and have an accuracy better than the finger prick method described above. There will be a large market for the instrument; *there are an estimated 387 million diabetics worldwide* (IDF6E 2014); that is, ~8.3% of the adult population. Type 2 diabetes make up ~90% of the cases. In the United States, diabetes care cost ~$245 billion in 2012 (ADA 2013).

Any accurate, truly NI blood glucose sensor would find a potential enormous market worldwide.

15.8 SEMI-INVASIVE, CONTINUOUS MEASUREMENT OF BLOOD GLUCOSE USING SUBCUTANEOUS SENSORS

15.8.1 Introduction

There are many theoretical and practical advantages to continuously monitoring a diabetic's blood glucose concentration [BG], not the least is to use the sensor's output as an input to a computer that continually adjusts the infusion rate of exogenous insulin to achieve normoglycemia.

To achieve continuous [BG] monitoring, the best solution appears to be a miniaturized, *implantable* sensor (Klonoff 2007). In this section, we will describe the latest efforts in developing a semi-invasive, subcutaneous interstitial fluid glucose [ifG] concentration-sensing system (Croce et al. 2013). We consider a subcutaneous sensor to be minimally invasive. Note that most physicians in the United States give [BG] in units of mg/dL, and researchers typically use units of mM/L; 1 mM/L = 18 mg/dL. 1 dL = 0.1 L.

Klonoff (2007) stated:

Subcutaneous glucose sensors are the ideal tool for measuring glycemic variability, which is a recently recognized risk factor for diabetic microvascular disease. Glycemic variability has been linked to oxidative stress which is linked to vasculopathy.... Continuous glucose monitoring is the best tool for assessing glycemic variability.

Some of the problems with implanted glucose sensors include: (1) The human body (immune system) generally treats implanted sensors as foreign objects and reacts accordingly. (2) The sensors require a DC power source: either a battery or an extra-corporeal source such as RF energy or light which is converted internally to DC power by the sensor's electronics. Another potential sensor power sources include piezoelectric current generated internally by body motion. DC power may also be obtained from implantable, nonenzymatic, glucose fuel cells. The body's [BG] itself was used in the prototype system devised by Onescu and Ekickson (2013), which could reach a volumetric power density of over 16 $\mu W/cm^3$. (3) Sensor operation is generally dependent on immobilized enzymes such as glucose oxidase or metallic oxide catalysts (Rahman et al. 2010, Kwon et al. 2012). Catalysts and enzymes can become "poisoned" and loose efficiency due to biological interference in long-term installations, requiring periodic recalibration, or sensor replacement.

The operating mechanism of most implanted glucose sensors is an electrochemical redox cell using glucose as a fuel, excess oxygen, and the enzyme glucose oxidase (GOx) as a catalyst. An amperometric glucose cell is held at a constant DC potential and supplied with dissolved O_2. The cell's current flowing to ground is an increasing function of the glucose concentration in the cell. The chemical outputs of the cell's reactions include gluconic acid (from glucose) and hydrogen peroxide.

15.8.2 Biorasis Inc. Glucowizzard™ Subcutaneous Continuous Glucose Monitoring

An early example of an implantable glucose sensor with a telemetry output was described by Beach et al. (1999). A contemporary prototype version of the system of Beach et al. has been described by Croce et al. (2013) and is being developed by *Biorasis Inc*. The Biorasis IC Glucowizzard sensor is a grain of rice-sized cylinder (0.5 × 10 mm) that is implanted subcutaneously using a 16-Gauge hypodermic needle; it uses CMOS circuitry. The amperometric glucose sensor has an area of 0.407 mm^2 and consumes ~108 μW of power. The Glucowizzard's signal processing circuitry has an area of 0.258 mm^2 and draws ~19 μA. There is a total power consumption of ~140 μW.

The Glucowizzard electrochemical amperometric glucose sensor cell described by Croce et al. (2013) has five functional layers: (1) Outermost layer 5 (75–100 μm thick) is a composite hydrogel membrane of polyvinyl alcohol (PVA) embedded with the anti-inflammatory steroid, dexamethasone-loaded, poly (lactic-co-glycolic acid) (PLGA) microspheres. (2) Next, layer 4 (5–10 μm) is glutaraldehyde-immobilized Catalase, designed to break down H_2O_2 to H_2O. (3) Layer 3 (1–3 μm) is a Glucose Flux-Limiting polyurethane (PU) membrane. (4) Layer 4 (75–100 μm) consists of glutaraldehyde-immobilized Glucose Oxidase (GOx) enzyme. Here, glucose and oxygen entering the cell react with GOx to form hydrogen peroxide (H_2O_2) and Gluconic acid (GA), which must leave the cell by diffusion. (5) The fifth and final layer (10 nm) consists of an Electropolymerized Poly(phenol) (PPh) film coating the platinum working electrode. A total of 0.7 V is maintained between the working electrode and an external Ag|AgCl reference electrode.

The amperometric output current from the glucose sensor cell (which is held at a constant 0.7 V potential) is fed to a VFC whose output pulse frequency is proportional to the interstitial fluid glucose concentration [ifG]. The VFC output frequency range spanned ~1.25–20 kHz given an input current range of ~0.1–1.5 μA. The sensor responds linearly well beyond the physiological [ifG] range (2–22 mM), over 0–25 mM (or 450 mg/dL). The entire sensor is coated with a PVA hydrogel and dexamethasone-loaded poly (lactic-co-glycolic acid) microspheres intended to provide continuous, localized delivery of the steroid *dexamethasone* to suppress immune inflammation and fibrosis.

Power for the implanted Glucowizzard is derived from periodic pulses of light energy from the readout device acting through the skin on photodiodes (operated as solar cells) on the sensor. Power is stored on a capacitor. The wrist-worn readout device is based on the Texas Instruments eZ430-Chronos™ development kit.

The sensor pulse output frequency drives a flashing on-board LED, the light from which is transmitted transcutaneously to a photodiode under the readout device. The photodiode's output pulse frequency is conditioned to drive a readout display showing the current history of a patient's [ifG] as well as be sent by a UHF RF link to a computer for processing and storage.

Note that there are several sources of inaccuracy for implantable, amperometric glucose sensors. These include but are not limited to changes in cell temperature, variations in local pO_2, the variable delay between changes in [BG] and [ifG], delay between a change in sensor [ifG] and sensor steady-state response (settling time), change in catalyst (GOx) efficiency, and bio-fouling of the cell's outer membrane.

Interstitial fluid glucose concentration [ifG] measured continuously subcutaneously follows the blood glucose concentration [bG] with a delay and a slightly reduced amplitude. Clinically, we are interested in [bG]; however, it is the [ifG] that is measured. It is possible to obtain a good estimate of [bG] if the transfer function relating [bG] to [ifG] can be estimated; this relationship can be expressed in the time domain as a continuous, real convolution integral:

$$[ifG](t) = \int_{-\infty}^{t} g(t-u)\,[bG](u)du = g(t)^{*}[bG](t), \qquad (15.89)$$

where * denotes the real convolution operation, g(t) is the impulse response (weighting function) of the [BG]-to-[ifG] system. In the Laplace (frequency) domain, we can write the convolution as: [ifG](s) = G(s) [BG](s). Thus [BG](s) = [ifG](s)/G(s). [ifG](t) is recorded and g(t) is estimated. G(jω) is generally low-pass in nature.

The problem of the [BG] to (interstitial) [ifG] transfer function (G(s)) dynamics was addressed by Guerra et al. (2012). They showed that these dynamics could be effectively compensated for by a deconvolution procedure operating on the sensor's output signal, [ifG](t), that relied on a linear regression model of the transfer function, g(t). The g(t) model could be updated whenever a pair of suitably sampled [BG] and [ifG] data records was recorded. The simple model used for the weighting function (impulse response) of the [BG] $\rightarrow$ [ifG] transfer function by Guerra et al. was: $g(t) = (\mu/\tau)\,e^{-t/\tau}$. Here, μ is a DC gain and τ is the model's time constant. Two optimum parameters (τ, μ) had to be determined in order to accurately calculate [BG] from the [ifG] record using discrete deconvolution. Note that another simple gain model could be: $[ifG](t) = \mu[BG](t - \delta)$, where μ is a static gain and δ is a transport lag (delay operation). The method of Guerra et al. can be applied to the output of any subcutaneous glucose sensor or the [BG]-to-AH glucose [ahG] system. (Note that the Fourier transform of g(t) is $\mu/(j\omega\tau + 1)$.)

One way to resolve uncertainty in sensor calibration is to use two or more sensors. With three sensors, output data can be averaged and a bad sensor spotted, removed, and replaced (Castle and Ward 2010). The functional, *in vivo* lifespan of the implanted Glucowizzard is not yet known.

15.9 PULSE OXIMETRY

15.9.1 Introduction

There are numerous medical procedures in which a knowledge of the percent saturation of arterial blood Hb with oxygen is important. Such procedures include but are not limited to childbirth (the baby and the mother), during surgical anesthesia where the patient is artificially ventilated, any open-chest surgery where a heart–lung machine is used, treatment of obstructive lung diseases including pulmonary emphysema and acute asthma, the treatment of drowning and smoke inhalation, and general intensive care and surgical recovery.

The molecular weight of Hb is ~64,400 daltons. The Hb molecule consists of four iron (Fe^{++})-containing heme rings (one is shown in Figure 15.25) joined to two pairs of unlike polypeptide chains (the globins) to form a tetramer. The chains undergo conformational isomerization when the Hb molecule binds with oxygen. Initial binding of oxygen to Hb causes an *autocatalytic process* that facilitates the binding of oxygen to the three neighboring heme rings in a *heme–heme* interaction (West 1985). About 15% of the blood by weight is Hb, contained inside the RBCs (also known as erythrocytes). The total Hb inside the RBCs (THb) can have one of the four forms: (1) *Reduced (nonoxygenated) Hb* (HbR). (2) *Oxyhemoglobin* (HbO_2). (3) *Carboxyhemoglobin,* where Hb has combined with carbon monoxide (HbCO). (4) *Methemoglobin* in which the iron in the heme rings has been oxidized to Fe^{+++} (metHb). In the first three forms, iron is bound in the ferrous oxidation state, Fe^{++}. Most of the THb is in the form of HbO_2 or HbR, the HbCO and metHb typically being <1% of the THb. Pulse oximeters typically ignore the small amounts of metHb and HbCO and measure the concentration ratio between HbR and HbO_2 (Brown 1980).

The Hb in normal arterial blood is about 97% saturated with oxygen (97% HbO_2), and normal venous blood returning to the lungs contains about 75% HbO_2 (Guyton 1991). Most pulse oximeters are ±2% accurate in the normal physiological 70%–100% oxygen saturation range. Pulse oximetry cannot distinguish between two pathological forms of Hb: carboxyhemoglobin (Hb combined with carbon monoxide) and methemoglobin. Pure carboxyhemoglobin (HbCO) reads 90% O_2-saturated Hb and methemoglobin tends toward 90% O_2 saturation. A history and detailed analysis of optical blood oximetry can be found in the papers by Takatani and Ling (1994), de Kock and Tarassenko (1993), and Brown (1980).

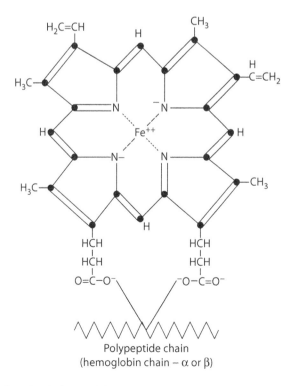

Polypeptide chain
(hemoglobin chain – α or β)

Figure 15.25 One-fourth of a hemoglobin molecule.

15.9.2 Pulse Oximetry Systems

Transcutaneous pulse oximetry (TPOX) is an NI means used to estimate the percent O_2 saturation of peripheral blood Hb using spectrophotometric techniques. Figure 15.26 illustrates the continuous optical absorbance (OD) spectra of 100% O_2-saturated pure Hb, reduced (deoxy-) Hb (0% saturation), and water in a 1 cm cuvette versus transmitted light wavelength. Note that at a wavelength of about 800 nm, there is an *isobestic* point where the absorbance is the same regardless of the % O_2 saturation of the Hb molecules. The isobestic absorption depends only on the path length, L, and the Hb concentration, C. To spectrophotometrically measure PsO_2 of Hb by transcutaneous, pulse oximetry, it is not necessary to measure the entire absorbance spectrum. Generally, two light-emitting diodes (LEDs) are used, one in the NIR near the isobestic wavelength at 800 nm and the other at ~650 nm (red). In some oximetry applications, (red 650 nm) and IR on the long side (950 nm) if the isobestic wavelength has been used (de Kock et al. 1993).

While pure Hb in a cuvette appears to obey the Beer–Lambert law governing optical absorption, Hb in erythrocytes (RBCs) in whole blood does not (de Kock and Tarassenko 1993), and nonlinear corrections must be made to obtain valid readings of the % HbO_2 saturation (SpO_2). There is much scattering and reflection by the RBC membranes.

Two types of transcutaneous oximetry are possible: (1) The *transmission* or *forward-scattered* mode in which light is passed through vascular tissue and collected at the other side with a photosensor. Tissues used for this application are the ear lobe, fingertips, or toes. Figure 15.27 illustrates transmission pulse oximetry (TPOX) schematically. (2) The *reflection* or *backscattered* mode in which backscattered light is measured. This type of oximetry is used on cheeks, the forehead, or the top of the head (infants during delivery). A schematic if reflectance pulse oximetry (RPOX) is shown in Figure 15.28. In order for either mode to work, the light must penetrate the skin, pass through layers of fat, connective tissue, muscle, capillary walls, and erythrocyte membranes, at least twice. In addition, the light impinges on RBCs carrying Hb at various degrees of SpO_2, depending on the capillary vascular anatomy, which can be variable among individuals, as is the blood flow rate through the capillaries. Thus, absorption is from an average of SpO_2 ranging from arterial inputs to venous outputs of the illuminated capillaries.

Most pulse oximeters are of the transmission type. As light propagates through the tissues, capillaries, and blood, it is attenuated and scattered. The useful information depends on the

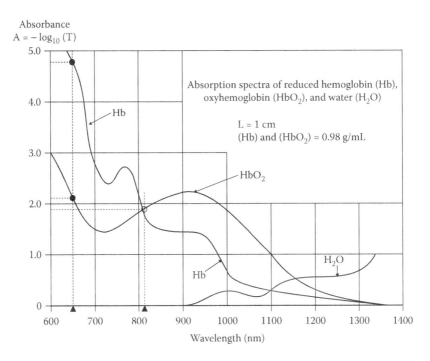

Figure 15.26 Optical absorbances of reduced- and oxy-hemoglobin (HbO_2) in the range from 600 to 1400 nm. Note that the isobestic wavelength is ~805 nm. See text.

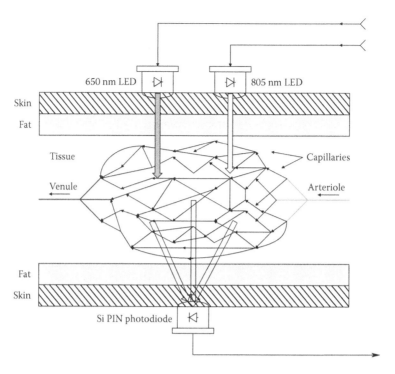

Figure 15.27 Schematic cross section of a body part showing representative rays in transmission pulse oximetry (TPOX).

wavelength-dependent absorption by the mixture of Hb and HbO_2. Absorption is also dependent on the erythrocyte packing density in the blood (*hematocrit*) and the volume of blood in the capillaries. It is this latter factor that gives pulse oximetry its name. At systole, peak blood pressure forces more blood (hence more RBCs) into the illuminated capillaries, thus absorbance varies in time, peaking at systole, and reaching a minimum at diastole at the capillary bed. In addition, at systole, RBCs carrying more HbO_2 enter the bed. Thus, in addition to a transient increase in absorber volume, there is a transient increase in HbO_2 at systole. Thus, the voltage output waveform from a pulse oximeter consists of a DC component plus a periodic wave that follows the systemic blood pressure with a slight lag due to propagation of the pressure

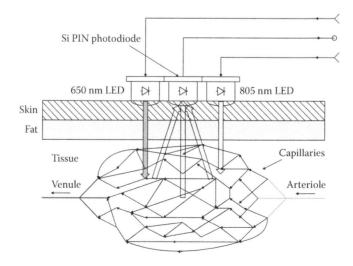

Figure 15.28 Schematic cross section of tissue showing representative rays in *reflection pulse oximetry* (RPOX).

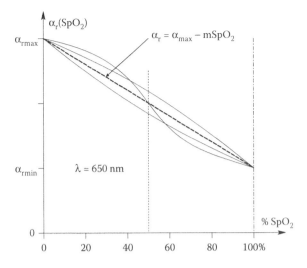

Figure 15.29 How the 650 nm extinction coefficient, α_{650}, of Hb varies with the % SpO$_2$.

wave through the arterial system. The components of optical absorption in tissues include: (1) Absorption due to skin, fat, bone, and tissue. (2) Absorption due to a fixed quantity of venous blood ($\sim$75% SpO$_2$). (3) A fixed component due to arterial blood ($\sim$97% SpO$_2$). (4) A variable, pulsatile, component due to arterial blood volume change. Components 2 through 4 are assumed to obey to the Beer–Lambert law at the red (650 nm) wavelength, and have SpO$_2$-independent absorption at the 800 nm isobestic wavelength. Figure 15.29 illustrates how, with the concentration, C, and path length, L, being held constant, the absorbance of Hb varies with SpO$_2$ at the red (650 nm) wavelength (i.e., essentially how the extinction coefficient, α_r, varies with SpO$_2$ at 650 nm). In the ideal case, it is a linear function of SpO$_2$ (dotted line), in practice it probably is not (solid lines). To simplify the heuristic analysis below, we will assume that α_r varies linearly with SpO$_2$. That is:

$$\alpha_r = \alpha_{r\,max} - m_r \overline{SpO_2}, \tag{15.90}$$

where m_r is the magnitude of the slope of the linear approximation line, SpO$_2$ is the average percent oxygen saturation of the illuminated, capillary blood, and $\alpha_{r\,max} = \alpha_{Hb}$.

In most transmission-type pulse oximeters, two LEDs are used as nearly monochromatic photon sources; one is red (650 nm) and the other is at the near infrared, isobestic, wavelength (805 nm). The diodes are alternately pulsed in the sequence: red, NIR, and dark. The dark interval is so that the oximeter can compensate for stray room light picked up by the photosensor. The photosensor is typically a silicon phototransistor or PIN photodiode which has a peak sensitivity at about 770 nm. Sensitivity at 650 nm is about 0.9 the peak sensitivity in mA/mW.

To understand how an oximeter works, we first consider the case where there is no pulse, that is, there is no time variability of the absorbance due to pulsatile blood flow into the capillaries. First, let the red LED be on. The light that exits the earlobe or fingertip is attenuated by nonwavelength-dependent physical factors such as absorption by bone and tissues, as well as wavelength-dependent absorption by HbO$_2$ in the RBCs in the capillaries. The intensity of light exiting the earlobe can be approximated by Beer's law:

$$I_{or} = I_{inr}10^{-(Br + \alpha_r CL)}, \tag{15.91}$$

where α_r is the extinction coefficient for HbO$_2$ for red light (650 nm), C is the effective concentration of HbO$_2$, L is the mean path length, and B$_r$ is the non-Hb absorption of tissues at 650 nm.

The transmitted 650 nm light is collected by the PIN photodiode, converted to a proportional voltage, V$_{ar}$, by an op-amp, and passed through a log$_{10}$(x) nonlinearity. These steps can be written as

$$V_{ar} = K_a I_{or} = K_a I_{inr} 10^{-(Br + \alpha_r CL)} \tag{15.92}$$

$$V_{Lr} = K_L \log_{10}(K_a I_{or}) = K_L \log_{10}(K_a I_{inr}) - K_L[B_r + \alpha_r CL].\tag{15.93}$$

Let us substitute Equation 15.89 in Equation 15.92:

$$V_{Lr} = K_L \log_{10}(K_a I_{inr}) - K_L[B_r + CL(\alpha_{max} - m_r \overline{SpO_2})].\tag{15.94}$$

Now the emerging light intensity from the 805 nm LED is attenuated but is independent of SpO_2. Its intensity can be written as

$$I_{oi} = I_{ini} 10^{-Bi}\tag{15.95}$$

The NIR light is conditioned by a log amplifier as well. I_{inr} is made $= I_{ini}$.

$$V_{ai} = K_a I_{oi}\tag{15.96}$$

$$V_{Li} = K_L \log_{10}(K_a I_{oi}) = K_L \log_{10}(K_a I_{ini}) - K_L[B_i].\tag{15.97}$$

The oximeter's output is formed by subtracting V_{Li} from V_{Lr}, sic:

$$V_o = (V_{Lr} - V_{Li}) = K_L \log_{10}(K_a I_{inr}) - K_L[B_r + CL(\alpha_{rmax} - m_r \overline{SpO_2})] - K_L \log_{10}(K_a I_{ini}) + K_L(B_i).\tag{15.98}$$

Collecting terms, we have

$$V_o \cong K_L(B_i - B_r) + K_L CL[m_r \overline{SpO_2} - \alpha_{rmax}].\tag{15.99}$$

Equation 15.98 suggests that if Beer's law holds, and the α_r extinction coefficient is a linear function of Hb SpO_2, then V_o will be a linear function of the average SpO_2 of Hb in the capillary beds. In practice these ideal conditions do not occur and V_o is a monotonically increasing, nonlinear function of $\overline{SpO_2}$. The actual $\overline{SpO_2}$ is found by a look-up table in the instrument's memory.

A second complication of TPOX is the effect of the arterial pulse on V_o. At local systole at the capillary bed being studied, the rising blood pressure forces new, more oxygen-saturated RBCs into the capillaries, momentarily dilating them and raising the average SpO_2 in the illuminated volume. This action raises the effective concentration, C, of HbO_2, and the effective length, L, of the light path also increases slightly because the illuminated tissue swells with blood pressure. Hence, the output voltage, $V_o(t)$, from a typical pulse oximeter follows the peripheral blood pressure waveform. Thus, it can be used to measure heart rate, estimate blood pressure (after calibration), as well as estimate peripheral SpO_2.

Direct, accurate measurement of arterial SpO_2 appears to be impossible using TPOX in a clinical setting unless blood samples are taken to calibrate it. As we have pointed out above, the effective SpO_2 in the illuminated capillary bed is an average of the levels of HbO_2 in the capillaries. This average is proportional to and lower than the arterial SpO_2. What can be relatively certain with a TPOX is that its sensitivity (i.e., output V/SpO_2) is known and remains constant. The useful medical information obtained from a TPOX is that the $\overline{SpO_2}$ has dropped so many percent from the initial (normal) value. Such a drop can be life-threatening and generally signals the need for immediate corrective procedures.

As the TPOX output is a periodic waveform that follows the brachial blood pressure waveform (assuming a fingertip is used), several algorithms have been developed to read the average SpO_2. A common one is to sample the V_o waveform at some fixed threshold and do a running average of the samples. Another is to detect and sample the V_o peaks and average. Still another is to sample the peaks and adjacent minima. A running average is calculated from the $(V_{opk} - V_{omin})/2$ series. As we pointed out above, the $V_o(t)$ waveform is due to volumetric and path length changes with BP as well as SpO_2 varying with the cardiac cycle.

Reflection mode pulse oximetry (RPOX) has been used on body parts too thick for light transmission. Takatani and Ling (1994) described reflection pulse oximetry used to measure the mean SpO_2 of an infant's brain. RPOX has also been used to determine the SpO_2 in the blood vessels of the retina (de Kock et al. 1993).

Increased *hematocrit* (**H**) (the percent of blood volume that is RBCs) also has the effect of raising C in Beer's law (normal hematocrit is about 40%). Schmitt et al. (1992) developed a prototype, NI, *hematocrit measurement instrument* using *two*, NIR, isobestic wavelengths of Hb and HbO_2: 800 nm and 1300 nm. Its operation is very like a pulse oximeter. By measuring the OD ratio, $\rho = OD_{800}/OD_{1300}$, of whole blood (*in vitro*), Schmitt et al. (1992) were able to plot a regression line:

$\rho = 0.781 + 0.007389$ **H**, with a correlation coefficient r = 0.995 for $0 \leq$ **H** $\leq 100\%$. The fit was even better in the **H** range from 20% to 60%. Schmitt et al. tested their transmission-mode hemocrit-meter on both a cuvette with whole blood and a more complex finger phantom. As in the use of pulse oximetry, their instrument was subject to uncertainties caused by skin pigmentation and other anatomical factors. Once this type of instrument is calibrated for a given individual, it would appear to be quite accurate.

15.9.3 Discussion

The modern pulse oximeter is a versatile, NI instrument. Often, an integrated oximeter front end containing the two LEDs, a silicon photodiode, and a connecting cable with connector is made disposable for clinical use. By adding a third LED emitting at 1300 nm, the oximeter can be adapted to not only measure SpO_2 but also hematocrit and pulse rate. We predict that the principle of measuring the absorbance of subcutaneous blood analytes at two or three wavelengths with eventually be extended to the transcutaneous measurement of analytes such as glucose, alcohol, heroin, etc. through the use of narrowband, laser diodes. Diode outputs can be conducted to the skin through fiber-optic cables, and the transmitted or reflected light containing the information can also be collected and transmitted to a remote sensor by a fiber-optic cable. The major problem with any transcutaneous optical system is individual variation in skin thickness and pigment, as well as variability in subcutaneous fat deposits and vasculature. This problems might be overcome if there were some blood analyte that is always fairly constant that could be used for normalization and calibration for an analyte such as glucose.

At this point in time, however, the state of the art is such that certain analytes can be measured transcutaneously with reasonable accuracy *on a given individual,* as long as the system is given a two-point, "gold standard" calibration using withdrawn blood samples (semi-invasively taken). As soon as the measurement interface is moved, or transferred to another patient, the system must be recalibrated.

15.10 NI MEASUREMENT OF CERTAIN BIOMOLECULES BY RAMAN SPECTROSCOPY

15.10.1 Introduction

Raman spectroscopy is based on the *Raman effect,* named for the Indian physicist, C.V. Raman, who was awarded the 1930 Nobel Prize for his discovery. In their seminal paper, published in the journal *Nature* in 1928, Raman and Krishnan observed that when light interacted with matter, some small amount of its energy was *scattered*, and the frequency of the scattered light was shifted in a complex manner from that of the incident beam.

Since its discovery, the Raman effect has been developed into a sensitive, analytical chemical tool with results that rival conventional spectroscopic techniques (UV, VIS, IR). The advent of monochromatic laser sources has expedited the rise of Raman spectroscopy as an analytical tool. In the past 20 years or so, Raman spectroscopy has been applied to various biomedical applications, such as measuring various important analytes in blood, urine, and serum, and detection of cancer in various tissues. A sampling of Raman applications in NI diagnosis and corresponding references follows: breast cancer diagnosis (Brozek-Pluska et al. 2012); general cancer diagnosis (Hanlon et al. 2000, Brauchle and Schenke-Layland 2013, Bakeev et al. 2013, Kong et al. 2015); cervical cancer diagnosis (Ramos et al. 2015); colorectal cancer diagnosis (Bergholt et al. 2013, Gaifulina et al. 2014); bladder cancer diagnosis (Kerr et al. 2014, Hanchanale et al. 2008); skin cancer (Zhao et al. 2010, Horiba 2011, ANDOR 2015); blood glucose measurement (Koo et al. 1999, Enejder et al. 2005, Lipson et al. 2009, Shao et al. 2012, Spegazzini et al. 2014); and general articles on diagnosis with Raman spectroscopy (Zeng et al. 2008, Tu and Chang 2012).

There are two kinds of Raman spectroscopy systems currently in use: *Conventional Raman* and *Stimulated Raman spectroscopy* (SRS). Figure 15.30 illustrates a typical, conventional, *in vitro* Raman system. A high-power diode laser emitting in the NIR, typically at 830 or 850 nm, is used as the source. Its beam is chopped or otherwise amplitude modulated to enable synchronous detection of the scattered light. NIR light is generally used to minimize any natural, background fluorescence from a complex, biological sample. (Recall that the shorter visible wavelengths and UV light excite fluorescence. See Section 15.3.) Most of the input light is elastically scattered (Rayleigh light) with no frequency shift by sample molecules. Inelastic (Raman) scattering in all directions occurs at about 10^{-8} times the intensity of the (input) Rayleigh scattered light. Energy from the monochromatic input beam is absorbed in the process of exciting vibrations of the various interatomic bonds of the analyte. The Raman scattered (output) light thus has a complex spectrum depending on the chemical structure of the analyte(s). In general, the Raman shifts of the output spectrum

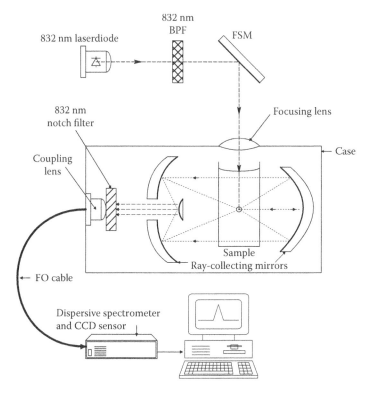

Figure 15.30 Schematic of an *in vitro* Raman spectrophotometer.

are given by $\Delta\nu_{Raman} = \nu_{in} - \nu_{scattered} = (1/\lambda_0 - 1/\lambda_1)$ cm^{-1}. $\Delta\nu_{Raman}$ is also called the *Stokes shift*. ($\lambda_0 = $ the excitation wavelength in cm, λ_1 is the Raman spectrum wavelength in cm. The excitation light frequency is just $f_0 = c/\lambda_0$ Hz.) The energy absorbed in the photon excitation of a particular, interatomic bond resonance is proportional to the $\Delta\nu_{Raman}$ of its spectral peak. That is, $E_{abs} = hc$ $\Delta\nu_{Raman} = hc\,(1/\lambda_0 - 1/\lambda_1)$ J.

To gather more of the weak, Raman-scattered light, often a parabolic mirror is used near the sample. An *optical, holographic notch filter* (HNF) is used to exclude the excitation light energy of wavelength λ_0. A HNF attenuates by $\sim10^{-6}$ at the center of its stop band, and passes 80%–90% of the input light at other wavelengths. (The spectral bandwidth of an HNF ranges from 10 to 20 nm between O.D. 0.3 or 50% transmission points.) (RamanRXN Systems 2001). The weak Raman light is passed through a dispersive spectrometer or monochromator that either projects the desired Raman spectrum on a linear, CCD sensor array, where the kth pixel intensity is proportional to $\Delta\nu_{kRaman}$, or light at a given $\Delta\nu_{Raman}$ is directed onto a single photomultiplier sensor or some photodiode. For *in vitro* Raman spectroscopy, relatively large input intensities are used, typically in the hundreds of mW. Such high input power cannot be used for *in vivo* Raman measurements because of potential heat damage to tissues, including the retina.

Raman spectra are generally displayed in units of WN in cm^{-1}, which is proportional to the Hz frequency of the light. Note that 1 cm^{-1} equals 3×10^{10} Hz, or 30 GHz. Thus, the frequency of 830 nm input light is $\nu_{in} = 3.61 \times 10^{14}$ Hz.

Figure 15.31 shows the Raman spectrum of ethanol *in vitro*. Note the sharp, signature peak at ~800 cm^{-1}, and the two small peaks around 980 cm^{-1}. The conventional IR absorbance spectrum of a substance has the same peaks and peak spacing as does the Raman spectrum. Additional information is available from a Raman system in the form of the polarization of the scattered light. Peaks from nonpolar chemical groups are generally stronger in Raman spectroscopy, while the converse is true for conventional IR absorbance spectroscopy of the same analyte. Figure 15.32 illustrates both Raman and IR absorbance spectra from methanol. Notice that in the two spectrograms, some congruent peaks are sharper and stronger than in the other spectrogram.

An SRS is a technique that avoids the nondirectional scattering of the frequency-shifted light emitted in conventional, single-source Raman spectroscopy. In an SRS, two lasers are used to

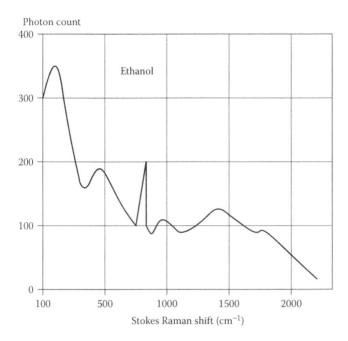

Figure 15.31 Smoothed sketch of the Raman spectrum of ethanol. (The actual curve has ca. ±5 count of random noise added to it.)

excite the analyte; a *pump laser* and a tunable *probe laser*. The intersection of their beams defines an analyte volume. When the frequency (or WN) difference between the two lasers equals the $\Delta\nu_{Raman}$ of a Raman-active mode, there is an increase in the irradiance of the transmitted probe beam and a corresponding decrease of the irradiance of the transmitted pump beam. In one SRS system designed to sense D-glucose in biological samples, the $\Delta\nu$ between the pump and probe lasers is made to be the $\Delta\nu_{Raman}$ of a major glucose Raman peak, that is, 518 cm^{-1} (Tarr and Steffes 1993, 1998). (Recall that $\nu\lambda = c$, and the WN in cm^{-1} = 3.333×10^{-11} ν, ν in Hz.) The actual frequencies of the pump and probe lasers are not as important as the $\Delta\nu$ between them. The pump frequency should be in the NIR if possible to avoid exciting intrinsic fluorescence of the specimen.

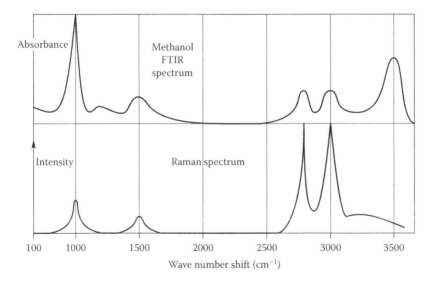

Figure 15.32 Sketch of the combined Raman emission and spectrometer absorbance spectra for methanol. Note wave number congruence in peak locations.

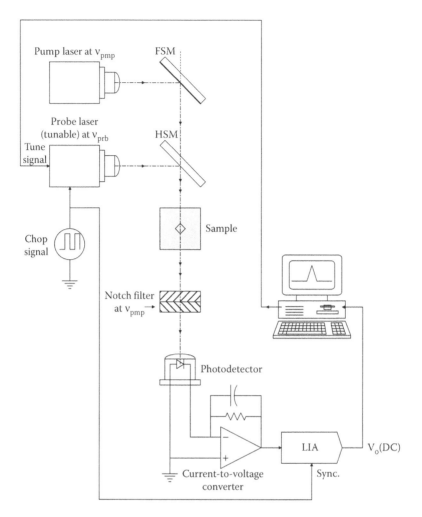

Figure 15.33 Schematic of a stimulated Raman spectroscopy system.

The advantage of the SRS technique is that no expensive monochromator is used. As shown in Figure 15.33, the probe laser's output is both wavelength tunable and chopped, either mechanically or electronically by switching the laser diode current on and off. The beams from the probe and the pump lasers are combined, either using fiber-optic mixing, or mirrors and a half-silvered mirror, and then directed into the sample. Light from the pump laser is greatly attenuated by an optical notch filter, letting through the modulated probe laser beam which is directed to a suitable photosensor. The sensor's output contains a modulated signal component consisting of the probe beam attenuated as a function of the Raman–Stokes energy absorbed by the analyte, as well as modulated components from sample background fluorescence, plus Raman emissions from the water solvent and from glass (cuvette, lenses, fiber optics). These latter components are artifacts with little $\Delta\nu$-dependence, and are easily subtracted from the desired signal following synchronous (lock-in) demodulation of the sensor output. Note that, in the SRS, the probe laser beam's frequency is not shifted, rather, its intensity is changed.

15.10.2 Diagnostic Applications of Raman Spectroscopy

Kong et al. (2015) commented: "The high chemical specificity, minimal lack of sample preparation and the ability to use advanced optical technologies in the visible or NIR spectral range (lasers, microscopes, fibre-optics) have recently led to an increase in medical diagnostic applications of Raman spectroscopy. The key hypothesis underpinning this field is that molecular changes in cells, tissues or biofluids, that are either the cause or the effect of diseases, can be detected and quantified by Raman spectroscopy."

Much of the early research and development to date on using Raman spectroscopy and the SRS in NI medical diagnosis has been in the form of *in vitro* studies on various biomolecules in solution, in blood and serum, and in excised, nonliving tissues. A comprehensive review of this early area of biomedical research can be found in the paper by Hanlon et al. (2000). For example, Salenius et al. (1998) did an *in vitro* study on the Raman spectra from the insides of samples of carotid and femoral arteries ranging from normal to those heavily affected by atherosclerosis. They looked for the Raman spectra from calcium deposits and cholesterol. Their results were well correlated with histological examination of the tissues, and demonstrated the feasibility of using the Raman approach *in vivo* as an invasive, diagnostic procedure. Raman light would be conducted to the intravascular sites with a fiber-optic catheter.

Because of its obvious importance in diabetes, the detection of glucose in blood, serum, and in the AH of the eyes has been approached by a number of workers using Raman spectroscopy. In the 1993 U.S. patent of Tarr and Steffes, and in their 1998 paper, the SRS is proposed to be used on the AH of the eye to sense glucose in the AH. It is known that the AH glucose concentration follows the blood glucose concentration with a lag and an attenuation factor. No one to date has done research on the dynamics relating AH glucose to blood glucose in humans, and how it may vary individually. What is assumed about this transfer function for humans has been induced from animal data from the 1980s (Arnold and Klonoff 1999). Thus, any measurement of AH glucose concentration, by whatever means, is an estimate of blood glucose based on a poorly known dynamic relation for a given patient. Once the transfer function is known, then past AH glucose readings can be deconvolved with the transfer function (assuming linearity, which I doubt) to more accurately find the present blood glucose concentration.

Tarr and Steffes (1993, 1998) proposed an SRS system to measure AH glucose concentration passed two, coaxial, SRS laser beams through the cornea from the side at an oblique angle so that they pass through the AH, across the front of the anterior chamber of the eye in front of the iris, and then exit obliquely. While not shown specifically in their patent and paper, the exit of the laser beams requires a coupling contact lens over the cornea with a refractive index greater than that of the cornea. Otherwise, the beams would remain trapped in the cornea because of the critical angle phenomenon (how fiber-optic cables work to trap light in their cores). The need for the coupling contact lens was first appreciated by March (1977) and later by March et al. (1982). The tangential, anterior chamber, optical path may permit the use of higher optical power than ordinarily permitted for laser irradiation of the eye for diagnostic purposes, because only a small amount of Rayleigh- and Raman-scattered light would reach the sensitive retina over a large area. However, optical irradiation standards set by OSHA, FDA, etc. are set for *any* laser light entering the eye, *regardless of path*. Apparently, a practical, approved, *in vivo* SRS system using the AH will have to use about 1/100th the power of an *in vitro* system operating on blood or serum.

Another approach to the beam geometry problem is to use the reflection off the front surface of the lens as described by Browne (1998). Although the emergent beams will have net power on the order of 10 s of nW, after filtering out the pump laser, the modulated probe beam can easily be measured with a photomultiplier sensor. Also by chopping both the probe and pump laser beams, more peak input power can be used.

The simplicity of the SRS approach to glucose measurement in the AH can be appreciated by the fact that glucose has a sharp peak in its stimulated Raman spectrum for a pump–probe laser WN difference of 512 cm^{-1} (Tarr and Steffes 1993). Since only the AH glucose concentration is sought, the lasers do not need to be tunable.

Application of Raman spectroscopy to the measurement of glucose, cholesterol, triglycerides, urea (BUN), total protein, and albumin in *in vitro* samples of human blood and serum (plasma) was described by Berger et al. (1999). The excitation was a powerful, 250 mW, 830 nm diode laser that was focused to a 50 μm diameter spot on the blood sample in a cuvette. The blood was stirred to reduce heating by the laser, but the samples were not cooled, nor were their temperatures measured. In spite of this casual attitude toward sample temperature, these authors obtained remarkably accurate results. One reason was that the Raman spectrum was dispersed into 1152 elements using a CCD array. The method of partial least squares was used to predict the concentration of each analyte. Further, they binned the CCD cells to form ~8 cm^{-1} spectral resolution, and only the portion of the Raman spectrum between 565 and 1746 cm^{-1} was used. These authors' results on *in vitro* blood and serum samples showed that measurement of the six analytes listed above was more accurately done on serum than on whole blood. The signal-to-noise ratio of serum measurements was about three times greater than for Raman spectrum measurements on whole blood. *In vitro* serum measurements were of acceptable accuracy for clinical use, however,

~5 min was required to acquire and average the CCD pixel data to reduce noise in each of the six Raman spectra computed.

Hanlon et al. (2000) summarized various Raman studies done on the detection of breast cancer. Hanlon et al. used principal component analysis in conjunction with logistic regression on spectra taken *in vitro* from biopsied breast tissue (normal, benign, malignant). They found that out of 14 normal specimens, 14 benign and 33 malignant tumors, 31 malignant specimens were classified malignant, 2 malignant specimens were classified benign, 13 benign specimens were classified benign, 1 benign specimen was classified as normal, and 14 normal tissue specimens were correctly classified as normal. Eventually these workers propose to develop a fiber-optic probe for invasive Raman breast tumor analysis.

Hanlon et al. (2000) also described the application of Raman spectral analysis in the diagnosis of Alzheimer's disease (AD). In their own *in vitro* studies of AD by Raman spectroscopy, Hanlon et al. found that by subtracting an average normal Raman spectrum from one from a brain with AD, two characteristic peaks were seen at 940 and 1150 cm^{-1}. By using principal component analysis techniques, Hanlon et al. were able to discriminate 12 AD specimens from five normal specimens. They proposed developing a Raman instrument to detect AD in which an NI, fiber-optic probe would be run up the nose ~7 cm to the olfactory epithelium. IR laser light would penetrate the epithelium and the cribriform plate in the roof of the nasal cavity to illuminate the olfactory bulb (part of the CNS), where the spectrum would be formed.

In a recent paper, Shao et al. (2012) reported the use of transmitted IR light (600–1650 cm^{-1}) through the ears of living mice and Raman spectroscopy to measure [bG]. In their study, no Raman signal was detected at glucose concentrations below 50 mmol/dL at 1125 cm^{-1}, even with integrating times ≤10 min. Note that human [bG] can be as low as 3–10 mmol/dL for normal individuals, and <30 mmol/dL for diabetics.

In the past 15 years or so, there have been many investigations and advances in the use of Raman and SRS for non- and semi-invasive medical diagnosis. The excellent review paper of Kong et al. (2015) described Raman diagnostic applications using tissues to detect brain cancer, breast cancer, lung cancer, skin cancer, esophagus cancer, prostate cancer, colorectal cancer, and bone diseases. Kong et al. (2015) also reviewed Raman applications using biofluids to quantify blood glucose, diagnose cancer, asthma, inflammatory responses, quantify coagulant and anticoagulant factors (INR) in blood, and malaria. Kerr et al. (2014) wrote an extensive review on the applications of Raman spectroscopy to the diagnosis of urinary bladder cancer. Another review of the state of the art of Raman spectroscopy by Brauchle and Schenke-Layland (2013) focused on NI, *in vitro* analysis of cells (including stem cells) and extracellular matrix components in tissues for detection of pathologies and diseases. Rubina and Murali-Krishna (2015) addressed the efficacy of Raman spectroscopy in diagnosing cervical cancers. Colorectal cancer diagnosis using Raman spectroscopy was described by Gaifulina et al. (2014). Tu and Chang (2012) and Bakeev et al. (2013) have given comprehensive reviews of the medical diagnostic applications of Raman spectroscopy.

15.10.3 Discussion

We have seen that good *in vitro* results have been obtained measuring certain analytes in water, and blood plasma or serum. Mildly invasive procedures such as cystoscopy, bronchoscopy, and colonoscopy provide a means to use Raman spectroscopy to examine lesions (candidate tumors) on the surface of the epithelium in these locations.

For NI, Raman spectroscopic, diagnostic applications, the pump or excitation laser's energy must be introduced transdermally, and the very weak, backscattered, Raman-shifted light must be collected and analyzed dispersively. An SRS could be used transdermally by shining the pump and probe lasers through a thin vascular tissue such as a finger web or an earlobe. A serious requirement in all forms of *in vivo* Raman analysis is to be able to operate it at laser power levels that will not damage the biological tissues being irradiated (by heating). As we have seen, this is very critical in ophthalmic applications of Raman spectroscopy.

In summary, applications of Raman spectroscopy and surface-enhanced Raman spectroscopy (SERS) in medical diagnosis include (Bakeev et al. 2013):

- Examination of biopsy samples

- *In vitro* diagnostics

- Cytology investigations at the cellular level

- Bioassay measurements

- Histopathology using microscopy

- Direct investigation of cancerous tissues

- Surgical targets and treatment monitoring

- Deep tissue studies

- Drug efficacy studies

15.11 CHAPTER SUMMARY

We have seen that there are many nonimaging applications of photon radiation in NI medical diagnosis, using wavelengths ranging from infrared through visible, UV, and x-rays. Many of the techniques are used to quantify specific biomolecules whose concentrations are abnormal in disease states. In Section 15.2, we saw how x-ray energy at two different wavelengths is used to measure the bone density and thus detect the osteoporosis. Tissue fluorescence in response to short blue and UV light was introduced in Section 15.3. Many important biomolecules fluoresce, and have unique, signature, fluorescence emission spectra. Thus, fluorescence can be used to sense abnormally high concentrations of certain molecules associated with the higher metabolism of cancer cells, and thus localize the lesions. Any point on the skin, or part of the body reachable by an endoscope can be probed for anomalous fluorescence.

Optical interferometric measurement of small displacements, covered in Section 15.4, is primarily a research tool looking for an application. Nanometer-sized vibrations on the skin surface and of a tympanic membrane have been measured. Interferometers are relatively delicate instruments and are sensitive to mechanical vibrations and optical path length modulations. If one is interested in measuring the peripheral blood circulation, LDV, covered in Section 15.5, is a preferred method.

TIR spectroscopies, both dispersive and nondispersive, have been shown to have promise for the measurement of molecules such as glucose, cholesterol, etc. Present problems with this type of spectroscopy, reviewed in Section 15.6, include repeatability and calibration. The reliable, robust, transcutaneous measurement of blood glucose by optical absorption at two or more discrete wavelengths still remains a pie in the sky.

Another physical technique for the measurement of blood glucose concentration makes use of the fact that solutions of D-glucose exhibit OR of LPL. An optically clear solution is required; the only one readily accessible by NI means is the AH in the eye. Section 15.7 describes the attempts to measure the OR of the AH caused by glucose dissolved in it. This is a challenging instrumentation problem because the ORs are typically in the tens of millidegrees, the light intensity used is limited by safety reasons, only a very small fraction of the incident light intensity is reflected out of the eye, and the eyeball is continuously in motion (micronystagmus), even when staring at a fixation spot.

In conclusion, there are no reliable, NI, FDA-approved, blood glucose-monitoring devices currently available. The search goes on.

In Section 15.8, we examined pulse oximetry. This is a mature instrumentation technique which, happily, does have wide clinical employment. Pulse oximeters are simple, low-cost devices that use a red and an NIR LED light source, and a common silicon photodiode to sense the backscattered light. They make use of the differential absorption of Hb versus oxyhemoglobin in the blood in the tissue under the device. Experimentally, the pulse oximetry principle has been modified to estimate the blood hematocrit.

Finally, in Section 15.9, the principles of Raman spectroscopy are described. Raman spectroscopy has the ability to identify various biomolecules *in vitro* and transcutaneously. It has been used experimentally to measure the dissolved glucose concentration *in vitro*, and it has been suggested that it may be suitable for measuring the glucose in AH. This may be another pie in the sky, because exiting light reflected off the front surface of the lens is about 1/1000 the input intensity, and of that, the actual Raman spectrum is ~1 part in 10 million. Also the eye introduces "optical noise" from its normal micronystagmus. However, there is no reason why Raman spectroscopy should not be effective on NI biofluid samples, such as saliva and urine (Hanchanale et al. 2008).

16 A Survey of Medical Imaging Systems

16.1 INTRODUCTION

Before the invention and application of simple x-ray shadow imaging in the early twentieth century, the only NI means of diagnosing diseases affecting internal organs was by palpation and visual observation of outward symptoms involving the skin (color, swelling, heat), gums, eyes, tongue, teeth, breath odor, breath sounds, urine, stool, patient complaints of pain, etc. In the past 46 years, NI medical imaging systems have gained tremendous sophistication and effectiveness, largely due to the evolution of 2- and 3-D digital signal-processing algorithms implemented on modern computers. In this chapter, we shall examine the operating principles and key features of modern, NI imaging systems. The mathematics of *tomography* are described and we show how it has been applied to various imaging modalities. Computer-assisted (x-ray) tomography, the so-called CAT scanner, is certainly familiar to healthcare professionals and to most students in biomedical engineering. The x-ray CAT scanner has been around the longest of modern imaging systems. The principles of tomography have been adapted to other imaging modalities, namely *ultrasound, positron emission tomography* (PET), *magnetic resonance imaging* (MRI), *single-photon emission tomography* (SPECT), *optical coherence tomography* (OCT), *electrical impedance tomography* (EIT), and *microwave tomography* (MWT). The ability of a modern medical imaging computer to stack the tomographic "slices" to generate an interpolated, 3-D image is now commonplace. Such 3-D views expedite diagnosis and aid in planning surgery. 3-D reconstructions in soft tissues are particularly useful in diagnosing lung, brain, breast, and liver cancers.

Although NI, the use of modern medical imaging techniques carries a small risk. X-rays, gamma rays, (and radioisotopes) are (or emit) ionizing radiations that have the potential to cause cell DNA damage and mutations. Ultrasound and microwaves generally do not carry risk in this form, but can damage cells and cell function by heating at high power levels. The small, high-frequency currents used in EIT are probably the most innocuous of the modalities used to probe the body's inner 3-D structure. Only infrared imaging of body surface is completely without risk. Extremely small skin temperature differences can be resolved which affect the body's blackbody radiation. IR imaging is a completely passive means of detecting local "hot spots" which might be due to cancer growing near the skin surface, or cold spots indicative of circulatory anomalies. (IR imaging is not a tomographic technique.)

The first topics we consider below are the generation and detection of x-ray images.

16.2 X-RAYS

16.2.1 Introduction

X-rays are a class of broadband, short wavelength, high photon energy, electromagnetic radiation. They were discovered by accident by German physicist Wilhelm Röntgen in November 1895. Röntgen was experimenting with cathode rays (electron beams) in a vacuum Crooke's tube, and noticed that fluorescence was produced on a screen far from Crooke's tube, and correctly guessed that a new type of radiation was involved. He went on to show that these unknown, "x-rays" had certain properties: They travel in straight lines, cast shadows of internal structures of opaque objects which they can penetrate, cause certain minerals to fluoresce, are not deflected by magnetic fields, and darken silver-halide photographic film. In fact, Röntgen made the first x-ray photograph of his wife's hand on December 22, 1895. He received the first Nobel prize in 1901 for his discovery and research.

16.2.2 Sources of Medical X-rays

The basic mechanism by which medical x-rays are produced has not changed since Röntgen's first discovery. In a vacuum, a collimated beam of high-energy electrons from a tungsten filament cathode are directed to hit a solid metal anode. To gain their energy, the electrons are accelerated through a potential of anywhere from 15,000 to 150,000 V from cathode to anode. There, the moving electrons interact with the metal atoms of the anode. Three forms of energy are produced: *x-rays, Auger electrons,* and a large amount of *heat* (LIR). The heat must be dissipated to prevent the temperature of the anode from rising to the anode metal's melting point. Various schemes are used to dissipate this thermal energy. One method is to keep the anode at ground potential, and liquid-cool it with circulating water or oil. Another common approach is to use a large, motor-driven, rotating disk anode so that the electron beam effectively has a larger target area, reducing the W/cm^2 on the anode. Anodes can rotate as high as 6000 rpm, and are water cooled as well. Figure 16.1 illustrates the design of an early twentieth-century Coolidge-type x-ray tube with a

309

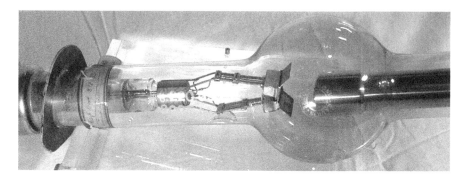

Figure 16.1 Photo of a Coolidge x-ray tube from the early 1900s. The cathode is on the left; it is heated by a filament and releases electrons which are accelerated to strike the anode (on the right) by an electric field setup by a potential difference of several thousand volts between cathode and (+)anode. The electrons release thermal and photon (x-ray) energy from the anode. The surface of the anode is angled so that the x-rays emitted are directed downward. (A public domain figure, available at: https://commons.wikimedia.org/wiki/File:Coolidge_xray_tube.jpg)

fixed Cu anode. Many modern medical x-ray tubes have tungsten (W) anodes; tungsten, also used for the cathode filament, has a high-atomic number of Z = 74, and a high-melting point (3370°C). Molybdenum is also used as an anode metal.

An x-ray tube requires two power sources: a low-voltage, high-current, AC source to heat the tungsten filament, and a high-voltage, low-current, DC source to supply the electron beam. Figure 16.2 shows a two-phase, high-voltage power supply. Note that this DC source *does not* have a filter capacitor to smooth the rectifier output. This is because the electron beam current is switched at the primary, and if a filter capacitor were present, the beam current would not stop abruptly, but would decay exponentially, making it difficult to control the x-ray dose and wavelength. Note that the beam current varies in the form of a full-wave rectified sinusoid; peak x-ray energy occurs at the peak anode–cathode voltage, 40 kV in the figure. For smoother, more monochromatic x-ray production, a three-phase AC supply and rectifier can be used. For really pure x-ray production, a DC beam current is required, calling for a filter capacitor to smooth the rectifier pulses. In this case, an expensive, high-voltage relay, or a silicon-controlled rectifier (SCR) is required to switch the beam current.

There are two mechanisms by which medical x-rays are produced. The first is called *bremsstrahlung radiation. Bremsstrahlung* is German for deceleration or slowing. The electrons striking the dense metal of the anode slow down abruptly, that is, they decelerate. When a charged particle accelerates or decelerates, it radiates electromagnetic energy. The power radiated by a decelerating electron, where velocity is parallel to the deceleration vector, is given by (Griffiths 2012):

$$P_x = \frac{q^2 \dot{v}^2 \gamma^6}{6\pi\varepsilon_o c^3} W, \tag{16.1}$$

where q is the electron charge, $\dot{v}$ is the deceleration, c is the speed of light, γ is the Lorentz factor, and ε_o is the permittivity of free space.

Because a single electron can collide with one or several anode atoms, and there are many electrons in the beam, bremsstrahlung radiation has a continuous energy spectrum similar to blackbody radiation, however, the peak energy is radiated in the range of wavelengths of 10ths of an Å. In a one electron–one atom collision, the shortest x-ray wavelength that can be produced is given by

$$\lambda_{min} = \frac{hc}{Vq} = \frac{6.624 \times 10^{-34} \times 3.0 \times 10^8}{V \times 1.603 \times 10^{-19}} m, \tag{16.2}$$

where h is Planck's constant, c is the speed of light, q is the coulomb electron charge, and V is the potential in volts through which the electron is accelerated toward the anode.

For example, if V = 40 kV, then λ_{min} = 3.1 m × 10^{-11} m = 31 pm = 0.31 Å. Thus, there is a sharp cutoff of the bremsstrahlung spectrum for λs shorter than λ_{min}. However, the spectrum has a long

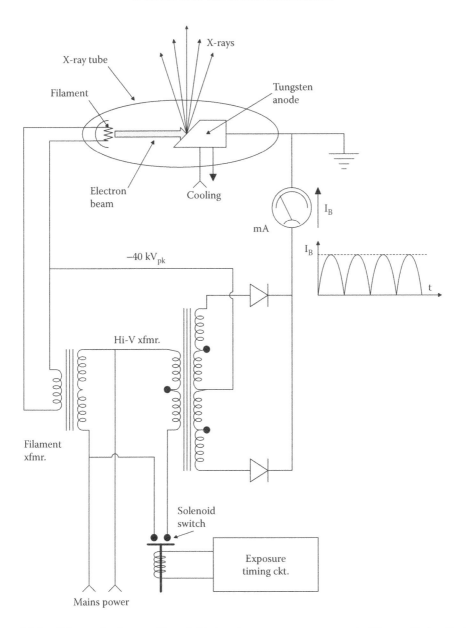

Figure 16.2 Schematic of an unfiltered, high-voltage x-ray power supply. The applied cathode potential is line frequency, full-wave rectified sine wave of −40 kV peak. Thus, the velocities of the electrons striking the anode range from near zero to $v_{max} = \sqrt{2}\, V_{pk}\,(q/m)$ m/s, producing a broad range of x-ray energies. Note that the anode is kept at ground potential to facilitate water cooling its mass.

tail over longer wavelengths. Only about 1% of the energy of the electron beam goes into making bremsstrahlung radiation; most of the beam energy is converted to heat.

The second source of x-radiation involves the interaction of the high-energy beam electrons with the deep shell electrons of the anode's metal. It is called the *characteristic radiation* of the anode metal. When the kinetic energy (KE) of the electron beam is above a threshold value called the *excitation potential*, electrons in the deep shells of the anode's atoms are knocked out, and outer shell, or loosely bound, conduction-band or valence electrons can fall into their place; in the process, x-ray photons are emitted having an energy equal to the energy difference between the displaced inner shell electron and the valence electron. As these energy gaps are quantized,

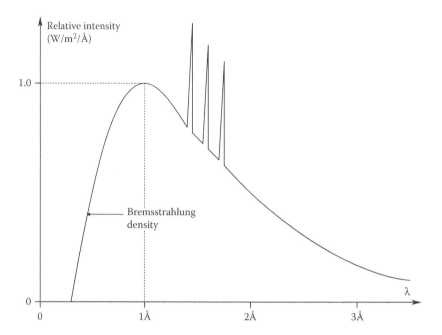

Figure 16.3 Normalized x-ray intensity spectrum for a 40 kV DC accelerating potential. The broad bremsstrahlung curve occurs even with constant energy electrons striking the anode.

narrow peaks of x-ray energy occur at certain wavelengths above the continuous bremsstrahlung spectrum. These peaks are the x-ray "signatures" of the anode metal used. For example, molybdenum has *characteristic radiation peaks* at 70.93, 71.35, 71.07, and 63.23 pm; copper has peaks at 154.05, 154.43, 154.18, and 139.22 pm wavelengths. Figure 16.3 illustrates a typical x-ray power spectrum, showing the bremsstrahlung and characteristic radiation peaks. Note that the dimensions of the spectrum are (W/cm²)/Å wavelength.

Many photons emitted in the characteristic radiation process interact with other atomic electrons in an *internal photo-electric* process. These electrons may gain sufficient energy to escape the metal surface as *Auger electrons*. When x-rays pass through free electrons (Auger or other electrons knocked loose by the beam), they experience the *Compton scattering effect* in which additional, longer wavelength x-rays are generated.

X-ray beams emitted from an anode have an angular distribution of energy which is dependent on the shape of the incident electron beam. As the angle of the x-ray departing from the anode increases, the peak of the bremsstrahlung spectrum shifts to longer wavelengths. The beam leaving at the shallow angle (3°) has the least total energy, but its peak spectral wavelength is the shortest, hence its photons have the highest available energy ($E = hc/\lambda$ eV).

Ideally, for imaging purposes, we would like to use monochromatic (single wavelength) x-rays focused in a tight pencil beam, or equivalently, an x-ray laser. Low-energy monochromatic x-rays have particular application in soft-tissue studies (e.g., mammography, detection of tumors in lung and liver tissue). For mammography, the optimal energy window ranges from ~15 to 25 keV. One way of generating narrow-spectrum x-rays is to add a monochromator to a conventional x-ray system output. Lawaczeck et al. (2005) described such a device; it consisted of a curved, highly oriented pyrolytic graphite (HOPG) crystal refractor and a slit collimator.

Another more complicated and expensive means of generating x-rays ranging from 15 to 50 keV consists of directing a collimated beam of electrons traveling at nearly the speed of light to hit head-on a beam of high-energy IR photons from a laser. The IR photons bounce off the high-energy electrons and gain the energy required to transform them into x-ray photons in a process known as inverse Compton scattering (Salisbury 2001). Carroll et al. (1991) described the details and physics of this process. At present, the complexity and cost of this system preclude it from common use in hospitals.

Monochromatic x-rays: Unfortunately, there is currently no economic way to create a low-cost, truly monochromatic, collimated, x-ray beam for medical purposes. However, conventionally generated x-rays can be filtered, diffracted by crystals, and focused to create narrow beams of limited wavelength range for imaging purposes.

Lawaczeck et al. (2005) described an experimental means of generating narrowband x-rays by inexpensive diffraction. A monochromator located at the output of the x-ray tube consisted of a curved, HOPG crystal and a simple slit collimator. For image generation, the object was moved through the fan-shaped monochromatic radiation beam. The beam size was ~35 mm × 200 mm in the object plane. In mammography, the object (breast under examination) must remain stationary, while the monochromatic beam is scanned.

The simplest collimator for stationary, shadow x-ray imaging is a simple adjustable, rectangular window or mask made of lead. The shadow of the collimator defines the active x-ray beam dimension. Other collimators are used to define narrow, pencil beams used in certain tomographic applications. A narrow beam collimator can be made from a small-diameter tube of an absorbing material such as lead. A second tube in line with the first is used to absorb any obliquely scattered x-rays from the first tube. In capillary tube collimators, lead glass or borosilicate glass capillaries are used. The diameter of these capillaries is generally ~10 μm. These capillaries apparently act like waveguides and capture obliquely directed photons and aim them straight along the capillary axes, increasing the intensity of the emerging, collimated beam by a factor of two to four (Padiyar et al. 2000, Sugiro et al. 2004, XOS 2008). Hasse et al. (2007) described an x-ray capillary collimator made from 10 μm diameter, 100 mm long, borosilicate glass capillaries set in a matrix of lead glass. The collimator outer diameter was 3 mm.

Also reported was an x-ray collimator made from a closely spaced array of small, closely packed tubes made in tantalum. The tantalum was ≥2 mm thick, and had an area of 110 mm × 70 mm. Holes were hexagonally close spaced, and had diameters of ~54 μm. Hole spacing was as small as 80 μm. The holes were drilled using an IR-pulsed disk laser in about 200 ms. Optimal pulse parameters for drilling 2 mm tantalum were: Pulse energy 5.5 mJ, Peak power 11 kW, pulse width 500 ns, pulse repetition rate (PRR) 8 kHz, drilling was done in nitrogen gas (Patwa et al. 2014).

X-ray absorbing grids are often placed over the flat-film case to block low-energy, oblique x-rays scattered by interaction with atoms in the object. An x-ray grid resembles an open Venetian blind in structure. By blocking the oblique rays, the image is made sharper. Figure 16.4 illustrates the use of a grid in a conventional, fixed x-ray system. First, the required area of the x-ray beam is defined by the collimator. Next, an aluminum plate is used to absorb low-energy x-ray photons which are less effective in imaging dense tissues. Their absorption reduces the overall dose of ionizing radiation to the patient. The lead grid is located between the patient and the film; as mentioned above, its function is to block low-energy, oblique rays that would degrade the image. A stationary grid casts its shadow on the film, which can be distracting for the radiologist interpreting the picture. When the grid is moved back and forth during the x-ray exposure, it no longer leaves its shadow, but is still effective at blocking oblique rays; such a moving grid is called a *Bucky grid* (Jacobson and Webster 1977). Pacific Northwest X-Ray Inc. (2105), Gresham, OR, markets grids in which aluminum strips are between the lead "slats." This design has dual functions: blocking oblique, low-energy rays and filtering out the direct, low-energy rays from the bremsstrahlung emission "tail."

16.2.3 X-ray Detectors and Recording Media

The original x-ray recording medium was a flat plate of ordinary silver bromide photographic film kept in a lighttight cassette. As the emulsion layer is thin, and AgBr is not a very efficient capturer of x-ray photons, a degree of darkening on the developed film caused by photons interacting with the AgBr crystals required a larger exposure than is required for modern, two-emulsion film backed with scintillator plates. In this embodiment, the emulsions respond not only to direct x-rays but also to visible photons emitted from the thin scintillation coatings pressed against the emulsions when x-rays excite the scintillator atoms. The scintillation is produced by high-atomic weight (high-Z) molecules such as calcium tungstate ($CaWO_4$). Laminated scintillation film is from 20 to 100 times more sensitive than plain x-ray film, permitting the use of lower x-ray doses in a given application; obviously, it is also more expensive than plain film (Webster 1992). An enlarged, cross section of a laminated scintillation film is shown in Figure 16.5.

Direct fluoroscopy was an early means of visualizing internal organs in the real time. In fluoroscopy, the radiologist stood behind a thin, fluorescent screen in line with the x-rays emerging from the patient. This radiation caused visible photons to be emitted from the screen; the higher the ray intensity, the brighter the image on the screen. Conversion efficiency of transmitted x-rays to visible photons is small; only about 7% of the photon energy is converted to light. Thus, the radiologist

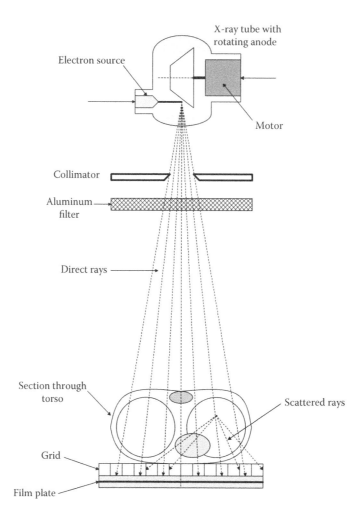

Figure 16.4 Schematic of an ordinary "shadow" x-ray system. The metal grid over the film plate is to eliminate oblique scattered photons and give a sharper image.

had to view the dim, green screen under low-light conditions using dark-adapted eyes which produce low-visual resolution. The technique was used to visualize the organs in motion, for example, the heart, its valves, and major blood vessels; often an iodine contrast medium was injected to improve the contrast on heart valves, coronary vessels, and aorta. Unfortunately, fluoroscopy resulted in high-radiation doses for both the patient and the radiologist. It also took considerable skill and experience to read or interpret the tachistoscopically presented fluorescent images.

Modern fluoroscopic techniques have led to both reduced patient radiation dose and no dose for the radiologist. The *image intensifier tube* (IIT) improves the conversion efficiency for real-time fluoroscopy. A cross-sectional schematic of an IIT is shown in Figure 16.6. Its operating principle is very much like the NIR night vision equipment used by the military. When an x-ray photon strikes the fluorescent screen, it emits photons. These photons stimulate an adjacent *photocathode* of the same size as the fluorescent screen to emit electrons, which are, in turn, accelerated by a ~25 kV DC potential to strike a phosphor anode, similar to that of a conventional, old-fashioned, black-and-white, TV CRT. The phosphor anode reemits bright, visible photons as a result of impact by the accelerated photoelectrons. To recapitulate, x-ray photons cause fluorescent screen molecules to emit visible photons which, in turn, generate photoelectrons. The photoelectrons are accelerated and focused, striking a phosphor screen, which emits high-intensity visible photons in the form of an x-ray shadow image. The IIT has a *brightness gain* which is the product of the *geometric gain* (ratio of the areas of the input fluorescent screen to the output phosphor screen) times the electronic gain (product of the accelerating potential, V, times the input fluorescent screen's quantum efficiency, η_i,

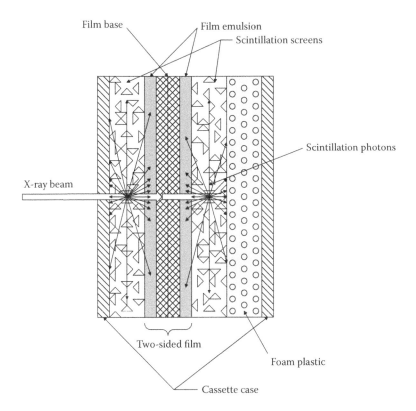

Figure 16.5 Cross-sectional detail through a laminated, two-sided, scintillation x-ray film.

the photocathode's efficiency, η_{pc}, and the output phosphor's efficiency, η_{op}). The intensified image on the phosphor can be viewed directly by eye using magnifying optics, or by a digital video camera. Thus, images can be stored, computer enhanced, then played back in slow motion, etc. Direct view of the phosphor screen should make use of a 45° mirror and telescopic optics to place the observer out of the x-ray beam path. Note that one drawback of fluorescent screen imaging is that the visible photons released by collision with an energetic x-ray photon depart in all directions; some are scattered by adjacent phosphor particles and still emerge, degrading the image quality.

Industrial Quality, Inc. (IQI 2015) developed a family of x-ray scintillating glasses under the U.S. Navy, Phase III SBIR contract. IQI claimed that the electronic images from their glass scintillators have less noise, and thus give a sharper picture. The glass can be made much thicker than conventional granular fluorescent screens, thus absorbing more x-rays and generating images that are less noisy and thus have a greater contrast range. There are no light scattering problems from clear glass.

Research and development is currently underway on semiconductor sensor arrays that permit direct conversion of transmitted x-ray energy to electrical outputs in submillimeter-sized pixel arrays. A major problem in these designs appears to be with the materials; an x-ray collision must liberate electrons in numbers proportional to the energy of the ray, and these electrons must be mobile and easily collected for charge-to-voltage conversion.

Tumer et al. (2009) described a high-resolution array for digital mammography and radiography operating in the current mode (TDI CCD) called MARY-N100 (MARY = **Ma**mmog**ra**phy), designed for 100 μm spatial resolution. MARY-N100 has a 64 × 192 array with 100 × 100 μ pitch. MARY-N50 and -N100 collect photoelectrons because they were designed for solid-state sensors that have higher electron than hole densities, such as $Cd_{0.9}Zn_{0.1}Te$ (CZT), CdTe, HgI_2, and Se detectors. A detailed, comparative description of the various types of position-sensitive semiconductor imaging detectors may be found in the 61 pp review paper by Russo and Del Guerra (2014).

In summary, medical x-ray technology is heading toward filmless imaging, where eventually all x-ray image data will be captured digitally and stored in ROMs or in DVD format. The ubiquitous CCD camera is playing a key role in this filmless technology in capturing images from scintillation plates. When perfected, large semiconductor x-ray imaging arrays promise to give better

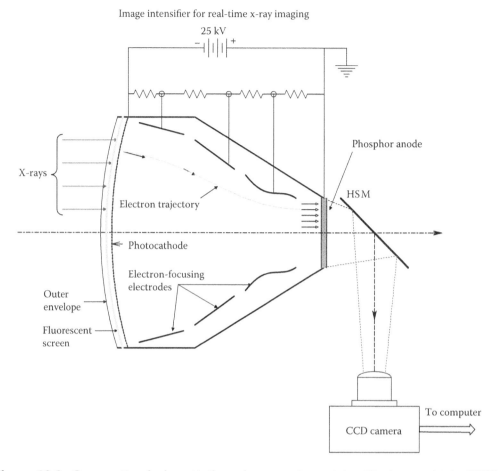

Figure 16.6 Cross-sectional schematic through an x-ray image intensifier (vacuum) tube (IIVT) used for real-time fluoroscopy in applications such as angiography. HSM = half-silvered mirror beam splitter.

resolution by eliminating the noise and scattering inherent in phosphors and scintillators, x-ray photons are directly converted to electrons in semiconductor arrays.

The *contrast* and *spatial frequency resolution* (e.g., in lines/cm) of x-ray images depends on many factors. Of great importance is the apparent size of the x-ray source spot. A large spot gives a fuzzy shadow of a sharp edge (density gradient) in the object. Image blurring is also caused by object motion (small motions from muscle tremor, heart action). Another source of fuzzy images comes from oblique, scattered rays that get through the Bucky grid. Photon scattering in phosphor screens can also degrade spatial resolution.

A practical, quantitative measure of the contrast and spatial frequency resolution of an entire x-ray imaging system or any component thereof is the *modulation transfer function* (MTF). Ideally, the MTF should be measured using an object having sinusoidal density for x-rays in 1-D. Because of the difficulty in constructing such a sinusoidal grid, the MTF is measured by using a lead spatial *square wave object* having a period of so many millimeters. In practice, it is better to use a series of grids each with a progressively smaller spatial period to test an x-ray imaging system. This is because the spatial frequency response of an image can be area and orientation dependent. For example, the highest spatial resolution might be at the center of the image, and drop off at the edges. At very low-spatial frequencies, the image of the grid is black (exposed) and clear (non-exposed) stripes. If film is the output medium, we can measure the *transmittance* of the clear and black areas. The *contrast* of the striped image is defined as

$$C(u) \equiv \frac{T_{max} - T_{min}}{T_{max} + T_{min}}, \tag{16.3}$$

where u is the spatial frequency of the object (and image) in lines/mm, defined as $u = 1/\lambda$. T_{max} is the maximum transmittance of the film (in a clear area under a lead stripe), defined as $T_{max} = I_{outc}/I_{in}$. I_{outc} is the intensity of white light emerging from the film, given an input intensity of I_{in}. Similarly, in a dark area on the film (under a gap between lead stripes) $T_{min} = I_{outd}/I_{in}$. For very low u, $C \rightarrow 1.0$.

As the spatial frequency of the striped lead object increases, the striped image becomes blurred at the edges of the stripes, and $T_{min} < 1.0$. For a very high u, the image appears to be a fuzzy sinusoid, derived from the fundamental frequency in the Fourier series describing the square wave object; thus, $C(u) \rightarrow MTF(u)$. In the limiting case, no periodicity is seen in the object; it is uniformly gray. The object's contrast is thus zero. Note that the spatial square wave object can be described by a Fourier series:

$$f(x) = f(x + \lambda) = F_o/2 + (2F_o/\pi) \sum_{k=1,\text{odd}}^{\infty} \sin(k2\pi x/\lambda) / k. \tag{16.4}$$

In the limit, as $\lambda \rightarrow \lambda_{co}$, only the first harmonic creates an image, so the effective object is:

$$f(x) \cong F_o/2 + (2F_o/\pi)\sin(2\pi x/\lambda) \quad k = 1. \tag{16.5}$$

Note that F_o is the maximum x-ray density of the lead stripes, λ is their spatial wavelength in mm, x is the direction of the stripes periodicity in mm, and λ_{co} is the minimum stripe period smaller than which, zero contrast is seen on the image.

Resolution of x-ray objects is complicated by the presence of noise in the image. Noise obscures the very small, high-spatial frequency, sinusoidal image of the grating. The noise appears as a fixed, 2-D, random pattern of low- and high-density areas on the film or intensifier screen. Thus, it is appropriate to talk about a *noise-limited (spatial) bandwidth* for x-ray objects.

Figure 16.7 illustrates typical MTFs for x-ray imaging by image intensifier and by film with fluorescent intensifier screens. In the latter case, the spatial cutoff frequency of the film with just the lead grid test object exceeds 10 cycles/mm. Noise from a living object overlying the lead grid

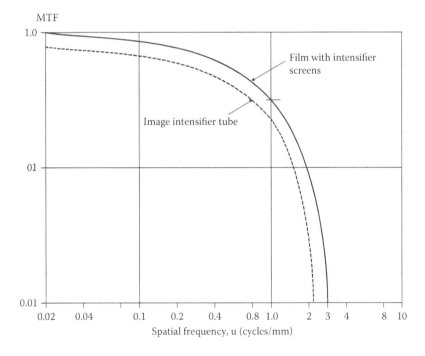

Figure 16.7 Typical modulation transfer function (MTF) for an ordinary x-ray system using two-sided scintillation x-ray film (*top curve*), and for readout by an image intensifier tube (IIT). Note that the spatial frequency cutoff lies between 2 and 3 cycles/mm.

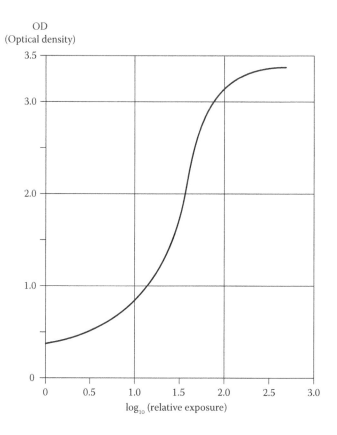

Figure 16.8 Sigmoid optical density versus relative exposure for developed ordinary x-ray film.

gives a noise-limited bandwidth of about 3 cycles/mm, which can be considered to be the practical bandwidth of this system when x-raying humans (Jacobson and Webster 1977).

Another factor in considering the MTF of film x-ray systems is the nonlinear optical density (OD) of exposed, developed film versus exposure (intensity × time). (OD $\equiv \log_{10}(1/T) = \log_{10}(I_{in}/I_{out})$.) Figure 16.8 illustrates a typical sigmoid curve for OD versus relative exposure for x-ray film. Note that the center of the OD versus relative exposure curve is fairly linear and can be approximated by

$$OD \approx \gamma \log_{10}(E/E_o), \tag{16.6}$$

where γ is the film's *gamma,* typically between 2 and 3, and E/E_o is the relative film exposure.

Common sense tells us that when the x-ray exposure is too high, nearly all of the film will be black, and very little spatial detail from the object will be visible. Similarly, if the film is underexposed, it will be too light, and a similar lack of contrast in the image will be present, ruining detail. In Figure 16.8, we see that the linear range is less than from $\log_{10}(E/E_o) = 1$–2. Thus, an object like a large bone (e.g., the femur) embedded in soft tissue (the leg muscles) may have the bone underexposed and lack detail, or the muscles overexposed and too dark if the x-ray exposure is not matched to the absorbency of the object. One way to avoid the problem of over- or underexposed film is to use a *dodger.* A dodger is a shaped, x-ray attenuator placed between the x-ray tube and the object to selectively reduce the exposure of soft tissue so that the entire film image is made in the linear gamma region, giving it maximum contrast and spatial frequency response (Jacobson and Webster 1977).

It is expected that modern x-ray imaging systems such as a scintillation glass screen imaged by a 1024 × 1024 pixel CCD camera can easily exceed the 2.3 cycle/mm cutoff bandwidth of an IIT shown in Figure 16.7.

16.2.4 X-ray Mammography

One of the great challenges in modern radiology is to be able to find lesions in soft tissues such as the breasts, lungs, or liver. Subtle differences in x-ray absorption in soft tissues are more apparent when the x-rays are generated with a lower electron accelerating voltage. Electron accelerating voltages from 10 to 40 kV are typically used for mammography applications. At lower x-ray photon energies (e.g., from 10 to 20 keV), there are larger differences in the mass attenuation coefficients of soft tissues (fat, muscle, connective tissue, blood vessel, cyst, tumor, etc.), hence greater contrast in the x-ray images of soft tissues. By using a tube with a 25 kV accelerating potential and a molybdenum anode followed by a filter of 0.8 mm Be and 0.03 mm Mo, the emitted spectrum is attenuated sharply for x-ray energies above 20 keV, and there is a tall, characteristic spike at ~18 keV energy.

Conventional X-ray mammography has not had outstanding results in detecting the breast cancers. In one Australian study (Howarth et al. 1999), researchers examined 155 women scheduled for breast cancer surgery. Multiple diagnostic modalities were used. Of 96 confirmed cancer cases, *scintimammography* correctly identified 81 while standard mammography correctly identified 61. Also, scintimammography failed to detect 15 existing cancers while standard mammography missed 31. X-ray mammography indicated that 6 out of 19 cancer-free patients had cancer, while the number of false positives with scintimammography was only 3 out of 19.

According to Komen (2015), overall, x-ray mammography has a sensitivity of 84%. This means mammography correctly identifies ~80% of the women who truly have breast cancer. Sensitivity is reported to be higher in women over 50 than in younger women. (Sensitivity is how well the screening test tells who truly has breast cancer; specificity is how well the screening test tells who truly does not have breast cancer.)

Scintimammography is demonstrably a better NI diagnostic technique for breast cancer than ordinary x-ray. Scintimammography makes use of the fact that cancer cells have higher metabolisms than other breast tissue, and will selectively take up a radioisotope-labeled metabolite, that is, Technetium-^{99m}Tc sestamibi (also known as *Cardiolite®*) (cf. Glossary). (The half-life of ^{99m}Tc is 6.0058 hours.) After a suitable time, any concentration of radioactivity in the breasts sensed with a gamma (scintillation) camera is suggestive of cancer which can be verified by needle biopsy. A low dose of about 4–8 mCi of the isotope is used for breast scans, which have a high sensitivity (91%) and a high specificity (93%) for breast cancer detection (Rhodes et al. 2011).

Digital mammography is another technique that offers an advantage over conventional x-ray/film mammography. In this technique, the film is replaced with a digital camera in which x-rays are sensed by a high-resolution microchannel system, each pixel of which converts x-ray photons to electron charge. The gain of each microchannel photomultiplier is from 10^6 to 10^8 electrons/photon. The charge from each pixel is integrated and converted to a voltage, thence to a digital signal. Digital mammograms taken with GE Medical Systems' Senographe 2000D® digital mammography camera have both high-contrast and high-spatial frequency detail, making it easier for the physician to interpret the image. Since the mammography image is in digital format, various linear and nonlinear spatial filtering algorithms can be applied to it to enhance suspicious areas of the primary image. In 2006, GE introduced the *Senographe Essential* digital mammography camera. It has the largest (24 cm × 31 cm) field of view available on the market, as well as stereotactic capability, allowing for a complete clinical solution (Middleton 2011).

An x-ray mammography technique was developed by researchers at the University of North Carolina Chapel Hill School of Medicine in collaboration with the Brookhaven National Laboratory's National Synchrotron Light Source, the Illinois Institute of Technology, and the European Synchrotron Radiation Facility in Grenoble, France. This innovative technique is based on phase-sensitive x-ray imaging, and is called *diffraction-enhanced imaging* (DEI) (Fitzgerald 2000); it may revolutionize medical radiography in the next decade. A synchrotron is the source of a very high-energy, highly collimated, electron beam which is aimed at an x-ray-generating target such as molybdenum. The emitted x-rays have the usual broadband, bremsstrahlung spectrum with characteristic emission spikes. They are directed to a silicon crystal x-ray monochromator which has the property of reflecting x-ray photons of nearly all the same wavelength at a particular angle. These "monochromatic" x-ray photons are next directed to the object to be imaged. As the synchrotron is a huge, immobile, particle accelerator, its beam geometry is fixed, and the target, monochromator, and analyzer crystal must remain fixed in order to function correctly. Thus, for the x-ray beam to scan the object, the object must be moved in relation to the beam.

The DEI method is sensitive to the *gradient of the refractive index* of the object. Recall that the simplest definition of the refractive index of a medium is that it is the ratio of the speed of light *in vacuo* to the speed of light in the medium. Because of the complex internal tissue structures, medical x-ray objects have complex (vector) refractive indices that are functions of position (x,y,z). In general, the complex refractive index can be written as: $\mathbf{n^*}(x,y,z) = n + j\kappa(x,y,z)$. The real part n is the *phase velocity,* and the imaginary part κ is called the *extinction coefficient* and indicates the

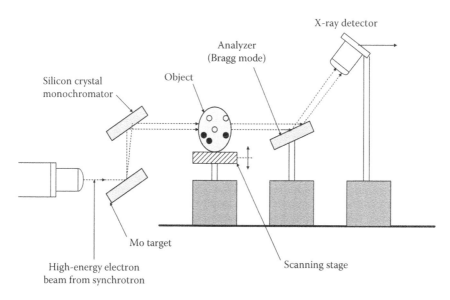

Figure 16.9 Schematic of a *diffraction-enhanced (x-ray) imaging* (DEI) system. Prototype DEI systems have exhibited phenomenal resolution of soft tissue details.

amount of attenuation as the EM wave propagates through the medium (Fitzgerald 2000, Hecht 2000). The DEI system is one means of visualizing object phase differences. Recall that the gradient of the complex scalar n*(x,y,z) is a vector defined by the vector operation:

$$\nabla n^*(x, y, z) = \mathbf{i}\frac{\partial n^*}{\partial x} + \mathbf{j}\frac{\partial n^*}{\partial y} + \mathbf{k}\frac{\partial n^*}{\partial z}. \tag{16.7}$$

Figure 16.9 shows the schematic of a DEI system. Insight into how the DEI system works may be found from the following quote from Fitzgerald (2000):

[The] radiation that emerges from a monochromator [crystal] is essentially parallel. As the X-rays traverse a sample placed between the monochromator and the angular filter (termed the analyzer), they can be absorbed, scattered coherently or incoherently (by milliradians or more), or refracted through very small angles (microradians) due to the tiny variations in the refractive index. X-rays emerging from the sample and hitting the analyzer crystal will satisfy the conditions for Bragg diffraction only for a very narrow window of incident angles, typically on the order of a few μradians. X-rays that have been scattered in the sample will fall outside this window and won't be reflected at all. Refracted X-rays within the window will be reflected, but the reflectivity depends on the incident angle. This dependence [is] called the rocking curve…

If the analyzer [crystal] is perfectly aligned with the monochromator, it will filter out any X-rays that are scattered or refracted by more than a few μrad. The resulting image at the X-ray detector will resemble a standard X-ray radiograph but with enhanced contrast due to scatter rejection.

If, instead, the analyzer is oriented at a small angle with respect to the monochromator—say by the half-width at half-maximum of the rocking curve—then X-rays refracted by a smaller angle will be reflected less, and X-rays refracted by a larger angle will be reflected more. Contrast is therefore established by the small differences in refracted angle of X-rays leaving the sample.

Thus, the image can show changes in diffraction angles and highlights the boundaries of fine, soft tissue structures in a breast. Preliminary studies have shown that the DEI technique has superior imaging properties; breast cancers are shown with detail increased by over an order of magnitude over conventional mammograms. A present and major disadvantage of the DEI technique is that it requires a synchrotron particle accelerator to produce the monochromatic x-ray photons required. Clearly, what is needed is a low-cost, portable source of collimated, monochromatic x-rays, such as an x-ray laser.

In the future, we can expect to see DEI x-ray imaging be developed and used for almost all types of conventional shadow x-radiography. X-ray interferometric imaging and phase-contrast radiography are also being investigated to exploit the high-image resolution that can be obtained given a collimated, monochromatic x-ray beam (Fitzgerald 2000). Instead of labeling cancers with radioactive metabolites and using a gamma camera, the labels can be metabolites labeled with radio-dense elements such as iodine or barium which may be easily seen on the DEI images. The DEI principle will also be extended to clinical, computed tomographic imaging (Dilmanian et al. 2000). (A mathematical description of DEI can be found in the Dilmanian reference.)

Positron emission mammography (PEM) is another new radiation modality used to detect potential breast cancers. PEM uses a pair of gamma radiation detectors placed on either side of the tissue under study to detect coincidence gamma rays following the administration of the radionuclide *fluorine-18 fluorodeoxyglucose* (^{18}F-FDG), a metabolite used in whole-body PET studies for the detection of cancers (Glass and Shah 2013). ^{18}F-FDG is taken up by a cancer cell's glucose transporter-1. Once inside the cell, the ^{18}F-FDG is phosphorylated and cannot be transported out of the cell; thus it accumulates in the cell. The radioactive fluorine nucleus is unstable, and as it decays, an energetic positron is emitted. The collision of the positron with an electron results in the production of two 511 keV gamma photons which are emitted 180° from each other. These two gamma photons are detected as a coincidence event (CE) by a pair of gamma cameras placed above and below the breast under study. Coincidence data from the camera detector cells are assembled by a computer into a set of 12 slices each in the right craniocaudal, left craniocaudal, right mediolateral oblique, and left mediolateral positions. PEM breast imaging has 1.5 mm resolution in-plane and 5 mm between planes (Glass and Shah 2013). (The Solo II High-Resolution PET Scanner used in PEM is marketed by *CMRNaviscan*, San Diego, CA.)

If there is any lesson to be learned from mammography, it is that no one test modality is completely without error. The current gold standard would appear to be needle biopsy, but this is an invasive procedure generally used to confirm results. Available, state-of-the-art, NI tests that are more accurate than x-ray/film mammography include digital mammography, scintimammography, PET scan, and MRI. And, as you will see in Section 17.2, there may be biochemical tests on blood or urine that can sense breast cancer before it becomes evident on any imaging modality. Certainly, a disease as important as breast cancer requires a multimodal approach to diagnosis to increase the detection probability.

16.2.5 Mammography with Ultrasound

An ultrasound scan of the breasts is an effective, NI means of detecting breast cancer. It is an important supplemental modality for the x-ray diagnostic procedures of conventional mammography. Ultrasound mammography by itself offers the advantage that there are no potentially harmful ionizing radiations used.

It has been reported that more invasive, node-negative (no lumps) breast cancers are found with ultrasound scans than by standard x-ray mammography (Doheny 2015). Using x-ray mammography, both a fluid-filled benign cyst and a solid tumor appear the same. Using ultrasound allows a radiologist to differentiate between solid tumors and cysts. However, ultrasound cannot resolve microcalcifications in the breasts, which are usually a first sign of breast cancer (Love 2015).

The relative merits of ultrasound screening versus x-ray mammography versus both means together are discussed in a Medscape article by Davenport (2014).

16.3 TOMOGRAPHY

16.3.1 Introduction

The etymology of the word *tomography* comes from the Greek *tomos*, a cut or slice, and -graphy from the Greek *graphein*, to write. Tomography has been applied in a number of imaging modalities in order to reconstruct images of internal "slices" of body parts: the brain, lungs, intestines, skeletal structures, etc. In its simplest form, a tomogram is generated by computer calculations done on sensor outputs when the source sends radiation through the body to sensors on the opposite side. Of consideration in the computation is the radiation pattern of the source, the radiation absorption characteristics of body organs, the directional sensitivity function (DSF) of the sensors, and the angle of the sources/sensors with respect to the body's axis. As you will see below, there are a number of possible geometric forms for scanning the object slice in order to obtain data to compute a tomographic image.

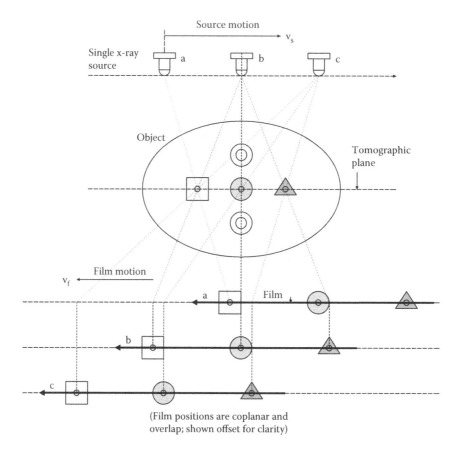

Figure 16.10 Schematic of a simple, *x-ray motion tomography* (XMT) system. Objects in the *tomographic plane* have the highest spatial frequency details. Objects out of the plane suffer lost high-spatial frequency response. Note that transverse linear film motion must be coordinated with the transverse linear x-ray source motion in the opposite direction.

Tomographic reconstruction of the structure of inner body parts is done with many modalities. The first and foremost is x-ray *computed tomography* (CT), or computed axial tomography (CAT) developed in the early 1970s in England by G.N. Hounsfield and A. McCormack. We also have PET, SPECT, *magnetic resonance imaging* (MRI), *ultrasound tomography* (UT), EIT, MWT, and OCT.

The *first and simplest* form of tomography is *x-ray motion tomography* (XMT); this is noncomputed tomography. A single, divergent-beam, x-ray source is used, and an x-ray film plate is generally the sensor. The first type of XMT system uses linear, parallel displacements of the x-ray source and films. As shown in Figure 16.10, the source and film are moved in a coordinated means so that when the source goes right by $+x$, the film plate moves left by a proportional amount, $-k\,x$. Due to the ray geometry, one plane in the object remains fixed in focus (the tomographic plane), while absorbers in other planes have their images blurred by (equivalent) spatial low-pass filtering caused by the uncoordinated motions of source and film (Macovski 1983, Chapter 7). In addition to linear motion, XMT can be carried out with radial and circular paths, depending on the application. In Figure 16.11, we see an XMT system devised by Ohno and Hayashi (1976), in which the camera moves in an arc around the center of the tomographic plane, while the film is moved in a flat plane. A variable aperture limits the spread of the x-ray beam to the area of the object; its aperture varies with the position of the source. Another type of XMT system is used to image the jaw and teeth in order to obtain detailed anatomical information relative to tooth implants. This dental system, called the Veraviewepocs® XMT system by J. Morita USA, Inc., rotates both the x-ray source and the film on circular sector paths around the patient's head (Morita 2011). Figure 16.12 shows the geometry of the Veraviewepocs XMT system.

However implemented, an XMT system can be used to image selected parts of the body inexpensively; for example, the spine or the lungs without showing the ribs. The mathematical details

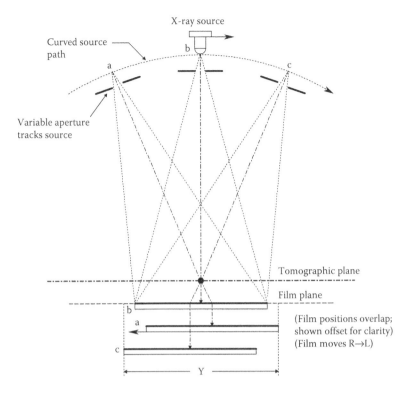

Figure 16.11 In the XMT system of Ohno and Hayashi (1976), the x-ray source follows a curved path. The x-ray beam is directed through a collimating window, which also moves with the source.

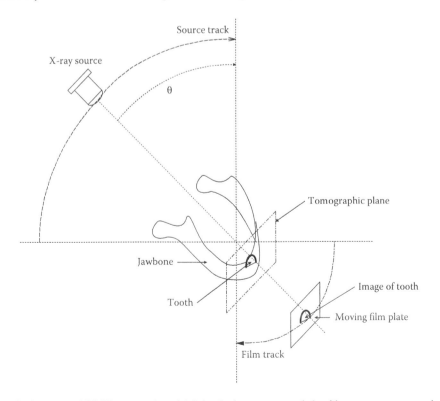

Figure 16.12 Dental XMT system in which both the source and the film move on curved paths.

of the projection geometry describing the resolution and spatial filtering of XMT systems can be found in Chapter 7 of Macovsky (1983).

Two disadvantages of XMT are cited by Macovsky (1983): (1) The radiation dose can be extensive if multiple planes are desired because the whole volume of interest is irradiated for each XMT. (2) The quality of the XMT image is no better than a standard x-ray. No spatial frequency enhancement occurs for simple x-ray film.

To illustrate how *computed tomographic* data are acquired, let us first examine the evolution of the x-ray CAT scanner. The first practical x-ray CT scanner was developed in England by Dr. G.N. Hounsfield in the early 1970s. This first-generation CT system used a single x-ray source emitting a highly collimated, pencil beam and a single x-ray sensor opposite the source. Data were gathered by linearly translating the beam and sensor across the patient and taking N intensity measurements (one every Δx cm) over a distance L spanning the patient. This data were digitized and stored in the 0° array. Next, the source and sensor were rotated some small angle, for example, $\Delta\theta = 1°$, and the linear scan of N points was repeated, and the digitized intensity data stored in the $1° - \Delta\theta$ array. This rotation by $\Delta\theta$ process was repeated a total of 179 times until an angle of $(180° - \Delta\theta)$ was reached, giving a total of 180 data arrays, each with an N intensity values in it. The scanning took approximately 5 min, and it took the computer ~20 min to reconstruct the data. This first-generation system used by Hounsfield was slow, and the patient was exposed to a relatively high dose of ionizing radiation. Still, it revealed for the first time the enhanced details in a tomographic slice of brain, or other soft tissue.

The *second-generation* x-ray CT scanner used a single-source emitting a uniform intensity, *fan beam* of x-rays. Multiple sensors were arranged in a fixed, linear array. The fan source and sensors were still translated linearly across the object then rotated $\Delta\theta$. $\Delta\theta$, in this case, could be larger, resulting in a ~30 s total scan time giving the patient shorter exposure to ionizing radiation. The image reconstruction algorithm was more complex than in the first generation because it had to deal with the angular fan-beam geometry.

A *third generation* of scanning geometry was introduced in 1976 that eliminated the need for translation. A single, fan-beam source of x-rays was used along with an arc-shaped sensor array opposite the source. The whole assembly rotated around the center of the patient. Patient scan time was now reduced to ~1 s.

In the *fourth generation* scanner, a fixed sensor array of from 600 to 4800 units (depending on the manufacturer) is arranged in a circle around the patient. A fan-beam x-ray source was rotated 360° around the patient. Again, scan time was ~1 s.

In *fifth-generation* scanners, the x-ray exposure (scan) time has been reduced to ~50 ms, fast enough to image a beating heart without excessive motion artifact. The fifth-generation system used a fixed, semicircular sensor array and a special x-ray tube with a semicircular tungsten strip anode. A high-energy electron beam is *electronically scanned* around the anode, producing a moving, fan-shaped beam of x-rays that rotates around the patient. There are no mechanical moving parts in the scanning process. Other designs of x-ray CT scanners are evolving, being driven by three factors: (1) Reduce the cost, (2) minimize the patient radiation dose, and (3) improve the resolution. Spirally (helically) scanned x-ray CT systems are being developed that will allow 3-D images to be acquired directly, instead of slice by slice.

In the following subsections, we introduce the reader to the complex mathematical processes required for CT image reconstruction.

16.3.2 Formation of Tomograms with the Algebraic Reconstruction Technique

We are all familiar with the simple, traditional, stationary "shadow" x-ray picture on film, such as a doctor might order to visualize a broken bone. A conical beam of x-rays is directed at the body part of interest, directly under which is a film plate. The tissues in the body part, for example, forearm, absorb x-ray photons according to Beer's law; thus, the x-rays emerging from the arm will have reduced intensities depending on the absorption coefficient of the type of tissue they pass through (e.g., bone, muscle, fat), and the path length they take through a particular type of tissue. Note that x-rays also can be scattered and emerge as secondary radiation, their photons traveling at an angle to the primary x-ray photons from the source. Often a 2-D grid is placed over the film or scintillation detector to exclude these oblique, secondary rays (Figure 16.4). Thus, the tissue under study essentially casts a sharp x-ray shadow on the film; tissue-like bone absorbs more energy, so the intensity of rays passing through bone are attenuated more than the rays emerging from only soft tissue. The more exposed an x-ray transparency plate is, the darker (more opaque) it is to light when developed. Thus, bones appear light on a conventional x-ray film, and a break in a bone shows up as a dark line.

Computed x-ray tomography allows us to see the fine structure of soft tissues normally hidden by bone in a conventional, shadow x-ray, including the brain and spinal cord, as well as the lungs, etc. Because of its greater pixel resolution, CT can locate lesions in soft tissues such as the brain, liver, pancreas, or breast not visible on conventional x-rays or XMTs. It is obvious that a real tissue is composed of a continuous mixture of absorbers, often arranged in layers or discrete geometries such as fat, blood vessels, and bones. In order to explore the anatomical details of a real tissue, we examine it by imaging contiguous, 2-D slices (tomograms). The absorbance details of the component tissues are measured on a discrete basis for instrumental and computational reasons. Each small area in a tomographic slice with the same computed absorbance is called a *pixel*; the smaller the pixels, the finer the resolution of the tissues. By processing the contiguous pixels in adjacent slices, we can define small, isoabsorbance volume elements called *voxels*.

To introduce the algebraic reconstruction technique (ART) to form tomograms, consider a 2-D model x-ray absorber, shown in Figure 16.13. Four regions (pixels), each having a different absorbance, are shown. We assume that Beer's law holds: that is, the transmittance along the jth ray path is:

$$T_j = I_{jout}/I_{in} = \exp\left[-\sum_{k=1}^{2}\mu_k\right], \tag{16.8}$$

where μ_k is the *absorbance* of the kth pixel.

When an x-ray beam passes through two pixels, the net absorbance is the sum of the two pixel's absorbances. Hence, the intensity of emerging beam 2 is $I_{2out} = I_{in} \exp[-(\mu_1 + \mu_2)]$, and the intensity of the diagonal beam 3 is $I_{3out} = I_{in} \exp[-(\mu_1 + \mu_4)]$, etc. The problem is to compute the $\{\mu_k\}$ from the intensities $I_{1out} \ldots I_{6out}$. By computing the natural logarithm of (I_{in}/I_{jout}), we have, for example, the absorbance, $A_3 \equiv \ln(I_{in}/I_{3out}) = \mu_1 + \mu_4$, etc. Note that A_j is in general, >1. Since six beams can be passed through the four-pixel absorber in a unique manner, there are six equations available to solve for the four unknown $\{\mu_k\}$:

$$A_1 = \mu_3 + \mu_4$$
$$A_2 = \mu_1 + \mu_2$$
$$A_3 = \mu_1 + \mu_4$$
$$A_4 = \mu_2 + \mu_4$$

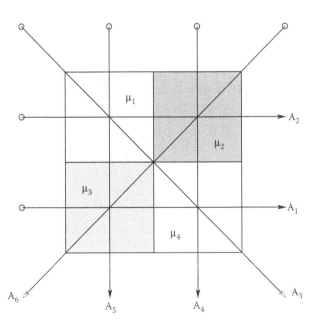

Figure 16.13 2-D, four-element x-ray absorber used to demonstrate the linear algebraic reconstruction technique (ART) of constructing a tomogram.

$$A_5 = \mu_1 + \mu_3$$

$$A_6 = \mu_2 + \mu_3.$$

With six equations and four unknowns, it appears that the system is overdetermined (four equations should be required to solve for four unknowns). However, solution for $\{\mu_k\}$ by using Cramer's rule to solve linear algebraic equations is impossible because the system determinant $\Delta \equiv 0$. Macovski (1983) showed that the $\{\mu_k\}$ can be estimated by an iterative, linear, ART, illustrated below:

$$^{q+1}\mu_k = {}^q\mu_k + \left[A_j - \sum_{k=1}^{N} {}^q\mu_k \right] / N, \tag{16.9}$$

where q is the iteration number, $^{q+1}\mu_k$ is the estimated absorbance of the kth pixel in the jth ray path after the qth iteration, N is the number of pixels in the jth ray path, $\sum_{k=1}^{N} {}^q\mu_k$ is the sum of the estimated absorbances for the pixels in the jth ray path, and A_j is the *measured* absorbance over the jth ray path.

Let us do a numerical example, following the procedure described in Macovski (1983): Let $\mu_1 = 2$, $\mu_2 = 8$, $\mu_3 = 5$, and $\mu_4 = 1$. Thus, $A_1 = 6$, $A_2 = 10$, $A_3 = 3$, $A_4 = 9$, $A_5 = 7$, and $A_6 = 13$. To obtain the q = 1 estimates, Macovski set all the (initial) q = 0, $\{\mu_k\}$ estimates to zero, and considered the two vertical rays. For A_5:

$$^1\mu_1 = {}^1\mu_3 = 0 + [7 - 0]/2 = 3.5.$$

For A_4:

$$^1\mu_2 = {}^1\mu_4 = 0 + [9 - 0]/2 = 4.5.$$

Thus, the q = 1 pixel estimates are: 3.5 4.5
3.5 4.5.

In the next (q = 2) iteration, the two horizontal rays were used. For A_2:

$$^2\mu_1 = 3.5 + [10 - 8]/2 = 4.5$$

$$^2\mu_2 = 4.5 + [10 - 8]/2 = 5.5.$$

For A_1:

$$^2\mu_3 = 3.5 + [6 - 8]/2 = 2.5$$

$$^2\mu_4 = 4.5 + [6 - 8]/2 = 3.5.$$

Now the trial absorbance values are: 4.5 5.5
2.5 3.5.

For the third iteration, Macovski used the diagonals: For A_3:

$$^3\mu_1 = 4.5 + [3 - 8]/2 = 2$$

$$^3\mu_4 = 3.5 + [3 - 8]/2 = 1.$$

For A_6:

$$^3\mu_2 = 5.5 + [13 - 8]/2 = 8$$

$$^3\mu_3 = 2.5 + [13 - 8]/2 = 5.$$

Thus, we see that in only three iterations for this simple example, the exact $\{\mu_k\}$ values were obtained. When j, N, and k are very large, convergence on the exact $\{\mu_k\}$ values can be very slow. Convergence can be tested by examining the magnitude of the normalized error for the jth path at the qth iteration.

$$\varepsilon_j = \left[A_j - \sum_{k=1}^{N} {}^q\mu_k \right] / A_j. \tag{16.10}$$

The linear ART process can be halted when the calculated ε_j reaches a preset minimum. Note that other nonlinear estimation techniques for the $\{\mu_k\}$ exist based on criteria such as the least MS error, etc.; however, their description is beyond the scope of this chapter.

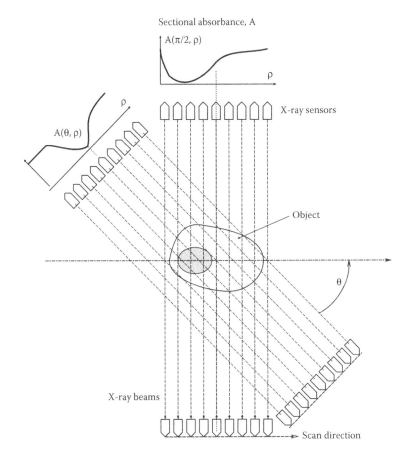

Figure 16.14 Parallel scanning geometry used in the first-generation CT scanners.

Current practice for finding the $\{\mu_k\}$ describing tomographic slices makes use of the *Radon transform* (RT), rather than an ART.

16.3.3 Use of the RT in Tomography

Figure 16.14 illustrates the geometry of a first-generation CT scanner. The pencil beam is linearly translated incrementally, then rotated some small $\Delta\theta$, and the process repeated until $k\Delta\theta = 180°$. Figure 16.15 illustrates the geometry of a third-generation CT system. In both cases, a family of plots of slice absorbance, $m(\theta, \rho)$ or $m(\theta, k\Delta\varphi)$, are made, shown as continuous functions in the figures. This absorbance data are used to reconstruct the absorbance or x-ray density of the object in discrete pixels. A summary of the mathematics of tomographic reconstruction follows:

The RT on Euclidean space was devised in 1917 by Johann Radon. Like many significant mathematical and physical discoveries, there was a substantial lag between its inception and a practical application. Not until the 1970s, following the development of the x-ray CAT scanner by EMI Ltd, was the RT found useful in computing the absorbencies of the pixels in a tomogram. Although the discrete RT is used in modern CT applications, it is easier to describe the significance of the RT using the continuous form. Thus, we can write the net absorbance seen by an x-ray beam passing through an object at an angle θ to the y-axis as the superposition of the differential absorbance elements in the ray path:

$$m(\rho,\theta) = \int_{(\rho,\theta\,\text{line})} \mu(x,y)\,d\sigma = \ln(I_{in}/I_{out}), \qquad (16.11)$$

where σ is the distance along the ray path in the object.

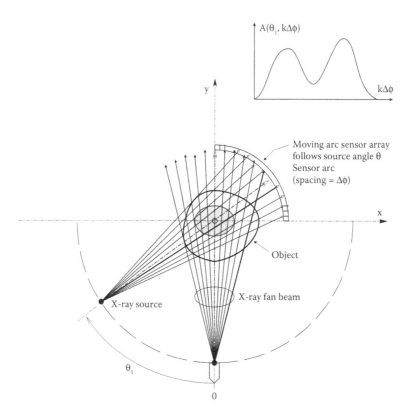

Figure 16.15 Fan beam scanning used in third-generation CT scanners.

Equation 16.11 can also be written using the *RT* of a *projection slice* through the object of absorbance, $\mu(x,y)$, using the delta function to define the path of integration:

$$m(\rho,\theta) = \int_{-\infty}^{\infty} \int_{-\infty}^{\infty} \mu(x,y)\delta(\rho - x\cos\theta - y\sin\theta)dx\,dy. \tag{16.12}$$

The delta function is ∞ for zero argument and zero for nonzero arguments. Its argument is the equation of a straight line in polar coordinates in the plane of $\mu(x,y)$, $\rho = x\cos\theta + y\sin\theta$. ρ is the perpendicular distance from the chosen line of integration to the x,y origin, and θ is the angle formed between the line over which the integration is done and the y-axis. Figure 16.16 illustrates this geometry.

Some properties of the RT are:

1. A $\mu(x,y)$ containing a straight line (not to be confused with the line of integration) or a line segment has an RT that exhibits an impulse or narrow peak at the RT coordinates ρ_0 and θ_0 which correspond to the parameters of the polar equation of the straight line (along which the segment possibly lies).

2. A $\mu(x,y)$ function that has a single point at (x_0, y_0) has an RT which is nonzero along a sinusoidal curve in Radon space of equation: $\rho = x_0 \cos\theta + y_0 \sin\theta$.

3. The RT satisfies: *superposition*: $R[\mu_1(x, y) + \mu_2(x, y)] = R_{\mu 1}(\rho, \theta) + R_{\mu 2}(\rho, \theta)$

    linearity: $R[a\,\mu(x, y)] = a\,R_\mu(\rho, \theta)$

    scaling: $R[\mu(x/a, y/b)] = |a|R_\mu(\rho a/b, \theta/b)$

    also, *rotation*, and *shifting*.

4. The RT is invertible.

5. A discrete, fast, RT algorithm exists, implementable in the frequency domain by FFT routines.

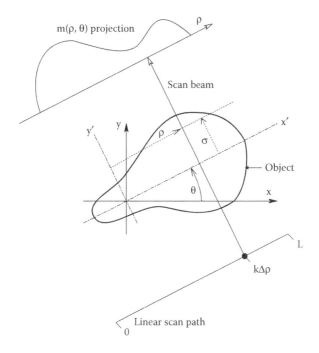

Figure 16.16 Scanning geometry relative to application of the Radon transform.

Computation of the *inverse Radon transform* (IRT) is used to estimate the original density image, $\mu(x,y)$. One way of finding the IRT is by application of the *Fourier slice theorem* (FST): "The 1-D Fourier transform of a projection taken at angle θ equals the central radial slice at angle θ of the 2-D Fourier transform of the original object." The FST states that if the 2-D Fourier space could be filled, the inverse, 2-D FT would recover the original object's x-ray density, $\mu(x,y)$. Filling can only be approximated using discrete, FFT implementation of the RT and FST. Interpolations are required, especially at high-spatial frequencies. To understand the FST, consider a rotation of the (x,y) coordinates by angle θ to become the (ρ,σ) coordinates. The rotation can be described by

$$\begin{bmatrix} \rho \\ \sigma \end{bmatrix} = \begin{bmatrix} \cos\theta & \sin\theta \\ -\sin\theta & \cos\theta \end{bmatrix}\begin{bmatrix} x \\ y \end{bmatrix} \quad \text{and} \quad \begin{bmatrix} x \\ y \end{bmatrix} = \begin{bmatrix} \cos\theta & -\sin\theta \\ \sin\theta & \cos\theta \end{bmatrix}\begin{bmatrix} \rho \\ \sigma \end{bmatrix}. \tag{16.13}$$

So $x = \rho\cos\theta - \sigma\sin\theta$, and $y = \rho\sin\theta + \sigma\cos\theta$, and the RT of $\mu(x,y)$ can also be written as

$$m(\rho,\theta) = \int_{-\infty}^{\infty} \mu(\rho\cos\theta - \sigma\sin\theta, \rho\sin\theta + \sigma\cos\theta)d\sigma. \tag{16.14}$$

Using Equation 16.14, the 1-D FT of $m(\rho,\theta)$ with respect to ρ is (at constant θ):

$$\mathcal{F}_1\{m(\rho,\theta)\} = M(\omega,\theta) = \int_{-\infty}^{\infty} m(\rho,\theta)\exp[-j2\pi\omega\rho]d\rho$$

$$= \int_{-\infty}^{\infty}\int_{-\infty}^{\infty} \mu(\rho\cos\theta - \sigma\sin\theta, \rho\sin\theta + \sigma\cos\theta)\exp[-j2\pi\omega\rho]d\rho\,d\sigma$$

$$= \int_{-\infty}^{\infty}\int_{-\infty}^{\infty} \mu(x,y)\exp[-j2\pi\omega(x\cos\theta + y\sin\theta)]\begin{vmatrix} \partial\rho/\partial x & \partial\sigma/\partial x \\ \partial\rho/\partial y & \partial\sigma/\partial y \end{vmatrix}dx\,dy$$

$$= M(\omega\cos\theta, \omega\sin\theta) = M(u,v),\text{in a 2-D, spatial frequency space,} \tag{16.15}$$

where $u \equiv \omega \cos\theta$, and $v \equiv \omega \sin\theta$, and the determinant is the Jacobean involved in changing from rectangular to polar coordinates.

Now the *inverse* 2-D FT is expressed in the polar coordinates, ω and θ in the (u,v) frequency space. Note that du dv $\equiv \omega$ dω dθ.

$$\mu(x,y) = F_2^{-1}\{M(u,v)\} = \int_{-\infty}^{\infty} \int_{-\infty}^{\infty} M(u,v)\exp[j2\pi(xu+yv)]du\,dv$$

$$= \int_{0}^{2\pi} \int_{-\infty}^{\infty} M(\omega\cos\theta, \omega\sin\theta)\exp[j2\pi\omega(x\cos\theta + y\sin\theta)]\begin{vmatrix} \partial u/\partial\omega & \partial v/\partial\omega \\ \partial u/\partial\theta & \partial v/\partial\theta \end{vmatrix} d\omega\,d\theta. \quad (16.16)$$

The angle integral above can be split into two integrals: one from 0 to π, and the other from π to 2π. We then get:

$$\mu(x,y) = \int_{0}^{\pi} \int_{0}^{\infty} M(\omega,\theta)\exp[+j2\pi\omega(x\cos\theta + y\sin\theta)]\omega\,d\omega d\theta$$

$$+ \int_{\pi}^{2\pi} \int_{0}^{\infty} M(\omega,\theta+\pi)\exp[+j2\pi\omega(x\cos(\theta+\pi) + y\sin(\theta+\pi))]\omega\,d\omega d\theta. \quad (16.17)$$

But it is known from FT theory that if $\mu(x,y)$ is real, then $M(\omega, \theta + \pi) = M(-\omega, \theta)$. This identity is used in Equation 16.17 to write (Rao et al. 1995):

$$\mu(x,y) = \int_{0}^{\pi} \left[\int_{-\infty}^{\infty} |\omega|M(\omega,\theta)\exp[j2\pi\omega(x\cos\theta \overset{(\rho)}{+} y\sin\theta)]d\omega \right] d\theta. \quad (16.18)$$

In Equation 16.18, the inner integral operates to filter each projection profile in frequency space. Now we define the 1-D, inverse FT of the filtered kernel, Λ:

$$\Lambda(\rho,\theta) \equiv \int_{-\infty}^{\infty} M(\omega,\theta)|\omega|\exp[j2\pi\omega\rho]d\omega. \quad (16.19)$$

Finally, we have the back projection by the real integration:

$$B\{\Lambda(\rho,\theta)\} = \int_{0}^{\pi} \Lambda(x\cos\theta + y\sin\theta, \theta)d\theta \cong \mu(x,y). \quad (16.20)$$

Multiplication by $|\omega|$ under the integral (in the frequency domain) serves as a high-pass filter applied to each projection profile in frequency space. Note that high-pass filtering accentuates noise, even if done over a finite ω range. Other band-pass filter functions can be used to minimize the effects of noise, and that filtering can also be done as real convolution in the spatial domain. The filtered profile, Λ, is summed along the ray paths in the image space.

Implementation of continuous, *filtered back projection* (FBP) requires infinite data to exactly reconstruct $\mu(x, y)$ of the object. In summary, the steps are (Rao et al. 1995):

1. Find the 1-D FTs of the projections.

2. Perform the filtering operation on the projections in the frequency domain, then do inverse FTs.

3. Find the back projections using Equation 16.20.

In practice, finite data are spatially sampled by the finite positions of the x-ray sensor array, and spatial antialiasing filtering is done to eliminate the effects of noise and high-spatial frequencies in the object's $\mu(x,y)$. FFT and IFFT algorithms must be used. A noisy, discrete estimate of $\mu(x,y)$ is found, and interpolation and smoothing is then used to estimate the x-ray densities of the discrete pixels of $\mu(p\Delta x, q\Delta y)$ in the tomogram. To minimize the effect of spatial noise in the FBP process, it is common to multiply the $|\omega|$ function inside the integrals of Equations 16.18 and 16.19 with a common Hamming or Hanning windowing function used with discrete data. The development of the mathematics for FBP applied to angularly scanned objects follows a similar course as above, but is too complex to examine in detail here. The reader interested in the mathematical details of discrete RT and FBP computation can consult the paper by Rao et al. (1995).

In summary, the reconstruction of the x-ray densities in each pixel of the tomographic image is a mathematically complex process. Many algorithms have been developed to interpolate and estimate $B\{\mu(x, y)\}$. Modern, parallel, multiprocessor, "supercomputers" can generate FBP density images in about 2–3 s (Rao et al. 1995).

16.4 POSITRON EMISSION TOMOGRAPHY

16.4.1 Introduction

PET is an imaging technique made possible by an amazing coincidence in nature. A PET image is basically a density map of radioactivity in a slice of tissue or organ viewed in 2-D. The radioactivity which comes from man-made isotopes is used to tag and identify certain types of living tissue, such as cancers, or to investigate tissue metabolism, such as in heart muscle and the brain.

When certain kinds of unstable, artificial radioisotopes return to a lower-energy level, one of their protons emits a *positron* (a particle with + electron charge and electron mass) and a neutrino, and thus becomes a *neutron* in the isotope's nucleus. The positron travels a short distance where it collides with an electron; the two annihilate each other in a matter–antimatter process that releases two energetic γ photons, each having an energy of 511 keV. The amazing coincidence is that the two photons originate at the same time and travel in opposite directions on nearly the same linear path (the *coincidence line,* or *line of response* [LOR]). The two photons exit the body and travel to two opposite sensors which are part of a multisensor, ring array that defines the tomographic plane. Other photons leave the body out of the plane of the sensor ring and are not detected; obviously, only photons with paths in the tomographic plane contribute to the calculation of radiodensity regions in the plane.

Because a variety of metabolites, drugs, and hormones can be labeled with positron-emitting isotopes, the chemical affinities of these tracer compounds to membrane receptors, cancer cells, specific gland tissues, myocardial infarction sites, etc. can be determined in the PET process. Some of the more common positron-emitting radioisotopes used in PET include ^{11}C (20.4 m, 4 mm), ^{13}N (9.97 m, 5.4 mm), ^{15}O (2.04 m, 8.2 mm), ^{18}F (110 m, 2.5 mm), and ^{120}I (81 m, NA). The first number in each parenthesis is the half-life of the isotope in minutes, the second number is the mean range of the positron in water. (The longer the range, the higher the initial positron energy.) The short-lived isotopes are produced in pure form in a cyclotron by high-energy bombardment with protons or deuterons. Then the isotopes must be incorporated into the tracer molecules by chemical reactions, and promptly transported to the PET scanner site where they are injected into the patient. Thus, a requirement for a PET scanner is a nearby cyclotron and radiochemistry lab.

An ^{15}O isotope is attached to tracer molecules such as carbon dioxide, molecular oxygen, and water. Ammonia is made with $^{15}NH_3$. ^{11}C is used to tag acetate ($H_3C–^{11}COO^-$), carfentanil, cocaine, diprenyl, *N*-methylspiperone, and raclopride. Methionine and leucine are tagged with $–^{11}COOH$. $^{18}F–$ is used with: haloperidol, fluorodeoxyglucose, fluorodopa, fluorouracil, and fluoroethylspiperone (Strommer 1996). The isotopically labeled compound is injected (usually IV) and within a few heartbeats is uniformly distributed in the blood. The concentration of the isotope in the blood then slowly decreases as it: (1) Is taken up by target tissues and organs, (2) is excreted, and (3) decays by positron emission. The isotope concentration rises to a peak in the target organ, then decreases to zero as it is metabolically destroyed and is eliminated from the site, and decays radioactively. Sometimes two different positron-emitting tracer compounds are given at once. For example, $^{15}NH_3$ and ^{18}Fluorodeoxyglucose are used to view myocardial perfusion and infarcted heart muscle in the same PET scan.

16.4.2 PET Process

Let us examine what happens to the two 511 keV photons emitted in the tomographic plane on a LOR. The two high-energy photons can interact with molecules in the body and undergo *Compton scatter* and *photoelectric absorption* (PA). In Compton scatter, the photon collides with an electron; the photon's direction is changed, the KE of the electron is increased, and the energy of the photon is decreased according to the formula:

$$E' = \frac{E_o}{1 + [h/(m_o c^2)](1 - \cos\theta)},$$
(16.21)

where E_o and E' are the photon's energy before and after the scattering collision, respectively, m_o is the rest mass of the electron, c is the speed of light, θ is the scattering angle, and h is Planck's constant.

Another way of describing what happens to the photon following the collision with the electron is:

$$\lambda' - \lambda = [h/(m_o c^2)](1 - \cos\theta), \tag{16.22}$$

where λ' is the photon's wavelength following the collision, λ is the photon's wavelength before the collision, h is Planck's constant, c is the speed of light *in vacuo*, m_o is the electron's rest mass, θ is the angle by which the photon's velocity vector changes following the collision. Note that a photon's energy is $E = hc/\lambda$, also, in general, $\lambda' > \lambda$.

In PA, a photon is absorbed by an atom and in the process, an electron is ejected from one of its bound shells. The probability of PA *increases* rapidly with *increasing* atomic number, Z, of the absorber atom. It also *decreases* rapidly with *increasing* photon energy. In water, the probability of PA decreases with approximately the third power of the photon's energy; it is negligible at 511 keV (Johns and Cunningham 1983).

The reduction of PET data begins with coincidence detection of the two photons traveling on the LOR. There are four categories of *CEs* caused by two photons arriving at two scintillation sensors in the sensor ring within the time window that defines a CE. Figure 16.17a illustrates a true CE. Two PE photons traveling straight on the LOR arrive at sensors within the event time window that defines the LOR. Exact coincidence is very improbable, because of path length differences and tissue interactions with the two 511 keV photons. Generally, the two photons arrive within several ns of one another, however.

In Figure 16.17b, we see how random coincidences can define a false LOR and thus contribute to a noisy PET scan. Two independent positron emissions release four photons, two of which strike sensors within the coincidence time window. The rate of random CEs is roughly proportional to the square of the concentration(s) of positron-emitting isotope(s) in the slice viewed by the sensors. The phenomenon of scattered coincidence is shown in Figure 16.17c. Here, a

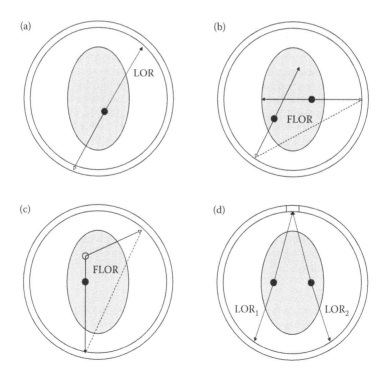

Figure 16.17 (a) A true PET event in the tomographic plane. (b) A coincidence event defining a false LOR (FLOR). (c) A false LOR caused by scattering of one photon of the pair. (d) Two valid LORs from two coincident events are rejected by the counting system.

false CE is caused by Compton scattering deflecting one or both photons emitted by a single positron–electron collision event. Scattered coincidence defines a false LOR that ultimately adds noise to the PET scan and also decreases its contrast. *Multiple coincidences* occur when two photons from two different positron–electron collision events strike the same sensor, while the other two photons strike a second and third sensor within the coincidence resolving time. Multiple CEs define two ambiguous LORs, and thus are rejected by the PET system; they are shown in Figure 16.17d.

The basic, high-energy photon detection sensor in a PET system is a fast photomultiplier tube (PMT) that is optically coupled to a scintillation crystal. Many such sensors are arranged in a ring surrounding the patient; the plane of the ring defines the tomographic slice that is imaged. The scintillation event is produced when an emitted, high-energy γ photon strikes the scintillator crystal and causes the emission of a high-energy electron, either by Compton scatter or PA. The high-energy electron passes through the crystal, exciting other electrons which loose energy in the form of radiated photons as they decay to their ground state energy.

A good scintillation crystal should have a high value of effective atomic number, Z. It should also generate a large number of scintillation photons when struck by a high-energy γ-ray photon. The crystal should have a low self-absorption factor for scintillation photons, and should have a refractive index close to that of the glass of the PMT to couple the scintillation light to the PMT's photocathode most efficiently. There are many materials suitable for scintillation detection; the scintillator of choice for PET sensors is *bismuth germanate* (BGO, or $Bi_3Ge_4O_{12}$), which has $Z = 74$, a linear attenuation coefficient (for scintillation photons) of 0.92 cm^{-1}, and a refractive index of 2.15. BGO emits 480 nm photons with a decay constant of 300 ns. Cerium-doped lutetium oxyorthosilicate (LSO) is another material that promises to be effective for PET sensors. LSO's $Z = 66$, its linear attenuation coefficient is 0.87 cm^{-1}, and its refractive index = 1.82. LSO emits at 420 nm and has a decay constant of 40 ns, giving an improved coincidence detection and maximum counting rate (Daghigian et al. 1993).

Pulses from each sensor's PMT are conditioned by a fast, *pulse-height window* circuit that has two adjustable threshold voltages: an *upper threshold voltage* (UTV) and a *lower threshold voltage* (LTV). PMT output pulses that do not exceed the LTV are not detected. These small pulses can be from weak scintillations from scattered and attenuated γ-rays that are not on an LOR, or even stray environmental radiation. Similarly, PMT output pulses that exceed the UTV originate from two photon coincidences at the sensor, and give no output. Pulses that lie in the voltage "window" between the LTV and UTV are probably from detection of a 511 keV emitted photon. If the output from a window circuit of another sensor across the diameter from the first also produces a pulse within τ seconds of the first, the coincidence circuit produces an output which establishes the LOR of that event between the two responding sensors. τ is typically about 12 ns for a PET system using BGO scintillators, even though the BGO decay time is ~300 ns. Figure 16.18 illustrates a block diagram of the pulse-height discriminator and time gate for LOR coincidence detection between two PET sensors defining an LOR. An output pulse at V_o indicates a one positron emission CE on LOR_{1k}.

The PET CE detection system has a finite limit to the number of CEs it can process per second. The decay time of the scintillator (300 ns) is the rate-limiting factor in identifying and processing the LORs. The maximum rate with BGO scintillators is about 10^6/s/scintillator. The PMT, pulse-height window, and logic can effectively function at well over 100 MHz. If the radioactivity level is too high in the object, some CEs can occur separated by so small an interval that they cannot be discriminated and identified as separate LORs. Under this condition, certain CEs do not get processed, and their LORs do not go into the tomogram computation. The missed LORs are known as *dead-time losses* (Badawi 1999).

Realization of the locations (or equivalently, the density) of the positron-emitting radioisotopes in the tomographic slice is accomplished by computing the intersections of the LOR vectors. The finite angle of acceptance of each sensor, $\delta\theta$, leads to ambiguity in the calculation of the density of PE events in a tissue. The intersection of two separate LORs in the sensor ring plane originating from two isotope molecules only nm apart does not necessarily define a point on the tomogram. Instead, there is a uncertainty area where the two atoms are located defined by the geometry shown in Figure 16.19. Also contributing to the uncertainty area is the fact that an emitted positron from a radioactive tracer molecule can travel in the tissue as much as 4–5 mm in any direction before the positron is annihilated by an electron, and the two γ ray photons are produced. The uncertainty area is on the order of 1 cm^2 in a 2-D PET tomogram.

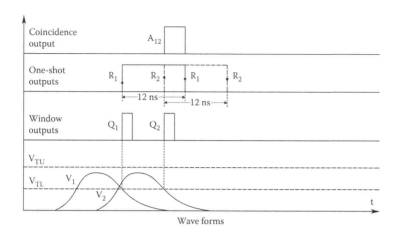

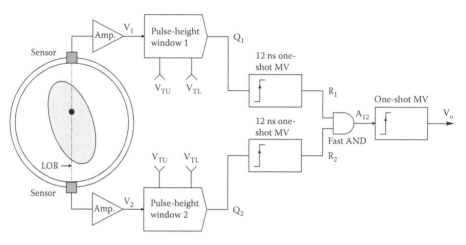

Figure 16.18   Timing diagram and block diagram of a PET pulse coincidence detection system.

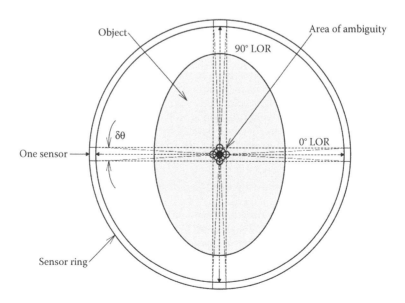

Figure 16.19   Ambiguity area defined by the finite acceptance angles of the photon counters when two events from the same point emit two intersecting LORs.

In computing a PET tomogram, the collected LORs are arranged in sets of parallel lines, each set at some angle θ with the y-axis. (The geometry is similar to the parallel beam approach to x-ray CT scanning.) θ is varied in small increments over $0°$ to $180° - \Delta\theta$. Just as in CT, a plot is made of the number of CEs on a given LOR path, $n(\theta, \rho)$ (Figure 16.20). Unfortunately, as we have seen above, there are several sources of noise and error in gathering $n(\theta, \rho)$. Some of these have to do with the random (Poisson) nature of radioactive decay, others have to do with the geometrical fact that the horizontal pacing between LOR lines becomes smaller going from the center of the ring toward its edges, and the fact that the sensors spatially sample the CE lines due to their finite number and spacing around the circle.

PET images are calculated using the RT and FBP as described in Section 16.3.3. Special attention has to be taken in the filtering to cutoff high-spatial frequencies in the data resulting from noise. An active research area in PET imaging is the application of statistical data reconstruction techniques to improve the image detail (increase its MTF cutoff frequency).

16.4.3 Some PET Applications

There is a large and growing list of clinical diagnostic applications of PET. PET has been used to evaluate the progression and severity of Alzheimer's disease (AD), Parkinson's disease, and traumatic brain injuries (Kitson et al. 2009, Magnoni et al. 2012, James et al. 2015). In addition, PET has been used in diagnostic cardiology, also in oncology (many types of cancer). PET responds to the isotopically labeled sugar, ^{18}F-2-deoxy-D-glucose (FDG), for which tumor cells have a higher affinity than do normal cells (Kumar 2008, Kitson et al. 2009, Kumar et al. 2010).

The PET scans are used in NI diagnosis of AD. As AD progresses, plaques of amyloid-β (Aβ) peptides form in the brain (see Glossary). An Aβ plaque is an aggregate of 36-43

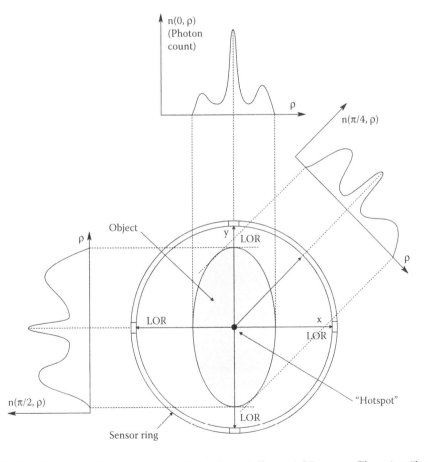

Figure 16.20 Representative photon counts for three different LOR arrays. There is a "hot spot" at the center of the slice.

AA peptides. These peptides are tagged (*in vivo*) with positron-emitting molecules of *Pittsburgh compound B* (PiB) (a radioactive analog of *thioflavin T*). Chemically, PiB is *2-(4'-[^{11}C] methylaminophenyl)-6-hydroxybenzothiazole.*

Unfortunately, detection and quantification of neurofibrillary (tau protein) tangles in the brain are generally done *in vitro* (Mavrogiorgou et al. 2011). However, MRI imaging in the NI assessment of AD Aβ plaques is now becoming more common (ICAD 2008, Bukhari 2013, Wagner 2014).

16.5 MAGNETIC RESONANCE IMAGING

16.5.1 Introduction

An MRI is also called *magnetic resonance tomography* (MRT) because one of the display modes is tomographic slices. An MRI scanner is basically a very large magnet with a hole in its center into which the patient is put. Before describing the physical details of how MRI works, let us examine some of the pros and cons of this NI imaging method. *MRI advantages include*: (1) MRI is totally NI and essentially risk free. Unlike PET and CAT methods, there are no ionizing radiations from within or without. (2) MRI gives excellent contrast for soft tissues including the brain, breasts, lungs, and liver. (3) MRI images blood vessels with high contrast because of the high-water content of blood. This feature enables the detection of aneurisms, stenoses, areas of high perfusion in parts of the brain during specific tasks, and the vascularization accompanying tumors. *Some disadvantages of MRI are*: (1) An MRI scan takes a long time; ~30 min, during which the patient must remain motionless to avoid image blurring. (2) MRI does not image bone well; tissue calcification is not easily seen. (3) MRI is acoustically noisy. The gradient magnets are switched on and off, producing loud "thunks" from magnetostriction. In some cases, this noise can reach 95 dB. A patient should wear earplugs to prevent possible hearing loss. (4) Because of the very high-magnetic fields involved, patients wearing pacemakers or cochlear implants, or having implanted metal joints, cannot undergo MRI. MRI is also avoided during the first trimester of pregnancy, although there are no reported harmful effects to the fetus. An MRT has pixel resolution between ~0.5 and 1 mm (Petridou et al. 2012).

16.5.2 MRI Physics

First, let us define the orthogonal axes relevant to MRI. The z-axis is the center axis of the main electromagnet, and also runs the length of the body, feet to head. The y-axis runs perpendicular to the z-axis, from the back to the front (chest) of the patient. The x-axis is perpendicular to the z- and y-axes, and runs from left to right.

MRI exploits the magnetic and electromagnetic properties of certain atoms in a very strong magnetic field. The main, z-axis, magnetic field used in MRI is called B_z. B_z is typically on the order of 0.3–1.5 Tessla (1 Tessla = 1 weber/m^2 = 10^4 Gauss). (By way of contrast, the earth's magnetic field is on the order of 0.5 Gauss.) A *superconducting,* solenoidal magnet is generally used to generate B_z. The magnet has niobium–titanium alloy windings, and is chilled with liquid helium to make it superconducting, making it easy to maintain the desired high DC current without generating heat. The patient is placed in the center of the magnet's coil where the field strength is maximum. It can be shown that the field strength in the center of the coil is (Sears 1953):

$$B_z = \frac{\mu_o NI}{L_c} \text{ Tesla,} \tag{16.23}$$

where μ_o is the permeability of vacuum ($4\pi \times 10^{-7}$ N s^2/Cb^2), N is the number of turns in the magnet coil, I is the coil current, and L_c is the coil's length in meters. At the ends of the coil, the magnetic field strength is about one-half than that at the center.

It is known that atoms with an odd number protons and/or neutrons possess a *nuclear spin angular momentum vector,* **M**, and thus exhibit the magnetic resonance phenomenon. Some of the atoms that are MR-active include [1]H (42.575, 1.000), [13]C (10.705, 0.016), [19]F (40.054, 0.830), [23]Na (11.262, 0.093), and [31]P (17.235, 0.066). The first number in parentheses is the (normalized) *Larmor frequency,* $f_L = \Gamma/2\pi$, in MHz/Tessla. The second number is the relative sensitivity versus hydrogen (^{1}H).

Figure 16.21 illustrates the vector relationships when a charged particle (proton) moves in a circular path at constant tangential velocity, **v**, at radius r. The *orbital magnetic moment vector,* **M**, is given by the vector cross product: $\mathbf{M} = \frac{1}{2} q (\mathbf{r} \times \mathbf{v})$, where **r** is the radius vector, and the *angular momentum* of the rotating particle, **L**, is defined by: $\mathbf{L} = m (\mathbf{r} \times \mathbf{v})$. Clearly, **M** and **L** are perpendicular to the plane of rotation of the proton.

When an atom's spinning proton interacts with an *external magnetic field* in the z-direction, **B**$_z$, a torque is experienced that causes its angular momentum axis to align with and precess about

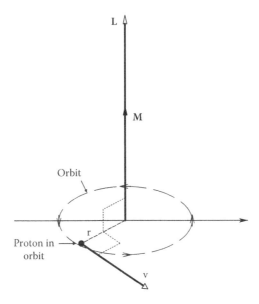

Figure 16.21   Vector magnetic moment, **M**, produced as the result of an orbiting proton.

$\mathbf{B}_z$. (The z-direction is defined as perpendicular to the plane of proton rotation.) The tip of the momentum vector describes a circle around $\mathbf{B}_z$. When $\mathbf{B}_z$ is first applied, it takes a finite *spin lattice relaxation time* for all the proton **M**s to respond. This response is characterized by an exponential equation of the form, $[1 - \exp(-t/T_1)]$, where T_1 is the *spin lattice relaxation time constant*. ($T_1 = 2$ s for urine, and 100–200 ms for fat.)

The steady-state frequency that the momentum vector revolves around $\mathbf{B}_z$ is called the *Larmor frequency,* given by

$$f_L = \Gamma |\mathbf{B}_z| /2\pi \text{ Hz,} \tag{16.24}$$

where Γ is the *gyromagnetic ratio,* given by the magnitude of the ratio of the orbital magnetic moment of the atom, **M**, to the *angular momentum* of the rotating proton, **L**. Γ can be shown to be equal to q/2 m, where q is the proton charge, and m is its mass (Murali 2015). Refer to Figure 16.22 for a description of the vectors.

It can be shown (Murali 2015) that the vector differential equation of motion for one, isolated magnetic moment subjected to $\mathbf{B}_z$ is:

$$\dot{\mathbf{M}} = \Gamma \mathbf{M} \times \mathbf{B}_z. \tag{16.25}$$

In an ensemble of many individual, precessing **M**s, $\mathbf{M}_e$ is the vector sum of the component **M**s. In a static, applied B field, $\mathbf{B}_z$, the phases of an ensemble of many precessing magnetic moments are random. That is, each individual, precessing **M** has a random position in its orbit (the dashed circle in Figure 16.22) induced by $\mathbf{B}_z$.

Because of this randomness, all of the x, y (or **i**, **j**) components of the individual **M**'s cancel out. Thus, the net macroscopic, magnetic moment of the magnetized ensemble is aligned with $\mathbf{B}_z$, even though individual protons are precessing around $\mathbf{B}_z$ at the Larmor frequency. Thus, the static net $\mathbf{M}_e = \mathbf{M}_z$, and $\dot{\mathbf{M}}_e = 0$.

The crux of detecting the number of molecules contributing to $\mathbf{M}_e$, hence the proton density in a volume element, is to perturb the individual **M**s by transiently changing the applied **B** vector's angle away from the z-axis (**k** unit vector). Because of the time-dependent motion of the x–y components of the tilted **M**s, and due to Faraday's induction law, an AC voltage at the Larmor frequency is induced in a suitably placed pickup coil. For a step change in the direction of B_z, $\mathbf{M}_{xy}$ does not persist; it decays exponentially to zero with a characteristic time constant called the *effective spin relaxation time constant,* T_2^*. T_2^* is about 100 μs for protons. Thus, the induced Larmor EMF also decays in amplitude.

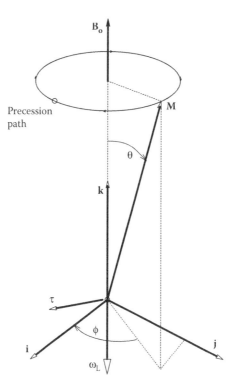

Figure 16.22 Vectors associated with a spinning proton interacting with an external magnetic field. The tip of **M** precesses around the **B₀** axis on the dotted line at the *Larmor frequency*.

16.5.3 How MRI Works

So where does the *resonance* in MRI come from? Instead of a stepwise, applied, DC, x–y component of **B**, let us apply an x–y component of **B** that rotates at the Larmor frequency, ω_L. That is, the net applied **B** vector is:

$$\mathbf{B} = \mathbf{B_z} + B_a[\mathbf{i}\cos(\omega_L t) - \mathbf{j}\sin(\omega_L t)]. \tag{16.26}$$

Thus, **B$_a$** rotates with angular frequency, ω_L, in the same sense as the individual **M** vectors precess around **B$_z$**.

The equation of individual **M** vector motion is now:

$$\dot{\mathbf{M}} = \Gamma \mathbf{M} \times (\mathbf{B_z} + \mathbf{B_a}). \tag{16.27}$$

When we substitute Equation 16.26 into Equation 16.27, the following two ODEs result:

$$\dot{\phi} = \Gamma[B_a \cot(\theta)\cos(\omega_L t + \phi) - B_z] \tag{16.28}$$

$$\dot{\theta} = -\Gamma B_a \sin(\omega_L t + \phi). \tag{16.29}$$

When $\omega_L = \Gamma B_z$ is substituted in Equation 16.28, we find the solution:

$$\phi = -\Gamma B_z t - \pi/2. \tag{16.30}$$

And from Equation 16.29, $\dot{\theta}$ will be maximal and is given by $\dot{\theta} = \Gamma B_a$. Thus, a circularly polarized magnetic flux density rotating at the Larmor frequency determined by **B$_z$** will maximize the rate of nutation. However, it is easier to generate a *plane-polarized* **B$_a$** than the circularly polarized one described above. The plane-polarized flux density vector can be written:

$$\mathbf{B_a} = \mathbf{i}B_a \cos(\omega_L t) = \tfrac{1}{2}B_a\{[\mathbf{i}\cos(\omega_L t) - \mathbf{j}\sin(\omega_L t)] + [\mathbf{i}\cos(\omega_L t) - \mathbf{j}\sin(\omega_L t)]\}. \tag{16.31}$$

The plane-polarized $\mathbf{B_a}$ is decomposed into right- and left-hand rotating components; the second term rotates opposite to the direction of precession and has negligible effect on nutation. It can be shown that when $\mathbf{B_a}$ rotates synchronously with the precessing magnetization vectors, a condition of *phase coherence* is induced in which the individual proton $\mathbf{M}$'s are all nutated coherently and thus have the same, fixed relationship around precessional orbits.

When the sinusoidal current producing $\mathbf{B_a}$ is gated on for about a microsecond, a peak *nutation angle* of ~90° is produced in proton (^{1}H) MRI. (The nutation angle is the angle $\mathbf{L}$ makes with the z-axis.) The amplitude of the RF pulse from this angle-shifted $\mathbf{M_e}$ decays exponentially with a *transverse relaxation time constant*, T_2 ($20 < T_2 < 300$ ms). T_2 is basically the phase memory time constant of the spin. T_2 is shorter in inflamed, edematous, or malignant tissues, and longer in fatty tissues. Note that $T_1 > T_2$ and T_2^*, implying that different physical mechanisms are involved between the initial response to $\mathbf{B_a}$ on, and $\mathbf{B_a}$ off. Many complex, interatomic magnetic reactions occur as the system goes from coherent spins to random phasing of the $\mathbf{M}$ rotations around $\mathbf{B_z}$. Note that the peak $|\mathbf{B_a}|/|\mathbf{B_z}|$ is typically ~0.005, a very small perturbation of $\mathbf{B_z}$. Control of the duration, period, and polarity of the $\mathbf{B_a}$ pulses and applied gradients are what give MRI images their exquisite contrast sensitivity. It can be shown that:

$$1/T_2^* = 1/T_2 + \Gamma \, | \Delta \mathbf{B_z} |/2, \tag{16.32}$$

where as before, T_2^* is the effective spin–spin relaxation time constant, T_2 is the actual spin–spin relaxation time, and $\Delta \mathbf{B_z}$ is the variation of the static magnetic field over the sample.

Three major types of pulse sequences are used in MRI: *Spin echo, inversion recovery,* and *gradient recalled echo.* T_E is the time from the 90° $\mathbf{B_a}$ pulse to the receipt of the spin echo. Following the 90° pulse, the body's $\mathbf{M_e}$ is tilted in a transverse direction. If the 90° pulse is followed with a stronger, 180° pulse, the individual $\mathbf{M}$'s swing back so that, initially, the slowest precessing protons now lead the change, and the faster changing $\mathbf{M}$'s are at the back of the group. The faster-responding ones catch up to the slow ones, so that they are back in phase; this causes the emitted signals to momentarily increase in amplitude. The fast and the slow responding $\mathbf{M}$'s then go out of phase again and the RF signal again decreases. This increase in signal following the 180° pulse is called the *spin echo.* The timing of the 180° pulse following the 90° pulse is critical; it must be optimized to differentiate tissues on the basis of their T_2 values, so-called T_2-weighted images.

An MRI offers the option of being able to magnetically and electronically select the plane of the slice. If the main DC field is given a gradient, $\mathbf{B} = \mathbf{B_z} + G_x x$, where the field still points in the z-direction, but its amplitude varies in the x-direction (G_x is just dB_z/dx), the Larmor frequency is a function of x: $\omega_L(x) = \Gamma(B_z + G_x x)$. Now if $\mathbf{B_a}$ with the excitation frequency $\omega = \Gamma B_z$ is applied, the slice $x = 0$ is selected. Spins in the y, z plane are tipped and emit RF signals, while other planes are not affected. The slice thickness, Δx, is controlled by the bandwidth of the band-pass filter acting on the RF signal from the pickup coil; a narrow filter bandwidth gives a thin slice. Use of a $\mathbf{B_a}$ frequency of $\omega = \Gamma(B_z + G_x x_o)$ allows the y, z plane of interest to be shifted along the x-axis to x_o. If a gradient $\mathbf{B_z} + G_y y$ is used, the x, z plane is selected and the slice thickness is Δy. Oblique planes of constant Larmor frequency can be generated by making the main flux density a function of x, y, and z.

Information from the amplitude and timing (T_1 and T_2) of the received, RF transients taken along with the pickup coil position and the $\mathbf{B_z}$ gradient-defined slice allow the RT and FBP to be used to form an MR image. As you can see, the process is much more complex than in forming a PET image. In PET we have discrete, all-or-nothing, CEs. In MRI, analog RF voltage waveshapes and timing, taken along with the magnetic conditions that produced them, are factored into the final image.

16.5.4 MRI Contrast Agents

When MRI is used to search for evidence of vascular anomalies (infarcts, aneurisms, ruptures, clots, etc.) in the brain, heart, and other organs, an injected contrast-enhancing agent is generally injected to more clearly show the vessel defect against background tissues. Contrast agents are paramagnetic or in the case of iron oxide, superparamagnetic. The most commonly used compounds for contrast enhancement are gadolinium based. MRI contrast agents based on ^{64}Gd^{+++} shorten the spin relaxation times of atoms within body tissues. The magnitude and duration of the spin polarization detected by the MRI RF receiver used to form the MR image decay with a characteristic time constant called the T1 relaxation time. Water protons in different tissues have different T1 values, which is one of the main sources of contrast in MR images. A contrast agent generally shortens, but in some instances increases, the T1 of water protons, enhancing blood vessel contrast in MR images. There are currently seven FDA-approved, Gd^{+++}-chelated MRI contrast agents in the United States (Everything 2015). These include:

- Gadiodamide (*Omniscan*®)

- Gadobenic acid (*Multihance*®)

- Gadopentetic acid (*Magnevist*®)

- Gadoteridol (*Prohance*®)

- Gadofosveset (*Vasovist*®, *Ablavar*®)

- Gadoversetamide (*OptiMARK*®)

- Gadoxetic acid (*Eovist*®)

When injected, the paramagnetic, trivalent, gadolinium metal ions ($^{64}Gd^{+++}$) are highly neurotoxic and nephrotoxic. In animals, the LD50 of injected free $^{64}Gd^{+++}$ is 100–200 mg/kg, but the LD50 is increased to ~10–20 g/kg when the Gd^{+++} is chelated (Penfield and Reilly 2007). Even when chelated with cyclic ionic compounds, there is some risk of release of the toxic trivalent Gd ion, hence possible complications of certain renal diseases. In 2009, the World Health Organization (WHO) issued a restriction on the use of several Gd MRI contrast agents (*OptiMARK Omniscan, Magnevist, Magnegita*, and *Gado-MRT ratiopharm*); these are contraindicated in patients with severe kidney problems, in patients who are scheduled for or have recently received a liver transplant, and in neonates up to 4 weeks of age.

Other MRI contrast agents include superparamagnetic iron oxide, superparamagnetic iron-platinum, and manganese. Some contrast agents can be administered orally to enhance MRI images of the GI tract. These include certain Gd chelates, Mn chelates, iron salts, $BaSO_4$, also natural products such as green tea and blueberry tea (Lee et al. 2003). *Perflubron*, a type of perfluorocarbon, has been used as a gastrointestinal MRI contrast agent for pediatric imaging (Bisset et al. 1996).

In spite of the small associated risks, $^{64}Gd^{+++}$ chelates remain the most commonly used MRI contrast agents.

16.6 SINGLE-PHOTON EMISSION TOMOGRAPHY

16.6.1 Introduction

The prototype *emission computed tomography* (ECT) device was developed by Kuhl and Edwards (1963). The first commercial SPECT device used a 32-channel gamma (Anger) camera and was called the *Tomomatic-32* (Jaszczak 1988). Since their inception, SPECT systems have steadily evolved; better, more highly collimated gamma cameras and improved DSP algorithms have improved image resolution (now ~3.5 mm) and turned the SPECT system into a valuable diagnostic tool. Some important applications of SPECT are the identification of tissues with low blood flow, specifically, the brain following a stroke, and the heart with coronary artery disease. Liver, kidneys, and other tissues are studied with SPECT, as well. A very important and promising application of SPECT is scintimammography—the detection of breast cancer by isotopic labeling.

Like PET, SPECT also involves the administration to the patient of a short-lived radioisotope incorporated into a drug, hormone, or metabolite with the object of measuring its density at target tissues relative to other tissues. However, the γ-ray emissions in SPECT occurs as single, random events (at random times and directions) rather than in the synchronous pairs of photons that define the lines of response in PET. The path of a γ-ray in the SPECT process must be estimated from the ray collimation properties and the relative position of the gamma camera used to count the γ emissions. In the SPECT process, the camera is slowly rotated around the target tissue (e.g., the head) a full 360°. It stops every $\Delta\theta$ and accumulates counts in its N channels. The information gathered is the number of counts originating along each of the N parallel rays defined by the collimator. Similar to PET, the raw data are K data sets, $n(j\Delta\rho, k\Delta\theta)$. K is the number of $\Delta\theta$ increments required to go from $\theta = 0°$ to 360°, and n is the number of discriminated radioactive events recorded in a given channel at a given camera angle. The K data sets, $n(j\Delta\rho, k\Delta\theta)$, are discrete Radon transformed, then FBP is used to reconstruct the density of radioactivity in the tissue being scanned. Figure 16.23 illustrates a schematic, top view of a human head being scanned by a SPECT system. Note that the lead tube collimator accepts only those γ photons that have paths

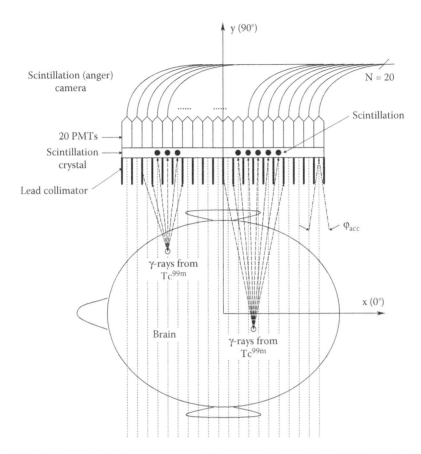

Figure 16.23 Schematic of a detector array picking up γ photons from ^{99m}Tc in the brain. Only those photons that enter a detector at less than its acceptance angle, φ_{acc}, are counted.

that lie inside a certain acceptance angle, ϕ. Oblique rays striking the camera at angles greater than $\pm\phi/2$ to the normal to the camera plane are absorbed by the lead sides of the collimator tubes and are not counted. All the gamma cameras used in SPECT use collimators of one style or another. A collimated gamma camera is called an *Anger camera,* after its inventor, Hal Anger, who developed it at the Lawrence Berkeley Laboratory in the 1950s (Anger 1964). Anger's original camera used a ½" thick, 11" diameter disk of NaI crystal as the scintillator, backed with 19 PMTs (Blazek et al. 1995). A lead tube collimator was used in front of the crystal. A spatial resolution of ~7 mm was claimed.

SPECT has a relatively poor resolution, partially due to the stochastic nature of the signals being counted, and partially due to the relatively large acceptance angles of the camera collimator tubes. However, the cost of a SPECT procedure is about one-fifth than that of PET. A SPECT system is technically simpler than a PET scanner. All it requires is a high-resolution Anger camera, a mechanical system to move it precisely, electronics to discriminate and count the camera's outputs, and a powerful workstation to compute the tomogram. A PET system requires a ring of photon counters, pulse-height discrimination circuitry, coincidence and detection electronics, and, of course, a computer to reduce the data.

As in PET, gathering the data sets, $n(j\Delta\rho, k\Delta\theta)$, takes more time than actually computing the tomogram by FBP. The SPECT data-gathering process is more efficient than for PET because an Anger camera can have a square array and gather data for a number of slices at one time.

16.6.2 Radiochemicals Used in SPECT

The radionuclide, Technetium-99 m was introduced in 1965 by P.V. Harper et al., as a labeling agent. It is the by-product of the radioactive decay of the radionuclide, ^{99}Mo, produced by neutron activation. ^{99}Mo decays by beta (electron) emission to Technetium-99 m (^{99m}Tc) (cf. Glossary), which is the most commonly used isotope used for tissue labeling. ^{99m}Tc has a half-life of 6.02 hours, and emits only 140.5 keV γ photons. The entire decay process may be diagrammed:

$$^{99}\text{Mo} \xrightarrow[\text{66 hours}]{\uparrow(\beta^- + v_e)} {}^{99m}\text{Tc} \xrightarrow[\text{6.001 hours}]{\uparrow\gamma 141\,\text{keV}} {}^{99}\text{Tc} \xrightarrow[\text{211,000 years}]{\uparrow\beta^- 249\,\text{keV}} {}^{99}\text{Ru}.$$

Depending on the type of SPECT diagnosis being attempted, the ^{99m}Tc is attached to a chemical that has an affinity to the tissue under study. Ceretec® and Neurolite® are ^{99m}Tc-labeled compounds used in the study of brain perfusion following the strokes. (Neurolite is also known as ^{99m}Tc-ECD and Ceretec as ^{99m}Tc-HMPAO.) Neurolite has a faster brain uptake and clearance than Ceretec. A dose of 30–30 mCi is given; imaging is done 30–60 min after the injection. Most of the ^{99m}Tc is excreted in urine.

^{99m}Tc has several properties that make it safer to use than other possible isotopes. Its gamma decay mode is easily detected by a camera. It has a short half-life (6 hours) in its decay into the low-radiation isotope, ^{99}Tc. This results in a relatively low-total radiation dose to the patient per unit of initial activity after administration, compared to other radioisotopes.

^{99m}Tc-pertechnetate (Technelite®) is used to image such tissues as brain lesions, gastric mucosa, thyroid gland, salivary glands, and blood. ^{99m}Tc can be bound to many organic compounds, for example, Cardiolite (also known as ^{99m}Tc sestamibi) which is used to investigate coronary blood flow in the heart. Miraluma™ is a ^{99m}Tc compound used in scintimammography. Other application of ^{99m}Tc-tagged pharmaceuticals includes the study of renovascular hypertension, urinary tract infections, testicular cancer, brain metabolism, cardiovascular tissue, hepatobiliary imaging, gastroesophageal reflux, etc. In fact, ^{99m}Tc is used in about 90% of all nuclear medicine studies.

Another radioisotope used in SPECT bone imaging and cardiac studies is Thallium-201. ^{201}Tl is produced with a cyclotron from ^{203}Tl. ^{201}Tl decays by electron capture to Mercury-201, a stable isotope. ^{201}Tl emits gamma photons with energies of 135 and 167 keV. It is a good thing if little is used; Tl and Hg salts are poisons.

Radioactive decay is a Poisson random process. That is, if the initial number of undecayed, radioactive nuclei in a volume is N_o, then after t time units (e.g., seconds, minutes, hours, etc.) the number, N, of undecayed nuclei in the volume is given by

$$N = N_o \exp[-\lambda t], \tag{16.33}$$

where λ is the *disintegration rate constant* characteristic of the radioisotope; its reciprocal is the decay time constant.

In fact, the rate of disintegration is simply:

$$\dot{N} = -\lambda N \text{ events/time unit}, \tag{16.34}$$

and the *half-life* of a radioisotope is simply:

$$T_{\frac{1}{2}} = \frac{\ln(2)}{\lambda} \text{ time units.} \tag{16.35}$$

16.6.3 Scintillation Crystals Used in Nuclear Medicine

In Table 16.1, the important properties of the most common scintillation crystals used for SPECT, PET, and nuclear imaging are given. Note that the scintillation decay time constant determines the event count rate of a given material. A high-effective atomic number, Z, material is more effective at trapping γ photons.

16.6.4 Gamma Cameras and Collimators

An essential component of modern gamma (Anger) cameras is a means to convert the 140 keV photons from ^{99m}Tc to electronic signals. Anger used a single, flat-plate crystal of sodium iodide (NaI) as a scintillation interface between the γ photons and an array of PMTs. The use of NaI has continued to the present. The NaI scintillator has the following properties: Effective atomic number, 50; linear attenuation coefficient, 2.2 cm^{-1} for 150 keV photons; optical index of refraction, 1.85; peak scintillation emission wavelength, 410 nm (violet); decay constant, 230 ns; mechanical NaI is fragile and deliquescent. The latter property means that NaI crystals must be hermetically sealed, either in vacuum or a dry inert gas. Modern, thallium-activated NaI crystals (NaI:Tl), such as those made and sold by Marketech International, Inc., come in various sizes and shapes; some

Table 16.1:   Properties of Some Important Scintillation Materials Used in Nuclear Medical Imaging along with PMTs

Properties	NaI(Tl)	BGO	CsI:Na	CsI:Tl	YAP:Ce	LSO:Ce
Chemical formula	NaI	$Be_4Ge_3O_{12}$	CsI	CsI	$YAlO_3$	$Lu_2(SiO_4)O$
Density (g/cm³)	3.67	7.13	4.51	4.51	5.37	7.40
Hygroscopicity	Yes	No	Slight	Slight	No	No
Refractive index, n	1.85	2.15	1.84	1.80	1.93	1.82
Peak emitted λ (nm)	410	480	420	565	365	420
Photons (meV)	41,000	9000	42,000	56,000	18,000	23,000
% of NaI:Tl	100	10	85	45	40	75
Scint. decay time (ns)	250	300	630	1000	27	40
Atten. length (cm) at 140 keV	0.408	0.086	0.277	0.277	0.697	0.107
Effective Z	50	83			36	

have been as large as a 17″ diameter disk, or a rectangular plate with a 38.5″ diagonal. Marketech also manufactures curved NaI:Tl crystals to conform more closely to the curvature of the human body. A typical thallium-activated NaI crystal used in SPECT is about 1 cm thick. Besides NaI:Tl scintillators, Marketech offers other scintillator materials, including CsI:Tl, CaF_2:Eu, BaF_2, Bi_4GeO_4, $Y_3Al_5O_{12}$, $YAlO_3$, Gd_2SiO_5, $CdWO_4$, $PbWO_4$, $NB(WO_4)_2$, ZnSe:Te, and $Lu_3Al_5O_7$ (Marketech 2015).

When a 140 keV γ photon from ^{99m}Tc decay penetrates the collimator and strikes the NaI:Tl crystal, its energy is absorbed and converted to 410 nm photons which propagate in various directions through the crystal. In classical Anger camera design, a closely packed array of glass-enveloped PMTs sits on the back of the single NaI crystal. The PMTs generally have hexagonal end profiles to permit close packing (such as the Hammamatsu R3336 and R1537) to better capture the emitted scintillation photons.

Because light is reflected and refracted at interfaces, some energy from the 410 nm scintillation is lost in going from the NaI:Tl crystal through the coupling medium to the PMT's glass envelope. In addition, absorption and attenuation of the oblique rays of 410 nm light occur in the crystal. In fact, some 410 nm light cannot leave the crystal because of *critical angle reflection*. If a 410 nm ray strikes the interface between the crystal and the coupling medium at more than the angle φ_c to the normal to the crystal surface, it will be totally reflected back into the crystal, where its energy will eventually be totally absorbed. From elementary optics, $\varphi_c = \sin^{-1}(n_1/n_2)$, where n_2 is the index of refraction of NaI at 410 nm (1.85), and n_1 is the index of refraction of the material outside the crystal but in intimate contact with it. The latter material can be a material such as microscope immersion oil with $n_1 = 1.515$, used to couple the scintillation light more efficiently to the PMT. With this n_1, $\varphi_c = 55°$, if air ($n_1 = 1$) is outside the NaI:Tl, then φ_c is only 32.7°.

When a burst of 410 nm light strikes the PMT's photocathode, electrons are released and travel through the electric fields of a series of dynode electrodes where they gain KE in a stepwise manner. The electron pulse grows in size as it approaches the anode because as each bunch of electrons strikes a dynode, its KE dislodges even more electrons, etc. The more the dynodes, the higher the PMT's current gain, but the longer it takes the initial photoelectron event to appear as a current pulse at the anode. A 10-dynode, hexagonal PMT used in Anger cameras, such as the Hamamatsu R3336, has an electron transit time of 47 ns and a rise time of 6 ns. On the other hand, the microchannel plate, R5916U series PMTs by Hammamatsu have a typical output pulse rise time of 188 ps and a pulse fall-time of 610 ps. The half-height pulse width is 345 ps. This speed would be wasted counting scintillations in a NaI crystal, however, because of its 230 ns pulse decay time for scintillation events. Figure 16.24 illustrates a cross-sectional schematic of a PMT with 10 dynodes.

As we have remarked above, good γ-ray collimation is a necessary condition for a high-resolution SPECT image. Collimators are generally an array of tubes through a lead plate located over the front surface on the scintillation crystal. Taken as a whole, the collimator comprises a 2-D spatial sampling array, not unlike the facets of an insect compound eye. And like a compound eye, resolution is linked mathematically to the field of view of each tube in the array. Each tube defines an acceptance angle, φ, for incident γ rays. Rays incident at angles greater than $\varphi/2$ strike lead and are absorbed. The geometry of this collimation is shown in Figure 16.23, and in more detail for one tube in Figure 16.25a. From the geometry in the latter figure, it is easy to show that the total

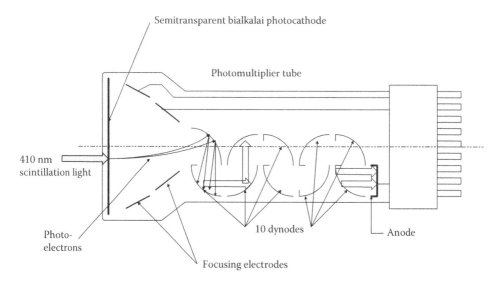

Semitransparent bialkalai photocathode

Photomultiplier tube

410 nm
scintillation light

Photo-
electrons

10 dynodes

Anode

Focusing electrodes

Figure 16.24 Cross-section of a photomultiplier tube with 10 dynodes (electron multipliers).

acceptance angle $\varphi = 2 \tan^{-1}(w/L)$, where w is the tube diameter and L its length. The smaller the φ, the more directional the collimator, and the higher the image resolution. In fact, we can describe a DSF, $f(\theta)$, for the tube based on the total intensity at the bottom of the tube (at the scintillation crystal's surface) as the function of angle θ made by an ideal, continuous, point source of radiation with the center line. $f(\theta) \equiv I(\theta)/I_{max}$, where $I(\theta)$ is the radiation intensity striking the bottom of the hole, that is, the scintillator plate, and I_{max} is the maximum intensity. It can be shown that $f(\theta)$ is the normalized, 1-D, *spatial impulse response* of the tube (cf. Section 5.2, Northrop 2001). Obviously, the intensity at the bottom of the tube is maximum when the point source is directly on axis ($\theta = 0°$), and must be zero for $|\theta| \geq \varphi/2$. For $0° < |\theta| \leq \varphi/2$, there is a crescent "shadow" formed by the wall of the tube on the bottom, as shown in Figure 16.25b. The 1-D spatial frequency response of the tube collimator is proportional to the Fourier transform of $f(\theta)$, $\mathbf{F}(u)$. $\mathbf{F}(u)$ is real and even in the spatial frequency, u, because $f(\theta)$ is real and even. Note that the narrower $f(\theta)$, the broader the collimator's spatial frequency response. However, there is a trade-off between a high-frequency response (small w/L ratio) and system sensitivity. With a small w/L, few of the γ photons will be counted in a given interval; most will strike the sides of the lead tubes and be absorbed. Thus, to obtain high-definition SPECT plots, a longer counting time is needed at each camera angle. (The $f(\theta)$ illustrated in Figure 16.25c is "typical"; no mathematical function was derived to describe it.)

A traditional Anger camera uses a flat collimator on a large, flat, NaI scintillation crystal, backed with an array of PMTs. As the object being imaged is generally oval or rounded in form, this means that the inherent ray geometry causes the image resolution at the edges of the camera to become degraded and distorted from that at the center. Center resolution is ~3.5 mm (Balzek et al. 1995).

16.6.5 Future Trends in Nuclear Medical Imaging

To reduce the cost and complexity of the traditional flat-plate Anger camera design, and to improve on its imaging resolution, several new design strategies for gamma cameras for SPECT are being explored. In one approach being developed at the Karolinska Hospital in Stockholm, a cylindrical NaI scintillation crystal is used to better fit human anatomy; the head or body part is placed in the center of the cylinder. γ photons from ^{99m}Tc are coupled to the cylindrical scintillator through four lead collimators. A length of 410 nm scintillation photons from the crystal are coupled to a radially oriented array of hexagonal PMTs, arranged in 4 rows and 18 columns, giving a total of 72 channels. U.S. Patent No. 5,783,829 (Sealock et al. 1998) described another gamma camera made with separate, curved sections of CsI scintillation crystals designed to better match the patient's geometry.

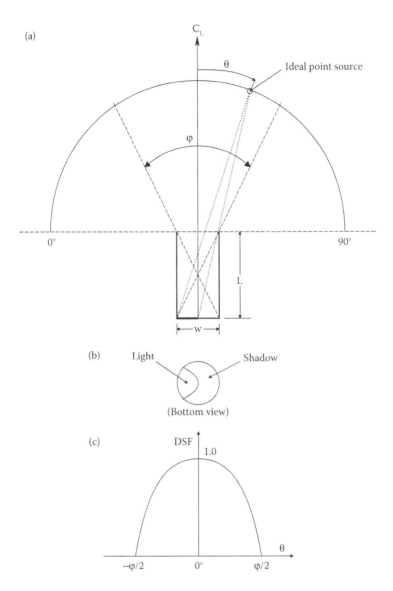

Figure 16.25 (a) Geometry of a system defining the acceptance angle of a γ photon collimator. Direct rays at angles $> |\varphi/2|$ do not strike the counter scintillator at the bottom of the tube; they are absorbed by the tube walls. (b) A crescent shadow is formed at the bottom of the collimator tube by a parallel bundle of rays striking the tube mouth from an angle to the right, as shown in (a). (The reader can verify this by shining a flashlight on a cardboard tube.) (c) A typical, normalized, directional sensitivity function for a tube collimator. In an array of such collimators, the narrower the DSF, the higher the spatial frequency resolution of the array.

Scientists at the *Instituto Nazionale di Fisica Nucleare* in Rome (INFN-Roma), group on High-Resolution Single-Photon Emission Tomography (HIRESPET) are taking two innovative approaches to improving the image quality in SPECT. One approach has been based on the innovative, Hamamatsu, *position-sensitive photomultiplier tube* (PSPMT). The single PSPMT replaces dozens of conventional PMTs as scintillation photon detectors. Photoelectrons are emitted from various positions of the large area photocathode, depending on the distribution of input photons from the scintillators. A proximity mesh dynode structure produces electron multiplication and preserves the initial spatial distribution of the emission from the photocathode. Hamamatsu makes several models of PSPMTs; The R8900U-00-02 series has a 30 mm square photocathode; the R3292-02 series has a 5″ diameter, circular, 12-stage, bialkalai photocathode (Hamamatsu 2012).

In the large, R3292 PSPMT, the anode is formed by an orthogonal grid of 56 nontouching wires, that is, 28 wires in the x-direction and 28 wires in the y-direction. The anode grids have a square area, whether the shape of the photocathode is round or square. In the large R3292 PSPMT, the grid measures 53.34 mm (2.1″) on a side. Between each wire on a side of the grid is a series of 1 k resistors, as shown in Figure 16.26.

To understand how the PSPMT works, let us first consider the y-axis wires. The gray dot represents a beam of multiplied photoelectrons striking the grid; it behaves like a current source, $i_s(n, t)$, where it strikes the nth y-grid wire. The op-amps are current-to-voltage converters. For example, i_{yb} flows into the op-amp's summing junction, a virtual ground, and $V_{yb} = -i_{yb} R$. At the nth wire ($n = 5$ in this example), the voltage, V_{yn}, can be shown to be:

$$V_{yn} = \frac{i_s Rn(K - n)}{K}, \quad (0 \le n \le K). \tag{16.36}$$

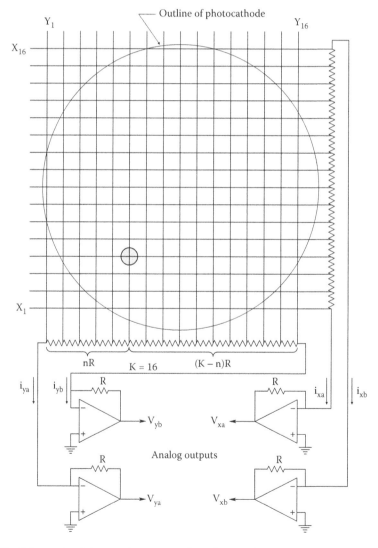

Figure 16.26 Schematic of the anode wires and analog readout electronics of a position-sensitive photomultiplier tube. The wires and photocathode are, of course, *in vacuo*.

And by Ohm's law, the current i_{ya} is:

$$i_{ya} = \frac{i_s Rn(K-n)/K}{nR} = i_s(1 - n/K).\tag{16.37}$$

And i_{yb} is:

$$i_{yb} = \frac{i_s Rn(K-n)/K}{(K-n)R} = i_s n/K.\tag{16.38}$$

Thus, $V_{ya} = -i_s(1 - n/K)R$, $V_{yb} = -i_s(n/K)R$, and $(V_{ya} + V_{yb}) = -i_s R$; that is, the sum signal gives the amplitude of $i_s(n, t)$. The difference, $(V_{ya} - V_{yb}) = -i_s R(1 - 2n/K)$. Thus, the four output voltages are sampled, and the ratio

$$\frac{(V_{ya} - V_{yb})}{(V_{ya} + V_{yb})} = (1 - 2n/K)\tag{16.39}$$

is calculated. Note that the ratio is a linear function of the wire position in the y-grid. A similar relation can be developed for the x-grid. Thus, a transient, amplified, photocurrent pulse $i_s(x, y, t)$ can be located in terms of the wire numbers in the x, y grid of the PSPMT by simple signal processing.

Blazek et al. (1995) described a prototype, high-resolution gamma camera. To take advantage of the PSPMT's high-spatial resolution, they used individual, small scintillator crystals, optically isolated from one another. Yttrium aluminum perovskit doped with cerium ($YAlO_3$:Ce or YAP:Ce) was formed into thin, square rods, 0.6 mm $\times$ 0.6 mm $\times$ 18 mm. An array of 11×22 of these YAP:Ce "needles" was used with an R2486 PSPMT. The prototype camera was tested with various ^{99m}Tc phantoms; it showed a resolution of $\sim$0.7 mm, a decided improvement over state-of-the-art, collimated, single-crystal Anger cameras.

A California company, *Gamma Medica-Ideas, Inc.*, has developed its LumaGem® gamma camera based on the same design strategy described in the paragraph above. The LumaGem system consisted of an array of $2 \times 2 \times 6$ mm^3 NaI:Tl pixels coupled to an array of PSPMTs. It has a 125×125 mm^2 field of view. A pinhole collimator was used on LumaGEM to acquire SPECT images of mice that had transgenic modifications to model various diseases. The preliminary images in the paper show detailed uptake in the mice, and are a convincing sign that animal SPECT can reach submillimeter spatial resolution (MacDonald et al. 2001). Another LumaGEM version used a $5'' \times 5''$, square array of $(75 \times 75) = 5625$ individual, "needle" scintillation crystals made from cesium iodide. The ends of the individual crystals are about 1.69 mm^2. The crystals are coupled to a high-resolution PSPMT. Because of its small size, the LumaGem camera is ideally suited for scintimmamography (FDA 2011) and thyroid studies, as well as eventual application for brain SPECT. The manufacturer claims a spatial resolution of 1.75 mm for the camera in imaging tissue.

In the future, there will be continuing development of smaller, high-resolution gamma cameras. Researchers at CERN (Geneva) and HIRESPET are developing an Imaging Silicon Pixel Array (ISPA) tube. The first version of this prototype device had geometry based on the venerable IR IIT (Figure 16.27). Instead of IR photons striking a photocathode and generating photoelectrons, the UV photons from a scintillator crystal hit the ISPA tube photocathode which emits photoelectrons. They are accelerated in straight lines, *in vacuo*, 20–50 mm by an electric field generated by a 20–25 kV potential. These high-energy photoelectrons strike a chip with a 16×64 (1024) matrix of biased diode sensors on it. The active chip area is 4.8 mm $\times$ 8 mm. Each diode in the array has a 75 μm $\times$ 500 μm area. Diode reverse current is proportional to the electron current striking it. In the basic system, no external lead collimator was used in front of the single-plate YAP:Ce ($YAlO_3$) scintillator. The 365 nm YAP:Ce scintillation photons were coupled to the ISPA tube's UV-sensitive photocathode through a quartz fiber-optic (FO) coupler. Resolution was tested using a lead plate collimator source with two 350 μm holes drilled in it 1.2 mm apart. The ISPA tube prototype with the FO window could resolve objects at $\sim$700 μm. In another version, YAP:Ce needles with 600 μm $\times$ 600 μm end areas were used to convert γ photons to 365 nm scintillation photons. The YAP needles are optically isolated from one another and together, act like a collimator. Resolution with the YAP needle ISPA tube was 310 μm (Puertolas et al. 1997).

A second-generation ISPA tube, shown schematically in Figure 16.28, uses an electric field lens to gather photoelectrons from a large photocathode (40 mm active diameter) and focus

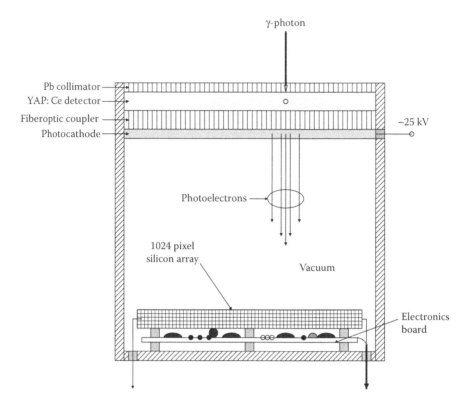

Figure 16.27 Section through a first-generation imaging silicon pixel array (ISPA) tube.

them on a smaller electron sensor chip. The demagnifying ratio of the prototype tube was 1/4.45 (D'Ambrosio et al. 1998, 1999). This cross-focusing (CF) ISPA tube will be studied using individual, 1 mm × 1 mm, column YAP:Ce crystals (YAlO₃) instead of the single YAP plate. The predicted resolution could be ~1 mm, suitable for scintimammography imaging and perhaps SPECT.

In summary, the ISPA tube approach detects photoelectrons arising from scintillations by a matrix of biased *pn* junctions. The PSPMT approach uses the crossed wire matrix of the PSPMT to sense the photoelectron current directly. However, the photomultiplier offers more photoelectron current gain and is more expensive.

16.7 OPTICAL COHERENCE TOMOGRAPHY

16.7.1 Introduction

OCT is a new, NI, laser-based, noncontact, imaging technique that can image tissue structures to a depth of 2–3 mm, *in vivo,* with a resolution of 5–15 μm (vs 110 μm for high-frequency ultrasound). OCT was first developed in 1991 at MIT's Research Laboratory for Electronics (RLE) by James Fujimoto (Fujimoto et al. 1995).

OCT has been used with endoscopes to examine cancers and lesions on the surfaces of human mucosa, including that of the inner esophagus, larynx, stomach, colon, urinary bladder, and the uterine cervix (Sergeev et al. 1997, Feldchtein et al. 1998). OCT has also been used in the study and characterization of skin melanomas, and it also has application in the study of wound healing, for example, for skin grafts in treating the burns. Another important application of OCT is in ophthalmology. The anatomical layers of the retina can be displayed, both radially and tangentially, and its thickness is measured. OCT has been found valuable in diagnosing diabetic retinopathy, macular holes, fluid accumulation, retinal detachments, etc. (Puliafito et al. 1996, EyeWiki 2015, OCT 2016). The study of the fine structure of tooth enamel, dentin, caries, and gums has also been made possible by OCT (Wang et al. 1999, Hsieh et al. 2013).

16.7.2 How OCT Works

The light source in OCT is generally a near-IR, *superluminescent light-emitting diode* (SLD or SLED) with a narrow bandwidth (e.g., 17 nm half-intensity around an 812 nm peak). *Optical coherence*

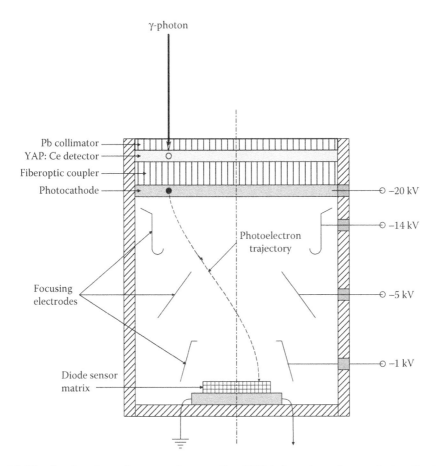

Figure 16.28 Section through a second-generation ISPA tube using a larger photocathode and focusing electrodes to direct photoelectrons from the photocathode of area A_p to the smaller diode detector array of area A_d.

length is purposely short compared to a laser diode, only about 30 nm. SLDs are multilayer devices; in the 800 nm region, they are fabricated from GaAs and AlGaAs. In the 1300–1500 nm range, they are made from InGaAsP and InP. Near-IR is used in medical OCT for better tissue penetration.

The SLD beam is directed to a *scanning Michelson interferometer* (Figure 16.29). The beam emerging from the interferometer is collimated into a small spot, or a narrow line (in the y-direction) which is mechanically scanned over the tissue under study; in x and y for the spot and x for the line. The reflected light is collected and directed back through the interferometer. The amount and phase of the reflected light depend on the refractive index of the microscopic anatomical components of the tissue under study, as well as their absorption in x, y, and z.

With the low-coherence SLD source, interference fringes are only generated if the absolute path distance between the two arms is very small (less than half the coherence length). The δz modulation effectively scans the object in the depth (z)-direction, once the coarse mirror position has been adjusted to balance the interferometer with the object. There is no fringe ambiguity problem such as would be caused with a highly coherent laser source. If the scanning mirror moves out of range of the SLD's coherence, the image vanishes. Thus, the OCT operator knows exactly the depth where the scanning is taking place.

The backscatter intensity output of the interferometer is a function of depth (z) and position (x,y) over the target. By adjusting the interferometer to keep z constant, a 2-D, x, y slice of tissue structure can be displayed. Or x can be held constant, and a 2-D, depth slice image in z and y can be generated (most common for retinal scans). The intensity output from the interferometer is directed to a single photosensor for the spot probe, and a CCD line-scan sensor for the line probe.

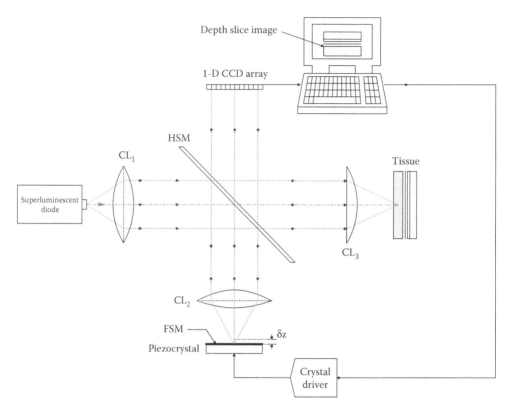

Figure 16.29 Schematic of an OCT system using a scanning Michelson interferometer. A short-coherence-length superluminescent diode (SLD) is used instead of a laser light source. The SLD is used to limit the thickness of the OCT image.

16.7.3 Applications of OCT

A commercial OCT system for ophthalmological scanning has been marketed by Humphrey Instuments. The Humphrey OCT system can reproducibly quantify retinal and nerve fiber layer thickness to better than 11 µm. Roche Diagnostics Co. in Germany developed an OCT system using a chromium fosterite, 1310 nm laser projecting a 4.5 µm spot. A single-mode, optical fiber, Michelson interferometer was used to condition the reflected radiation. Most OCT systems to date are experimental because the technology in the field is evolving so rapidly. The trend today is away from the classical, straight-beam, Michelson interferometer to the use of single-mode, optical fiber, Michelson interferometers, such as illustrated in Figure 16.30. Note that a visible LED is used for targeting. The probe in this configuration produces a single, small spot.

An important enhancement of OCT being developed is Doppler optical coherence tomography (DOCT). DOCT is based on coherence gating. It combines laser Doppler flowmetry (LDF) (see Section 15.5 of this text) with OCT. Heterodyne mixing of the superimposed source light with the Doppler-shifted, backscattered light at a photodiode surface yields a lower RF sideband whose frequency, f_D, is proportional to the velocity of moving scatterers parallel to the incident, collimated beam. Because of the small beam diameter and low coherence of the source, a Doppler frequency can be determined for all of the *moving* reflectors in an OCT image pixel. Colors can be assigned by the imaging computer to give qualitative velocity information on pixels containing the moving scatterers. The frequency of the detected Doppler shift was shown in Section 15.5 of this text to be:

$$f_D \equiv (\nu_s - \nu_r) = (2\nu_s/c')\,|\mathbf{v}|\cos(\theta) = (2/\lambda_s)\,|\mathbf{v}|\cos(\theta)\,\text{Hz}, \tag{16.40}$$

where $\mathbf{v}$ is the velocity vector of the moving scatterer, c' is the speed of light in the medium containing the moving scatterer, ν_s is the frequency of the incident light of wavelength λ_s, ν_b is

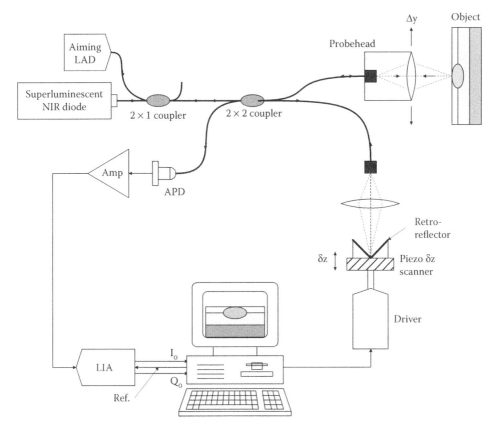

Figure 16.30   Fiber optic Michelson interferometer used with an SLD for OCT.

the frequency of the backscattered light, and θ is the angle between **v** and the line between the
scatterer and the source/pickup.

Yazdanfar et al. (1997) studied DOCT on living, *Xenopus laevis* tadpoles, and were able to observe the
structure of and blood velocity in the tadpole's beating heart in real time. They found that the majority
of Doppler shifts came from the motion of the ventricle itself; blood velocity was harder to measure
because of turbulence in the ventricle. (Recall that the Doppler shift is caused by the reflector particles'
velocity components parallel to the incident light.) The reader should consult Yazdanfar et al.'s paper
for details of how they acquired and processed images. It appears that DOCT is well suited for experimental studies on microcirculation in tumors, the retina, the heart, healing wounds, burns, etc.

Another variation on basic OCT exploits the *birefringence* in the tissue being scanned. That is,
how the polarization vector of incident polarized light is changed by certain tissues at scattering. These changes provide additional information on the optical fine structure of the object's
tissues including refractive index and absorbance. *Polarization-sensitive optical coherence tomography*
(PSOCT) has been carried out by several means. Figure 16.31 illustrates an air-path, Michelson
interferometer adapted to measure the polarization state of the selected OCT voxel (de Boer et al.
1999). de Boer et al. used an 856 nm, 0.8 mW superluminescent diode with a spectral half-peak
intensity bandwidth (FWHM) of 25 nm. The beam from the SLD was linearly polarized horizontally by passing it first through a Glan–Thompson polarizer before the spectrophotometer. The
beam was then split into two equal intensity arms by a polarization-preserving beam splitter
(PPBS). In the upper (reference) arm, the light was passed through a zero-order quarter-wave plate
(QWP) oriented at 22.5° to the incident polarization, reflected off a moving 45° mirror and reflected
from a retroreflector reference mirror. The reflected light was again directed to the moving mirror
and again passed through the QWP, gaining a total E-vector rotation of 45° with respect to the horizontal. The moving mirror modulated the length of the reference channel path length by 20 µm to
generate a carrier frequency. A neutral-density filter (NDF) was used to reduce the intensity noise
in the image by a factor of 50 (the OD was not given). Light in the sample arm passed through a

second QWP oriented at 45° to the incident horizontal linear polarization; this produces circularly polarized light that is incident on the sample. The backscattered light passed again through the focusing lens, and again the QWP. This light had an arbitrary (elliptical) polarization due to interaction with the sample. This light was recombined with the 45° polarized light in the reference arm and directed to a polarizing beam-splitting prism that separated the mixed beams into orthogonal polarization components which were directed to photodetectors. The optical theory that describes the detection process is too complex to pursue in detail here. The interested reader should refer to the papers by de Boer et al. (1999), and Saxer et al. (2000) for details. Results in these papers showed that the OCT images made with polarization sensitivity had greatly increased contrast and detail. Pixel sizes in the range of 5–10 μm^2 were demonstrated in the Saxer et al.'s paper.

Still another version of the OCT system was described by Sticker et al. (2000). These workers developed a variation on the birefringence-measuring OCT system described above called *differential phase-contrast OCT* (DPC-OCT). Their system was evaluated using a nonliving, optical test sample, and was shown to be responsive to the optical phase changes in the light returned from the object. It could display images based on very small optical path differences that were invisible

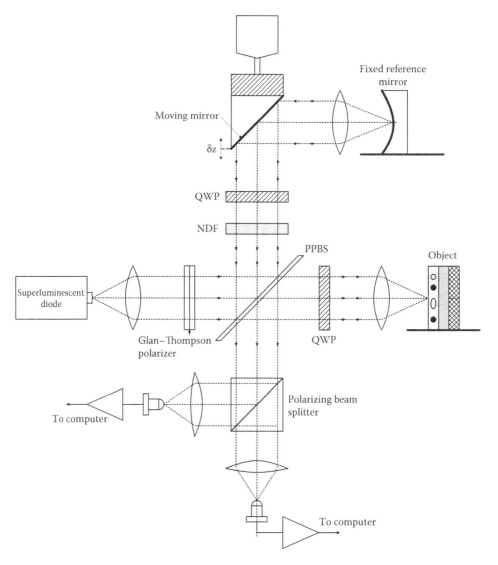

Figure 16.31 Michelson interferometer adapted to measure the polarization state of the object in generating an OCT image. (System similar to that described by de Boer, J.F. et al. 1999. *IEEE J. Sel. Top. Quantum Electron.* 5(4): 1200–1204.)

in conventional, intensity-based OCT imaging. Such path differences can be due to refractive index fluctuations and/or geometrical path variations.

An FO, Michelson interferometer version of the polarization-sensing OCT has special problems because the optical fibers themselves exhibit birefringence when moved or subjected to mechanical strain. It is possible to compensate for these problems, however at the expense of some optical and signal-processing complexity.

Perhaps in the future, polarization *and* Doppler enhancements can be combined in the same FO OCT system.

16.8 ULTRASOUND IMAGING

16.8.1 Introduction

Ultrasonic imaging is a popular, widely used form of NI medical imaging that carries negligible risk to the patient. No ionizing radiations are used, nor are ultra-strong magnetic fields required; the sound pressure levels in medical ultrasound are too low to cause cell damage by heating or cavitation. Ultrasonic imaging is used on all major internal tissues, including the brain, eyes, heart, liver, intestines, breasts, uterus, testes, the fetus, placenta, etc. Pixel resolution in ultrasound imaging depends, among other factors, on the sound wavelength used. As with electromagnetic radiation (e.g., light), the wavelength $\lambda = f/c$, where the sound frequency applied to the tissue is f, and c is the speed of sound in the tissue (typically about 1540 m/s in "soft tissue"). Medical ultrasound frequencies range from ~1 to 50 MHz. Thus, λ (*in vivo*) for 10 MHz ultrasound is ~154 μm, and for 50 MHz ophthalmologic ultrasound, $\lambda = 30.8$ μm. While pixel resolution increases with increasing frequency, so does energy absorption by the ensonified biological tissue.

By combining Doppler ultrasound with imaging, it is possible to view major blood vessels in the body and quantitatively measure their blood velocity at the same time the image is made. Doppler ultrasonic imaging is invaluable in diagnosing kidney failure, coronary stenoses, pulmonary embolisms, and strokes.

Obstetric ultrasonic imaging is useful in determining such things as the number of fetuses, the sex of a fetus, critical fetal dimensions indicating normal growth and fetal age, possible birth defects; and before delivery, how the fetus is lying, the head size (is a cesarean section indicated), the placental location, the amount of amniotic fluid, fetal heart rate, and is the umbilical cord lying normally.

When it is impossible to view the retina of the eye through the cornea because of trauma (e.g., to the cornea, or blood in the eyeball), ophthalmologic ultrasound can be used to diagnose a detached retina, or locate imbedded foreign objects. True OCT gives at least an order of magnitude better resolution of the retina and its pathologies than does ultrasound, but there must be a clear, undistorted optical path to enable its use.

16.8.2 Physics of Ultrasound Propagation in Solids and Liquids

Ultrasound is basically sound of frequencies exceeding 20 kHz, up to 100 s of MHz. In biological systems, sound propagation is generally in solids and liquids (e.g., blood, extracellular fluid, amniotic fluid, CSF, urine, etc.), and sometimes in air (in the lungs). The sonic energy is introduced into the body by a transmitting transducer in intimate contact with the skin so that its vibrational displacements introduce sound waves through the skin into the body. Ultrasound propagates in the body by *longitudinal pressure waves* in which tissue elasticity allows a "particle" fixed in the volume to move back and forth longitudinally around a common center. Its motion is in the z-direction (direction of propagation of an acoustic plane wave). To describe the particle motion mathematically, consider it has a differential element of mass, $dm = \rho\,A\,dz$. The acceleration of dm is $a = d^2\xi/dt^2$, where ξ is the particle displacement in the z-direction. A Taylor's series can be used to find the differential force on dm:

$$F(z+dz) - F(z) = \left[F(z) + \frac{dF(z)}{dz} dz + \cdots \right] - F(z) = \frac{dF(z)}{dz} dz. \tag{16.41}$$

So by Newton's second law,

$$\frac{dF(z)}{dz} dz = \rho A\, dz\, \frac{d^2\xi(z)}{dt^2}. \tag{16.42}$$

353

Equation 16.42 reduces to

$$\frac{dp}{dz} = \rho \frac{du}{dt},$$ (16.43)

where in the above equations, $p = F/A$ in N/m^2 (Pa), $u = \dot{\xi}$ the particle velocity in the z-direction in m/s, and ρ is the medium's density in kg/m^3.

The *specific acoustic impedance* of the medium is defined as $Z_s \equiv p/u$. The fundamental dimensions of Z_s are $ML^{-2}T^{-1}$, and its units are *Rayls*. (For example, the Z_s of muscle is about 1.70×10^6 kg $m^{-2}s^{-1}$, or 1.70 M Rayls.) Another version of acoustic impedance is used in describing the properties of wind instruments. This definition is more analogous to Ohm's law for electricity. Here, $Z_{ac} = p/\dot{q}$. That is, Z_{ac} is equal to the pressure in Pascals at a point divided by the volume flow rate in m^3/s. It is easy to show that the fundamental dimensions of Z_{ac} are $ML^{-4}T^{-1}$; its units are often given as Pa s/m^3 (Smith et al. 2000).

The following is a heuristic development of the *wave equation* for longitudinal particle motion in one dimension (z) in a nonlossy, elastic medium. Assume that a plane acoustic wave is propagating in the +z-direction in a tube of area A. The medium has a uniform, equilibrium density, ρ_o, kg/m^3. (Note that, in reality, ρ_o is a function of position in the ensonified object, that is, $\rho_o (x,y,z)$.) Now the mass of a small slice of medium is: $\Delta m = \rho_o A \Delta z$. Now consider a particle displacement from z to $z + \Delta z$. The acceleration of this point at $z + \Delta z/2$ can be approximated by

$$a \cong \frac{\partial^2}{\partial t^2} \left[\frac{\xi(z) + \xi(z + \Delta z)}{2} \right].$$ (16.44)

Thus, by Newton's second law of motion:

$$A(\Delta P_1 - \Delta P_2) \cong \Delta m \frac{\partial^2}{\partial t^2} \left[\frac{\xi(z) + \xi(z + \Delta z)}{2} \right].$$ (16.45)

The left-hand term has the dimensions of force. ΔP_1 is the pressure change in the volume elements between $z - \Delta z$ and z; ΔP_2 is the pressure change in the volume elements between $z + \Delta z$ and $z + 2\Delta z$ due to medium deformation. These ΔPs follow from the definition of the *adiabatic bulk modulus of elasticity* of the medium, B:

$$\Delta P_1 \cong -B \left[\frac{\xi(z) - \xi(z - \Delta z)}{\Delta z} \right]$$ (16.46)

$$\Delta P_2 \cong -B \left[\frac{\xi(z + 2\Delta z) - \xi(z + \Delta z)}{\Delta z} \right].$$ (16.47)

Substituting the relations above for the ΔPs, we can write:

$$B \left\{ \frac{\xi(z + 2\Delta z) - \xi(z + \Delta z)}{\Delta z} - \frac{\xi(z) - \xi(z - \Delta z)}{\Delta z} \right\} \cong \rho_o A \Delta z \frac{\partial^2}{\partial t^2} \left[\frac{\xi(z) + \xi(z + \Delta z)}{2} \right].$$ (16.48)

Now we take the limit as $\Delta z \to 0$. The result is the one-dimensional wave equation:

$$\frac{\partial^2 \xi(z,t)}{\partial z^2} = (\rho_o/B) \frac{\partial^2 \xi(z,t)}{\partial t^2}.$$ (16.49)

In 3-D, the wave equation has the more general form:

$$\nabla^2 \xi(x,y,z,t) = \frac{1}{c^2} \frac{\partial^2 \xi(x,y,z,t)}{\partial t^2},$$ (16.50)

where ∇^2 is the (scalar) Laplacian operator: and c is the wave velocity: $c = \sqrt{B/\rho_o}$ m/s written as

$$\nabla^2(*) = \frac{\partial^2(*)}{\partial x^2} + \frac{\partial^2(*)}{\partial y^2} + \frac{\partial^2(*)}{\partial z^2}.$$ (16.51)

Note that the wave equation can also be written in terms of the *instantaneous excess pressure,* p(x,y,z,t):

$$\nabla^2 p(x,y,z,t) = \frac{1}{c^2} \frac{\partial^2 p(x,y,z,t)}{\partial t^2}. \tag{16.52}$$

The *characteristic acoustic impedance,* a property intrinsic to the medium, is defined as

$$Z_c \equiv \rho_0 c = \sqrt{B\rho_0} \ \ kg/m^2 s. \tag{16.53}$$

When an acoustic plane wave (with wavelength much smaller than the interface dimensions) strikes the interface between two media having different characteristic acoustic impedances, two things happen analogous to a light ray striking the boundary between two media with different refractive indices (Figure 16.32): (1) *Reflection.* If the propagation axis is at an angle θ_i with the normal to the interface, a portion of the incident wave is reflected at an angle $\theta_r = \theta_i$. (2) Transmission with *refraction* follows Snell's law: $\theta_t = \sin^{-1}[(c_2/c_1)\sin(\theta_i)]$. From boundary conditions, it can be shown that at the interface, the reflected wave has an intensity given by: $p_r = R\,p_i$, where:

$$R = \frac{\rho_2 c_2 \cos(\theta_i) - \rho_1 c_1 \cos(\theta_t)}{\rho_2 c_2 \cos(\theta_i) + \rho_1 c_1 \cos(\theta_t)} = \frac{Z_{c2}\cos(\theta_i) - Z_{c1}\cos(\theta_t)}{Z_{c2}\cos(\theta_i) + Z_{c1}\cos(\theta_t)}. \tag{16.54}$$

Similarly, the pressure of the transmitted wave front is given by: $p_t = T\,p_i$, where for normal incidence:

$$T = 1 + R = \frac{2Z_{c2}}{Z_{c1} + Z_{c2}}. \tag{16.55}$$

R is typically ≤ 0.01 for soft tissue interfaces, thus very little of the transmitted ultrasound energy is reflected back in pulse echo imaging.

The *intensity* of an acoustic wave, I, is defined as the energy per unit time (power) that flows across a unit area perpendicular to wave propagation. Its units are $J/s \cdot m^2$ or W/m^2, or in CGS units, $ergs/cm^2 s$. For the simple case of an infinite, 1-D, plane wave, it can be shown that:

$$I = 2\pi^2 f^2 (\rho_0 c)\xi^2 = \omega^2 Z_c \xi^2 / 2 \ W/m^2. \tag{16.56}$$

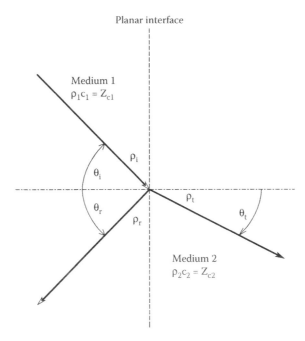

Figure 16.32 Vectors showing the reflection and refraction when acoustic plane waves strike a plane interface between two media having different characteristic acoustic impedances.

All of the foregoing mathematical descriptions are based on the assumption that the propagating medium is *perfectly elastic*, that is, energy put into particle displacements is recovered, none is lost. In reality, all real propagation media are lossy; they are *viscoelastic*. Some of the acoustic energy put into particle displacement is lost as heat. Thus, an acoustic wave looses energy as it propagates; its pressure and particle velocity decrease with propagation distance. Assuming that a sinusoidal plane wave is propagating in the +z-direction, the excess pressure can be written as

$$p(z,t) = P_o \exp(-\alpha z) \exp[-j(kz - \omega t)], \tag{16.57}$$

where α is the absorption coefficient (actually, $\alpha(x,y,z)$), and the intensity as a function of p is given by

$$I = \frac{|p|^2}{\rho_o c} \text{ W/m}^2. \tag{16.58}$$

The intensity is attenuated with distance according to

$$I(z) = I_o \exp(-2\alpha z). \tag{16.59}$$

$\mu \equiv 2\alpha$ is defined as the *intensity absorption coefficient*. In general, μ has an approximately linearly increasing function of frequency, that is, $\mu(f) = \mu_o + \beta f$, so the cost of using higher-frequency ultrasound to get better resolution is that its useful penetration depth is limited. This is not a problem, for example, for 50 MHz ophthalmic ultrasound, which only needs to penetrate to the depth of the eyeball to resolve retinal structure. To image deep tissues such as the liver, 3–10 MHz ultrasound is used.

16.8.3 Ultrasound Transducers

Recall from Chapter 14 that a piezoelectric material possesses the dual properties of generating a voltage (or equivalently an internal charge displacement) if it is physically strained (compressed, twisted, bent, sheared, etc.); or, if a voltage is impressed across it producing an internal electric field, the transducer will exhibit a strain ($\Delta L/L$). An important descriptor of piezo-transducer behavior is the *short-circuit charge sensitivity to applied stress*, or *d-parameter*, which has the dimensions of (Cb/m²)/(N/m²) = Cb/N. d is also called the *piezoelectric strain constant* (Shung and Zipparo 1996), or the *piezoelectric charge coefficient*. An alternate and dimensionally consistent interpretation of d when the transducer is used as a *motor* is (strain developed)/(applied, internal E-field) (Germano 1961).

A given transducer has three or more d-parameters, d_{jk}. j and k refer to the orthogonal axes in which the transducer lies. The 3-D is the same as the z-axis along which the stress is developed (or stress is applied). The 2-D and 3-D are the same as the x- and y-axes. Thus, the *direct charge coefficient*, d_{33}, describes the charge/m² displaced along the z-axis of a *thickness-expander* transducer when the stress (N/m² units = Pa) is also applied along the z-axis. d_{31} describes the behavior of a *length-expander* transducer which produces displaced charge density in the z-direction when the stress is in the x-direction. d_{33} is an important d-parameter in that it gives the number of picocoulombs of charge, q, effectively separated in the transducer in the direction the stress is applied. The separated charge produces a voltage across the electrodes of an open-circuited transducer given by $V_o = q/C$, where C is the *capacitance* of the transducer. For a simple disk or plate transducer, $C = \kappa \, \varepsilon_o \, A/L$, where ε_o is the permittivity of space, κ is the piezoelectric material's dielectric constant, A is the area of the electrodes, and L is the distance separating the electrodes (the transducer's thickness). The charge separated by a constant stress gradually leaks back to its equilibrium distribution in the transducer, allowing $V_o \to 0$.

There is also a *piezoelectric voltage coefficient* set, g_{jk}, that gives the strain ($\Delta L/L$) produced by a mechanically unloaded transducer "motor" as the result of an applied, charge density in Cb/m². Alternately, when a transducer is acting as a generator, it is useful to describe g units as the (open-circuit E-field produced)/(applied stress in N/m² or Pa). In general, the g_{jk}-parameters are related to the d_{jk}-parameters by: $g_{jk} = d_{jk}/(\kappa_j \, \varepsilon_o)$ (strain developed)/(applied charge density). κ_j is the dielectric constant of the transducer material in the j-direction.

Note that the d- and g-relationships for transducer behavior described above only apply for electrical and mechanical frequencies below the natural, *mechanical resonant frequency* of the transducer. At and near mechanical resonance, the transducer's behavior can be modeled by a complex R,L,C, transformer equivalent circuit, the behavior of which will not be considered here.

Early piezoelectric transducers were naturally occurring materials such as used in World War II sonar systems, such as quartz, Rochelle salt ($NaKC_4H_4O_6 \cdot 4H_2O$ = sodium potassium tartrate), or ammonium dihydrogen phosphate ($NH_4H_2PO_4$ = ADP). The first synthetic, piezoceramic material was barium titanate ($BaTiO_3$). Synthetic, *ferroelectric,* piezoceramics are not naturally piezoelectric; they must be *poled* by exposing them to a very strong internal electric field (~20 kV/cm) as they cure. There are now many different piezoceramics; for example, many formulations of lead zirconate titanate (PZT, $Pb(Zr, Ti)O_3$), lead zirconate, lithium metaniobate ($LiNbO_3$), and lead metaniobate ($PbNb_2O_6$). One advantage to the use of piezoceramics is that they can be made in any desired shape to suit the application (disks, rods, bars, hollow cylinders, half-cylinders, hollow spheres, hemispheres, etc.).

An important consideration in the design of ultrasound transducer systems is the fact that all transducer materials, with the exception of polyvinylidene fluoride (PVDF), exhibit natural mechanical resonance at frequency $f_n = \omega_n/2\pi$ Hz. This means that the efficiency of the ultrasound output (and input) is greatest when the AC-driving frequency is at f_n, or when the acoustic wave impinging on the transducer is near f_n. In pulsed ultrasound, the transducer can be excited by a short burst of AC at f_n. The rate that the transducer oscillations buildup and decay is governed not only by the AC pulse envelope but by the internal mechanical damping, ξ, of the loaded transducer. Decay is generally governed by an envelope of the form, $\exp(-\xi\omega_n t)$. If a transducer is excited by a single, narrow, DC pulse, the sound pressure produced at the transducer surface will be of the general shape of a damped sinusoid, sic:

$$p(t) = P_o \exp(-\xi\omega_n t)\sin\left[\omega_n\left(\sqrt{1-\xi^2}\right)t + \varphi\right]. \tag{16.60}$$

The Q or quality factor of a second-order, damped resonant system can be shown to be: $Q = 1/(2\xi)$.

The electrical equivalent circuit of an ultrasound transducer near and at resonance is complex, its R,L,C, transformer parameters depend not only on the mechanical properties of the transducer itself but also upon its front- and rear-face acoustical loading. The rear face can be loaded with a material that will lower the overall Q of the transducer, and the front (driving) surface must be acoustic-impedance matched to the tissue load for efficient energy transfer. Reflections occur at the interfaces of the matching media, and the tissue. The tissue also absorbs far more sound energy than it reflects. In general, the loaded transducer *at resonance* presents a series or parallel R-C circuit to the driving power amplifier (Shung and Zipparo 1996).

In order to measure the voltage generated by the piezo-transducer, or apply an internal electric field to cause it to move, thin metal electrodes are vapor-deposited on its active surfaces. Silver, gold, or aluminum are generally used. Wires making contact with the thin electrodes are generally attached with silver-filled epoxy; the heat from soldering can damage the coating and/or the transducer. Contacts are also made with thin spring electrodes that press on the metallized transducer faces.

Because modern ultrasound imaging systems generally work in the pulsed mode, it is important that the transducer be adequately mechanically damped to prevent excess "ringing" when excited by a pulse of RF excitation. Damping is implemented by backing the transducer with a high-frequency energy-absorbing material, and/or can be an intrinsic property of the transducer material. Lead metaniobate has a mechanical Q of 15 compared to LZT transducers, where the Q is typically in the 100 s. The Curie temperature (above which the material looses its piezoelectric properties) for lead metaniobate is 550°C, versus a typical maximum operating temperature for LZTs of 150°C.

An unusual and versatile piezoelectric material is the plastic PVDF. PVDF is a polymer composed of long molecular chains having the repeat unit, $-CH_2-CF_2-$. When the polymer is *poled* with a strong electric field, the polymer chains line up in parallel. Unlike a vitreous piezo-material, PVDF has an extremely low Q. In fact, its frequency response runs from 0.005 Hz to a GHz. The basic half wavelength thickness of a 28 μm thick PVDF transducer is ~40 MHz. PVDF has been successfully used at 50 Mz for ophthalmological investigations (Lockwood et al. 1966). As a consequence of its high-internal damping, PVDF cannot handle high, average radiated sound intensities without heating. Unfortunately, PVDF has a low-maximum operating temperature of 100°C. PVDF is flexible and can adhere to body contours; it also has a low Z_c of 3.9×10^6 kg/m²s (3.9 M Rayls), close to the Z_c of water (1.48 M Rayls) and of soft tissue (~1.63 M Rayls). Thus, it is easier to couple acoustic energy from PVDF to the body than from a hard piezoceramic like PZT which has a Z_c ~24×10^6 kg/m²s.

Let us consider the case of a single, cylindrical, piston radiator launching ultrasonic vibrations into a uniform medium, such as water. It can be shown (Liley 2001) that the excess pressure magnitude varies *along the z-axis* according to

$$|p| \, (2\pi A/k) \left\{ 2 - 2\cos\left[k\left(\sqrt{r^2 + z^2} \right) - z \right] \right\}^{1/2} , \tag{16.61}$$

where $k = 2\pi/\lambda$, A is a constant of proportionality related to the source pressure at the transducer face, and r is the transducer's radius.

For P of the z-axis at some angle ϕ in the near-field, the expression for $|p|$ is sufficiently complex that we will not consider it here. The typical behavior of $|p|$ on-axis is shown in Figure 16.33a. The z-value where the last peak occurs in the $|p|$ versus z plot marks the boundary between *near-field*

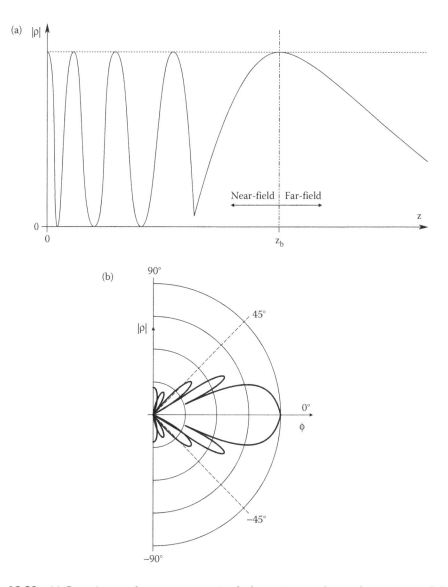

Figure 16.33 (a) On axis sound pressure magnitude for a piston radiator showing near-field ($0 < z \le z_b$) and far-field ($z > z_b$) behavior. (b) A typical constant intensity contour for a piston radiator in its far-field as a function of angle away from the z-axis. Note the complex side lobes.

and *far-field* radiation behavior. z_b is given by: $z_b = r^2/\lambda - \lambda/4$. In the far-field, the excess pressure *off axis* can be modeled by

$$|p| = \frac{A\pi r^2}{\rho}\left\{\frac{2J_1[kr\sin(\phi)]}{kr\sin(\phi)}\right\}, \quad \rho > z_b, \tag{16.62}$$

where $J_1[*]$ is a Bessel function of the first kind, and r, ρ, ϕ, A, k have been defined.

Figure 16.33b illustrates a typical polar plot of *far-field* $|p|$ versus ϕ. It can be shown that the angle at which $|p|$ first becomes zero is: $\phi_o = \sin^{-1}(0.61\ \lambda/r)$ (Shung and Zipparo 1996). Side lobes are undesirable in ultrasonic imaging because they produce spurious return signals which decrease image resolution. Good transducer design requires a narrow main lobe, and a large ϕ_o with weak sidelobes. Also, it is often desirable to have a focal point of the transducer closer than would be normally set by z_b. One answer to this design problem is to use an *acoustic lens* between the transducer and the tissue being scanned. An acoustic lens basically brings the radiated ultrasound energy to a sharp focus at a $z_b' < z_b$ at the expense of a rapidly expanding beam beyond z_b'. Acoustic lenses must have dimensions larger than λ to be effective refractors. Some materials used for acoustic lenses are silicone elastomer (Sylgard™), polyurethane, and Plexiglas.

The trend with modern ultrasound transducers is to use *multielement arrays*. Such arrays allow the beam to be focused and steered electronically by varying the phases and amplitudes of the excitation signals to the individual array elements. A transducer array can be made in the shape of concentric, annular, piezoelectric rings, spaced with an appropriate inert material to acoustically isolate the transducers. This type of array produces a beam with circular symmetry; its focal point (point of maximum intensity and minimum cross section in z) can be set by adjusting the excitation to the ring transducers. Still another design, used in such applications as fetal imaging to image slices, uses a *linear array* of narrow, rectangular transducers laid in parallel, separated by narrow *kerfs* of absorbing material for electrical and acoustic isolation. The sound beam from a linear array can be scanned laterally by exciting subgroups of transducers in sequence, or as a *phased array* where all the piezo-elements are excited simultaneously, and the focused beam is steered at an angle ϕ from the array's center. By moving the head of a linear array slowly, perpendicular to its long axis, a "book" of slice images can be generated. Holding the array fixed and tilting it with respect to the body generates a set of fan images, and rotating around its vertical axis while perpendicular to the body generates a set of perpendicular sections at various angles. The length of one linear array marketed by Parallel Design, Inc., is 50 mm; 128 piezo-elements are used, spaced 0.390 mm on centers. Each element is ~1 cm in length and ~0.2 mm wide. The array elements' center frequency is ~8 MHz.

Rectangular, 2-D, multielement arrays also are used. They, too, can be focused and the beam steered in two angular dimensions, ϕ and θ. Transducers in the rectangular array are long rods or posts, the diameters or end dimensions of which are much less than their lengths. A $42 \times 42 = 1764$ element, 2.5 MHz array has been investigated at Duke University. Among the problems faced with such large arrays are making physical electrical contact with the inner elements, and low signal-to-noise ratio due to poor acoustical isolation and small element size (Shung and Zipparo 1996, Smith et al. 1996).

It is mathematically difficult to calculate the spatial distribution of the sound pressure magnitude, $|p|$, at some point P at a radial distance, ρ, from the center of an array (O) and at an angle ϕ with the z-axis, and angle θ with the x-axis by a projection of ρ into the X–Y plane (Figure 16.34). The calculation involves the superposition of the $|p|$s from each element of the array at P. Such design predictions are generally left to computer modeling.

16.8.4 Doppler Ultrasound Imaging

Doppler ultrasound imaging combines traditional ultrasound imaging with Doppler velocity detection of moving scatterers. The scatterers are red blood cells (RBCs) in blood, or moving tissues such as heart valves or aneurisms. Recall from Chapter 14 that the Doppler frequency *shift* in reflected, CW ultrasound is given by $f_D = 2|v|f_T\cos(\theta)/c$ Hz, *where* f_T is the transmitted frequency, **v** is the scatterer velocity, θ is the angle a line from the transducer to the scatterer makes with **v**, and c is the speed of sound in the medium surrounding the scatterer. Thus, the returning waves from the moving scatterers will have frequency $f_r = f_T \pm f_D$. (+ for scatterers approaching the transducer.)

As the modern Doppler imaging systems work in the pulsed mode, the Doppler effect can also be expressed in the time domain. The velocity **v** can be estimated from δt, the time difference in signal returns from successive pulses. See Figure 16.35 for a description of the geometry. The

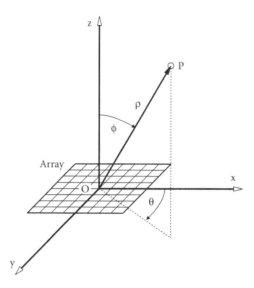

Figure 16.34 Spherical coordinates above a transducer array relevant to calculating its radiation pattern.

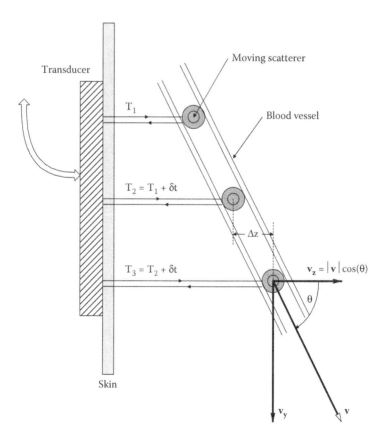

Figure 16.35 Diagram illustrating how a pulsed Doppler array can be used to find object velocity. At each successive pulse, the time for the return echo increases by an amount, δt, given by Equation 16.62 in the text. δt is then used to find $|\mathbf{v}|\cos(\theta)$.

ultrasound pulse repetition interval (PRI) is the reciprocal of the PRR. (Note that the PRR is not f_n.) In the time interval PRI, the moving, reflecting object moves away from the transducer by Δz. That is, $\Delta z = (PRI)|\mathbf{v}|\cos(\theta)$, which means that the next ultrasound pulse must travel *double* this extra distance, taking an extra time, δt. Clearly,

$$\delta t = 2(PRI)|\mathbf{v}|\cos(\theta)/c. \tag{16.63}$$

Thus

$$|\mathbf{v}|\cos(\theta) = (c\delta t)/[2(PRI)], \tag{16.64}$$

where c is the average sound velocity in the tissue between the transducer and the moving object. One can also think of the fractional time shift in terms of phase, that is, there will be a phase lag between successive returning pulses, φ, given by $\varphi = 2\pi\,\delta t/(PRI)$ radians. If this relation is solved for PRI and substituted into Equation 16.64, we find:

$$|\mathbf{v}|\cos(\theta) = c\varphi/(4\pi)\,m/s. \tag{16.65}$$

The moving objects are generally RBCs; there are $\sim 5 \times 10^6$ RBCs in a cubic mm of blood. Each RBC is a flattened disk of $\sim 7.5\,\mu m$ diameter and $\sim 1.9\,\mu m$ thick on the edge and $\sim 1\,\mu m$ thick in the center. Thus, RBC dimensions are $\ll \lambda$ of the ultrasound, which means they are way too small to present ultrasound images. Also, in blood vessels with laminar flow, the blood velocity has a parabolic profile, maximum at the center and zero at the vessel walls. In the great arteries and in the chambers of the heart, flow can be turbulent over parts of the cardiac cycle. Thus, the reflected Doppler signals from blood are a superposition of many, many small, scattered signals from moving RBCs with different cross sections and velocities. In general, the intensity of the Doppler-shifted backscatter from moving RBCs is $\sim 40\,dB$ less than that from surrounding tissues (Routh 1996).

Doppler information is generally presented in ultrasound slice images of organs such as the heart, kidneys, aorta, carotid arteries, etc. as *colors*. For example, starting at $+30\,cm/s$ velocity, yellow to orange to red to black at 0 velocity, then violet through blue to green as the velocity reaches $-30\,cm/s$. Doppler information is more qualitative than quantitative in this mode of display. Still, if there is a heart valve problem such as mitral regurgitation, it will show up well on the Doppler image, and can be correlated with another NI modality such as sonocardiography (Section 3.3) (Routh 1996).

The processes whereby the Doppler information is inserted into the slice image are complex both in terms of hardware and software, and will not be covered here.

16.9 OTHER IMAGING MODALITIES

16.9.1 Introduction

In this survey of medical imaging methods, it is appropriate to briefly describe some of the less frequently encountered imaging methods and evaluate them for medical diagnostic utility and/or research potential. As we have seen, not every modality is without risk. Every imaging modality carries a cost–benefit ratio. The cost includes the dollar cost to the patient as well as risk of harm from radiation, contrast agent, anxiety, etc. The benefit of an imaging system lies in its resolution and its ability to diagnose specific, important diseases such as various types of cancer, atherosclerosis, heart valve damage, etc.

Those imaging modalities involving ionizing radiations such as x-ray, x-ray CT, PET, and SPECT certainly carry more risk than MRI, ultrasound, impedance tomography, and MWT. In the sections below, we briefly describe *long-wave infrared thermal imaging, MWT,* and *impedance tomography.* Only LIR thermal imaging is risk-free; it is noncontact, NI, and puts no energy or radioactivity into the body. However, it is pretty much limited to detecting superficial circulatory defects, soft-tissue injuries, and breast cancer.

16.9.2 LIR Thermal Imaging of Body Surfaces

We know from Figure 6.2 in Section 6.32 that the IR blackbody radiation curve at 310 K peaks at $9.34\,\mu m$ wavelength. Thus, sensors used to map and image surface IR radiation from human skin should cover from ~ 2 to over $100\,\mu m$. Because of practical considerations, including infrared imaging optics, most IR cameras for body temperature imaging cover from 2 to $14\,\mu m$ of source wavelength. The optics for IR thermographic imaging generally make use of materials that are opaque in visible wavelengths. Diamond-turned lenses of ZnSe (also known as *Irtran-4*) are effective from 0.6 to 16 μm. The other Irtran materials are: *Irtran-1* (MgF$_2$, passes 1–9 μm); *Irtran-2* (ZnS, passes 0.9–20 μm); *Irtran-3* (CaF, passes <0.3–8 μm). Germanium passes from 2 to 14 μm, silicon passes from 1.2 to 8 μm, and KRS-5 passes from 0.6 to 50 μm. Mirrors (plane and spherical) are generally gold coated. LIR Camera imaging optics can also be done entirely with mirrors to eliminate the need for exotic lenses, but such designs are generally bulky.

Two general classes of LIR detectors exist: *thermal detectors* and *photon detectors*. Thermal detectors work by blackbody absorption of LIR radiation causing a minute increase in the sensor's temperature, ΔT. Thermal detectors include *thermopiles, bolometers,* and *pyroelectric sensors.* Thermopiles are arrays of miniature thermocouples that output microvolt-level signals.

The resistance of a bolometer increases with a slight rise in temperature; the ΔR is generally sensed with a bridge. Pyroelectric materials are special piezoelectric materials that generate voltages in response to thermally induced surface strain. Pyroelectric sensors must be used with a chopper. (See Section 6.3 for a detailed description of pyroelectric IR detection.) Thermopiles, bolometers, and pyroelectic sensors are broadband in their IR wavelength responses (exclusive of limitations placed by the focusing optics). Photon detector sensors include *photodiodes* and *photoconductors* that work by incident LIR photons generating electron-hole pairs that cause increased current to flow. The longest wavelength detectable by a photon detector is given approximately by

$$\lambda_{max} = 1.24 / E_G \, \mu m, \tag{16.66}$$

where E_G is the material's bandgap energy in eV.

An advantage of photodiodes over photoconductors is that they can be operated at zero bias as photocurrent generators; also, they have no appreciable dark current, unlike voltage-biased photoconductors.

As might be expected when trying to measure small differences in Kelvin surface temperature around 300°K, thermal (Johnson) noise (and shot noise for photodiodes) is a problem. One way of reducing noise and enhancing thermal sensitivity is to operate the sensor array at reduced temperature. Heat extraction by boiling liquid nitrogen (LN$_2$), or liquid argon (LA) is often used to cool IR sensor arrays. (NB: LN$_2$ boils at 77.35°K, and LA boils at 87.45°K.) Ricor Ltd., Lichud, Israel developed a miniature Stirling cycle cooler for LIR camera cooling (Ricor 2015). These compact devices will cool the detector array from 300 to 80°K in less than 8 min, and have steady-state cooling capacities of 0.25 to 0.5 W at 80 K. Typical input power for a 0.5 W cooler is 35 W at 24 Vdc. Carting around several small, rechargeable, gel cell, lead acid batteries, or Lithium ion batteries is considered less cumbersome than a Dewar of LN$_2$, and having to fill the camera's cryo-chamber every hour or so.

Recently, IR imaging cameras have come on the market that operate at room temperature, eliminating the need for cumbersome cryogenic enclosures and an expensive LN$_2$ supply.

Some materials for IR photodiodes include mercury cadmium telluride (MCT) and mercury manganese telluride (MMT); the latter material is useful from about 2 to 12 μm. Other materials used in photon-capture thermal imaging include indium antimonide (IA), $Pb_{1-x} Sn_x Te$(In) and gallium arsenide.

Modern gallium arsenide IR cameras that run at 77°K can resolve temperature differences on human skin of ±0.001°C in a 5 mm^2 patch of skin. Furthermore, 10–50 mK modulation of skin temperature can be followed at up to 10 Hz, enabling observation of skin temperature variations during the cardiac cycle, a good indicator of hemodynamics (Anbar 1998).

The *L-3 Cincinnati Electronics Corp.*, Mason, OH, makes several state-of-the-art, portable LIR thermography, focal plane array cameras (e.g., *Night Conqueror 640 100/500, Night Warrior 640, Night Conqueror CMI,* etc.). They claim the ultra-compact Night Warrior 640 is one of the smallest, high-resolution (640 × 512, 15 μm pitch) mid-wave infrared (MWIR) (3.5–5.0 μm) cooled cameras in the world. Sensing is by a cooled, InSb focal plane array. The Night Warrior 640 consists of an integrated detector/dewar/cooler assembly (IDCA) and camera electronics. Cooling uses a closed-cycle Stirling system (L3 Cincinnati 2015).

Digatherm (2015) of Ocala, FL, offers two veterinary thermal imaging tablets, each consisting of a laptop computer, software, and a room temperature vanadium oxide sensor camera. Their IR Tablet 640® has a 17 μm FPA (VO$_x$) 640 × 480 Pixel Array with a 7–14 μm spectral response. This system has a 30 Hz frame rate and a 14 bit dynamic range, and a −40°C to 80°C operating range. These systems have application in veterinary medicine in spotting local hot spots due to strains and sprains in race- and show-horses' legs.

Portable IR cameras are finding increasing popularity in NI diagnosis of medical problems in ambulatory large animals including, but not limited to, horses, cattle, zoo animals, etc. See, for example, the chapter by Stelletta et al. (2012) in the book by Prakash (2012) on *IR Thermography,* also the review paper by Robson (2010).

An uncooled, broadband, bolometer, LIR imaging array was described by Butler and Marshall (2004) at Lockheed Martin IR Imaging Systems in Lexington, MA. A bolometer is a thermal (IR) sensor heated by incident, absorbed IR radiation, which undergoes a temperature rise that causes its resistance to increase. The bolometer array contains 327×245 micromachined bolometer elements, each about 46 µm square. Each microbolometer sensor consists of a silicon nitride microbridge that lies above a CMOS silicon substrate and is supported by two silicon nitride legs. A vanadium oxide (VO_x) film, which has an approximately 2% temperature coefficient of resistance at ambient temperatures, is deposited on the bridge to form the bolometer resistor element. Each of the microbolometer sensors is connected to an underlying unit cell in the silicon CMOS readout integrated circuit (IC) substrate via two holes in the passivation layer on the top of the IC. The detector's thermal time constant was 14 ms and the detector resistance was 15–30 kΩ. The array had a spectral response of ~7.5 to 14 µm, a frame update rate of 60 Hz, and a noise-equivalent differential temperature (NEDT) $< 0.1°K = 100$ mK. Again we see a trade-off between the convenience of room temperature operation and lower thermal resolution because of noise. Second-generation imagers provide an NEDT of ~20 to 30 mK with $f/2$ optics. A goal of third-generation imagers is to bring the NEDT down to ~1 mK (Rogalski 2009).

As the main source of heat exchange from the body's core to the skin is the peripheral circulation, the spatiotemporal distribution of skin temperature is closely associated with the behavior of the vascular system including the cardiac cycle and the functioning of the autonomic nervous system which controls vasodilation and contraction, and regulates the blood flow in surface veins and arteries. "Hot spots" on the skin indicate either increased blood flow to the region, for example, caused by local inflammation due to arthritis, infections or Paget's bone disease. Increased local blood flow can also be due to a highly vascular cancer near the skin surface (e.g., breast cancer). The neuromodulator, *nitric oxide* (NO), is a potent relaxor of vascular smooth muscle, causing vasodilation and increased blood flow. NO is known to be produced by a number of immune system cells involved in inflammatory reactions, as well as chondrocytes; osteocytes; and different lines of cancer cells, including breast cancer, melanomas, squamous cell carcinoma, and colorectal cancer. NO is also produced by the vascular epithelium in response to nervous stimulation. Cancer-induced NO may enhance angiogenesis in the cancer and NO-induced regional vasodilation may also lead to metastasis (Anbar 1998). Thus, the detection of a hot region on one breast not seen on the other indicates a high probability that a cancer may be present, and other more definitive tests should be done (e.g., ultrasound, x-ray, scintimammography, biopsy, etc.). *Deep venous thrombosis* (DVT) in a leg can also cause anomalous heating on the back of that leg. Normally, the temperature of the back of the legs has a smooth gradient of about 3° from the upper thighs to the lower calves. If DVT is present, the temperature of the calf will be significantly raised. Thermographic diagnostic sensitivity to DVT is 97%–100%, however, thermography cannot localize the exact site of the thrombosis (Harding 1998), and other means must be used to locate it.

Cold spots indicate anomalous, reduced vascular perfusion of an area. This can have a nervous origin (extreme vasoconstriction signaled by sympathetic nerves that release norepinephrine which causes the vascular smooth muscle to contract (Guyton 1991)). Local, reduced perfusion can also have a mechanical cause such as injury, phlebitis, arteritis, or arteriosclerosis. Examination of a thermogram of the face that shows an asymmetric cold side can be due to reduced flow in the common or external carotid artery on that side. Such a hypothesis can be verified by Doppler ultrasound, or more invasively, by x-ray angiography.

As medical imaging systems go, thermography is one of the safest and least expensive. Its major medical uses appear to be in the detection of breast cancer and other skin cancers, arthritis, infections (inflammation), and circulatory system dysfunctions. As camera designs are perfected, expect to see larger arrays and lower NEDTs.

16.9.3 Microwave Imaging

We normally think of microwaves in conjunction with radar and microwave ovens for cooking. However, microwaves penetrate living tissue, and like other electromagnetic radiation, experience absorption, reflection, scattering, and refraction as they interact with various tissue components. As in the case of ultrasound, if the intensity is kept low, heating is negligible, and there are no known, long-term, adverse effects to medical microwave exposure. Microwaves are nonionizing radiations. As in the case of ultrasound, there is a trade-off between short wavelength (high resolution) and increasing absorption as wavelength decreases. One property that makes microwave imaging attractive is the fact that microwave absorption is a function of the (complex) dielectric constant of tissues. At a frequency of 2.5 GHz, dielectric permittivity varies from about 5 for fat to 56 for normal myocardium at body temperature. By comparison, the contrast range for soft tissue for x-rays is ~2%, and is less than 10% for ultrasound (Semenov et al. 1996). In air, a 10 GHz source has a 3 cm wavelength; in the body, this falls to ~3.4 mm because of the much slower speed of microwave radiation, *in vivo*, being proportional to the reciprocal of the square root of the dielectric constant. The effective speed of EM radiation in tissue is $v = (0.34/3) \times 3 \times 10^8 = 4.4 \times 10^7$ m/s.

Semenov et al. (1996) stated:

> In microwave tomography there are extremely difficult mathematical problems connected with image reconstruction. The linear optics approximation which is used for X-ray tomographic image reconstruction cannot be used in the case of microwave tomography. For microwave tomographic image reconstruction it is necessary to solve the Maxwell equations or their scalar approximations. In the past few years this problem has been extensively investigated.

Microwave imaging has great potential for the detection of breast cancer because of the greater contrast caused by the high-dielectric constant of the cancer due to its higher water content. Several university laboratories are working to develop prototype microwave imaging and tomographic systems for mammography. An experimental MWT system studied at the Kurchatov Institute in Russia used a power density of no more than 0.1 mW/cm². The Russian system and several in the United States use a tank of distilled water or other liquid into which the transmitting and receiving antennas are immersed along with the specimen. The water serves the same purpose as ultrasound coupling gel, that is, impedance matching, to maximize energy transmission into the specimen.

State-of-the-art resolution in experimental microwave medical imaging systems is ~1 cm. This in itself is not exceptional, and one could argue at this point, why bother? Certainly, other imaging modalities have better resolution. However, as we have indicated above, the strength of the method may lie in its ability to pick up as high-contrast images, structures that have large gradients in dielectric constant compared with surrounding tissue, for example, breast cancers and brain cancers.

Much of the future development of effective medical microwave imaging systems will be focused on perfecting the design of antennas and their radiation patterns. Semenov et al. (1996) suggest that at least 128 transmitting and 128 receiving antennas will be required for accurate scattered field detection. Higher transmitted frequencies will be able to be used for microwave mammography because the overall transmission path is shorter and a greater absorption rate can be tolerated. Thus, resolution can be higher.

Semenov and Corfield (2008) used a physical modeling study to evaluate the efficacy of MWT for brain imaging and feasibility assessment for stroke detection. They concluded that MWT of deep brain tissues and stroke detection presents a significant technical challenge, because the objects of interest are located inside a high-dielectric contrast shield, that is, the skull and CSF. They found that at the level of MWT imaging technology used, the smallest imaginable area of acute stroke is estimated to be ~2 cm. They suggested that the use of multifrequency MWT has potential for significantly improving brain imaging results.

16.9.4 EIT in 2-D Imaging

EIT is an NI, nonhazardous, portable imaging technique suitable for outpatient screening and bedside use, especially in the ICU. EIT can be used for the detection of lung problems such as accumulated fluid or a collapsed lung; it also can be used to detect anomalies in blood flow (e.g., DVT), pelvic fluid accumulation, determination of the boundary between dead and living tissue, screening for breast cancer, etc. (Harikumar et al. 2013).

EI tomograms generally have poor spatial resolution compared to other imaging techniques such as MRI and x-ray CT. It is also noisy and subject to anatomical distortion due to breathing, heartbeats, and patient motion. EIT displays can use *admittivity magnitude* or *impedance magnitude* as a function of position (x,y,z) (Nguyen et al. 2012). Examples of EIT plots can be found in the review papers by Adler (2008), Pikkemaat et al. (2012), and Harikumar et al. (2013).

One can think of the inverse problem (IP) in EIT as the ultimate problem in multiport circuit analysis. The object of the IP analysis is to describe the electrical parameters of a circuit distributed in a 3-D volume, or tomographic slice. The circuit is a "black box," and electrical access is by a finite number of electrode pairs distributed uniformly around its periphery. Furthermore, the circuit is continuous, rather than being composed of discrete *conductances* and capacitive *susceptances*. That is, there is a continuous, 3-D internal distribution of many complex *impedivity vectors*, $\mathbf{z}(x,y,z) = \rho + j\gamma$ ohmmeters. The real *resistivity*, ρ, is a function of (x,y,z), and complex γ is a function of the radian frequency ω of the applied AC current, and also is a function of the spatial distribution of the *permittivity*, $\varepsilon(x, y, z)$ in the tissue. The central problem is how to estimate the vector magnitude $|\mathbf{z}(x, y, z)|$ from a finite number of voltage measurements, given an AC current of a few mA, and frequency from 10 Hz to 100 kHz, injected at each electrode pair in turn, and how to relate the estimated $|\mathbf{z}(x, y, z)|$ to medically important factors in the electrified volume, such as edema, ischemia (lack of blood), lung volume, swollen and inflamed organs, etc.

Typically, there are N = 16 (or 32), equally spaced, skin electrodes used in a 2-D "belt" array, encircling the patient's chest, head, or abdomen (Harikumar et al. 2013). An adjacent pair of electrodes in the array is used for the AC current source stimulus; the other N − 2 electrodes are used to sense body potentials (magnitude and phase) caused by the applied AC current. In turn, each of the adjacent electrode pairs is used for the current stimulus. Figure 16.36 illustrates the N = 16 electrode "belt," how the AC current is injected and how the N − 3 = 13 differential voltages are measured. In the *Adjacent Drive Method* (Harikumar et al. 2013), the AC current injection port is cyclically advanced from electrodes 1 and 2 to electrodes 2 and 3, thence 3 and 4, etc. until 16 and 1 are reached. All of the (N − 3) electrode pairs not associated with current injection are used to measure the differential voltages produced by a particular current injection electrode pair. Harikumar et al. (2013) also described the *Opposite Method,* in which current is applied, in turn, between pairs of opposite electrodes on the "belt." The N − 4 potentials in this method are measured between the electrode adjacent to the current ground and the remaining electrodes, excluding the current injection electrode. "Thus the *Opposite Method* suffers from the disadvantage that for the same number of electrodes, the number of available current injections that can be applied is less than for the *Adjacent Method*" (Harikumar et al. 2013). Note that there is yet another pattern of current injection described by Harikumar et al. (2013) the *Cross Method,* which we will not consider here.

Because EIT uses innocuous levels of high-frequency, sinusoidal currents, and does not involve ionizing radiation, it is safe. Compared to other imaging modalities, it is also inexpensive, requiring only electrodes, a voltage-controlled sinusoidal current source, N − 3 differential voltage preamplifiers, phase-sensitive rectifiers, multiplexors, A/D boards, and a powerful computer.

Much of the ongoing research today on EIT is on the algorithms with which to permit rapid and accurate estimation and mapping of the resistivity vector magnitude, $|\mathbf{z}(x, y, z)|$, in a tissue "slice." Early EIT systems, using the finite element approach, assumed a circular boundary for the tissue being investigated. The EIT system of Edic et al. (1995) used 32 electrodes to apply 31 different, 28.8 kHz current patterns to the body (torso) (one electrode was always the current return or ground). A total of 32 electrodes were used to measure the in-phase and quadrature voltages resulting from each current applied. A 496-element "Joshua tree," *finite element model* (FEM), was used to model the admittance of the body. Edic et al. (1995) used a fast implementation of Newton's one-step error reconstructor (FNOSER) to calculate the static, absolute, conductivity, and permittivity distributions in the finite elements. Their study demonstrated the efficacy of their mathematical approach, but in this writer's opinion, gave no results on which to base a diagnosis. Clearly, more electrodes will improve resolution.

Better results were obtained in an EIT modeling study by Jain et al. (1997). They used a 6017-node mesh FEM with 512 boundary nodes to solve the *forward problem*, in which the voltages on the boundary nodes of the object are calculated given the known interior admittance distribution and currents applied to the boundary. The governing, continuous equation for the potential distribution in the object $\phi(x, y, z)$, given $\gamma(x, y, z)$ is the Laplace equation for the area, Ω:

$$\nabla \cdot (\gamma \nabla \phi) = 0 \qquad (16.67)$$

and the boundary equation for points x,y,z on the electrode boundary, Γ, is:

$$\gamma(x, y, z)\frac{\partial \phi}{\partial \eta} = \mathbf{J}, \qquad (16.68)$$

where the partial derivative is the vector *directional derivative* of the potential on Γ, $\mathbf{J}$ is the current density vector applied to the surface, and $\gamma(x, y, z)$ is the admitivity. Note $\mathbf{z} = [\gamma(x, y, z)]^{-1}$.

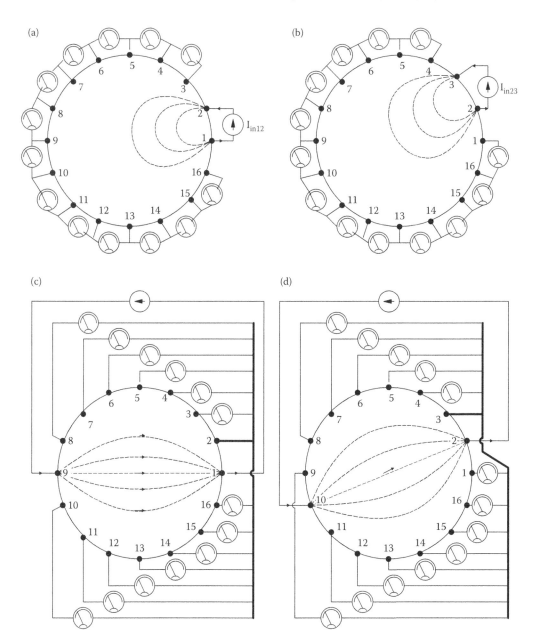

Figure 16.36 Two electrode array architectures for determining EIT slice tomograms: (a) First current projection of an adjacent current source-driven array. (b) Second current projection. (c) First current projection of an opposite current source-driven array. (d) Second current projection. (After Harikumar et al. 2013. *Int. J. Soft Comput. Eng.* 3(4): 193–198.)

We are after an estimate of $\gamma(x, y, z)$. Jain et al. also used the boundary element method (BEM) to generate the voltage data for inhomogeneous conductivity distributions inside object areas with noncircular (e.g., elliptical) boundaries with success. Phantoms with controlled distribution of σ and β were used in their study.

The future success in EIT as a useful, NI, diagnostic imaging modality will depend on the development of better algorithms to estimate $z(x, y, z)$, and also on the ability to cram more electrodes into a finite circumference. It should be possible to place 250 electrodes in a 1 m circumference, and use two at a time for AC current injection, and the other 249 to record the voltage at points on the periphery, Γ. At present, EIT needs further refinement before it can compete effectively with any of the established imaging modalities in a particular diagnostic mode.

Note that Polydorides and Lionheart (2002) have developed and released a free Matlab Toolkit of routines that can be used to solve the forward and inverse EIT problems in 3-D, based on the complete electrode model along with some basic visualization utilities.

16.10 CHAPTER SUMMARY

As you have seen from this introductory chapter on medical imaging, there are a large number of imaging modalities that allow visualization of internal organs and their pathologies. Imaging had its beginning with the invention of the stationary shadow x-ray, and then evolved to simple motion tomography, thence to various forms of computed tomography. X-ray imaging relies on differences in the x-ray photon absorbency of tissues, which can be very small in soft tissues such as the breast and brain. Contrast agents can be injected in blood vessels for x-ray angiography used to detect conditions such as coronary artery blockage or carotid artery stenosis.

Along with the inception of x-ray CT imaging, the mathematics of tomographic reconstruction has evolved making use of the RT, FBP, and other image reconstruction algorithms. Imaging modalities such as MRI, PET, SPECT, etc. all use variations of these techniques.

MRI has evolved into a high-resolution imaging modality that is primarily sensitive to the water density in tissues, and which can be used to locate tumors with greater resolution than x-ray CT.

The use of radioisotopes and radionuclides attached to molecules that have affinity to particular tissues has enabled PET and SPECT to locate tissues such as cancers. The high-energy γ-photons in PET and SPECT are generally detected using collimators with scintillation sensors.

Ultrasound is the major NI, nonionizing imaging modality. The amplitude, phase or time delay, and frequency of reflected and backscattered sound waves are used to construct tomographic images of internal organs, and resolve details of fetuses *in utero*. This chapter has also considered EIT, IR thermographic imaging (of the body surface), and microwave imaging.

A promising, very high-resolution imaging modality currently under development is x-ray diffraction imaging. A beam of highly coherent, monochromatic x-rays is required, which are generated with the aid of a synchrotron. An invention which would really revolutionize medical imaging would be a compact, low-powered x-ray laser.

Lower resolution, NI imaging techniques described include LIR camera detection of body surface temperature variations useful in diagnosing circulatory system anomalies caused by inflammation, clots, or sclerotic plaque buildup in blood vessels. Microwave Imaging was seen to have application in screening for breast cancer. Microwaves are not ionizing radiations, and carry far less angiogenic risk than conventional x-rays. Finally, we considered EIT, in particular, the IP, where a large number of electrode pairs are placed on a body part (e.g., the chest), and one electrode pair of the N pairs is excited with an AC test signal at a time. The voltage amplitudes and phases across the other (N − 1) electrode pairs are then used to reconstruct a map of the electrical impedance of the volume of interest, enabling detection of anomalous structures. Low-current AC excitation in the range of 20–30 kHz carries no ionizing risk.

17 Innovations in Noninvasive Instrumentation and Measurements

17.1 INTRODUCTION

Cancers are generally detected in the body after they reach a critical size where they can be seen on an imaging system (~1 cm diameter in the case of breast cancer), palpated, disrupt some normal physiological process, or cause pain, discomfort, or bleeding. The *latency period of a cancer* is the interval between its initiation and clinical detection. For some slow-growing cancers, the latent period can be 5 years or more. A major objective in oncology is early detection because it is easier to fight an identified small cancer than a large one, especially before it has had a chance to spread (become metastatic).

For some types of cancer, the body's immune system (IS) recognizes the tumor as foreign tissue early in its growth because of abnormal damaged or mutated cancer cell surface proteins, and the IS mounts an attack on the tumor cells. The attack may prove ineffectual because the tumor grows faster than the IS can fight it, or the tumor cells may secrete substances that suppress IS's actions. Still, there will be circulating antibodies (Abs) in the blood against signature tumor cell surface proteins. The problem is to detect these Abs and use them as a sign that a particular type of cancer is growing in an otherwise asymptomatic body. The mitochondrial DNA (mtDNA) of cancer cells may also be mutated, and can serve as a basis for cancer detection. The use of mtDNA to identify cancers in the normal latency period is described below.

Cancers growing in the body also produce shifts in the normal concentrations of certain biochemical components of saliva, sputum, urine, and blood. Detection of these concentration shifts also holds promise for early NI asymptomatic cancer detection, and is discussed in the sections below.

Certain hereditary diseases can also be identified by DNA analysis; either there are DNA base sequences that code one or more abnormal (enzymes) proteins, or the coding for an enzyme is missing. Other hereditary diseases involve DNA coding for bad or missing cell membrane receptor proteins. Again DNA analysis can point to such diseases.

Fluorescence analysis is another growing field that combines immunology, molecular biology, and biophotonics. Fluorescent molecular "probes," made by attaching fluorescent molecules (a *fluorophore*) to a specific antigen (Ag) (or Ab) can be used to physically locate specific proteins on cell surfaces, or circulating molecules (including Abs) in the blood. Fluorescent *in situ* hybridization (FISH) is an important technique for genetic analysis and cancer detection and characterization. FISH works in the following manner: A DNA double-stranded helix from the nucleus (nDNA) or from mtDNA of cells is enzymatically cleaved into single (complementary) strands exposing many nucleic acids. A DNA probe molecule is prepared with a desired base sequence which is complementary to, and which will mate up with the bases of one of the cleaved single DNA strands. The probe is tagged throughout its length with fluorescent molecules bound to its deoxyribose-phosphate side. Thus, a specific chromosome target can be tagged and made uniquely visible under short-wavelength general illumination. Shorter, specific, gene regions that code for specific proteins can also be selected and marked. FISH is not at the present an *in vivo* technique. Cells whose DNA is to be studied can be obtained by NI cheek swabs or in sputum, or semi-invasively by needle biopsy. FISH requires histological techniques in which a cell of interest is fixed and mounted on a microscope slide; its DNA is then cleaved by heating with formamide at 70°C. The fluorescent probe molecules are then introduced by a micropipette, and the preparation is covered with a cover glass and incubated for several hours at 37°C. After incubation, the excess probe molecules are washed away, and all of the cell's DNA can be highlighted with a general stain fluorescing at a wavelength different than the probe. The fluorochrome molecules used emit at characteristic wavelengths which are selected by a band-pass filter or monochromator attached to the viewing microscope (Katzir et al. 1998).

Five different fluorochrome probes each fluorescing at a different wavelength (one green, two red, two IR) can be used at the same time for complex human chromosomal (24) analysis by FISH (Speicher et al. 1996). A SpectraCube® system (described below) was used to perform the multicolor, M-FISH analysis. Note that mtDNA, RNA (messenger RNA and retroviral RNA) can also be marked with complementary, fluorescent probes.

Spectral karyotyping (SKY) is a powerful research tool enabling researchers to follow chromosomal rearrangements in mouse cancer cell lines (SKY is a variation of FISH). *Spectral pathology* (SPY) is a spectral imaging technique used with bright-field microscopy. Typically, chromogenic dyes such as hematoxylin and eosin are used to stain the tissue slices. By spectrally decomposing the image with a system like SpectraCube, the information can be used to identify and characterize cancers. We describe the innovative SpectraCube system, and show some of its applications in diagnosis.

In this chapter, we also describe the "DNA Biochip," an integrated circuit approach to chemical sensing in which sections of genetically engineered, complementary strands of DNA "probe" molecules are bound to test cell sites on a silicon or glass substrate. When the sought-after single-strand DNA analytes appear in the test solution, they bind with the specific complementary DNA bases in the test cells. In one type of biochip, the binding of analyte to probe molecules causes an electrical current to flow for that cell which is proportional to the number of analyte molecules bound; this direct current is amplified and displayed. The DNA biochip principle is not limited to DNA and RNA analysis; Ag and Ab binding can also be used to gate current.

17.2 DNA ANALYSIS BY POLYMERASE CHAIN REACTION

The *polymerase chain reaction* (PCR) is a molecular biology/biochemical protocol used to exactly replicate (amplify) a single piece of DNA (oligo) from a sample to create thousands to millions of copies of that particular DNA sequence (Riley 2005). These copies allow other analytical techniques to more easily identify the base sequences of the oligo. The PCR allows the DNA from a sample as small as a fraction of a genome, a single-cell nucleus, or a mitochondrion to be characterized in terms of its base sequences. The PCR has many applications, ranging from criminal science to genomics. However, in this section, we will address the PCR applications in medical diagnosis.

The PCR was developed ca. 1983 by Kary Mullis. The history of PCR development has been described by Bartlett and Stirling (2003). The basic PCR process requires:

- A *DNA template* that contains the DNA region or target to be amplified.

- *Two primers* that are complementary to the 3′ ends of each of the sense and antisense strand of the dsDNA target.

- *Taq polymerase* (or another DNA polymerase, e.g., *Pfu*) with an optimum working temperature around 72°C.

- *Deoxynucleoside triphosphates* (dNTPs), the building blocks from which the DNA polymerase synthesizes a new DNA strand.

- A pH *buffer solution* to provide a suitable chemical environment for optimum enzyme activity.

- *Bivalent cations;* generally Mg^{++} is used.

- K^+ ions.

The PCR process is typically carried out in a reaction volume of 10–200 μL in small reaction tubes with 0.2–0.5 mL volumes in a *thermal cycler*. The thermal cycler alternately heats and cools the reaction tubes to obtain the temperatures required for each step of the PCR process. Typically, the process consists of a series of 20–40 repeated temperature changes, called cycles, with each cycle commonly consisting of three discrete temperature steps. Operations 2, 3, and 4 described below are done in a single cycle.

The PCR procedure consists of the following operations:

1. *Initialization step:* (only required for DNA polymerases that require heat activation by hot-start PCR). The reactants are heated for 1–9 min to 94–98°C.

2. *Denaturation step:* This step is the first regular thermal cycling step, and consists of heating the reaction to 94–98°C for 20–30 s. It causes separation of the DNA helix by breaking the hydrogen bonds between complementary bases, yielding single-stranded DNA molecules.

3. *Annealing step:* The reaction temperature is lowered to 50–65°C for 20–40 s, allowing annealing of the primers to the single-stranded DNA template. This temperature needs to be low enough to allow for hybridization of the primer to the DNA strand, but high enough for the hybridization to be specific, that is, the primer should only bind to a perfectly complementary part of the template. The polymerase binds to the primer–template hybrid molecule and begins DNA formation.

4. *Extension–elongation step:* In this step, the reaction temperature is made 72–80°C, an optimum for the DNA polymerase (*Taq polymerase*) to function. In this step, the DNA polymerase assembles a new DNA strand complementary to the DNA template by adding dNTPs that are

complementary to the template in its 5′–3′ direction, condensing the 5′ phosphate group of the dNTPs with the 3′-hydroxyl group at the end of the growing DNA strand. The growth time depends both on the DNA polymerase used and the length of the target DNA fragment being duplicated. As a rule of thumb, at the optimum temperature, the DNA polymerase will add 1000 bases per minute. Under optimum (ideal) conditions, at each extension step, the amount of DNA target is doubled, leading to exponential amplification of the specific DNA target fragment.

5. *Final elongation*: This single step occasionally may be performed at a temperature of 70–74°C (this is the optimal temperature for most polymerases used in PCR) for 5–15 min after the last PCR cycle to ensure that any remaining ssDNA is fully extended.

6. *Final hold*: This step is held at 4–15°C for an indefinite time and is used for short-term storage of the reaction product.

7. *Check*: To check whether the PCR process generated the anticipated DNA fragment (also known as the *amplimer* or *amplicon*), agarose gel electrophoresis is employed for size separation of the PCR products. The size(s) of the products is determined by comparison with a DNA "ladder" (a molecular weight marker), which contains DNA fragments of known size, run on the gel alongside the PCR products.

PCR has several important medical applications. The DNA to be analyzed is obtained from cells in a blood drop, from a cheek swab, a hair follicle, or from a minimally invasive tissue biopsy. Some of the medical applications include, but are not limited to

■ PCR testing of a person's genome for heritable genetic diseases is one important application. Prospective parents' DNA can be tested for being carriers of a recessive gene or genes that might be expressed in their children.

■ PCR can be used as part of a sensitive test for tissue typing, critical information for organ transplantation or donation.

■ Many forms of cancer involve base alterations to *oncogenes*. By using PCR-based tests to study these mutations, therapy regimens can sometimes be individually customized to a patient.

■ With highly infective viruses, PCR tests have been developed that can detect as little as one viral genome among the DNA of over 50,000 host cells (Kwok et al. 1987). (Note that HIV is a retrovirus whose ssRNA genome is copied into its host cell's DNA.)

■ PCR-based tests allow the detection of small numbers of hard-to-culture disease organisms (both dead and alive) in body fluids. *Mycobacterium tuberculosis* divides once every 15–20 hours under ideal conditions, which is very slow compared to other bacteria. The *M. tuberculosis* genome was sequenced in 1998.

■ PCR testing is used to track the mutations of a disease pathogen in time, and identify new, virulent subtypes that emerge in an epidemic, or alternately, evolve into more benign strains.

Besides medical applications, the PCR has found application in forensics; genetic "fingerprinting" of a suspect or victim can provide positive identification. All that is needed is a single-nucleated cell or in some cases a single mitochondrion. PCR DNA "fingerprinting" can help in parental testing.

Note that ~26 variations on the basic PCR protocol described above have been reported in the literature. (cf. the April 2016 *Wikipedia* article: "Polymerase chain reaction.")

17.3 DNA SEQUENCING WITH NANOPORES

The use of nanopores for sequencing single, single- or double-strand DNA oligos allows a single DNA oligo to be characterized electrochemically by a series of current pulses as the DNA strand rapidly threads itself though the nanopore at a rate of ~1–3 μs per base (i.e., A, G, C, and T) (Ayub and Bailey 2012). This means that a single strand of DNA having 8000 bases can be characterized in ~20 ms. If the DNA sample is the result of PCR, then 99 more identical DNA analyses for noise reduction may take a total of ~20 s. Nanopore diameters are ~1–5 nm in internal diameter depending on the material, and they have been made from materials including, but not limited to, silicon nitride, graphene, single-layer MoS_2 (SLMS), alpha hemolysin (αHL), and *Mycobacterium smegmatis* porin A (MspA). αHL is a bacterial protein that normally causes lysis of erythrocytes.

Its pore is ~10 nm long and has two distinct 5 nm diameter sections. The MspA pore is funnel shaped, with a 1.2-nm hole at the bottom. SLMS has ~1 nm thickness with a 2.3-nm diameter pore. It has a high SNR >15 in sequencing dsDNA oligos (Farimani et al. 2014).

When a DC electrical potential difference of 100–600 mV is established across the nanopore axis, the resultant electric field in the nanopore causes an ionic current (in the range of single nAs) to flow through the pore. ssDNA or dsDNA strands can be passed through the nanopore by attracting them by electrophoresis, or by the use of enzyme "guides" attached to the "mouth" of the nanopore to attract the DNA. As the DNA strand passes through the nanopore, each base molecule (A, G, C, and T) (or base pair) modulates the steady-state ionic direct current in a characteristic manner because of its size and surface charges, giving a unique pulse-height signature as each particular base passes through.

Ongoing research seeks to optimize the nanopore DNA and RNA sequencing process. Recently, DiFiori et al. (2013) reported that shining low-power green laser light on a silicon nitride nanopore increased the electric charge near the walls of the pore, which was immersed in saline water. By modulating the surface charge, it is possible to control the amount of *electroosmotic flow* through the nanopore, which affects the speed of translocating nucleic acids. A few mW of green light can slow the translocation speed of dsDNA by more than an order of magnitude. Slowing the translocation enables a more accurate reading of the passage of each nucleotide pair (Benowitz 2014).

In summary, rapid nucleic acid sequencing with nanopores is an exciting, new analytical technology. The best nanopore material at this writing appears to be MoS_2. Research is needed to improve the reliability, accuracy, and precision of the technique. Note that DNA (and RNA) samples can generally be obtained by NI means: for example, cheek swabs, saliva, urine, a blood drop, a hair follicle, etc. Also be aware that while analysis speed for a single oligo is fast (~20 ms), there are many, many oligos composing a genome with over 20,000 genes, and a computer is required to sort them all out.

17.4 FLUORESCENCE TESTS FOR BIOMOLECULES: FISH AND SKY

In Section 15.3, we described the use of fluorescence to detect cancers and other lesions noninvasively, *in vivo;* that is, using endoscopes to directly examine the fluorescent properties of the cells in the surface of a lesion. In this section, we further explore this topic, including how the use of fluorescent dyes bonded to probe molecules can reveal chromosomal, gene, and oligonucleotide structures. The ability to probe the structure of DNA and RNA base sequences is currently an extremely active research topic in oncology and genetic medicine. Cancer cells exhibit mutations not only in their nuclear DNA (nDNA) but also in their mtDNA, providing possible early tests for cancers, and aiding researchers to understand the causes of various types of cancer.

Generally, fluorescent tests on DNA can be done on prepared cancer cells taken by biopsy (an invasive procedure) using fluorescent nucleic acid labeling techniques and confocal laser scanning fluorescence microscopy. Alternately, the cells and mtDNA to be analyzed can be found in specimens of urine, saliva, and sputum (NI procedures). DNA fragments (oligonucleotides) can be "amplified" or reproduced enzymatically by the PCR technique, so many more, identical molecules are available to study, *en masse.*

FISH is a molecular labeling technique which is used to detect the chromosomal location (and presence) of a specific genomic target. FISH was invented at the Lawrence Livermore National Laboratory in the mid-1980s by J.W. Gray and D. Pinkel. The FISH technique involves the selective binding of one or more probe molecules, each labeled with a separate, unique fluorescent dye (fluorochrome) to target single strands of DNA or RNA. The single-strand, labeled, DNA (or RNA) probe molecules are synthesized in lengths dependent on the application. Multiple complementary probes can be synthesized from all of the fragments from a single, long strand of DNA of a particular chromosome. These probes can label the total target chromosome. Alternately, chromophore-labeled probes can be made for a single gene, or can use a relatively short oligonucleotide, composed of as few as eight nucleotides. Short oligonucleotide probes can be used to find and label the complementary target sequences in any single-strand, chromosomal DNA or RNA.

The FISH can be used to distinguish all of the chromosomes; five or more unique fluorescent markers (fluors) must be used in various combinations to effect unique marking of all 23 chromosomes. The use of multiple fluors is called M-FISH. A sixth fluor can be used to give banding patterns. M-FISH has great potential for cancer research for the diagnosis and evaluation of treatments, particularly for various leukemias where the chromosomes can be "jumbled." M-FISH will aid in the identification of recurrent chromosome changes and rearrangements. Speicher et al. (1996) developed epifluorescence wavelength filter sets and software that allows the detection and discrimination of 27 different DNA probes hybridized simultaneously to human chromosomes. The perfection of this technology led to the development of SKY which enables the simultaneous differentiation of all 24 human chromosomes in 24 colors. Sharma and Sharma (2001) pointed out that SKY takes advantage of the fact that spectral Bioimaging, in contrast to traditional filter systems, is not influenced by intensity variations which often impair the results of FISH experiments, or simply not make them analyzable. The analysis of multicolor FISH experiments by a SpectraCube system provides a high number of measurement points along the spectral axis for each point (pixel) of the image which yields an extremely high signal-to-noise ratio.

For SKY, all 24 flow-sorted human *chromosome painting* probes are combinatorically labeled with a set of five different fluorochromes (one green, two red, and two IR). Each chromosome is assigned with a unique combination of fluorochromes and thereby a highly characteristic emission spectrum, which is used for definite chromosome recognition. Image acquisition is achieved with the SpectraCube system (cf. Section 17.4), which is a combination of an interferometer (used as a Fourier spectrometer) and a CCD camera, which can be mounted on nearly every existing fluorescence microscope.

Mitochondria are cell organelles that are responsible for the synthesis of adenosine triphosphate (ATP) (largely from oxygen and glucose) in a complex series of enzymatically controlled chemical reactions. ATP is a ubiquitous molecule, used by the body's cells as a common energy currency; it drives many of the chemical reactions in the body including various *ion pumps* used by neurons, muscle cells, kidney tubule cells, etc. as well as powering the synthesis of glucose from lactic acid, the synthesis of fatty acids from acetyl coenzyme-A (acetyl Co-A), the synthesis of cholesterol, phospholipids, hormones, and many other substances. Mitochondria are unique because they have a double-walled membrane isolating them from the cytosol, and they have their own circular, 16.5 kb DNA chromosome that codes for 13 proteins and several regulating enzymes. There are about 10 copies of the genome in each mitochondrion, and up to 10^4 mitochondria in a cell. Damage to mtDNA (e.g., from ionizing radiation) is more common than to nDNA; mutations occur most frequently in the NADH dehydrogenase subunit 4 gene and in the displacement loop region (Hochhauser 2000). About 90% of the mitochondrial proteins are coded by genes from DNA in the cell nucleus (nDNA), however, suggesting that in the process of evolution, genes have been lost from the mtDNA. Human mtDNA is inherited from the unfertilized ovum, hence everyone's mtDNA comes from their mother.

When a cancer cell dies (undergoes apoptosis or is attacked by the IS's natural killer cells), cell fragments and mtDNA enter the surrounding medium (urine, saliva, etc.). In a key pilot study, Fliss et al. (2000) found that mtDNA isolated from the urine of patients having bladder cancer showed mutations. The same mtDNA mutations were found by direct examination of biopsied cells from the cancer. Similar results were found for head, neck, and lung cancers using saliva and lung lavage samples from the respective patients. Mutations were also found in cancer cells' nDNA, as might be expected, but the mtDNA mutation tests are many times more sensitive because a cancer cell only has one nucleus with nDNA, and thousands of mitochondria, each with up to 10 copies of its mtDNA. (See *Cancer mortality* in the Glossary for an overview of the U.S. and worldwide death rates from various kinds of cancers.) Thus, the screening of fluids obtained noninvasively (urine, saliva, sputum) for mutations in mtDNA using FISH, SKY, spectral imaging techniques, or a DNA biochip hold promise for rapid and inexpensive cancer screening in the future. For more on cancer mortality statistics, see Glossary.

17.5 SPECTRACUBE SYSTEM

The SpectraCube system, a product developed and patented by Applied Spectral Imaging Co. in Israel, is a unique imaging system which allows the detailed wavelength (spectral) information associated with each pixel of an illuminated object to be determined and displayed (Garini et al. 2006, Huttenberger et al. 2008, Hieber et al. 2011). The object can be a length of fluorescently tagged DNA in a cell nucleus, a tissue probed with a Raman laser, an autofluorescent tissue such as a growing cancer viewed by an endoscope, or varieties of DNA tagged with fluorescent oligonucleotide probes bound to a DNA biochip. (The SpectraCube system can also be used in geological and natural resources image analysis [remote sensing], it is not limited to medical diagnosis.) U.S. Patent No. 5,539,517 (Cabib et al. 1996) describes the optical technology used in the SpectraCube system. U.S. Patent No. 5,784,162 (Cabib et al. 1998) elaborates on applications of the SpectraCube system in biomedicine. U.S. Patent No. 5,995,645 (Soenksen et al. 1999) illustrates how the SpectraCube system can be used to find cancerous cells. Suspect cancer cells from a biopsy are stained with two dyes, one of which binds preferentially to cancer cells. Spectral imaging is used to detect those cells imaged in certain pixels that are cancerous. The SpectraCube system can not

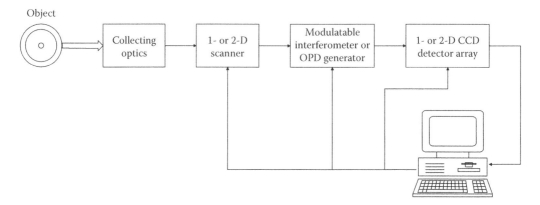

Figure 17.1 Block diagram of the SpectraCube system.

only give gray-scale intensity information for every pixel but can also measure the spectrum of each pixel in a predetermined range.

At the heart of the SpectraCube system is an *interferometer* that allows computation of the spectrum of the light reflected or emitted from each object pixel using the *Fourier transform* (FT) *spectrogram method* (described in detail in Section 8.2.2 of this book). Note that the use of an interferometer and the FT method replaces the need for a monochromator or many narrow band-pass filters for spectral decomposition. Cabib et al. (1996) showed that several different kinds of interferometer can be used to derive the spectrum of the light from each object pixel. They showed that both interferometers with moving mirrors to vary the optical path distance (OPD), and also interferometers with fixed mirrors (where the OPD is varied by the angle of incidence of rays from object pixels) can be used. For illustrative purposes, Cabib et al. (1996) described embodiments of their invention with internally modulated Fabry-Perot and Michelson, and fixed Michelson and Sagnac interferometers.

Figure 17.1 shows a block diagram of the SpectraCube system covered by U.S. Patent No. 5,995,645 (Soenksen et al. 1999). An optical schematic diagram of a typical SpectraCube configuration is shown in Figure 17.2. Note that in this embodiment, a *Sagnac interferometer* with fixed

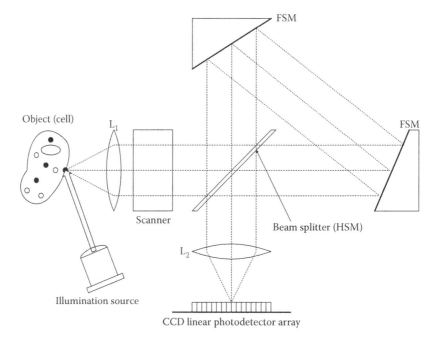

Figure 17.2 Schematic of a SpectraCube system in which the interferometer is a Sagnac type with fixed mirrors.

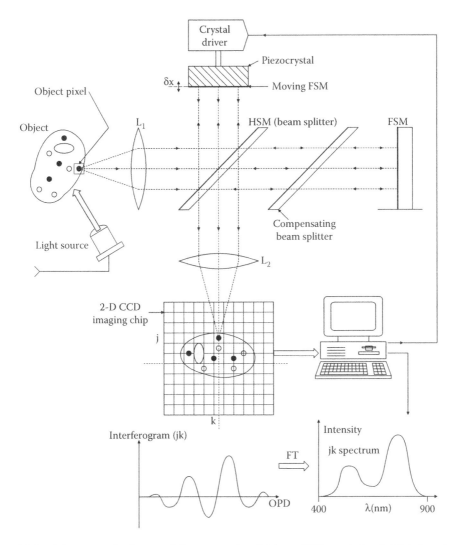

Figure 17.3 Schematic of a SpectraCube system in which an OPD-modulated Michelson interferometer is used to find the spectrum of each pixel using Fourier transform (FT) calculations.

mirrors is used. The OPD required to form an interferogram is inherent in the angle of incidence, β, of the incoming rays. It is shown in Cabib et al. (1996) that the OPD in the Sagnac interferometer is proportional to β. Figure 17.3 illustrates a Michelson interferometer with an OPD varied by a mirror mounted on a piezoelectric crystal transducer. Horizontal scanning is not required in this embodiment because a square CCD photosensor array is used, rather than the CCD linear array shown in Figure 17.2. Quoting Cabib et al. (1996):

In all the embodiments of the invention described below (in the Patent text), all the required optical phase differences are scanned simultaneously with the spatial scanning of the field of view in order to obtain all the information required to reconstruct the spectrum, so that the spectral information is collected simultaneously with the imaging information.
A method and apparatus according to the present invention may be practiced in a large variety of configurations. Specifically, the interferometer used may be of either the moving [mirror] or the non-moving type and the detector array may, independently of the type of interferometer, be one- or two-dimensional. When the interferometer is of the moving type and the detector array is two-dimensional, no scanning (of the object) is required, except for movement of the interferometer which is an OPD scan. When the interferometer is of the moving type and the detector array is one-dimensional, spatial scanning (of the object)

in one dimension is required. When the interferometer is of the non-moving type and the detector array is two-dimensional, OPD scanning in one dimension is required (to vary β, hence the OPD). When the interferometer is of the non-moving type, and the detector array is one-dimensional, scanning in two-dimensions is required, with one dimension relating to a spatial scan while the other relates to an OPD (β) scan.

In the internally modulated Michelson interferometer of Figure 17.3, the output is directed to a 2-D CCD photodetector array. Note that no external scanning is required. Once the image and the spectra of each of its pixels have been computed, the information can be used to screen tissue samples (generally obtained by biopsy) for cancer cells. Cancer cells have different affinities for various fluorescent dye molecules than normal cells, and the pattern recognition software used with a SpectraCube system can be programmed to "recognize" cancer cells by their spectral signatures. The same technique can be used in DNA analysis using multiple fluorescent tags on probe oligonucleotides, either on chromosomes on a prepared microscope slide, or on a DNA biochip, as described in the next section. SpectraCube systems enable efficient, rapid, and accurate SKY to be done, where genetic aberrations in both nuclear DNA (nDNA) and mtDNA can be located and characterized. SKY is useful in research on genetic diseases and on the causes of cancer.

Another application of the SpectraCube system is in ophthalmology. The ophthalmic applied spectral imaging system (OASIS) has been developed by the Applied Spectral Imaging Co. The OASIS system is a sophisticated fundus camera that allows resolution of chemical as well as structural details in the retina. For example, the processor can be programmed to map regions of low-oxygen saturation (see Section 15.8 on Pulse Oximetry) in the retina, a condition relating to vascular disease caused, for example, by diabetes (i.e., diabetic retinopathy). OASIS can also detect drusen by their spectral characteristics. (Drusen can be present in retinas affected by age-related macular degeneration; see Section 2.2.1.) The OASIS system uses a modified and cooled Hamamatsu C4880-81 CCD camera with 640×480 pixel resolution. The interferometer used in the OASIS system has fixed mirrors; the OPD length is modulated by parallax angle to get ~100 data points in the interferogram for each pixel. Each pixel's interferogram is FFTd to give a corresponding spectrogram. The system's computer is programmed to analyze each spectrogram, and assign a (pseudo)color to each pixel, depending how it matches the property sought (i.e., oxyhemoglobin) (Curran 2000).

17.6 ANALYTICAL MICROARRAYS

17.6.1 Introduction

A microarray is a 2-D array of recessed cells (pits) etched into a solid substrate (usually an etched glass slide, a silicon plate, a plastic planar surface, a nitrocellulose membrane, or a hydrophobic polystyrene surface). In early versions, cells were organized into rectangular arrays, typically $20 \times 20 = 400$ in a 1 cm square area. In modern cell spot microarrays (CSMAs) made by contact printing, a microarray can be given 200 μm spot diameters spaced 500 μm on centers, giving 3888 spots in an area of 18×54 mm on a single, polystyrene, microplate-sized vessel (this is 900 spots/cm^2) (Rantala et al. 2011, VTT 2015). CSMAs are being used for systematic RNAi screening, identifying large sets of siRNA molecules. Each spot can bind as much as ~50 pg siRNA plus detection reagents (Rantala et al. 2011).

Readout of CSMAs is typically by selective staining of target molecules bound to the cell spots, then using automated microscopic analysis to measure the wavelengths and intensities of the bound analytes.

As you will see below, microarrays are being used for Ab–Ag tests of blood microsamples, analysis of DNA and RNA oligos, protein structure analysis, and quantifying carbohydrates, sugars, glycans, etc. in blood microsamples. Their major advantages include the ability to run multiple tests in parallel (simultaneously), low sample volume requirements, and high-speed automated optical readouts.

17.6.2 Ab Microarrays

An Ab microarray (AbMA) is used to detect specific Ags; a set of Abs is spotted on a microarray plate. Next, a solution containing various Ags is introduced, and some will bind with their target Abs. Next, the AbMA plate is washed. Then fluorescent Ab tags specific to the Ags are introduced; they also bind to the Ags already bound to their specific Abs attached to the AbMA plate. Fluorescent microscopy is used to quantify the Ags bound to known Abs on the plate.

Early AbMAs devised by Chang (1983) used 400 spots on a 1 cm² plate. Chang's invention can be used to quantify certain leukocyte cell surface Ags, such as CD proteins (e.g., CD3, CD4, CD8, etc.). Also, HLA allotypic Ags, Ags from viral and bacterial membranes, and various soluble Ags, Ags from cancer cell membranes, etc. Chang has three patents on AbMA technology.

17.6.3 Nucleic Acid Microarrays

DNA microarrays, also known as DNA biochips, come in many embodiments; they are actively being developed by many corporations and university laboratories around the world. There are several forces driving their invention; one is the economy resulting from the speed of analysis they permit, which effectively makes use of molecular parallel processing. They require fewer personnel than do conventional analytical techniques, and they offer high-analytic accuracy. DNA microarrays are used to determine the molecular structure of chromosomes, genes, and other oligonucleotides (oligos). They also can be used to analyze proteins, including Ags, Abs, and receptors on cell surfaces. They have many applications in the fields of genetic medicine, cancer diagnostics, and pharmaceutical development. For example, they provide genetic analysis of bacterial strains, showing how mutations can lead to drug resistance.

A DNA microarray is composed of a rectangular grid of open compartments or "cells" formed on a flat substrate such as silicon or glass. The cell dimensions of DNA microarrays are on the order of 10 s to 100 s of μm, at least two orders of magnitude larger than features on a typical electronic microcircuit. Much art and ingenious surface chemistry have been invested in attaching probe molecules to an array's cells. In one scheme, developed at Rockefeller University in NY, Shivashankar and Libchaber (1997) used an atomic force microscope and laser "tweezers" to graft a single strand of DNA to a 3 μm diameter latex bead and then bond this complex into a microarray cell so that the DNA could be probed with fluorophore-labeled oligos in solution. Another approach has used an electric field applied to the target cell to attract charged probe molecules to that cell; the process is repeated until all the cells are filled with different probes. The company *Affymetrix* in Santa Clara, CA, has adapted a photolithographic process to assemble various oligonucleotide fluorescent probes in the array's cells. Experimental microarrays with over 96,000 cells containing different oligos have been built as gene probes (ACGS 2015). Note that probe DNA oligo molecules generally have known base sequences and are labeled with fluorescent molecules; probes can be in solution, or be tethered to substrate molecules in the cells. The target molecules are the analytes; their base sequence is unknown and to be determined. If the probe molecules are tethered, the target analytes are in solution, and vice versa.

There are three basic detection or readout schemes that are currently used with DNA microarrays: The most common is based on fluorescent labeling of probe molecules that bind with target molecules in the microarray's "cells." Fluorescence can be read out by interrogating each cell sequentially with a collimated laser beam that excites the fluorescence in a particular cell, if any. Band-pass filters are used to read each type of fluorescence. Alternatively, the entire microarray can be illuminated with the UV-exciting light, and a SpectraCube system can be used to analyze simultaneously all the fluorescent signatures of the cells.

Radioactive labeling of probe molecules in solution is a second means of detecting probe–target ligands. The target molecules are bound to cells in the array. Autoradiography with film is used to detect bound complexes on the array; a more qualitative than quantitative approach.

A third type of readout is electrical. *Clinical MicroSensors, Inc.* (CMS) (now Genmark Diagnostics, Inc., Pasadena, CA, which was Osmetech Molecular Diagnostics, was a subsidiary of Motorola) developed a charge-based method in which various oligonucleotide probes are bound to array cells. When a target complementary DNA section binds to an oligo probe on a cell, a third molecular probe carrying iron can bind to the ligated probe and DNA. The presence of the iron is sensed electronically by the altered E field around the cell, and a current flows for that cell proportional to the amount of third probe molecule attached in the cell. Thus, a DC current readout is possible from each cell, the magnitude of which is indicative of the amount of target DNA bound to a given cell's probe oligo.

Another electronic detection means for detecting probe–target binding was described by R.B. Lennox in U.S. Patent No. 6,107,180, *Biosensor Device and Method*. 22 Aug. 2000. Lennox's invention uses conductivity-based phenomena as well as a field effect. Figure 17.4 illustrates a cross section through the simplified array cell of Lennox's system. In one embodiment of Lennox's biosensor, a monolayer of 8–22 carbon-saturated hydrocarbon (SHC) chains are bound to the conductive substrate by sulfhydryl linkages. The chain density is 3–5 per nm². Ligand (probe) molecules are then attached to the distal ends of a small fraction of the chains. In the absence of target analyte

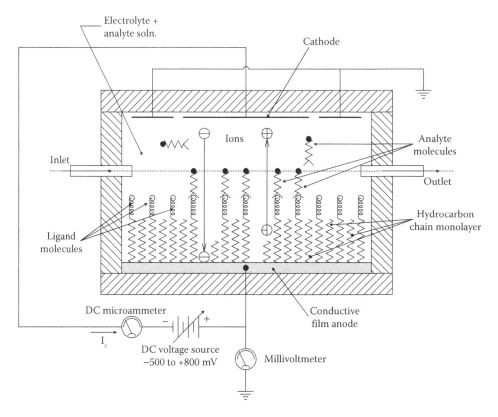

Figure 17.4 Lennox 2000 biosensor system. When an analyte molecule binds with the target site on a ligand molecule, the underlying dense hydrocarbon monolayer parts and allows ions to flow. DC cell current is proportional to the bound analyte concentration.

molecules, the dense, ordered packing of the SHC chains forms an effective, high-resistance barrier to electron flow through the cell. When a target molecule forms chemical bonds with a probe molecule, the ordered geometry of the SHC chains is perturbed, allowing certain ions from the bathing solution capable of undergoing a redox reaction to react at a noble metal electrode surface. A typical redox ion could be $Fe(CN)_4{}^-$, or $Fe^{+++} \rightarrow Fe^{++}$ (reduction). Lennox (2000) claimed that only one binding event (probe to analyte) triggers 10^2–10^6 redox events (and electrons) to flow per second, thus is highly multiplicative. A cell's electron current is proportional to the number of reacted probe molecules in the cell. Quoting Lennox:

> By analogy to a [field effect] transistor, the redox solution serves as the "source," the monolayer as the "gate," and the underlying electrode as the "drain." Current flow in a transistor is initiated by applying a threshold voltage to the gate. In the *biosensor* of the invention, current flow is initiated by a stimulus—in this case, a ligand receptor binding event—to the monolayer "gate."

Of course, a suitable DC potential must be maintained to support the redox reaction used.

Electrical readout of DNA microarrays is especially attractive because no expensive lasers and fluorescence imaging CCD cameras are required; only N current-to-voltage converters, an analog multiplexer, and an analog-to-digital converter to interface with the computer used to manage data. The N cells on a biosensor "chip" require noble metal electrodes (gold or platinum) for the redox reactions. A drawback of the electrical DNA microarray is that this type of system has very high-temperature sensitivity; the electrical conductivity of ionic solutions, and redox reactions have very high-positive tempcos. This means that the temperature environment of an electrical DNA biosensor must be strictly regulated. The mean-squared value of thermal noise voltage sources is proportional to the Kelvin temperature.

A future readout system for microarrays can make use of *surface plasmon resonance* (SPR) (Section 8.2.4). A rectangular matrix of probe molecules, each having an affinity to a particular target molecule, will be deposited in cells on the surface of an SPR grating or prism. When the probe molecule in any one cell binds to its target molecule, the dielectric constant and refractive index change in the chemical layer, affecting surface plasmon generation. We have seen in Section 8.2.4 that the binding reaction affects the absorption of input photon energy and its conversion into plasmons. In one way, this binding can be detected by shining a beam of monochromatic, linearly polarized light (LPL) on the metal film on the grating directly under the cell in question. The intensity of the reflected beam is monitored. Binding causes a shift in the reflected light beam *angle* at which maximum absorption (minimum reflection) occurs, as shown in Figure 8.14.

In an alternate readout approach, the light beam is kept at a fixed angle and a wavelength is chosen that will give minimum intensity of the reflected light beam shined on the unreacted cell in question. When target molecules bind to the probe molecules in the cell, the wavelength for maximum absorption (minimum reflection intensity) will shift. This alternate readout approach requires a monochromator to vary the λ of the input beam at constant intensity and angle. Figure 8.15 illustrates this wavelength-dependent absorption shift at constant incidence angle as binding occurs.

If the *variable angle method* is used, a simple diode laser can be used to test for probe binding with a single photomultiplier detector. The mechanical design in this case is more complex; for N cells, the laser and detector have to be moved to systematically cover each cell, and also scanned in angle. Using the *fixed angle method*, the entire SPR cell array can be illuminated with one beam at a fixed angle and λ. Detection can be by a square array CCD camera, also at a fixed angle with respect to the SPR microarray. The wavelength of the illuminating beam can be repetitively swept over the λ range of interest, and each of the CCD outputs averaged to improve SNR and to measure the binding dynamics. The λ of the input beam can be varied continuously with a monochromator, or discretely with a bank of narrow band-pass filters acting on a white light source. I believe the latter method will be simpler and less expensive because nothing moves (except the gratings in the monochromator, or the filters).

Applications of molecular biosensors are growing with the number of designs available. As we have described above, cancer screening through genetic mutation detection of nDNA and mtDNA is very important. The DNA microarray is also finding application in drug design. As various kinds of bacteria become resistant to older antibiotics, it is possible to track the mutations that lead to changes in internal enzymes, etc. that confer this resistance. Thus, new antibiotics can be designed to exploit weaknesses in the more stable parts of a bacterium's genome. The DNA microarray is not limited to DNA. RNA from retroviruses such as HIV can be analyzed for mutations as well.

Simple cells with bound *protein Ags* can be designed to test for particular Abs in the blood or other body fluids; conversely, monoclonal Abs can be bound as probes to detect a particular bacterial Ag such as on *Escherichia coli, Streptococcus, Pneumococcus*, etc., and even read out the subtype to facilitate antibiotic selection. They can facilitate detection of *PLA2*, a protein produced by prostate cancer cells and *melastatin*, a protein produced by melanoma cancer cells.

17.6.4 Peptide and Protein Microarrays

Peptides are short chains of amino acid (AA) monomers linked by peptide (amide) covalent bonds. Chain length is typically 2–20 AAs. Peptides can be formed by breaking up larger protein molecules. A peptide microarray (PmA) is a collection of diverse peptide aptamers attached to a solid glass or plastic surface. There are many applications for PmAs, such as mapping an Ab's epitope, finding key residues for protein binding, profiling an enzyme (e.g., kinase, phosphatase, protease, acetyltransferase, histone deacetylase, etc.). They can also be used diagnostically to profile-changing humoral immune responses during a disease or infection, monitoring the course of therapeutic interventions, development of new vaccines, etc.

After attaching a set of peptides to a chip, it can be incubated with a variety of different biological samples such as purified enzymes or Abs, patient or animal sera, cell lysates, etc. After several washing steps, a secondary Ab with the needed specificity is applied. The secondary Ab is tagged with a unique fluorescent label for parallel optical detection, or the secondary Abs can be tagged with chemiluminescent, colorimetric, or radioactive isotope markers (for autoradiographic detection).

Protein and PmAs are established as a promising tool for a wide variety of applications, including, but not limited to the identification of protein–protein interactions, protein–phospholipid interactions, small molecule targets, and substrates of protein kinases. As in the case of PmAs, they can also be used for clinical diagnostics and monitoring disease states (Hall et al. 2007, Chandra et al. 2011). The three major categories of PmAs are analytical microarrays, functional microarrays, and reverse-phase microarrays. AbMAs are the most common analytical PmA (Bertone and Snyder 2005) (cf. Section 17.5.2 above).

Analytical protein microarrays are typically used to examine a complex mixture of proteins in order to quantify binding affinities, molecular specificities, and protein expression levels of the mixture.

Functional protein microarrays (FPmAs) differ from analytical microarrays in that the FPmAs contain full-length functional proteins or protein domains. The FPmAs are used to investigate the biochemical activities of an entire proteome in a single experiment. They can be used to study protein–protein, protein–DNA, protein–RNA, protein–phospholipid, and protein–small molecule interactions (Hall et al. 2007).

Reverse-phase protein microarrays (RPPmAs) use cell lysates from cells of interest (e.g., cancer cells). The lysate is immobilized on a nitrocellulose slide using a contact pin microarrayer. The slides are then exposed to Abs against the target protein of interest. The bound Abs are typically detected with fluorescent, chemiluminescent, or colorimetric optical assays. Reference peptides are also printed on the array slide for quantitative calibration of target lysates. RPPmAs permit the detection of altered proteins (from genetic mutations or posttranslational modification causes) caused by disease.

17.6.5 Glycan Microarrays

Glycan molecules are found on the surfaces of all living cells. They comprise highly diverse structures that participate in cell physiology through glycan-binding proteins (GBPs) that recognize them as ligands (Rillahan and Paulson 2011). They are critical for the complex web of intercellular communications (C^3).

A glycan microarray uses multiple glycans or glycocojugates spot-printed on a single slide, and is used for screening GBPs. GBPs include lectins, Abs, and those GBPs on the surfaces of bacteria and viruses (Song et al. 2012, 2014a,b, Stowell et al. 2014).

Glycan microarrays, since their inception in 2002, have evolved into a powerful and still-developing tool for glycobiology research. Although the glycome is generally acknowledged to be larger than the genome and the proteome, the libraries that have been developed for DNA and Protein microarrays are currently larger than the glycan libraries; there is much work underway.

17.6.6 Lectin Microarrays

Lectins are proteins that have specific binding activity toward the carbohydrate residues of glycoproteins and glycolipids such as those found on cell surface membranes. On example of a glycated protein is HbA1c (glycated hemoglobin (Hb) in erythrocytes), an indicator of present and past blood glucose levels. Over 300 lectins have been identified in a variety of species, ranging from viruses and bacteria to plants and animals. The lectin sugar-binding proteins can be classified into five groups according to the monosaccharide to which they have the highest affinity: (1) *Mannose*; (2) *Galactose/N-acetylgalactosamine*; (3) *N-acetylglucosamine*; (4) *Fucose*; and (5) *Sialic acid*. "These proteins, which function as recognition molecules in cell–molecule and cell–cell interactions, have been implicated in a number of essential biological processes including cell proliferation, cell arrest, apoptosis, tumor cell metastasis, leukocyte homing and trafficking, and especially microbial (viral and bacterial) infection" (Hu and Wong 2009).

C-type lectins are the largest family of GBPs. They are prominently expressed on the leukocytes of the IS, and have become increasingly recognized as pattern recognition receptors (PRRs) that mediate both innate and adaptive immune responses to pathogens (Rillahan and Paulson 2011).

The lectin microarray is a new analytical technology in which a panel of various lectins is immobilized on a planar substrate, such as a *PhotoChip*™ which is a thin-film slide coated with a dextran-based polymer. Once the lectins are printed on the PhotoChip's slide, high-intensity, 365 nm UV radiation is used to photoactivate the covalent bonding between the lectin proteins and the dextran polymer on the slide. Several other technologies have been described for the creation of lectin microchips (Hu and Wong 2009).

One readout method of the lectin microarray to sense bound glycoproteins uses fluorescence. A biotinylated Ab is incubated with the bound target glycoprotein, then incubated with fluorescent-labeled streptavidin. Different fluorescent molecules were used to permit unique identification of different glycoproteins. Readout is optical.

Hu and Wong commented: "…the purpose of lectin array analysis is not to identify accurate glycan structures, but rather to obtain information of functional glycans that are recognized by a panel of lectins." Some applications of lectin microarrays include the identification of different pathogen strains from their unique cell-surface glycans (Hsu and Mahal 2006). Protein glycosylation has been shown as a key event in certain disease development, such as cancer cell invasion and metastasis; many glycosyl epitopes are tumor-associated Ags. "Lectin microarrays may turn out to be a promising tool for high-throughput analysis of minute clinical samples towards the identification of glycoprotein biomarkers for cancer detection" (Hu and Wong 2009).

17.7 NI CHEMICAL TESTS FOR CANCER NOT INVOLVING DNA

17.7.1 Introduction

With the rise of new methods in analytical biochemistry, and cost- and health-driven goals for the early detection of cancer, researchers have found a number of substances in blood, urine, saliva, and sputum (other than DNA) that are well correlated with the diagnosed presence of various cancers. Many of these substances may be present as the result of the increased metabolism of cancer cells, or may be the result of substances secreted by cancer cells as they grow, or can be the result of biochemical signals secreted by GM bacteria growing in close association with tumor cells. Changes in some IS proteins can also occur as cancers grow.

One of the earliest reports was by Faraj et al. (1981). These workers observed significantly elevated concentrations of *L-dopa, dopamine,* and *3-o-methyldopamine* in the urine of patients having diagnosed malignant melanoma. An enzyme-radioimmunoassay was used to quantify the concentrations of these substances. There was no significant rise in the concentrations in normal patients, and the elevated concentrations in melanoma patients decreased after surgery to remove the melanomas.

17.7.2 Melatonin and Cancer

Melatonin (MEL) is a hormone secreted by the pineal gland in the brain. Control of pineal secretion of MEL is from nerve stimulation that has origin in the body's biological clock (zeitgeber) located in the suprachiasmatic nucleus. The secretion rate of MEL follows a circadian rhythm, being higher at night during the period of sleep and lower in the daytime. Figure 17.5 illustrates its structural formula. MEL is a pleiotropic hormone, that is, it has multiple effects on different target organs in the body. MEL is known to influence nearly all glandular secretions of the endocrine system (Bartsch et al. 1992, Goldman 1999). It has become popular to take exogenous MEL at night to promote deep sleep, and to aid recovery from jet lag. MEL has also been found to have an antioxidant effect similar to vitamin C. That is, it destroys free radicals before they can cause cell damage and possible cancer. Exogenous MEL has also been used in high doses with interleukin-2 (IL-2) to treat cancers; in some cases, it has been found effective (NTP 1996).

Our interest here is how cancers growing in the body affect the MEL concentration in urine and plasma. Following extensive clinical studies, Bartsch et al. (1992) reported that initial growth of the cancer (breast cancers with estrogen receptors and prostate cancers) is associated with an

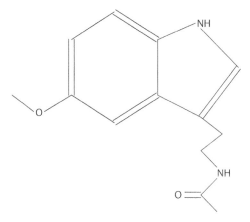

Figure 17.5   Melatonin molecule.

increased nocturnal secretion rate of MEL; as the tumor grows, nocturnal MEL secretion is markedly suppressed. Nocturnal MEL secretion rate returns to normal when the cancer metastasizes or when the patient is treated with antiestrogen therapy with tamoxifen. Although the relationship between cancer growth and nocturnal MEL secretion rate seems well established, apparently no work has been done to see how sensitive the MEL test is in detecting occult breast or prostate cancers.

17.7.3 Pteridines and Cancer: Other Chemical Tests

It is known that certain cancer cells produce an excess of a class of molecule known as pteridines. Figure 17.6 illustrates the structural formulas of three common pteridines (pteridine, pterin, and biopterin). Pteridines are a class of bicyclic heterocyclic molecules, the more important of which are folic acid, biopterin, and their derivatives. Biopterin in its tetrahydro form participates in the enzymatic conversion of the AAs phenylalanine, tyrosine, and tryptophan by various hydroxylation reactions to different members of the catecholamine family, important neurotransmitters. Tetrahydrobiopterin (THBP) is also an essential factor in the three forms of nitric oxide (NO) synthase. NO is an important cell-signaling substance.

Capillary electrophoresis was used to separate the pteridines in urine. Concentrations in various pteridine components were measured by counting photons from laser-induced fluorescence as the various electrophoretic components migrated past the laser beam. Preliminary studies have shown that there is a significant increase in certain pteridines in the urine of cancer patients. Future research may show that "signatures" based on the concentrations of the various pteridine components have a potential to detect cancers in their latency period, and possibly discriminate between different kinds of cancers (Han et al. 1999).

Yet another potential cancer screening modality may make use of the ratio between two different subgroups of immunoglobulins in blood associated with the IgG class of Abs. Research by Schauenstein and Schauenstein (1998) on the subgroups of the IgG class of Abs has shown that the ratio of concentration of the subgroups, [IgG$_1$]/[IgG$_2$], was found to decrease in patients with various cancers. Schauenstein and Schauenstein stated:

> Originally based on a biochemical assay to detect a reactive inter-heavy chain disulphide group (SS*) in the hinge region of IgG$_1$, it turned out accidentally that the majority of human sera

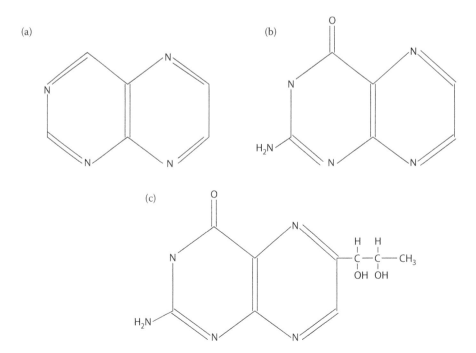

Figure 17.6 (a) Pteridine molecule, (b) pterin molecule, (c) biopterin molecule.

derived from patients suffering from cancer of various organ systems exhibited significantly decreased values of SS*, indicating a selective decrease in the percentage of IgG_1 as compared with the total IgG fraction, whereas the percentage of IgG_2, containing the only accessible free SH group of IgG, tended to increase. Later these initial findings were substantiated with larger numbers of patients afflicted with malignant diseases of selected tissues, such as the female breast, the female genital tract, and the prostate gland. These first studies revealed that benign proliferative or inflammatory diseases of the same organs did not exhibit a similar phenomenon. With breast cancer, it was shown that the decrease of SS*, that is, the percentage of IgG_1, occurs very early and becomes highly significant at tumor stages where conventional serological markers such as CEA, CA 15-3, and TPA are largely still in the normal range. Furthermore, as shown for the first time for gynecological malignancies, the drop in the percentage of IgG_1 turned out to be useful in the postoperative monitoring of tumor patients." ... "The mechanism(s) of this tumor mediated dysregulation of $[IgG_1]/[IgG_2]$ is (are) still undetermined.

These authors went on to state that clinical trials are being done to evaluate the effectiveness of this serological marker as a sensitive diagnostic tool for cancer screening. Time will reveal its effectiveness.

Transferrin is an 80 kDa glycoprotein found in the blood plasma. Transferrin has the role of transporting iron in the ferric form (Fe^{3+}) from the gut, and from its storage form bound to ferritin in liver cells to red blood cells (RBCs), where the transferrin binds with RBC membrane receptors in the process of transferring the iron into the cell where it is incorporated in Hb. At any given time, about 0.1% of the total iron in the body is bound to transferrin, 66% is in Hb, 3% is in myoglobin, 30% is stored intracellularly in ferritin, 1% is chelated, and 0.1% is in heme enzymes (cf. Transferrin 2001).

Baker (2000) reported on the *Transferrin Receptor Red Cell Assay* (also called the E-Tr test) developed by Dr. Joseph Gong at U. Buffalo. Gong's test reveals the extent of cumulative bone marrow stem cell damage from x-ray exposure, other ionizing radiation, and from certain chemicals that mimic ionizing radiation exposure (Gong and Glomski 1997, 2000). Gong said:

All cancers develop from a pool of mutated cells that are "turned on" by one or more triggers. The larger the pool of mutated cells, the greater the risk. Cancer can take years to develop, depending on the type. This test provides a way to measure the [radiation] damage before the first sign of cancer appears. It can also determine if cell mutations from ionizing radiation are increasing over time. If so, the individual can take steps to stop the increase, perhaps through a change in job, diet or environment. It gives people more control over their health.

Gong and coworkers found that the number of RBCs with transferrin receptors increases monotonically with ionizing radiation exposure. Thus, the simple bioassay for the RBC ferritin receptors in a drop of blood can give an accurate, physiological indication of a person's recent radiation exposure and cell damage. The E-Tr test is functionally better than the conventional fogged film badge or electrometer dosimeter which merely measure radiation, *per se*. Gong's test is covered by U.S. Patent #5,691,157 (Gong and Glomski 2000, 1997). Fluorescent-labeled Abs are used to bind with those RBCs with a radiation-induced increase in transferrin receptors. In their patent, Gong and Glomski show a very linear increase in RBCs with transferrin receptors versus radiation dose over a range of 0 to ~2 Gy (Gray; 1 Gy = 100 rad).

We have seen that cancers perturb the biochemical milieu around them in subtle ways, perhaps leading to the development of NI screening tests based on the changes in certain biochemical constituents in blood, urine, saliva, or sputum. Growing cancers also have altered metabolic needs, generally because they are growing faster than the tissues surrounding them. This property also makes them vulnerable for NI diagnosis. Researchers at the Mayo Clinic and at the University of Minnesota have recently developed a technique for diagnosing latency period breast cancer that uses radioisotope-labeled vitamin B_{12} (cyanocobalamin) (^{57}Co-cyanocobalamin). Vitamin B_{12} is preferentially taken up by breast cancer cells, and also by lung cancer in patients with metastases; the cancer's radioactivity is above the body's background radioactivity and is detected with a gamma camera. Vitamin B_{12} is involved in the production of genetic material in dividing cells, and also is essential for the metabolism of certain AAs and fats. It is also required for the conversion of inactive folate to active form.

The AA *homocysteine* is formed by the demethylation of the natural AA, methionine (Figure 17.7). A number of workers (Boushey et al. 1995, Perry et al. 1995, Verhoef et al. 1996, Bronstrup et al. 1998, Chao et al. 1999) have found that a high level of homocysteine in the blood is a potent risk signal for cardiovascular disease (atherosclerosis), heart attack, and stroke. It may

(a)

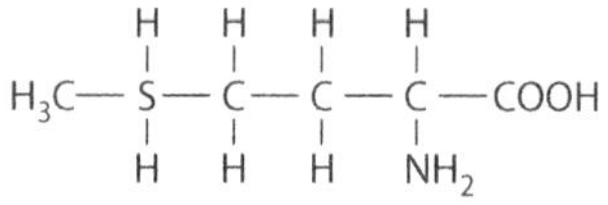

$$H_3C - S - C - C - C - COOH$$

(b)

$$HS - C - C - C - COOH$$

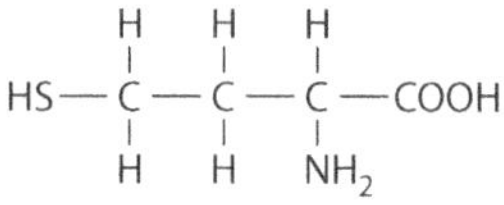

Figure 17.7 (a) Amino acid methionine. (b) Amino acid homocysteine.

also be associated with kidney disease, psoriasis, breast cancer, and acute lymphoblastic leukemia (Follest-Strobl et al. 1997, Moghadasian et al. 1997). The exact cause for elevated homocysteine concentration is not clear; it may be related to disease-caused stress, and it undoubtedly has a complex biochemical explanation. The administration of vitamins B_{12} and B_6 brings the level of homocysteine down, presumably reducing the risks. Thus, it appears that the measurement of elevated blood homocysteine concentration does not have specific, predictive diagnostic value, but is indicative of a spectrum of possible future and/or ongoing health problems.

17.7.4 GM Bacteria for NI Tumor Detection

Recently, Danino et al. (2015) published a seminal paper describing, using a mouse model, an innovative test for liver cancer using fluorescence in the urine generated by harmless GM bacteria interacting biochemically uniquely with liver cancer cells. It was discovered in the early 1900s that certain bacteria selectively colonize tumors. Danino et al. used a harmless probiotic bacterium, *E. coli* Nissle 1917 (EcN) to develop their liver cancer metastases detection system. EcN robustly colonized tumor tissue in mouse models of liver metastasis, but did not colonize healthy livers or fibrotic liver tissues.

EcN was engineered to overexpress a LacZ reporter. *LacZ* is a gene that encodes the protein enzyme, β-*galactosidase*. The GM EcN is introduced orally, and passes through the portal system to invade the liver. The mice were also given LuGal, a combined luciferin and galactose signaling molecule. When the LuGal reaches the bacteria in the tumors, the bacterial β-galactosidase enzyme breaks it down to form luciferin, which is then excreted in the urine, where it can be quantified photooptically as proportional to the liver cancer density.

Work is currently underway to adapt the GM EcN/LuGal method to early, NI, liver (and other) cancer detection in humans. The method of Danino et al. (2015) can detect liver tumors in mice larger than ~1 mm³. It showed no harmful side effects on known cancerous mice and was shown to be harmless (over 12 months) when given to noncancerous animals. "Testing as little as 1 μL of the collected urine was sufficient to elicit a positive luciferase signal, … Thus we were able to detect the presence of metastatic tumors within 24 hours of oral PROP-Z administration."

17.7.5 *In Vitro* Magnetic Levitation of Single Cells for Cancer Detection

In a recent paper, Durmus et al. (2015) described a novel, minimally invasive method for discriminating normal cells from malignant cells from the same organ. Their method makes use of magnetic levitation of single cells in a paramagnetic medium: The cell being studied is suspended in a fluid in a chamber having a 1 mm × 1 mm cross section, 50 mm length, and a 0.2 mm wall thickness. The fluid can be a Gadolinium-based paramagnetic solution. Two permanent magnets (50 mm long × 2 mm wide and 5 mm height), with the same poles facing each other, surround the test chamber. (Maximum magnet **B** was given as 1.45 T.) Two tilted mirrors were used to observe the cell's motion in the test chamber, one for illumination and one for observation with a microscope. When a cell reached equilibrium in the **B** field, it was found to be levitated inside the chamber at a position where the magnetic force ($\mathbf{F_{mag}}$) equals the buoyancy force ($\mathbf{F_b}$), that is, where $\mathbf{F_{mag}} = \mathbf{F_b}$. A cell is equilibrated at a unique levitation height (z) dependent on its density, independent of its volume. The equilibrium height of a cell along the channel height can be modeled by Equation 17.1, which equates magnetic with gravitational force. Durmus et al. gave the equilibrium force equation:

$$(\Delta \chi / \mu_o) \left\{ B_x \frac{\partial B_z}{\partial x} + B_y \frac{\partial B_z}{\partial y} + B_z \frac{\partial B_z}{\partial z} \right\} - \Delta \rho g = 0, \tag{17.1}$$

where $\Delta\chi = \chi_c - \chi_m$, χ_c is the magnetic susceptibility of the cell, χ_m is the susceptibility of the surrounding medium, μ_o is the permeability of free space, g is the acceleration of gravity, $\Delta\rho$ is the volumetric density difference between cell and paramagnetic medium (i.e., $\rho_c - \rho_m$), and x, y, and z are the coordinates of a cell in the channel.

At force equilibrium, cells with the same density as the paramagnetic medium are at the middle of the channel (z = 0), and cells with densities different from that of the medium are at equilibrium above (if $\rho_c < \rho_m$), or below (if $\rho_c > \rho_m$) midchannel. Fine "tuning" of the equilibrium height of cells was effected by changing ρ_m.

A highly concentrated medium allows for the differentiation of cells of similar densities, while a less concentrated medium can be used to examine a heterogeneous population of cells. An alternative tuning method could be by varying **B** by use of a DC electromagnet.

Durmus et al. "… identified unique differences in levitation and density blueprints between breast, esophageal, colorectal, and non-small cell lung cancer cell lines, as well as heterogeneity within these seemingly homogenous cell populations." They also demonstrated "… that changes in cellular density and levitation profiles can be monitored in real time at single-cell resolution, …."

To be an effective NI or minimally invasive cancer detection method, cells to be tested using the MagDense platform of Durmus et al. must be easily obtained; both malignant cells and neighboring normal cells are needed for comparison. Unfortunately, acquisition of mixed normal and tumor cells in most cases appears to involve some sort of invasive biopsy.

17.7.6 Use of Circularly Polarized Light for NI Cancer Detection

Over the past 4 years, a new endoscopic modality for cancer detection in surface mucosa is being developed that uses reflected polarized light (Novikova et al. 2012, Kunnen et al. 2014, Cherry 2016). In the method described by Cherry (2016), synthetic biomarker particles are coated with a gold nanolayer that is responsive to circularly polarized light (CPL). The coated biomarkers are added to a small blood sample from the patient where they bind to the target molecules, if present. This *increases* the reflectivity of CPL in the labeled sample, indicating the presence of molecules associated with cancer cells.

A good, nontechnical description of the use of polarimetric imaging of suspected cancers in *ex vivo* colon mucosa samples (biopsies) may be found in the paper by Novikova et al. (2012). These researchers used a CCD camera with 256×256 pixels to create 4×4 Mueller matrices of the target tissue using four wavelengths from 500 to 700 nm, and four different polarization settings. They stated: "Our research demonstrated that cancerous areas that are both budding (earlier stage) and ulcerated (less thick and more advanced) depolarize less than healthy tissues at short wavelengths. However, the level of depolarization is not homogeneous within the ulcerated region." They went on to report that in the cancerous layer, there was an increase in cellular density and vascularization with respect to the healthy zone, as well as the formation of stroma and the destruction of the natural order of the tissue. They noted that: "At all wavelengths, the budding zone is always less depolarizing compared to all other parts." They concluded: "We found that Mueller matrix polarimetric images of *ex vivo* human colon specimens with a specific form of colon cancer (Liberkühn adenocarcinoma) revealed enhanced contrast between healthy and cancerous sections." Their work paved the way for possible *in vivo*, NI biomedical diagnostic applications of the Mueller matrix imaging technique, with particular applications for:

- The early detection of cancer

- Improving the performance of biopsies

- Cancer staging before surgery

- Detecting residual tumors after radio-chemotherapy (sic) treatment

- Detecting and monitoring tumor recurrence

The 2014 paper by Kunnen et al. is on the same topic of optical tumor detection using CPL, but is more technical, using Mueller matrices, Stokes vectors and Poincaré spheres, as well as illustrating optical pathways. They concluded: "This provides a good foundation for further work implementing the noninvasive circularly/elliptically polarized light based diagnostic approach for early disease detection, as many forms of cancerous growths alter [optical] properties such as anisotropy and density of scattering sites."

Note that it is relatively easy to generate (and sense and detect) a source of CPL. When LPL, such as from a laser, passes through a quarter-wave plate (QWP) at a 45° angle to the plate's fast and slow axes, it can be shown that the emergent ray is circularly polarized (otherwise elliptically polarized). Conversely, passing CPL through a QWP yields LPL, providing an easy means of detecting CPL intensity using another linear polarizer (see the figure at CPLFig 2015).

While the use of reflected CPL to detect cancers noninvasively is still in its developmental stages, results so far indicate that it will have great utility in applications such as colonoscopy.

17.8 MINIMALLY INVASIVE SENSORS USING DROPS OF BLOOD

17.8.1 Introduction

There is a growing trend, nurtured by new analytical technologies, to obtain diagnostic information by analyzing a single drop or two of the patient's blood, obtained semi-invasively (by finger prick). An example of a U.S. company that has specialized in a broad-range low-blood volume diagnoses is *Theranos,* a Palo Alto, CA-based medical laboratory service company founded in 2003 by Elizabeth Holmes. Theranos (2015) offers many tests (a total of 213) using a single blood drop; one example is the *Comprehensive Medical Panel* which includes tests for albumin, alkaline phosphatase, alanine aminotransferase, aspartate aminotransferase, total bilirubin, blood urea nitrogen (BUN), creatinine, and the blood concentrations of [Ca^{++}], [Cl^-], [K^+], [Na^+], [CO_2], [Glucose], and total protein. Theranos offers other comprehensive test panels, for example, the STI Comprehensive Panel, which includes tests for Chlamydia DNA, Gonorrhea DNA, HBsAg, a HCV Antibody Screen, a Herpes Simplex Screen, a HIV 1:2 Antibody Screen with reflex to HIV-1/HIV-2 Antibody Differentiation, and a Syphilis Screen (TP Antibody).

Beginning in 2013, Theranos began to offer testing services directly to consumers in Theranos Wellness Centers located in Walgreen stores; as of January 2015, one was located in Palo Alto, CA, and there are 40 locations listed in various Arizona cities (Theranos 2015).

Traditional, mid-twentieth-century laboratory chemical and toxicology tests, with the exception of blood glucose concentration, have required withdrawn venous blood samples on the order of 10–20 mL (Sunshine and Jatlow 1982). Blood chemical components are generally given in concentrations (e.g., serum potassium of 3.5–5.0 mEq/L, BUN 10–20 mg/100 mL) (Collins 1968).

With modern DNA sequencing machines, only a drop is needed to obtain enough nuclear material to characterize pathogen DNA if the pathogens in the blood or their nuclear material are present in sufficiently high densities. If not, one strategy is to repeat the test several times to beat the odds, or take a larger, IV sample, concentrate it, and run the DNA test. Physiologically important ions in the blood can be measured by micro-ion-selective electrodes without harming the sample. Note that the volume of a drop is variable, depending on the fluid parameters of the liquid (viscosity, density, dissolved solids, surface tension, etc.). A "drop" is now defined by pharmacists as exactly 0.05 mL = 50 µL or 20 drops/mL; a drop is abbreviated gtt, plural: gtts (from Latin: *gutta*).

17.8.2 Malaria Parasite Detection Using Magnetic Resonance Relaxometry of Hemozoin in Blood

Malaria is a deadly disease caused by *Plasmodium* spp. parasites that are transmitted by the bites of infected *Anopheles* spp. mosquitoes. It is endemic to the tropics worldwide. In 2013, according to the WHO (2014a), there were worldwide ~198 million cases of malaria, and ~584,000 deaths, about 90% of which were young children. This is an approximate mortality of 29.5%, comparable to Ebola. It is important in malaria, as with most diseases, to effect early diagnosis before the *Plasmodium* parasites multiply, causing the debilitating symptoms that lead to death. Also according to the WHO (2014b), if the annual rate of decrease over the past 13 years (2015–2002) is maintained, malaria mortality rates are projected to decrease by 55% globally and by 62% in the WHO Africa Region. Malaria mortality rates in children aged under 5 years are projected to decrease 61% globally, and by 67% in the WHO Africa Region.

Conventional diagnosis of malaria involves a number of modalities: Clinical analysis relies on a history of fevers measured by signs such as rectal temperature, nailbed pallor, splenomegaly, malarial retinopathy, etc. Conventional tests on a putative patient's blood include light microscopic examination of thick blood films for free parasites and infected erythrocytes. Over 20 malaria Ag tests on blood samples can be used to detect *Plasmodium* spp. For example, *Plasmodium falciparum* expresses a unique lactate dehydrogenase enzyme (pLDH) that can be detected. Also, the *Plasmodium* glutamate dehydrogenase (pGluDH) enzyme is a signature product of the parasites. However, in this section, we will describe a new, minimally

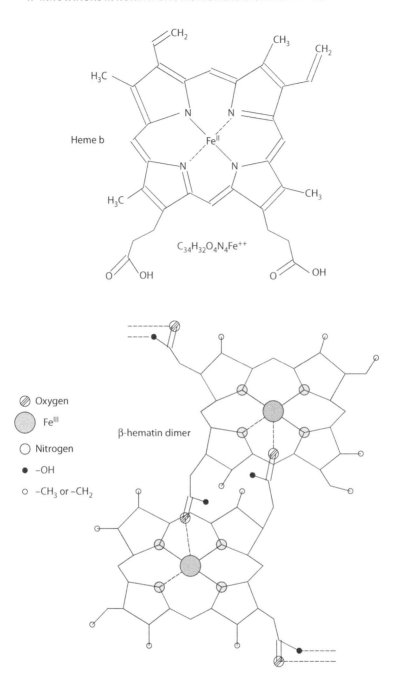

Figure 17.8 *Top*: The heme-b molecule. *Bottom*: The β-hematin dimer molecule.

invasive blood test for malaria that makes use of a nontoxic metabolic by-product made by plasmodium parasites as they metabolize the Hb in the erythrocytes that they invade. This by-product is called *hemozoin* or a polymer of β-*hematin crystals* (Figure 17.8 illustrates Heme-b and the β-hematin dimer). Hemozoin is seen in electron micrographs as insoluble crystals in the cytoplasm of the *Plasmodium* spp. that are feeding on RBCs. The parasites evidently cannot metabolize the heme-b molecules of Hb, and therefore convert it biochemically to hemozoin, a hydrogen bond-linked polymer of β-hematin molecules in which the Fe^{++} iron of Hb has been oxidized to Fe^{+++} by the parasite. Hemozoin is formed by hydrogen bonds formed between hematin units and coordinate bonds between iron atoms and carboxylate groups.

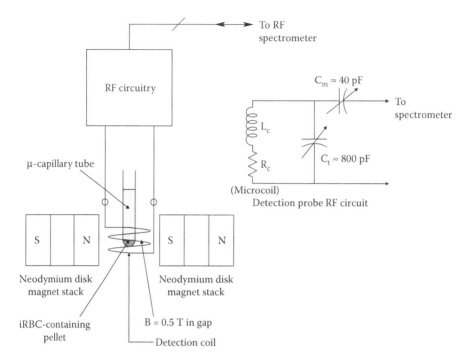

Figure 17.9 Schematic of system of Peng et al. (2014) used to quantify the concentration of hemozoin in microliter samples of blood.

For a comprehensive review about the biochemistry and physiology of heme, hematin, and hemozoin, see the paper by Sullivan (2005).

The fact that Fe^{+++} is highly paramagnetic means that hemozoin crystals in the *Plasmodia* that are feeding on RBCs can be sensed using sensitive micromagnetic resonance relaxometry (MRR) on microliter samples of blood and RBCs containing *Plasmodia*. A very ingenious electronic system that can detect minute masses of hemozoin in microliter blood samples from malaria victims has been developed by Peng et al. (2012, 2014). A schematic of their system is shown in Figure 17.9.

The MRR hemozoin detection process of Peng et al. begins with the withdrawal of <1 mL of the patient's blood. About 10 μL of blood is placed in each of several microcapillary centrifuge tubes and the tubes are spun at 3000 *g* for 3 min. A pellet of consolidated RBCs with a hematocrit near 100% forms at the bottom of the microcapillary centrifuge tube. The pellet has an effective volume of ~1 μL.

The capillary tube tip with the spun-down RBCs is placed in a ~0.5 Tessla permanent magnet's B field (Peng et al. 2014), also inside an RF excitation coil and a tuned RF pickup coil. In the paramagnetic hemazoin in the DC magnetic field, protons spin with a resonance frequency of 21.65 MHz (proton transverse relaxation). A periodic train of 21.65 MHz AC excitation pulses is applied to the sample. Each applied RF excitation pulse elicits a short 21.65 MHz proton spin "echo" RF burst. Following the initial spin echo, each succeeding transverse echo pulse has a successively smaller peak amplitude, given a constant excitation rate and amplitude. The amplitudes of the echo series follow an approximately exponential decay envelope. It is this rate of decay of peak RF responses that is sensitive to the amount of paramagnetic hemozoin present in the RBCs (hence *Plasmodia*) in the capillary tip. Uninfected RBCs have a long decay time (like a time constant), while the presence of Fe^{+++} in hemozoin causes a faster decay rate of the pulse echo envelope, and thus serves as a quantitative measure of the density of hemozoin, hence the number of *Plasmodia* present.

Peng et al. (2014) claimed their MMR system has a threshold detection level of fewer than 10 infected *Plasmodia* per microliter in a volume below 10 mL of whole blood. Ideally, this system might be made truly NI if it could be adapted to sense *Plasmodium* hemozoin Fe^{+++} in capillary blood vessels in thin membranes or tissues, such as finger webs, ear lobes, or lips. Early detection of malaria by MMR promises to be less expensive than the Ag tests for *Plasmodium* spp. and also microscopic tests of blood using stains. The prototype MMR systems of Peng et al. (2014) and Vo et al. (2014) are fast, and require no stains, reagents, or Abs. However, the treatment for infected patients depends on the species of infecting *Plasmodia*, and this information requires Ab or DNA tests.

17.8.3 Colorimetric and Redox Blood Glucose Sensors

Although systems for noninvasively measuring blood glucose concentration [BG] using IR light spectrometry on whole blood, or the amount of polarization rotation by glucose in a clear medium (e.g., urine, aqueous humor, plasma) have been developed and tested, the state of the art (in 2015) is still linked to the physical use of a sample drop of blood or plasma.

Early (ca. 1980) methods of estimating glucose concentration in blood, serum, or urine used test strips that changed color proportionally to the concentration of glucose, [G]. Test strips were impregnated with a several chemicals, including glucose oxidase which catalyzed the oxidation of glucose in a blood drop to gluconolactone, or the enzyme, glucose dehydrogenase. In addition to the oxidizer enzyme, the strips contained a benzidine dye derivative which is oxidized to a blue polymer by the hydrogen peroxide (H_2O_2) formed in the oxidation reaction. The test strip had to be "developed" for a precise interval to ensure the reaction had completed before washing off the blood drop and then reading the intensity of the blue spot in a colorimeter. The intensity was proportional to [BG].

Most modern glucometers used today for self-testing still use a drop of blood or serum obtained through the skin, and operate electrochemically, making use of the electrical energy associated with electrons shifted in redox reactions involving glucose. Using a reproducible amount of blood, the blood glucose reacts with an enzyme electrode containing *glucose oxidase* (or *–dehydrogenase*). The enzyme is reoxidized with an excess of a mediator reagent, for example, ferricyanide ion ($Fe^{+++}[CN]_6^{\equiv}$), or *ferrocene monocarboxylic acid* ($Fecp_2R$). The mediator, in turn, is reoxidized by a reaction at the anode electrode (cf. Glossary (*Redox reactions*) for the half-cell reactions).

The Abbott FreeStyle© Home Glucometer uses test strips that contain a printed circuit electrochemical cell that responds to the [bG] in a single, 0.3 μL blood drop sample obtained by skin prick. The test strips contains a microcapillary channel around the electrodes. A larger, working electrode is coated with glucose oxidase and the ($Fecp_2R$) mediator is used to reoxidize the reduced glucose oxidase. The mediator, in turn, must itself be reoxidized. In operation, a 160 mV voltage from the meter is applied between the reference and working electrodes, and the current in μA is measured 5–15 s after applying the blood drop to the test strip. The current is linearly proportional to the [BG] in mM/L or mg/dL. (To convert from mM/L to mg/dL, multiply by 18.) For example, in a typical FreeStyle test strip, about 9 μA flows through the biased cell when the [BG] = 10 mM or 180 mg/dL, and ∼4 μA is read when the [BG] = 100 mg/dL. The reading range of the FreeStyle meter is 20–500 mg/dL (plasma equivalent glucose concentration).

17.8.4 Blood Clotting Time (INR) Measurement

The coagulation or clotting of blood is a complex biochemical process whereby blood changes from a liquid to a gel. Coagulation is normally a process that causes the cessation of blood loss from an externally damaged blood vessel through the formation of a clot. Clotting can also occur internally as the result of severe bruising of blood vessels. Medical conditions such as atrial fibrillation (AFib) can lead to the formation of microclots in the atrium of the heart as the result of static blood flow condition. Deep vein thromboses (DVTs) are large clots that form in leg veins as the result of static venous blood flow conditions resulting from leg vein compression (e.g., due to prolonged sitting in a bad posture) and/or defects in the venous valves that prevent them from blocking retrograde flow. There are many risk factors for the formation of DVTs and atrial clots.

A patient at risk for blood clots is generally treated with the drug, *warfarin* (also known as *Coumadin, Jantoven, Marevan,* and *Uniwarfin*). Warfarin and related *4-hydroxycoumarin*-containing compounds decrease blood coagulation by inhibiting the enzyme, *vitamin K epoxide reductase,* which leads to the reduction of vitamin K, necessary for the clotting process. (Vitamin K is found naturally in certain foods in two forms: K_1 = *phylloquinone* and K_2 = *menaquinone*.) Vitamin K_2 is the main storage form in animals; it has several subtypes which depend on the isoprenoid "tail" chain length. Vitamin K_1 is found mainly in green leafy vegetables, brassicas, grapes, etc. K_2 is found in liver pâté, cheeses, chicken livers, egg yolks, etc. Because of unintentional, random dietary inputs of vitamin K, a person subject to embolism formation who is being treated with chronic warfarin may find his/her propensity to form clots variable in time. Because of this variability, patients being treated with warfarin are generally required to periodically monitor their clotting time as described by the *international normalized ratio* (INR), using a minimally invasive electronic instrument that uses a drop of blood on a proprietary test strip.

INR is defined as

$$\text{INR} \equiv \left\{ \frac{\text{PT}_{\text{test}}}{\text{PT}_{\text{normal}}} \right\}^{\text{ISI}},$$ (17.2)

where the ISI exponent is the International Sensitivity Index, usually between 1 and 2. PT_{test} is the measured prothrombin (clotting) time, $\text{PT}_{\text{normal}}$ is the mean prothrombin time for normal persons *not* under warfarin medication. Prothrombin time is the time it takes plasma to clot after addition of *tissue factor* (cf. Glossary).

The mean INR of 18 normal subjects measured professionally on capillary blood was 1.10 with an SD of 0.09 (8.18% CV). The mean INR of 155 subjects under well-regulated warfarin therapy was 2.85 (SD = 0.17, %CV = 5.84). The mean INR of 46 patients using a capillary (blood drop) self-tester was 2.78 (SD = 0.18, %CV = 6.32) (appn 2014).

Several manufacturers have developed small, portable, instruments for home INR monitoring. These include but are not limited to the Roche Coaguchek XS©, the iLine microsystems© Micro INR device, and the Alere INRatio©2 PT/INR Monitoring System. These instruments use a single drop of capillary blood to make their INR measurements, and are classified as minimally invasive.

As an example, we will summarize the function of the Alere INRatio2 PT/INR Monitoring System. The instrument is powered with 4 AA alkaline batteries (7.5 V DC), has an internal memory to store data, and also a data output port to connect with a PC. Its measurement range is 0.7–7.5 INR units and it requires a 15 μL drop of capillary blood, generally from a fingertip, deposited on its test strip. An Alere test strip has three pairs of electrodes that plug into the meter. A test strip at room temperature must be used within 15 s of unwrapping. The blood drop flows into three microchannels in the test strip by capillary action. A test takes ~60 s before the monitor presents INR data to the user (FDA 2014). A microchannel in the test strip contains a clotting factor. The blood in this channel clots in about 1 min. As the clot forms, its electrical resistance, measured between two electrodes, increases. When the resistance reaches a steady-state value, its value is used by the meter to calculate the patient's INR.

17.8.5 Scanning Confocal Microscopy

Scanning confocal microscopy (SCM), in particular, scanning fluorescent confocal microscopy (SFCM), was devised by Marvin Minsky at Harvard University (Minsky 1988). A confocal microscope can create sharper images than an ordinary light microscope; that is, it can provide higher-image contrast and higher resolution (higher-spatial frequency response), all things being equal (object, magnification, etc.) (Shotton 1989, Webb 1996, Semwogerere and Weeks 2005, Rappaz et al. 2008). An SCM allows higher resolution of cellular components in blood drop samples. An SCM achieves its high resolution by using a short wavelength, monochromatic light source (e.g., a laser), and excluding most of the light from the specimen that is not from the object (voxel) in the microscope's focal plane. Consequently, the image has less haze and better contrast than that of a conventional light microscope. Using an SCM, it is possible to build a 3-D reconstruction of a thick specimen by assembling a series of high-resolution slices taken in a defined focal plane along the specimen's vertical (**z**) axis. An image-processing computer is required to control the **x–y** scan, assemble the data from the photomultiplier, perform additional numerical spatial filtering, and then display the high-resolution image in pseudocolor on a monitor. A simplified schematic of an SFCM is shown in Figure 17.10. Figure 17.11 illustrates a dual-mirror scanning mechanism for an SFCM.

Applications of the SFCM in medical diagnosis include examination of blood drops for anomalies. Blood contains erythrocytes (RBCs), leukocyctes (WBCs), platelets, and can have things that shouldn't be there, such as free bacteria and blood-borne parasites. Protozoans of particular interest include *Plasmodium* (~200 species) (*P. falciparum, P. vivax, P. knowlesi,* and *P. malariae* cause malaria in humans). The spirochete bacterium, *Borrelia burgdorferi,* causes Lyme disease, and the spirochete bacterium, *Treponema pallidum* (an obligate intracellular parasite), causes syphilis. (There are ~31 *Treponema* spp.) Also parasites such as *Schistosoma* (26) spp. (*S. mansoni, S. intercalatum, S. haematobium, S. japonicum,* and *S. mekongi*) can infect humans and cause schistosomiasis.

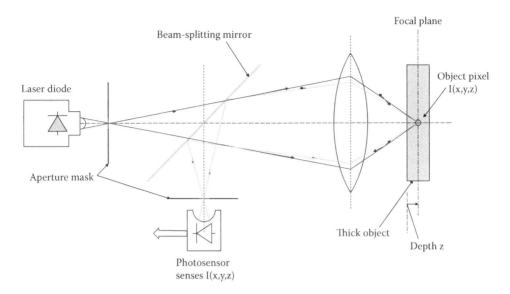

Figure 17.10   Schematic of the optics of a scanning fluorescent confocal microscope (SFCM).

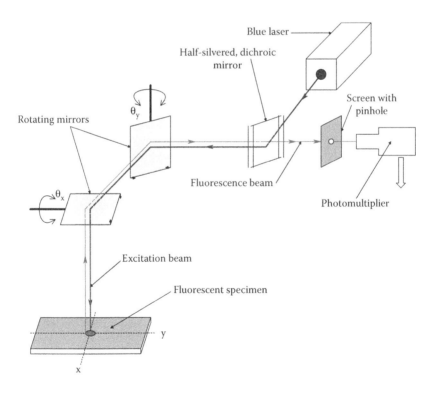

Figure 17.11   Schematic of a dual-mirror scanning mechanism for an SFCM.

The parasitic nematode, *Trichinella* (8) spp. *(T. spiralis, T. nativa,* and *T. britovi*), can infect humans and cause trichinosis. The parasite *Trypanosoma brucei* and *T. brucei gambiense* are responsible for East and West African Sleeping Sickness, respectively. The disease known as babesiosis is caused by a protozoan blood parasite, *Babesia* (14) spp. *B. microti, B. duncani,* and *B. divergens* infect human erythrocytes. The physical symptoms of babesiosis are often confused with Malaria. Babesiosis is spread by tick bites.

SCFM can allow visualization and identification of these blood-borne pathogens with high resolution, and also provide more positive identification using fluorescent molecular tags to determine the species and varieties of these organisms. DNA gives the last word, however.

17.8.6 Liquid Biopsies and the Detection of Cancer

Tumor cells shed fragments of their signature DNA and proteins into the bloodstream that potentially can be used to noninvasively screen for early-stage cancers and monitor progress in treatment (Karachaliou et al. 2015).

The blood for liquid biopsies is obtained minimally invasively by hypodermic withdrawal from a blood vessel, or by taking a few drops from a finger prick. Circulating blood contains tiny amounts of free-floating DNA (oligos), called circulating free DNA (cfDNA). The major source of this cfDNA is from the nuclei and mitochondria of cells that die (generally from natural or therapeutically induced cell apoptosis). These destroyed cells can include epithelial cells whose lifetime has expired, cells that have been infected by microorganisms, and, most importantly, cancer cells attacked by the IS or anticancer treatments (e.g., radiation, drugs). Since cancer is a genetic disease, rapid detection and characterization of cfDNA by modern sequencing methods can be used to noninvasively detect and type dying cancer cells that shed circulating tumor DNA (ctDNA). This characterization can lead to the identification of therapeutic targets and drug-resistance-conferring gene mutations on ctDNA from tumors as well as circulating (metastatic) tumor cells (CTCs). This blood sampling and DNA characterization process has been called a "liquid biopsy" (Heitzer et al. 2015, Heitzer et al. 2013, Alix-Panabières and Pantel 2013a,b,c, Diaz and Bardelli 2014). On the other hand, Gorski 2015 argued that "… it's way, way too early to consider using them, [that is, liquid biopsies] as screening tests for cancer in asymptomatic patients. … The potential of genomic tests is huge, but such tests need to be validated by science before being offered to patients on a large scale."

It is important to note that the human IS is good at "cleanup chores"; the cfDNA tends to be phaged up and recycled as nucleotides. Because of this cleanup activity, each cfDNA oligo can have an *in vivo* half-life of ~2 hours (Diaz and Bardelli 2014). However, Pinzani et al. (2010) reported the half-life of fetal cfDNA to be 16.3 min, so the actual half-life of cfDNA probably lies in the range of 16–120 min, depending on the physiological states of the patient's IS, liver, bone marrow, kidneys, etc. The fact that the concentration of ctDNA from patients with metastatic breast cancer varies substantially indicates one difficulty in using ctDNA as a diagnostic tool (Heidary et al. 2014).

Alix-Panabières and Pantel (2013a) commented: "Early during the formation and growth of a primary tumor (e.g., breast, colon, or prostate cancer), cells are shed from the primary tumor and then circulate through the bloodstream. These circulating tumor cells (CTCs) can be enriched and detected via different technologies that take advantage of their physical and biological properties. CTC analyses are considered a real-time "liquid biopsy" for patients with cancer." The paper by Alix-Panabières and Pantel (2013a) describes technologies for CTC enrichment, CTC detection, and characterization. Alix-Panabières and Pantel (2013c) have pointed out that characterization of tumor genomes from free tumor DNA oligos in the blood offers a technical challenge because the presence of "normal" DNA in the blood creates a signal-to-noise problem. They underscored the fact that isolation and genomic characterization of isolated, identified CTCs gives a more rapid and certain analysis than using ctDNA. Using whole CTCs also permits characterization of the cell coat proteins, necessary for anticancer drug development.

Liquid biopsy, coupled with the new nanopore analytic technologies for DNA sequencing, is developing into one of the more promising tools in diagnostic oncology.

17.9 BLOOD ALCOHOL CONCENTRATION ESTIMATION BY BREATHALYZER

There are several means of noninvasively estimating a person's blood alcohol concentration (BAC) without direct access to the subject's blood. An NI instrument in common use is the breathalyzer, which can use several technologies to quantify ethanol vapor in the breath (BrAC). When a person drinks an alcoholic beverage, some alcohol (EtOH), not metabolized by the liver, appears in the blood. Blood passing through the lungs releases CO_2, water vapor, and ethanol vapor into the exhaled breath. It is this exhaled alcohol vapor that is sensed by a breathalyzer. The concentration of ethanol vapor in the breath is proportional to the ethanol concentration in the blood, assuming steady-state conditions. This means that a breathalyzer of any type must be calibrated with ethanol vapor of known concentration, and the ratio of breath alcohol to BAC must be known for "typical" subjects (given sex, age, body weight). Taylor (2015) reported that one study reported that breathalyzer estimates vary at least 15% from actual blood alcohol (BAc) levels. Also, at least 23% of all individuals tested will have breath results in excess of true BAc levels. The bottom line is that breathalyzers provide a noisy estimate of true BAc levels, and in important situations, direct BAc measurement should be made using withdrawn blood samples.

The current (no pun intended) technology for measuring ethanol vapor concentration in breath makes use of a redox fuel cell into whose liquid electrolyte, breath with alcohol vapor is bubbled: The reactions are carried out at a constant DC redox cell potential and the direct current is measured. Note four electrons are released for each EtOH molecule oxidized:

At the anode, ethanol is oxidized to acetic acid:

$$\underset{\text{Ethanol vapor}}{CH_3CH_2\overset{\downarrow}{OH}(g)} + H_2O \overset{\text{Oxidation}}{\rightarrow} \underset{\text{Acetic acid}}{CH_3COOH(l)} + 4H^+(aq) + \overset{\uparrow}{4e^-}. \tag{17.3}$$

At the cathode, atmospheric oxygen is reduced:

$$O_2(g) + 4H^+(aq) + \overset{\downarrow}{4e^-} \rightarrow 2H_2O(l). \tag{17.4}$$

The overall reaction is the oxidation of ethanol to acetic acid (HAc) and water:

$$CH_3CH_2OH(l) + O_2(g) \rightarrow CH_3COOH(l) + H_2O(l). \tag{17.5}$$

The current (electron flow) in this redox reaction is measured; it is proportional to the concentration of the limiting reagent, ethanol. The redox reaction should be carried out at a constant temperature.

A colorimetric technology was used in earlier breathalyzers. An acid solution of potassium dichromate, $K_2(Cr_2O_7^=)$, was used:

$$\underset{\text{(orange)}}{\overset{\text{dichromate}}{2Cr_2O_7^=}} + \overset{\text{EtOH}}{3C_2H_5OH} + \overset{\text{acid}}{16H^+} \rightarrow \underset{\text{(blue-green)}}{\overset{\text{chromium}}{4Cr^{+++}}} + \overset{\text{HAc}}{3CH_3COOH} + 11H_2O. \tag{17.6}$$

The degree of the color change can be quantified electronically using differential absorption of two light wavelengths from LEDs (similar to a blood oximeter), or by visual comparison with colored test strips.

Another possible means of quantifying the concentration of ethanol vapor on the breath is to use a spectrophotometer. The dominant gases in exhaled breath are CO_2, water vapor, dioxygen (O_2), and ethanol vapor. Inspection of the optical absorbance (or transmission) spectra for these gases shows a clear "window" at $\nu = 2850\text{-}3000$ cm^{-1} ($\lambda = 3333\text{-}3509$ nm) for ethanol absorbance (or transmittance), without interference from the visible and NIR absorbances of O_2, water vapor, and CO_2. However, a spectrophotometer is generally a massive, benchtop instrument, unsuitable for field estimates of BAc from a suspect's breath. The hand-portable breathalyzer with an electrochemical, redox cell is the most effective means of estimating BAc at this time because of its field portability. Of course, the "gold standard" for BAc determination is blood, not ordinarily withdrawn by a law enforcement officer in a field situation. The blood sample requires a qualified medical person to withdraw it, and laboratory preparation before analysis for ethanol by a spectrophotometer, a gas chromatograph, or by electrochemical means.

Musselman et al. (2013) described the use of a Perkin-Elmer AutoSystem™ headspace-gas chromatography (HS-GC) to quantify EtOH in blood samples. Comparison was made with other volatile substances mixed with the blood sample, that is, methanol, acetaldehyde, isopropanol, acetone, N-propanol, and toluene. These authors found that the HS-GC system readout gave a clear, separate EtOH peak, and had an ethanol LOD = 0.005%, and a LOQ = 0.010%. (LOQ is limit of quantitation.)

A (NI) urine sample can also be used to estimate BAc and test for alcohol abstinence (Wojcik and Hawthorne 2007). Ethyl glucuronide (EtG) is a nonvolatile, water-soluble metabolite of ingested alcohol. It appears in the urine immediately after the consumption of alcohol. EtG can stay in the urine for up to 80 hours past the time of alcohol consumption. Thus, its presence can denote that a person has had alcohol at least 3 days ago. Detection of EtG in urine is an unreliable quantitative estimator for recent alcohol consumption and BAc. EtG is formed from exposure to small amounts of alcohol found in common hygiene products (e.g., 21.6% in Listerine™ mouthwash), cosmetic and household products, as well as some foods and medications.

Quoting from Alcoholism (2014): "The EtG test is simply not reliable by itself to determine alcohol consumption. According to the SAMHSA advisory: "Currently, the use of an EtG test in determining abstinence lacks sufficient proven specificity for use as primary or sole evidence that an individual prohibited from drinking, in a criminal justice or a regulatory compliance context, has truly been drinking."

"Legal or disciplinary action based solely on a positive EtG … is inappropriate and scientifically unsupportable at this time. These tests should currently be considered as potentially valuable clinical tools, but their use in forensic settings is premature."

17.9.1 BAC Estimation by Measuring Transdermal Alcohol Concentration Using Wearable Sensors

17.9.1.1 Introduction

Much attention has been paid recently to the development of wearable, NI, continuous measurement systems to estimate BAC by measuring secreted transdermal alcohol. When a person drinks an alcoholic beverage, ~95% of the input (CH_3CO_2OH) is enzymatically metabolized by the liver into *acetaldehyde* (CH_3CHO), thence to *acetate* (CH_3COO^-) and water. About 4% of the total intake is secreted as alcohol vapor through the lungs, and as liquid in the urine. Only about 1% is secreted through the skin as vapor and/or liquid in sweat. It is this 1% that is the focus of bioengineers developing wearable transdermal alcohol measuring (TAM) devices. Over the first decade of the twenty-first century, several NI transdermal glucose sensors have been developed (Hawthorne and Wojcik 2006, Marques and McKnight 2007, Webster and Gabler 2007, Dougherty et al. 2012). Some, such as the *Secure Continuous Remote Alcohol Monitoring* (SCRAM) devices, are large, bulky systems designed to be worn 24/7 under court order by chronic alcoholics. SCRAM devices not only monitor transdermal alcohol concentration but also contain GPS and output telemetry capability. Their attachment straps can be locked on a subject's ankle.

From data provided by Marques and McKnight showing plots of actual BAC(t), WrisTAS (a wrist-worn, transdermal alcohol sensor) output, and a SCRAM device output, it is clear from a system's engineering perspective that when we treat the alcohol input to the subject as a bolus (impulse input), the BAC(t), the WrisTAS(t), and the SCRAM(t) represent the outputs of low-pass-type transfer functions with increasingly large time constants. The BAC(t) waveform reached its peak in ~10 min. The WrisTAS(t) peaked in ~45 min, and the SCRAM(t) output peaked after ~40 min. Both WrisTAS(t) and SCRAM(t) decayed toward zero concentration much more slowly than BAC(t). Both WrisTAS(t) and SCRAM(t) readings go to negligible readings about 3 hours *after* the BAC(t) does following a bolus input.

To find the transfer function relating BAC(t) to the observed WrisTAS(t), one can *deconvolve* the linear relation between BAC(t) and WrisTAC(t). WrisTAC(t) is given by the convolution:

$$\text{WrisTAC(t)} = \int_0^t \text{BAC}(\tau)H_2(t-\tau)d\tau,$$

where $H_2(t)$ is the transfer function relating BAC(t) to WrisTAC(t).

17.9.1.2 BACtrack Skyn®

The *BACtrack Skyn* is a new, compact, wrist-wearable, transdermal instrument that electrochemically measures the alcohol vapor that escapes through the skin and uses this measurement to estimate actual BAC. The device can sample TAC as frequently as once a second, and display these data for the wearer, and also transmit the data via *Bluetooth* to an *iOS* device. It permits the wearer to passively track their alcohol consumption in real time, with, of course, the compartmental transfer delays from BAC(t) noted above. The transduction mechanism used by TAC devices is generally the constant-potential, redox fuel cell. The chemical reactions supported in the cell are shown above in Equations 17.3 through 17.5. The cell current is proportional to the ethanol vapor concentration.

Not known at this time are whether the *Skyn* device must be calibrated for each individual, and to what extent the time lag in the BAC-to-TAC transfer function will complicate accurate measurements of BAC(t). Also, since the *Skyn* device is worn on the wrist, it may be subject to interference from alcohol vapors in cosmetics, or even from held drinks, not-yet imbibed. Hawthorne and

Wojcik (2006) observed: "…this suggests that TAC measurements are not a direct replacement for BAC or BrAC measurements in terms of a quantitative real time result."

The *BACtrack Skyn* device is not yet FDA approved at this writing (May 2016).

17.10 CAPSULE ENDOSCOPY

Capsule endoscopy (CE), also known as wireless CE, is arguably a truly NI diagnostic imaging system that allows real-time, color imaging of the interiors of the esophagus, the stomach, and the small and large intestines (Toennies et al. 2009, ASGE 2013). Note that the interiors of the esophagus, stomach, and the large intestine are accessible by conventional fiber optic endoscopes, but the small intestine is not. Hence, one important application of the CE is to survey the health of the components of the small intestine (duodenum, jejunum, and ileum). The clinician looks for images of lesions, polyps, impacted foreign objects, etc.

The endoscope capsule is swallowed; no anesthesia or medication is required, however a fasting period of 10–12 hours is required before its use. After passing through the alimentary canal (a typical distance of ~9 m), the endoscopy capsule is passed in the stool and generally not recovered. A typical time of passage of a capsule through the entire alimentary canal is ~8–10 hours, with ~1 hour spent in the stomach, 4 hours in the small intestine, and 5 hours in the colon. The capsule takes many, many high-resolution photographs; one thing a CE cannot do is take biopsies. Typically, the maximum frame rate of CEs is about 4 frames/s (Toennies et al. 2009). In many capsule designs, the frame rate can be set by RF telemetry to match the capsule's transit speed through the alimentary canal in order to optimize performance and save battery energy.

A schematic cross section of a CE is shown in Figure 17.12. The components include an illumination source (four or six white LEDs); a wide-angle image-focusing lens with a short focal length; a CMOS or CCD color imaging chip; control electronics to manage lighting, image frame rate, image buffer storage, image transmission by UHF radio, etc.; the capsule's batteries (must hold effective charge for the duration of the capsule's journey through the alimentary canal, ~12 hours or more); permanent magnets (to aid location of the capsule in the alimentary canal); a radio transmitter chip and antenna. Typical transmission frequency is 432 MHz. External (receiving) antennas are worn by the patient and feed into a video receiver and are stored in a video recorder. Typical capsule dimensions are LOA, 25–27 mm; diameter, 11 mm. The ends are rounded with a radius of ~5.5 mm.

Images are of excellent resolution and typically have 1:8 magnification. In video capsule endoscopy (VCE), the capsule moves passively with normal peristalsis, no gas inflation of the bowels is required, and the mucosa and villi are imaged in their collapsed state. According to Cave (2015), the U.S. FDA first approved the CE made by Given Imaging™, Yoqneam, Israel in August 2001. In October 2007, the U.S. FDA approved a second small bowel capsule (*EndoCapsule*™ by Olympus

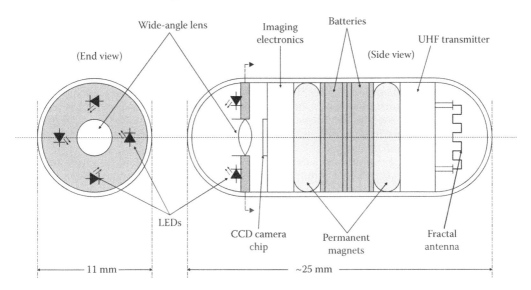

Figure 17.12 Cross-sectional schematic of a telemetering capsule endoscope.

Corp., Allentown, PA); it uses a CCD camera chip instead of a CMOS chip. Some capsules have been equipped with data receivers to enable operators to reset the capsule's frame rate, *in situ*.

If a medically significant feature is imaged by the capsule, it must be located immediately. This can be done by sensing the permanent magnetic field of the capsule's magnets with a Hall sensor array, using a directional UHF antenna to locate the capsule transmitter, or even by x-ray imaging. The magnetic approach appears to be the most accurate (Toennies et al. 2009).

Lastly, there is a possible medical risk associated with the use of radio endoscopy capsules. This has to do with possible interaction of the low-power UHF video signals broadcast by the capsule with the electronic circuitry of implanted cardiac pacemakers and defibrillators. The U.S. FDA and capsule manufacturers recommended that CE not be used on patients with cardiac assist devices. Bandorski et al. (2011) in a recent review article described these concerns and reported, in five *in vivo* studies on the effect of UHF-transmitting endoscopy capsules on implanted cardioverter defibrillators, that there was no interference. However, in one *in vitro* study, interference did occur.

17.11 USE OF DIFFUSE REFLECTANCE IMAGING TO DETECT ORAL CANCER

17.11.1 Introduction

Diffuse reflectance is a spectroscopic modality normally used for characterizing finely powdered and crystalline materials. It makes use of the fact that a fraction of a spectrometer beam focused on a translucent sample surface not only undergoes specular (mirror) reflection at the surface but also penetrates the surface and is diffracted and reflected by compressed crystalline particles of the powder sample. Some of the rays that interact optically with the subsurface layers of particles are reflected back through the surface sample as diffuse reflection; others are absorbed and dissipated in deeper layers of the sample. The luminous intensity of the diffuse reflected rays varies spatially according to Lambert's cosine law for an ideal diffuse reflector. Spectrographic analysis of the diffuse reflected rays yields a characteristic diffuse reflectance spectrum.

By scanning a 2-D surface with different input wavelengths, and analyzing the diffuse reflected light, it is possible to build up a colorized picture characterizing the material. Such a diffuse reflectance imaging system (DRIS) can be used to noninvasively analyze the living tissue for the detection of cancers (Andor 2014).

17.11.2 DRI System Design and Applications

Diffuse reflectance imaging (DRI) has been used successfully for the location of sites for guided biopsy of suspected malignant tissue (Jayanthi et al. 2012), the detection of premalignant and malignant changes in the oral mucosa (Stephen et al. 2013), also, the determination of the health of epithelial tissues using a fiber optic probe (Yu et al. 2014), characterization of breast tumor margins (Nichols et al. 2015), and detection of cervical intraepithelial lesions (Fernandes et al. 2015).

A basic DRIS consists of a collimated white light (tungsten) source focused on the tissue under analysis at an angle to the normal to the tissue surface. Directly over the source spot is a scanning zoom lens that collects the diffuse, back-scattered rays, followed by two monochromators in an imaging spectrograph which, in turn, feeds into a CCD camera, the output of which interfaces with a camera control, then an image-processing computer and display screen. The DRIS imaging process may be described as follows: {2-D Monochrome DR images of the tissue are acquired at 545 nm and 575 nm} → {Image enhancement by removal of specular reflection} → {Image registration} → {Computer generates DR intensity ratio image (545/575 nm)} → {Pseudo-color pixel mapping of DR ratio image is generated} → {Clinician identifies the site for biopsy or treatment from the colorized DR ratio image.}

In the DRIS described by Stephen et al. (2013), the DR light images of oral mucosa were analyzed at 545 and 575 nm, using white light illumination. A DR ratio image was computed for each pixel (545/575). Stephen et al. found that normal, healthy oral tissue had a median pixel ratio value of 0.87, premalignant tissue had a median pixel ratio of 1.35, and malignant lesions had a median pixel ratio value of 2.44. These workers concluded: "We find DR imaging to be very effective as a screening tool in locating the potentially malignant areas of oral lesions with relatively good diagnostic accuracy while comparing it to the gold standard [of] histopathology."

17.12 COREGISTERED PHOTOACOUSTIC AND ULTRASOUND IMAGING

With the goal of providing a higher resolution imaging modality that will enable the early detection of ovarian and other types of cancers, workers in the University of Connecticut

Department of Biomedical Engineering (Alqasemi et al. 2014, Salehi et al. 2014, Wang et al. 2014) are developing a photoacoustic tomography (PAT) system to characterize the microanatomy of ovarian tissue. Their PAT system uses focused, pulsed, NIR laser light to elicit a photoacoustic (PA) response from the scanned tissue. Transient acoustic waves are generated from thermoelastic expansion resulting from the transient temperature rise in the tissue from the absorbed photon energy of the laser pulses.

For every optically excited pixel, the PA response is sensed by one or more ultrasound transducers. The acoustic transducer array output is used to reconstruct the optical absorption distribution, which is directly related to the microvessel density of tumors and tumor angiogenesis (Alqasemi et al. 2014). According to these authors, "In the diagnostic frequency range of 3–8 MHz, the penetration depth of PAT in tissue can reach up to 4 to 5 cm using NIR light, which is comparable with the penetration depth of conventional transvaginal US." "Though the resolution of PAT is excellent compared with a pure optical imaging modality, such as DOT, it lacks signal [from] inside homogeneous structures and detects signals mainly from the surface due to US transducer bandwidth limitations. This makes the coregistration of PAT with conventional US inevitable for better mapping of light absorption to the corresponding anatomical structure."

The paper by Alqasemi et al. (2014) described in detail their US/PAT system hardware and their data acquisition structure. In summary, their system prototype probe consisted of a commercial 128-element transvaginal U.S. array having a 6 MHz central frequency and an 80% bandwidth, also thirty-six 200 μm core fibers to illuminate the object with pulsed NIR laser light. They tested their system on three objects: (1) A thin black thread to test system lateral resolution and axial sensitivity. (2) A live, tumor-bearing mouse to demonstrate the real-time imaging capability of the system. (3) A third set of tests were done on *ex vivo* normal and malignant human ovaries to demonstrate the diagnostic imaging capability of the system. The ultimate goal of the US/PAT system development is to make a reliable NI instrument to be used transvaginally for early diagnosis of ovarian cancer, and, ultimately, for general use in early cancer detection.

17.13 CHAPTER SUMMARY

The two disciplines that will contribute the most to the next generation of NI diagnostic instrumentation are photonics and molecular biology. We have seen how photonics in the embodiment of FT spectroscopy, as in the SpectraCube system, can analyze the spectral absorption of biological surfaces at the pixel level. Such analysis will make the detection of skin cancer more reliable.

The use of fluorophore-tagged molecules with affinities for various Ags, Abs, biomolecules, and nucleic acid fragments has opened up another growing group of modalities for NI, photon-based diagnosis, including FISH and SKY. DNA biochips are emerging as a potent diagnostic tool. In some designs, the readout is electric, in others, readout is by fluorescent taggants scanned by a blue laser.

We might also expect to see the development of reliable transcutaneous, spectrophotometric measurement of critical blood analytes, including glucose, certain hormones, opioids, drugs, etc. (At present, the percent oxyhemoglobin and hematocrit can be measured transcutaneously by spectrophotometric analysis.)

Microliter (drop) volumes of blood now can be used for a wide range of laboratory diagnoses of diseases and medical conditions including diabetes, malaria, kidney failure, blood glucose, etc. Contributing to this rise in microliter analytical technology is the development of instruments that use test strips with IC-printed circuit redox fuel cells, and photophore-labeled Abs and Ags.

New, more reliable instruments to estimate BAc noninvasively are being developed. CE permits NI inspection of the linings of the stomach, duodenum, cecum, jejunum, ileum, and colon; it uses RF transmitted through the body wall to give a continuous image readout. To underscore the importance of photons in NIMD, we described the use of diffuse reflection spectroscopy imaging to locate precancerous growths in epithelial tissues.

18 Introduction to Noninvasive Therapies

18.1 INTRODUCTION

In this chapter, we consider certain candidate noninvasive therapies (NITs) for medical conditions that initially may not require surgery or other invasive procedures. Other NITs described are well established and FDA approved.

The NITs we will cover are technical in nature; they *do not* involve massage, surface ointments, acupuncture, exercise regimens, braces, swallowed medicines and drugs, or diets. However, they do include photon radiation modalities (e.g., IR, x-ray, γ-radiation) and mechanical energy radiation (ultrasound [US]). Also, electric currents include transcutaneous electric nerve stimulation (TENS), interferential current therapy (ICT), transcutaneous magnetic stimulation (TMS), other electromagnetics, tumor-treating fields (TTF), and enhanced external counterpulsation (EECP). Also described are pneumatic respiratory therapies including continuous positive airway pressure (CPAP) (ventilation), and intermittent positive-pressure ventilation (IPPV).

The possible future use of US to treat Alzheimer's disease (AD) in humans is considered. Recent work on mouse models has given promising results.

Hearing aids (HAs) are described along with their role in mitigating hearing loss (HL) through advanced digital signal processing (DSP) algorithms.

Smart wound dressings that release targeted antibiotics, and vacuum wound dressings are described.

Lastly, we consider whether the modern advances in *Gene Editing* with CRISPR-Cas9 and CRISPR-Cpf1 can become NITs for certain genetic disorders.

18.2 BRAIN STIMULATION THERAPIES

18.2.1 Introduction

There are three basic NITs that can be used to treat what broadly considered are "brain problems." The first therapy, described in the following section, is called repetitive transcranial magnetic stimulation (rTMS). As the name suggests, rTMS uses an externally applied, time-varying magnetic field to induce electric currents and fields in the volume conductor that is the brain. These induced currents and fields can modulate the activity of cortical and other brain neurons.

The second NI brain therapy, transcranial DC stimulation (tDCS), involves passing a milliamp-level DC current through the brain using two or more scalp electrodes. The applied DC current and E-field in the brain also can modulate neuronal activity, affecting behavior and sensory experiences.

The third brain therapy is called electroconvulsive therapy (ECT). ECT has had a long history, going back to 43 AD, where electric torpedo fish (also known as marbled electric rays; *Torpedo marmorata*) were used on the patient's head to treat gout (presumably the pain) and headaches (Siever 2013). *T. marmorata* can produce bursts of underwater voltage pulses at 230–430 pps, (10–64 pulses), at 60–80 V in seawater. It uses this output to frighten away predators and capture prey by electrocution. I am not sure how the early Roman patients reacted. ECT was formerly known as electroshock therapy; modern ECT makes use of esthesia and muscle relaxants to prevent convulsions, a grim side effect of early twentieth-century ECT.

18.2.2 Repetitive Transcranial Magnetic Stimulation

rTMS has been shown to produce complex neuronal activity in the brain volume under the excitation coil(s). This is typically a brain region that is implicated in mood regulation, such as the prefrontal cortex. The transient magnetic pulses pass through the skull and into the brain; here they induce brief electric fields that affect the activity of neurons underlying the coil. The frequency of pulse delivery influences whether brain activity is increased or decreased by an rTMS session. Recent studies also suggest that stimulation over the left and right sides of the brain can have opposite effects on mood regulation (Hopkins Medicine 2015a).

rTMS (and transcranial magnetic stimulation [TMS]) are NI methods used to treat certain CNS dysfunctions, ranging from migraine (Misra et al. 2012), treatment-resistive major depressive disorder (McGirr et al. 2015), neuropathic pain secondary to malignancy (Khedr et al. 2015), negative symptoms of schizophrenia (Prikryl and Kucerova 2013), and loss of function caused by stroke. As of 2014, all other investigated uses of rTMS have only possible or no clinical efficacy.

In rTMS, a single plastic-encased, multiturn, solenoid coil is placed on the scalp over the brain region to be stimulated. See Figure 18.1 for an illustration of this system. Typically, several (e.g., 10)

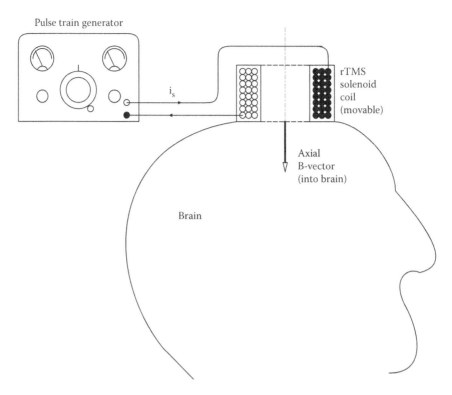

Figure 18.1 Schematic of an rTMS coil on the head.

10–20 Hz, 10–60 s trains of current pulses are used in rTMS coils in a therapy session (Khedr et al. 2015, McGirr et al. 2015, Misra et al. 2015). Therapy sessions are generally repeated. Some of the side effects of rTMS include temporary mild headaches, painful scalp sensations, facial twitching, and very rarely, seizures (Hopkins Medicine 2015a).

Basic physics (Sears 1953) tells us that the magnetic flux density at a point on the center axis of a single, N-turn, solenoid coil at the end of the coil is

$$B = \mu_o \frac{Ni}{l} \, Wb/m^2, \tag{18.1}$$

where l is the axial length of the coil, N is the number of turns, i is the instantaneous current in the coil, and μ_o is the permeability of space. B is directed axially by the RH screw rule. For a coil on the skull, the permeability is that of the brain, which is generally taken as μ_o.

Alternately, if the coil has a large radius to axial length, the magnetic field magnitude B at the center of the coil (d = 0 on the axis) can be written:

$$B = \mu_o Ni / (2r) \, W/m^2, \tag{18.2}$$

where r is the coil's radius.

B decreases with distance from the coil's center as d^{-3}. It is well known that a time-varying magnetic flux will induce an electromotive force (EMF), E, in another coil or conductive pathway lying perpendicular to the current-carrying coil's axis at some distance d from the current-carrying coil's center. This EMF is given by

$$E = -d\Phi / dt = -A \, dB/dt \, V, \tag{18.3}$$

where Φ is the total magnetic flux in Webers passing through the area of a hypothetical, closed, conductive pathway in the brain. If the pathway has a resistance R ohms around its circumference, a current i = e/R will flow in the pathway, affecting neural functioning. Note that $\Phi = BA$, where A is the area of the pathway and B is the magnetic flux density from the coil, through the pathway.

When a pair of so-called butterfly excitation coils is used for rTMS, the flux through the closed conductive pathways in the brain is the result of the vector superposition of the time-varying Bs from the two excitation coils. This superposition can be calculated using the finite element method, allowing optimum coil positioning (coil size, separation, angle, position on the head) to be investigated to permit optimum deep brain stimulation (Deng et al. 2014). The net result of the butterfly coil is a sharper peak in the induced electric field in the brain directly under the coils than is caused by a single solenoid TMS coil.

18.2.3 Transcranial DC Stimulation

We have seen in the previous section how certain brain volumes can be noninvasively stimulated by time-varying, transcranial magnetic fields that cause the creation of electric fields and circulating currents in the underlying, nonhomogeneous volume conductor formed by cortical neurons. In this section, we will describe the NI stimulation of brain tissues by DC applied through electrodes directly attached to the scalp. tDCS is used for safe neurostimulation therapy for the treatment of depression, obsessive–compulsive disorder, migraine, insomnia, and chronic pain (e.g., caused by fibromyalgia) (Mendonca et al. 2011, Mueller 2015). A typical tDCS therapy consists of five 20 min sessions over five consecutive days, Monday through Friday. Sometimes a second series of five sessions may be necessary (Mueller 2015). tDCS affects brain activity: measured with FMRI or PET, it has been found that cortical neurons under the DC (+) anode have their activity raised by ~20%–40% when the current density under the anode exceeds 40 μA/cm^2. At the (−) cathode, at the same current density, brain function is reduced by 10%–30% (Siever 2013).

Just as the induced currents and electric fields generated by rTMS have been modeled in a volume conductor using finite element techniques, the distributions of DC currents and fields in the brain resulting from tDCS scenarios have been studied by Oostendorp et al. (2008).

Brunoni et al. (2012) reviewed the neuromodulatory effects of studies using tDCS. They specifically addressed four topics: (1) mechanisms of action of tDCS; (2) methodological aspects related to clinical research of tDCS; (3) ethical and regulatory concerns; and (4) future directions regarding the novel approaches, novel devices, and future tDCS studies.

tDCS has been realized as a useful research tool to study brain–behavior relationships in healthy subjects by Pope (2015). tDCS in humans normally involves delivering a low (e.g., 1–2 mA) DC for 15–20 min through saline-soaked, inert metal electrodes attached to the scalp. A typical tDCS electrode configuration for brain stimulation might involve the anodal (+) electrode being placed on the head over the brain region of interest, and the cathodal (−) electrode being placed on the cheek or shoulder on the contralateral side of the body. In the case of cerebellar tDCS stimulation studied by Pope (2015), intracerebral current flow between the two electrodes had relatively little functional spread to nearby brain regions (e.g., the visual cortex), and is thought to excite or inhibit Purkinje neurons in the cerebellar cortex, leading to neurophysiological and behavioral changes. There is both functional and anatomical evidence for a neural connective pathway between the cerebellum and the prefrontal cortex. Pope reported that cathodal tDCS over the right cerebellar hemisphere (depressing cerebellar activity) could influence cognitive processes involving language, learning, and memory, functions involving prefrontal cortex neurons.

The bottom line concerning tDCS and rTMS is that the human brain has awesome complexity, and these brain stimulation techniques have been shown to have some useful, therapeutic effects, but not on all subjects; exactly how they work remains to be clarified. Mueller (2015) stated: "The exact mechanism of tDCS is not clear but extensive neuro- physiological research has shown that direct current (DC) electricity penetrates the skull and outer layers of the cortex to modify neuronal cross-membrane resting potentials and thereby influence the level of neuronal excitability and modulate firing rates."

18.2.4 Electroconvulsive Therapy

While tDCS uses low milliamp-level DC currents for therapeutic effects, NI ECT brain stimulation originally used line-frequency AC current, and more recently, short bursts of narrow ($\leq$1 ms) rectangular pulses with peak current values around 800 mA are being used. This high current generates a high-transient E field in the brain, producing convulsions, as well as therapeutic effects. More will be said about ECT stimulus parameters below.

ECT can provide significant, rapid improvements (sometimes temporary) for the following psychiatric disorders (Mayo Clinic 2012):

- *Severe depression*, including thoughts of suicide and/or severe *anorexia nervosa*

- *Treatment-resistant depression*, where medications are not effective

- *Severe mania*, a state of intense euphoria, agitation, or hyperactivity that occurs as part of bipolar disorder

- *Catatonia*, characterized by lack of movement, fast or strange movements, lack of speech, etc.

- *Agitation and aggression in patients with dementia*

An actual ECT treatment session takes only 5–10 min. However, time is required for preparation, including anesthetization and injection of other pharmaceuticals including a muscle relaxant, plus recovery time, bringing the entire procedure to about an hour. An ECT therapy session can often be done as an outpatient procedure. A usual course of ECT involves multiple administrations, generally given two or three times per week until symptoms are gone, or have been satisfactorily mitigated. ECT is administered under an anesthetic, and with a muscle relaxant to suppress the ECT-induced seizures.

The side effects of ECT may include the following:

- *Confusion*: This may last from a few minutes to several hours.

- *Memory loss*: This can include retrograde amnesia. Some patients have trouble recalling events that occurred during the weeks of treatment, or events after ECT has stopped.

  These memory problems usually improve within a couple of months.

- *Physical side effects* that directly follow an ECT session. These may include nausea, vomiting, headache, jaw pain, muscle aches, or spasms.

- *Medical complications*: During ECT, heart rate and blood pressure increase. This could lead to heartproblems.

An ECT stimulation (or a tDCS) session's intensity is generally specified as the electrode current, rather than a voltage. That is, the ECT or tDCS source generator must be a *current*, rather than a *voltage source*. If a low output-impedance voltage source was used, the actual current through the brain could be individually highly variable because of the variability of the impedances of the two electrodes, the underlying scalp tissue, the skull, the meninges, the cerebrospinal fluid, and, of course, the brain tissue in the subjects. Presumably, it is the voltages induced in the brain volume conductor caused by the ECT current densities interacting with the brain tissue impedances therein that are important. We traditionally think of neurons responding to voltages across their membranes at their spike generator loci (SGLs). The normal DC resting potential (EMF) across a neural membrane is about 60 mV, inside negative. Thus, any electrical stimulus (such as ECT pulses) that causes the transmembrane potential to momentarily become less negative, that is, go in a positive direction, can bring an *SGL* closer to its transmembrane voltage firing threshold where it can generate an action potential, sending one or more nerve impulses down its axon to either stimulate or inhibit other target neurons. Prolonged neural depolarization can also be the result of local changes in the concentrations of extracellular cations (e.g., Na^+, K^+, Ca^{++}) and anions (e.g., Cl^-) caused by the mobility of these ions in the transient ECT-caused electric field in the brain. Note that conversely, induced hyperpolarization of a nerve's SGL membrane will inhibit a neuron's propensity to fire in response to an excitatory input stimulus. Of course, ions in the brain also migrate in the DC field set up during tDCS.

Metal ECT electrodes are relatively large, $\sim$2–5 cm in diameter, and generally use electrolyte-soaked gauze pads between them and the skin on the scalp. The electrodes must be of a redox-resistant metal, such as carbon, gold plate, a platinum alloy, stainless steel, or titanium. An ion-containing conductive paste or gel, such as the *Redux Paste* and *Gel* made by Hewlett-Packard, can also be used to coat the clean skin under the electrodes, and also directly cover the electrode surface before its application to the skin. The conductive paste forms an interface where electrons leaving the metal anode (+) electrode react with ions in the conductive paste, with a complementary scenario occurring at the metal cathode (−). These ions, principally Na^+, K^+, and Cl^-, penetrate the skin, scalp tissue, skull bone, and brain, setting up an electric current and field in the brain volume conductor. The E field in the brain is strongest just under the electrode sites.

As mentioned above, the peak ECT electrode current required depends on the individual treatment, and typically can be set to around 500–900 mA. If alternating positive and negative pulses are used, or an AC sinewave, there is no net ion migration from around the electrodes. If unipolar (positive) pulses are used, there will be some electrode polarization, and net redox reactions in the paste or saline electrode coupling fluid; some (+) cations will be lost by electrochemical reduction.

A measure of the *dose* of pulsed ECT is the net charge in coulombs delivered by the electrodes (Peterchev et al. 2010). If a short, unipolar, rectangular pulse train is used, this charge can be found from:

$$Q = \underset{Cb/s}{(peak\,current)} \times \underset{s}{(pulse\,width)} \times (number\,of\,pulses\,given) \quad Coulombs\,(Cb). \qquad (18.4)$$

For example, if the peak current is 800 mA, the pulse width is 0.5 ms, and a total of 20 pulses is given, the net charge is Q = 8 milli Coulombs (mCb). If alternating positive and negative pulses are given having the same current magnitude, there will be zero net charge supplied by the ECT generator. However, the net charge moved back and forth is simply 2Q from Equation 18.4. Another parameter useful for quantifying ECT dose is the total energy in joules supplied by the stimulus pulse train. This energy, U, can be found for a pulse train as the time integral of the power delivered during the pulse train, which is equal to the product of the net charge, the current amplitude, and the dynamic head resistance (Peterchev et al. 2010):

$$U = Q \times (peak\,current) \times (dynamic\,head\,impedance)\ Joules\,(J). \qquad (18.5)$$

Measurement of the dynamic head impedance, Z_h, can be approximated by using Ohm's law. Using an oscilloscope, one measures the peak pulse voltage at the electrodes, V_{pk}, and divides it by the peak current, I_{pk}. $Z_h = V_{pk}/I_{pk}$. In current ECT practice, the individual dose is typically adjusted by setting the total charge of the stimulus, Q. The clinician has a control over the pulse width, the pulse rate, the number of pulses, and the peak current. A critical stimulus parameter generally not considered is the DC current density in the brain, directly under the electrodes.

18.2.5 Summary

The human brain is an extremely complex system. Early estimates of the number of neurons in the adult human brain have ranged as high as 100 billion (10^{11}) with 10 times as many glial cells (Herculano-Houzel 2009); however, a recent estimate gives the total in the adult male brain a total of 86.1 ± 8.1 billion neurons, and 84.6 ± 9.8 billion "nonneuronal" cells (Azevedo et al. 2009).

Just as the Human Genome Project set out to unravel the complexity of the human (and other organisms') genetic code, the *White House BRAIN Initiative* (Brain Research through Advancing Innovative Neurotechnology) initiated by President Obama on April 2, 2013 has set out to create an in-depth, dynamic understanding of brain function (NIH 2015). Proposed initial government expenditures were a very modest $110 million from DARPA, the NIH, and the NSF. By September 2014, the BRAIN initiative total support had grown to over $300 million, with five participating federal agencies (Whitehouse 2014).

The complexity faced by the BRAIN projects is orders of magnitude greater than the Human Genome Project, and they promise to spend orders of magnitude more funds on the research which could generate as much as ~300 exabytes (3×10^{20} bytes) of data every year. Nevertheless, it is only by understanding brain function, physiology, biochemistry, and anatomy will clinicians understand how rTMS, tDCS, and ECT actually work. The brain must be taken from "black box" status to a set of understood "modules," and their interconnectivities, to make NI brain therapies more effective.

18.3 TREATMENT OF OSTEOARTHRITIS WITH US

18.3.1 Introduction

Osteoarthritis (OA) is a common, painful, degenerative disorder of the articular cartilage associated with hypertrophic bone changes. Risk factors include but are not limited to advancing age, genetics, female sex, past joint injury, obesity, and diet. Diagnosis is based on family history, a history of joint pain aggravated by movement, and x-ray imaging. OA affects major load-bearing joints, for example, the hips, shoulders, knees, spine, and finger joints. Treatments for OA include taking NSAIDs to reduce pain and inflammation (e.g., aspirin, ibuprofen, naproxen), appropriate exercise, corticosteroid injections, dietary supplements of glucosamine and chondroitin, and hyaluronic acid injections (Sinusas 2012). Note that something as simple as weight loss in overweight and obese adults with OA can reduce knee and hip joint loads, mitigating pain, and increasing mobility (Messier et al. 2005).

However, in the following section, we will examine the efficacy of noninvasive application of US to the affected joints.

18.3.2 US Treatment of OA

There have been a number of studies on the use of US therapy to manage OA. Significant in many of these studies is the omission of the details of the US treatment parameters, that is, the frequency, waveform, intensity level in W/cm^2, and treatment time. The US energy is quantified as W/cm^2. Low-intensity US uses US with intensities less than 3 W/cm^2, which can stimulate cell proliferation and tissue repair. High-intensity US uses focused US transducers that concentrate wave energy in a smaller tissue volume; they reach intensities higher than 5 W/cm^2, which causes cavitation, coagulative necrosis of tissue due to heat absorption. It is normally used as an ablative agent to destroy target tissues (Leong et al. 2013). In tissues treated with low-intensity pulsed ultrasound (LIPUS), nonthermal effects dominate. Overall (cumulative) US doses are measured in J/cm^2. Note that US energy is coupled from the transducer to the skin with a thin layer of gel that acts to match the acoustic impedance of the transducer to underlying tissue.

In their *Review Article*, Leong et al. (2013) cited the US frequencies, waveforms used, intensities, and durations of treatment used in four studies of the use of US as OA therapy. Table 18.1 summarizes some of these data.

According to Leong et al. (2013):

> Recent clinical trials suggest ultrasound improves OA-associated symptoms, including pain and joint dysfunction. … Furthermore, while disease-modifying effects of ultrasound have not been reported in OA patients, supportive data from *in vitro* and *in vivo* studies suggest a chondroprotective role of ultrasound, which includes enhancing anabolic activity, lowering levels of catabolic activity, and preventing apoptosis in chondrocytes. … In summary, therapeutic ultrasound may exert effects not only on symptom-modification but also has a strong potential for chondroprotection and disease-modification in OA.

To summarize, therapeutic ultrasound (TUS) has the following inhibiting or downregulating effects: (1) It suppresses proinflammatory cytokines such as IL-1β and TNF-α. (2) It downregulates adipokines, leptin, adiponectin, visafatin, and resistin (all which act to increase IL-1β and TNF-α). (3) TUS acts to reduce OA-associated pain, chondrocyte apoptosis, and cartilage degradation (Leong et al. 2013).

18.4 RADIATION THERAPY VERSUS CANCERS

18.4.1 Introduction

Radiation therapy (RT) is used as a supplementary NIT to control or kill malignant (cancer) cells. Chemotherapy and surgery are invasive procedures used to fight cancer, and will not be considered in this section. Unfortunately, RT can also damage normal cells in the periphery of the radiated tumor. RT uses ionizing radiation to destroy DNA and other critical biomolecules in tumor cells causing cell death. Ionizing radiations can damage vital intracellular molecules (e.g., DNA, RNA, protein enzymes, etc.) by breaking hydrogen bonds and destroying the molecular 3-D structures necessary for molecular function. Intracellular molecular signals from a radiation-damaged cancer cell can cause the cell to undergo programmed cell death, or apoptosis (Northrop and Connor 2009, Section 2.5.2).

Table 18.1: Therapeutic Ultrasound Therapy for Osteoarthritis

US Frequency	Waveform	Intensity	Dose	Subject	Reference
1 MHz, CW	NA	0.8 W/cm^2	3–4 min/session, 2 d/week; over 12 weeks	Man	Mascarin et al. (2012)
1 MHz, LIPUS	1:4 Pulsed-mode duty cycle	2 W/cm^2	5 min/session	Man	Tascioglu et al. (2010)
3 MHz, LIPUS	20% duty cycle pulses	40 mW/cm^2	20 min/session, 6 d/week for 6 weeks.	Rabbits	Li et al. (2011)
1 MHz, LIPUS	20% duty cycle pulses	300 mW/cm^2	10 min/day, for 2 weeks	Rabbits	Zeng et al. (2012)

Ionizing radiation includes high-energy photon sources including cosmic rays, gamma rays, x-rays, and short-wavelength ultraviolet light (UVC, $\lambda = 290$–100 nm, E = 4.43–12.4 eV). Also capable of causing damage to important intracellular molecules are high-energy particles from radioisotope decay and particle accelerators. These include but are not limited to: *Alpha particles* (^{4}helium nuclei), *Beta particles* (electrons), and *neutrons*. Both natural and man-made ionizing radiations can cause cancers. Natural radiations include particles from the decay of natural radioisotopes in the earth, as well as cosmic ray photons from space. Particle and photon energy is generally given in electron-volts (eV) (1 eV = 1.6033×10^{-19} J). The U.S. FCC defines ionizing radiation as that with a photon energy of greater than 10 eV (equivalent to ultraviolet C photons with $\lambda = 124$ nm). Ionization of a typical water molecule requires 33 eV. The generation of medical x-rays is described in detail in Section 16.2 of this book.

The energy range of diagnostic x-rays is 20–150 keV. Orthovoltage and Supervoltage energy x-rays span 200–1000 keV in energy. X-rays in this energy range are typically used to treat cancers at, or close to, the skin surface. There are many other sources of superhigh-energy photon beams. For example, linear electron accelerators (linacs) can be used to produce electrons and also x-rays with energies from 4 to 25 MeV. The shape and intensity of the electron beam produced by a linac can be modified or collimated by several means.

Certain electron-emitting radioisotopes such as $_{77}Ir^{192}$ (β^- at 0.240 MeV), $_{27}Co^{60}$ (β^- at 0.315, 0.663, and 1.488 MeV), and $_{55}Cs^{137}$ (β^- at 0.511 and 1.176 MeV) can also be used to make x-rays.

18.4.2 Radiation Therapy

Deep tumors in the body can be treated by beams of ionizing radiation (generally x-rays), or brachytherapy (BrT), to induce cancer cell apoptosis. In the case of beam RT, to minimize the effects of the ionizing radiation on healthy tissues, collimated radiation beams are sequentially directed from several angles to intersect at the deep, internal tumor site, maximizing the radiation dose in that volume. 3-D conformal RT is becoming the standard treatment for a number of tumor sites that can be well defined by imaging scans. This form of external beam RT is also called stereotactic radiation (SR). An advantage of stereotactic treatments is that they deliver the right amount of radiation to the tumor in a shorter amount of time than traditional treatments which can often take 6–11 weeks. Also, the SR treatments are given with high accuracy, which limits radiation damage to healthy tissues.

While the RT is itself painless, it has delayed side effects that include fatigue and skin irritation resembling a mild-to-moderate sunburn. If rectal, anal, prostate, bladder, uterus cancer, etc. is given RT, side effects include soreness, diarrhea, and nausea. Because of radiation-induced tumor cell apoptosis, there can be general inflammation and soreness in the radiated volume as the patient's immune system "tidies-up" the debris from dead cells.

BrT (also known as sealed-source radiotherapy) is a moderately invasive treatment for deep, soft tumors (e.g., cervical, prostate, breast, and skin cancers). It involves the precise, surgical placement of small, short-range, radioisotope sources ("seeds") directly at or in the site of the cancer. To chemically isolate the isotope from body fluids, it is enclosed in a protective capsule. One advantage of BrT is that it the cancer can be treated with very high doses of localized radiation; it allows the patient to be ambulatory which is not possible with external beam radiotherapy (EBRT). A course of BrT can often be completed in less time than other RT techniques. This may reduce the chance for surviving cancer cells to divide and grow in the intervals between each RT dose. Also patients typically have to make fewer visits to the oncologist compared with EBRT. Also, BrT is generally performed on an outpatient basis.

Some of the radionuclides used in BrT are listed in Table 18.2.

18.5 TTF: LF AC ELECTROMAGNETIC FIELD STIMULATION TO FIGHT GLIOBLASTOMAS

Glioblastoma is a deadly, rapidly growing form of brain cancer that is resistant to most conventional antitumor therapies (e.g., radiation, chemotherapy, surgery) (Bruce 2014). One NIT that has shown promise is the use of induced low-frequency (LF) electric fields, called TTFs, in the tumor to inhibit cancer cell mitosis and induce their apoptosis. The use of TTF was initially described by Kirson et al. (2004). Kirson et al. examined the effect on growing *Glioblastoma multiforme* (GBM) cells *in vitro*, and located intradermally in mice. Low-intensity, LF electric fields (100–300 kHz) were used, applied to mice through intradermal, 10 mm long, insulated wire electrodes. The electric field strength in tissue was calculated to be <2 V/cm in the mice, and measured to be <2 V/cm *in vitro*.

Table 18.2: Some Radionuclides used in Brachytherapy*

Radionuclide	Radiation Type	Half-life	Energy
Cesium-137	β⁻	30.17 years	0.663 MeV
Cobalt-60	β⁻	5.26 years	1.17 and 1.33 MeV
Iridium-192	γ-rays	73.8 days	0.38 MeV (mean)
Iodine-125	*Electron capture, ε	59.6 days	27.4, 31.4, and 35.5 keV
Palladium-123	*Electron capture, ε	17.0 days	21 keV (mean)
Ruthenium-106	β⁻	1.02 years	3.54 MeV
Radium-226	α	1599 years	4.78, 4.60, 4.34, 4.19, 4.16

*See Glossary.

The physiological effects of TTFs on normal and cancer cell lines have been described by Davies et al. (2013). The predominant effect of TTFs is on dividing cells (undergoing mitosis). There was no effect on quiescent cells, but in dividing tumor cells, there was interference with mitosis, with apoptosis as the formation of the cleavage furrow approached the stage of cell separation, and finally rupture of the cell membrane and membrane blebbing. Two mechanisms of action of TTFs were proposed: (1) an antimicrotubule effect (inhibiting mitotic spindle formation) and (2) a dielectrophoretic effect.

A review of the efficacy of TTF on human *Glioblastoma* patients found that TTF was as beneficial as standard chemotherapy, but had different side effects. The adverse effects of TTF were topical skin rashes caused by prolonged electrode use; standard chemotherapy causes severe nausea, hair loss, weight loss, digestive and blood problems. Regardless of treatment mode, the mean survival time was 6.3–6.4 months (Calzón and Llanos 2013). Note that the side effects of chemo are more severe than TTF. However, TTF costs about $21,000 per month. Note that Medicare and many private health insurers have declined to cover TTF treatment on the grounds that it is still investigational.

The Novocure® TTF100-A TTF System was approved by the U.S. FDA in 2011 for treating patients with recurrent GBM. The name of the Novocure system was changed to Optune® on November 14, 2014. In the Optune system, four "transducer arrays" (antennas) are placed on the scalp to target the underlying tumor with "crossed fields" (the tumor is located by MRI imaging).

18.6 TRANSCUTANEOUS ELECTRICAL NERVE STIMULATION

Transcutaneous electrical nerve stimulation (TENS) uses a pulsatile electric current to stimulate peripheral nerves for therapeutic purposes such as relief of chronic back or sciatic nerve pain (Physiopedia 2015b). A typical portable, battery-operated TENS unit has adjustable pulse frequency, pulse width, and height. Generally, TENS stimulation is applied through two or four electrodes stuck to the skin over the tissue volume(s) to be treated. Adhesive, pregelled, conductive electrodes are generally used. LF stimulation (50–100 pps) with an intensity below motor contraction (1–2 mA pk), or a very LF (1–5 pps) with a higher intensity (15–20 mA pk) that produces motor contraction, can be used.

A recently FDA-cleared, upper calf-wearable TENS device was marketed in mid-2015. Called Quell™, it costs ~$250; a month's supply of electrodes costs ~$30. The electrode pair goes on the skin under the elastic support band for the Quell device on the upper calf. A description of the Quell device and how it works can be found at Indiegogo (2016), and Quell (2015).

Mechanisms of TENS therapy include two primary, neural, pain relief mechanisms which can be excited by TENS stimulation: (1) Activity on the **Aβ** sensory (nonnociceptive) nerve fibers activates the pain gate control mechanism; that is, it reduces the transmission of a pain signal on the "C" nerve fibers, through the spinal cord, thence to the brain. **Aβ** fibers are best stimulated at a high rate (90–130 pps). (2) An alternate approach is to use an LF stimulation (2–5 pps) to stimulate the fast **Aδ** pain fibers which activate opioid pathways in the CNS. These provide pain relief by causing the release of endogenous opioids (enkephalins) in the spinal cord and CNS which reduces the activation of the noxious sensory pathways. Alternately, burst-mode TENS stimulation can be used: A train of 100 pps current pulses is periodically interrupted with a train of LF (5 pps) pulses, ensuring both **Aβ** and **Aδ** afferent fibers are stimulated (Physiopedia 2015b).

TENS therapy is not always effective for a given class of pain. This may be due to incorrect electrode placement, bad setting of pulse parameters (frequency, pulse width, and current magnitude), or individual variance in neuroanatomy. TENS has been used effectively for analgesia in certain cases of chronic neck, shoulder, joint and back pain (e.g., from compressed spinal disks), also, in the prevention of migraine headaches. A benefit of TENS analgesia is that it can permit the patient to perform therapeutic exercises to mitigate the underlying causes of the pain (i.e., strengthen particular muscle groups).

A unique head-mounted TENS device, *Cefaly®*, was approved by the U.S. FDA March 11, 2014 for the *prevention* of migraine headaches. The Cefaly device is worn on the patient's forehead. It was the first specialized TENS system having FDA approval for pain prevention, rather than pain suppression. The electric currents from the Cefaly TENS device interact with the (bilateral) **V1** (sensory) branches of the fifth cranial nerve (trigeminal) under the skin of the forehead. Out of a sample of 2313 migraine patients, 54% were satisfied with the relief it provided (Magis et al. 2013, ACHE 2014).

18.7 HEAT THERAPY

Heat therapy, also called *thermotherapy*, is a noninvasive means of mitigating internal pain arising from a number of sources. The heat is applied in the form of infrared radiation to the skin, or by direct conduction to the skin, thence underlying tissues. There are a number of external therapeutic heat sources including, but not limited to

- Disposable heat patches, pads, or belts available at most drugstores (the heat is from a chemical reaction)

- Warm bath, shower, hot tub, or pool (These are conduction sources for the whole body, or an arm or leg.)

- Microwaveable hot pack

- Hot water bottle (wrapped in a towel)

- IR incandescent lamp (essentially a blackbody emitters)

- IR high-powered LEDs

When heat comes from a direct contact source, it has to warm the external layer of skin to a temperature several degrees above the internal tissue temperature for heat to be conducted to deep tissue layers (at 37.1°C) and then warm them. The maximum safe skin surface temperature is ~42°C (107.6°F). IR radiation is more useful than visible radiation because the skin absorbs most of it. IR penetration depth (hence heating effects) depends on the wavelength range used: IR-A ($\lambda = 0.78$–1.4 μm) reaches several millimeters; IR-B (1.4–3.0 μm) penetrates into the dermis (~1 mm). IR-C (3 μm–1 mm) is mostly absorbed in the external layer of the epidermis (*stratum corneum*). The optical absorption coefficient of skin, μ_a, in cm^{-1}, and scattering coefficient, μ_s, in cm^{-1}, were given by Lee et al. (2011). μ_a values at different wavelengths were μ_a (660 nm) = 0.29 cm^{-1}, μ_a (750 nm) = 0.13 cm^{-1}, μ_a (830 nm) = 0.12 cm^{-1}, μ_a (980 nm) = 0.37 cm^{-1}, μ_a (1064 nm) = 0.8 cm^{-1}. The scattering coefficients at corresponding wavelengths were μ_s (660 nm) = 260 cm^{-1}, μ_s (750 nm) = 210 cm^{-1}, μ_s (830 nm) = 180 cm^{-1}, μ_s (980 nm) = 150 cm^{-1}, μ_s (1064 nm) = 130 cm^{-1}. Thus, it would appear that the most effective heat lamps are IR-A emitters. Lee et al. (2011) examined the wavelength dependence of energy penetration depth in tissue. They found that the greatest amount of heat generation was observed in deep tissue using $\lambda = 830$ nm. They concluded: "The [HbO$_2$] concentration was significantly increased in the laser-irradiated group and these findings suggest that LLLT using $\lambda = 830$ nm may be of benefit in accelerating recovery of [from] muscle spasticity. … this system may also be applied to back-pain treatment/monitoring, ulcer due to paralysis, and various myotonic conditions."

Kitabayashi et al. (2010) reported on their fabrication and testing of a new 940 nm, 5 mW, IR LED. This device was unique in having a full-width of half-maximum (FWHM) wavelength span of 25 nm, which is less than half that of a 940 nm, 2 mW, IR LED currently available. Such a device promises to have application in thermotherapy as well as other NI IR-A LED applications.

Some of the other NI, transcutaneous, IR-A LED applications (other than thermotherapy) use 850–940 nm, IR-A LED light because of its deeper penetration properties: For example, it has application in the NI recharging the batteries of implantable prosthetic devices (Song, Hao et al. 2014). Also, Hartmann et al. (2015) described four different NI lipometers that use reflected NIR light from deep tissue to estimate subcutaneous fat content. These include: (1) The *Futurex*™ device that uses 940 and 950 nm IR-A LEDs. Four to six LEDs are used; a photodiode (PD) collects reflected IR light. (2) The *Lipometer*™ device uses 660 nm, deep-red LEDs, and a single NIR PD. (3) The *NIR Technologies* device uses a Fourier transform-NIR spectrometer, an NIR laser source, and a PD detector. (4) The *Dermalog*™ system uses a wideband, IR-A LED source (800–1000 nm). The detector is a 2-D spectrometer with a slit-shaped aperture that senses the reflected light.

The therapeutic effects of heat include, but are not limited to

- Increasing the extensibility of collagen connecting tissues

- Decreasing joint stiffness

- Reducing arthritis pain (WebMD 2015)

- Relieving muscle spasms

- Reducing inflammation and edema

- Increases local blood flow (heat-induced vasodilation). This provides proteins, nutrients, and oxygen for expedited healing.

In closing, we briefly describe a wearable, NI, thermotherapy, analgesic device called the *Willow Curve*™ currently being advertised on TV (February 25, 2016) (Willow Curve 2016). The purpose of this device is to provide temporary pain relief for many acute and chronic conditions, including pain associated with shoulders, elbows, the neck, hands, knees, and feet. The parent company is *Physicians Technology, LLC,* Monroe, MI. The Willow Curve device costs $599 plus S&H (2016). Instead of using IR-emitting lamps for thermotherapy, the device has a concave curved array of 24 red LEDs (of unspecified wavelength range) that provide thermal energy to the underlying skin which causes a beneficial vasodilation of blood vessels. Also, imbedded in this LED matrix are solid-state IR sensors to sense skin temperature. The on/off duty cycle of the LEDs is modulated by the device's digital controller in order to maintain a safe, maximum, measured surface skin temperature and the desired input power setting. The manufacturers claim that the device causes *increased lymphatic flow; reduced rate of production of inflammatory immune cells; slowed nerve response time reducing the perception of pain; release of pain-mitigating endorphins; specific pain receptors are blocked which promotes pain relief; toxic debris* [sic] *in the joint, a cause of inflammation and pain, is cleared away with increased circulation.* None of these claims have been independently verified for the Willow Curve device. Note that the blackbody photon emission spectrum of an ordinary tungsten lamp can contain proportionally more IR-A,B,C energy than a monochrome red LED of the same power; it is a better blackbody IR source than the red LED which is a relatively narrowband red and IR-A photon emitter. Summary comments by Hall (2015) on the *Science-Based Medicine* website included: "Willow Curve makes a lot of claims (cf. Treatable 2016), but there is no credible evidence to back them up. There are a lot of unanswered questions and red flags. Even if the effect is significant, it appears to be small in magnitude. Willow Curve appears to be unlikely to cause direct harm, and I don't doubt that anything that delivers heat might help relieve pain: but I'm not persuaded that the Willow Curve has any unique advantage over other, much less expensive products."

The more conventional, time-tested heat sources appear to be more cost-effective. Certainly, power level and dose time must be carefully monitored in any kind of thermotherapy to prevent thermal damage to the affected skin and underlying tissue.

18.8 INTERFERENTIAL CURRENT THERAPY

18.8.1 Introduction

ICT was initially described by Nemec (1959) and Goats (1990); it uses two constant-amplitude and frequency, kilohertz-frequency, alternating currents from two pairs of electrodes placed on the skin to stimulate subdermal tissues (nerves, muscle, bone, blood vessels, lymph ducts, etc.). The electrodes are placed so that the two current paths through the subdermal tissue cross. They must interact nonlinearly within the target tissue conductive volume to form an LF, interference or beat frequency (Δf) component voltage. The magnitude **b** in Equation 18.6 of the deep tissue, square-law, resistive nonlinearity acting on the two ICT currents is not known. Figure 18.2 illustrates the "X" placement of two pairs of ICT electrodes on a patient's lower back. Presumably, the alternating currents from the two pairs of interferential electrodes interact nonlinearly with the ions involved in deep tissue neuromuscular control (Na^+, K_+, Cl^-), effectively causing a mathematical multiplication of the currents. This multiplication basically generates a double-sideband,

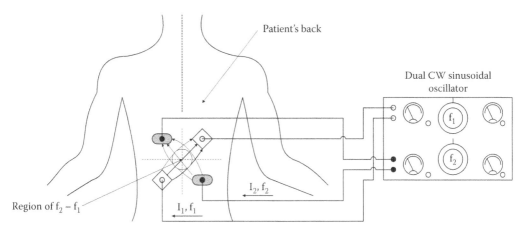

Figure 18.2 Illustration of the "X" placement of two pairs of ICT electrodes on a patient's lower back. Δf is generated in small volume where I_1 and I_2 currents cross.

suppressed-carrier modulation (DSBSCM) voltage signal, proportional to $i_m(t)$. (cf. Section 2.8.2 in Northrop 2014). Mathematically, this square-law modulation is shown in Equations 18.6 and 18.7:

$$i_m(t) = \mathbf{b}[i_1(t) + i_2(t)]^2 = \mathbf{b}\left[i_1^2(t) + 2i_1(t)i_2(t) + i_2^2(t)\right], \tag{18.6}$$

where $i_1(t) = A\cos[f_1(2\pi t)]$, and $i_2(t) = B\cos[f_2(2\pi t)]$.

The square-law part of the nonlinearity generates squared cosinusoidal terms yielding two double frequency terms, two DC terms, and a desired cross-product term, illustrated in the trig identity Equation 18.7.

$$i_m(t) = \overbrace{A\cos[f_1(2\pi t)]}^{i_1(t)} \times \overbrace{B\cos[f_2(2\pi t)]}^{i_2(t)} \equiv (AB/2)\{\cos[(f_1 + f_2)2\pi t] + \cos[(f_1 \overset{\Delta f}{-} f_2)2\pi t]\} \tag{18.7}$$

Let: $f_1 = f_2 + \Delta f = 4100$ Hz, $f_2 = 4000$ Hz; so $i_m(t) = (AB/2)\{\cos(2\pi 8100\,t) + \cos(\overset{\Delta f}{2\pi 100t})\}$. $\tag{18.8}$

Note that the multiplication can be the result of any nonlinear electrochemical resistive process having a square-law characteristic (e.g., $r = \mathbf{a}u + \mathbf{b}u^2 + \mathbf{c}u^3 + \cdots$, $u = i_1 + i_2$). The resultant LF (e.g., 100 Hz) component is more physiologically active, and is accepted as the basis for ICT; the 8.1 kHz component presumably has little physiological effect. The amount of LF voltage generated will depend on the amount of undefined, square-law, nonlinear resistivity (the $\mathbf{b}$ term) that the i_1 and i_2 alternating currents encounter in the tissues. Note that the beat frequency increment, Δf, can be scanned over 0 to several hundred Hz to generate a desired effect. It is not known how the current density vector, $\mathbf{J_m}(t, x, y, z)$, is directed with respect to the various tissues, in particular the nerve and muscle fibers in the IFC treatment volume.

Some ICT systems use only two electrodes, and premix (premodulate) $i_1(t)$ and $i_2(t)$ in the machine, rather than in the tissue (Ozcan et al. 2004). Thus, the ICT electrode voltage is given by $v_m(t)$ in Equarion 18.9. The 8.1 kHz (KA) component "sees" a low-skin impedance, and the 100 Hz (Δf) (KB) component sees a much higher-skin impedance. Hence, the putatively more therapeutically effective 100 Hz current is much smaller than the larger, 8.1 kHz component, assuming A = B.

$$v_m(t) = K\{A\cos[(f_1 + f_2)2\pi t] + B\cos[(f_1 \overset{\Delta f}{-} f_2)2\pi t]\}. \tag{18.9}$$

where K, A, and B are real constants. (It is not known whether A = B in the premodulated ICT study of Ozcan et al. (2004).)

Using a small-sample number (12) of patients, Ozcan et al. compared the analgesic effects of two, parallel, single-electrode-pair, premodulated AC ICT currents with the conventional crossed current, four-electrode ICT configuration. They were of the opinion: "Our findings suggest that the use of premodulated IFC (ICT), delivered through two large electrodes on either side of the target area [a total of 4 electrodes, two parallel current paths were used], is likely to be more effective than the traditional true IFC arrangement in terms of depth efficiency, torque production, and comfort."

A simplified, linear circuit model for total skin impedance ($\mathbf{Z_s}(j\omega)$) uses a resistor R_T in series with a parallel resistor R_S and capacitor C_S. This basic skin impedance model can be written (see Section 4.2 in this text):

$$\mathbf{Z_s}(j\omega) = R_T + \frac{R_s}{j\omega C_s R_s + 1} \text{ ohms.} \tag{18.10}$$

Using superposition, the total electrode current supplied by the machine can be written in phasor notation:

$$\mathbf{I_e} = \mathbf{V_m}/\mathbf{Z_s} = \frac{K}{R_T + R_s/\{j[2\pi(f_1 + f_2)C_s R_s] + 1\}} + \frac{K}{R_T + R_s/\{j[2\pi\Delta f C_s R_s] + 1\}} \tag{18.11}$$

Mixing the two VLF (4100 Hz and 4000 Hz) sources in the tissues is preferred, rather than using a single LF AC source of frequency Δf is that the impedance of the skin decreases with increasing applied frequency. This simple skin impedance model, of course, does not include the deep tissue resistive nonlinearity. At very high frequencies ($\omega \gg 1/R_sC_s$), $|\mathbf{Z_s}|$ reduces to R_T. By using 4.1 kHz and 4.0 kHz sources, the electrode–skin interface impedance is made lower, hence there is less heating of the skin for a given deep tissue current, $i_m(t)$. At 50 Hz, the total skin impedance magnitude is ~3200 ohms, while at 4 kHz, $|\mathbf{Z_s}| \cong 40\ \Omega$.

Note that using premodulated, two-electrode ICT, the total AC power loss in the total skin impedance (as heating) can be written:

$$P_{tot} = K^2 A^2/\text{Re}\{\mathbf{Z_s}(j2\pi(f_1 + f_2))\} + K^2 B^2/\text{Re}\{\mathbf{Z_s}(j2\pi\Delta f)\}\ \text{Watts} \tag{18.12}$$

Note that $\text{Re}\{\mathbf{Z_s}(j2\pi(f_1 + f_2))\} \ll \text{Re}\{\mathbf{Z_s}(j2\pi\Delta f)\}$.

18.8.2 Applications of ICT

ICT has been shown to be useful for the following applications (Noble et al. 2000, Hurley et al. 2001, Cheing and Hui-Chan 2003, ISEAPT 2015, Physiopedia 2015a):

- *Relief and management of acute and chronic pain,* in particular post-traumatic pain, sympathetically maintained pain as in shoulder–hand syndrome, lower-back pain, and Raynaud's phenomenon (spasm of the digital arteries). An ICT Δf of ~100 Hz stimulates pain gate mechanisms.

- *Stimulation of skeletal muscles*: Here, ICT electrode placement and Δf is used to stimulate motor nerves.

- Δf is made 10–50 Hz to cause prolonged (tetanic) contraction; Δf of 1–10 Hz will give twitches. Targeting muscles, ICT can be used for relaxation of muscle spasm, prevention and retardation of atrophy from muscle disuse, muscle reeducation, and maintenance of range of motion.

- *Increase of blood flow*: Increased vasodilation is produced following ICT due to its effect on the parasympathetic nerve fibers regulating the local blood flow. Increased blood flow aids healing.

- *Reduction of edema*: Chronic post-traumatic edema can be reduced by the use of ICT. This effect is probably due to the electrically induced smooth muscle contractions in the local lymphatic ducts and veins. Δf is made ~15 Hz, or a swept Δf of 10–25 Hz is used.

- *Stimulation of soft tissue healing and repair, and bone fracture healing.*

18.8.3 Other Forms of ICT

In classic interferential therapy, we have seen that the effective component of the applied current in the tissue is thought to be the low (Δf) component of the effective product of two cosinusoidal currents, one of medium frequency f_1, and the other of frequency $f_2 = f_1 + \Delta f$.

An alternate form of burst-modulated alternating current (BMAC) is called *Russian current*. In its defined form, Russian current is a 2.5 kHz AC current that is applied in 20 ms rectangular bursts with a burst duty cycle of 50%. That is, the externally applied current is $i_1(t) = A$ $\cos(2\pi 2500\ t)$ *multiplied by* an $i_2(t)$ that is a 0–1 amplitude square wave with a 50% duty cycle and a period of 40 ms. Another version of Russian current was described by Ward (2009); in this example, the stimulation carrier is 1 kHz, and the 0–1 modulating square wave is 50 pps with a 4 ms/20 ms duty cycle. Ward concluded: "Both the historical evidence and more recent findings indicate that the stimulation parameters commonly used clinically (Russian and interferential currents) are suboptimal for achieving their stated goals and that greater benefit would be obtained using short-duration 2- to 4-millisecond bursts of kilohertz-frequency AC, with a frequency chosen to maximize the desired outcome." Ward went on to recommend that for maximum muscle torque production, a frequency of 1–2.5 kHz should be used, with a burst duration of ∼2 ms.

Also, for minimal discomfort and less muscle torque, a frequency of 4 kHz should be used with a 4 ms burst duration.

18.8.4 Electrode Placement for ICT

In all electrotherapy modalities, and in ICT in particular, electrode placement is a critical parameter. The therapist must have a comprehensive knowledge of neuromuscular anatomy, spinal neuroanatomy, and the neurophysiology of pain. Because ICT involves two intersecting current pathways in a particular volume of deep tissue, electrode placement is critical if one is to maximize the effect of the stimulation (Hurley et al. 2001).

18.9 ELECTRICAL AND MAGNETIC STIMULATION IN BONE HEALING

18.9.1 Introduction

Bone has a complex physiology and anatomy; on a weight basis, bone is stronger than aluminum, it is a composite material of approximately equal amounts of hydrated proteins and minerals. Three major bone cell classes are *osteoblasts, osteocytes,* and *osteoclasts*. Osteoblasts are single-nucleus cells that synthesize bone, functioning in groups of connected cells called an osteon. Osteoblasts synthesize a very dense, cross-linked, Type I collagen, plus several other specialized proteins in smaller quantities (e.g., osteocalcin and osteopontin) which form the organic matrix of bone. Parathyroid hormone (PTH) from the parathyroid gland is an important regulator of blood calcium ion concentration [Ca^{++}], and also the activity of osteoblasts. Osteocytes are star-shaped cells found in all mature bone; they are not capable of mitosis. Osteocytes are long-lived; they do not divide, and have a half-life of ∼25 years. They are derived from osteoprogenitor stem cells, some of which also differentiate into osteoblasts. When osteoblasts become trapped in the matrix they secrete, they become osteocytes. Osteocytes are networked to each other by long cytoplasmic extensions that occupy tiny canals (canaliculi), which are used to exchange nutrients and waste through cellular gap junctions. Osteocytes are actively involved in the routine turnover of bony matrix, through various mechanosensory mechanism. They destroy bone through a rapid, transient mechanism (relative to osteoclasts) called ostocytic osteolysis. Hydroxyapatite [$Ca_{10}(PO_4)_6(OH)_2$], calcium carbonate, and calcium phosphate are deposited around the cell.

Osteoclasts are a type of multinucleated bone cell that has the function of resorbing bone tissue. Immune system macrophages are transformed into osteoclasts through the action of receptor activator of nuclear factor κβ ligand (RANKL) and macrophage colony-stimulating factor (M-CSF). These hormones are produced by neighboring stromal cells and osteoblasts; this requires direct contact between these cells and osteoclast precursors. Osteoclasts are regulated by several hormones, including PTH and interleukin-6 (IL-6) (Northrop and Connor 2009, Table 7.1). Osteoblasts secrete IL-6.

It has long been known that bone growth and load-bearing strain in bone have been associated with ionic phenomena in which both transient and DC potentials are generated (Fukada and Yasuda 1957, Friedenberg and Brighton 1966, Onibere and Khanna 2008, Fintek 2015). In 1964, Becker et al. reported that bone is most electronegative in areas of growth where osteoblasts are active, such as fractures and epiphyseal plates.

Most tissues in the human body are capable of self-repair when injured by accident or surgery. Included in this list are the bones: Once a break in a bone occurs, natural bone repair that assures a strong union normally occurs within several months. Occasionally, the formation of new bone is slow, and the break fails to heal properly, usually because scar tissue has filled the gap where the new bone was expected to form, or blood circulation to the injured area has been compromised. A number of modalities have been found useful to exert some level of effect on bone growth and healing. These include mechanical forces (compression, distraction osteogenesis, and shear), electrical currents and fields, magnetic fields (DC, AC, and pulsed [PEMF]), and US energy. All of these have been found to exert some effect on bone growth and healing (Kuzyk and Schemitsch 2009, Behrens et al. 2013).

Our focus in this section is on the use of NI electric currents and fields and magnetic fields in the enhancement of bone healing and treating the nonunion of fractures. As in the case of the use of ICT on deep tissues, there is general agreement that electrical bone healing (EBH) in its several modalities is effective. What is lacking is general agreement on how effective they are, and standard protocols for administering EBH and evaluating its effects (Griffin and Bayat 2011).

From basic physics, we know that a charged particle (e.g., an ion) at rest at a point (**x,y,z**) in a static electric field has a vector force $\mathbf{F_e}$ exerted on it given by $\mathbf{F_e} = q\,\mathbf{E}$ N, where q is the particle's charge in coulombs, and **E** is the electric field vector at the point in V/m. Likewise, an ion moving with vector velocity **v** m/s in a magnetic field with flux density vector **B** experiences a vector force given by $\mathbf{F_m} = q\,(\mathbf{v} \times \mathbf{B})$ N. X denotes the vector cross-product operation (cf. Glossary). $\mathbf{F_e}$ and $\mathbf{F_m}$ figure in the use of electric and magnetic fields to expedite bone healing, relief from deep bruising, injury pain, and ICT. As an additional complication, the EMF V induced in a closed circuit is given by the relation: $V = -d\psi_m/dt$ V, where ψ_m is the total magnetic flux linking the circuit (in Wb). The complex factors governing exactly how applied **E, B,** and d**B**/dt affect the physiology of healing remain to be fully understood.

18.9.2 Electrical Stimulation Modalities for Bone Healing

In 1968, Jahn concluded that a secondary source of endogenous DC bone potential comes from the migration of inorganic ions within the bone matrix. In 1971, Friedenberg et al. insightfully and successfully applied a DC to heal the nonunion of a malleolar fracture. A short history of the many approaches to bone healing by electrical stimulation may be found in the comprehensive review by Onibere and Khanna (2008).

Currently, electrical stimulation to expedite bone healing has three major forms (Onibere and Khanna 2008): (1) *Invasive*: DC using electrodes surgically implanted at the fracture site. (2) *Semi-invasive*: A DC is applied to the nonunion through a Teflon-coated, stainless steel cathode that is inserted percutaneously into the affected site. The cathode must be anchored to the bone to hold it in place. An adhesive anode electrode is placed anywhere on the skin surface. (3) *NI*: Capacitively coupled (C-C) AC or pulsed electric fields use skin electrodes placed over the injury site (Scott and King 1994, Beck et al. 2008). An AC or transient (dV/dt) current flows in the conductive tissues. (4) (Also *NI* treated in the section below.) An inductively coupled (AC) electromagnetic field exists from coils on the skin surface. These AC EM fields induce alternating currents in the damaged tissues.

18.9.3 Pulsed Magnetic Stimulation for Bone Healing and Other Medical Conditions

First, we consider the mathematics associated with the production of a therapeutic magnetic field: When a current i is passed through an N-turn coil, a magnetic field (flux density) **B** Wb/m² is set up. Physics texts generally derive an expression for **B** generated by a current-carrying coil at a point P, given the coil's dimensions. For example, at the end of an N-turn solenoid coil of radius r and length l, it is easy to show that **B** is directed along the coil's axis and is given by

$$\mathbf{B_0} = \mu_o Ni\,/\,2l \quad \text{T (also known as 1 Wb/m}^2\text{).} \tag{18.13}$$

If the coil has $l \ll r$ (i.e., it has negligible length compared to its radius, i.e., becomes a ring coil), the **B** field at its center can also be shown to be:

$$\mathbf{B_0} = \mu_o Ni/(2l) \quad \text{T.} \tag{18.14}$$

The **B** vector on the coil's center axis at a distance d from the center of the ring coil can be shown to be (Sears 1953):

$$\mathbf{B}(d) = \frac{\mu_o Nir^2}{2(d^2 + r^2)^{3/2}} = \frac{\mu_o Nir^2}{2[\sqrt{d^2 + r^2}]^3} = \frac{\mu_o Nir^2}{2h^3} \quad \text{T,} \tag{18.15}$$

where z = d and $h \equiv \sqrt{(d^2 + r^2)}$, from the geometry in the figure.

More generally, **B**(x,y,x) at a point P at a distance R far from the thin ring coil's center can be shown to be the vector sum of $\mathbf{B_R}$ and $\mathbf{B_\psi}$ given in polar coordinates (Sears 1953):

$$\mathbf{B_R} \cong \mu_o Nir^2\cos(\theta)/(2R^3) \quad (\mathbf{B_R} \text{ is in-line with R.})$$
$$\text{T; approximately, when } R \gg r. \tag{18.16}$$

$$\mathbf{B_\theta} \cong \mu_o Nir^2\sin(\theta)/(4R^3) \quad (\mathbf{B_\theta} \text{ is perpendicular to R.),} \tag{18.17}$$

where θ is the angle R makes with the z-axis.

Note that when $R \gg r$, $\mathbf{B}(x,y,z)$ falls off with $1/R^3$, not $1/R^2$. If P lies on the z-axis, $\theta = 0$, $\mathbf{B}(x,y,z) = \mathbf{B}_R = \mu_o Nir^2/(2R^3)$. See Figure 18.3 for illustrations of the solenoid and thin-coil B-field geometries.

Another effect of applied EMFs is seen in the interaction of a charged particle (e.g., an ion) moving with velocity vector $\mathbf{v}$ in a magnetic field $\mathbf{B}$ Wb/m² and an electric field $\mathbf{E}$ V/m. The force vector in newtons on the ion, $\mathbf{F}$, is given by the Lorentz equation:

$$\mathbf{F} = q\mathbf{E} + q(\mathbf{v} \times \mathbf{B})N. \tag{18.18}$$

When a moving conductive fluid intersects a magnetic field, an EMF, E_f, is induced given by the Faraday's law of induction equation (Northrop 2014):

$$E_F = -\int_0^d [(\mathbf{v} \times \mathbf{B}) \cdot dL] \text{ volts}, \tag{18.19}$$

where X is the vector cross-product operation (see Glossary) and · denotes the vector dot product operation. The net result in the brackets is a scalar.

When $\mathbf{B}$ and $\mathbf{L}$ are mutually perpendicular to the fluid velocity, $\mathbf{v}$, Equation 18.19 reduces to: $E_F = B v d$. d is the distance in m between the electrodes contacting the moving fluid; it is the length of the $\mathbf{L}$ vector connecting the centers of the electrodes.

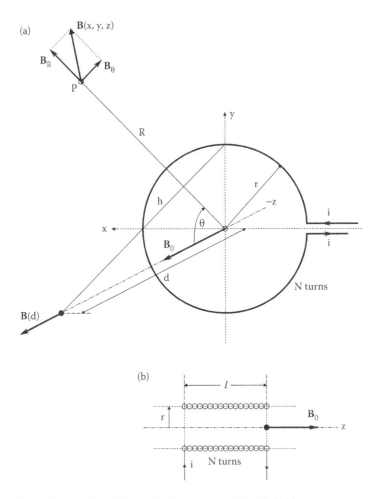

Figure 18.3 Illustrations of the thin-coil (a) and solenoid (b) B-field geometries.

Time-changing magnetic fields can also induce an EMF in a closed circuit of area **s** enclosing time-varying flux lines according to the relation:

$$E_i = -\int_s \partial \mathbf{B}/dt \cdot d\mathbf{s}, \tag{18.20}$$

where no charges are moving in the area s, $\mathbf{B}$ = flux density (Wb/m^2), d$\mathbf{s}$ = vector element of area (m^2), t = time, · denotes the vector dot product operation.

To summarize, magnetic fields exert forces on moving charges creating concentration gradients; they also generate EMFs and electric fields when they interact with moving conductive fluids (e.g., blood in blood vessels), EMFs are produced when magnetic fields vary in time while intersecting a conductive circuit.

The effect of the $\mathbf{B}$ field from the therapy coils is usually felt in tissues at a depth of several cm. Fortunately, the relative magnetic permeability, $\mu_r = \mu/\mu_o$, of biological tissue (blood, bone fat muscle, etc.) is very close to unity, and the $\mathbf{B}$ field penetrates all tissues without significant distortion or attenuation from the tissue. For example, some μ_r values given by Collins et al. (2002) are water, 0.99999096; fat, 0.99999221; bone, 0.99999156; blood, 0.99999153; brain white matter, 0.99999120, empty space, 1.00000000. $\mu_o \equiv 4\pi \times 10^{-7}$ (N-s^2)/C^2. Unless differences in relative permeability are being used for imaging, for calculations, use $\mu = \mu_o$.

In *NI bone healing* stimulation from magnetic flux density, one or more external coils are placed surrounding the nonunion region in a bone or injury site, and AC, DC, or pulsed (time-varying) currents are passed through the coil(s) to generate $\mathbf{B}$ fields that penetrate the tissue. Markov (2007) stated: "It has been shown that at least three amplitude windows [for AC, DC, and PMF therapy] exist: at 50–100 µT (5–10 Gauss), 15–20 mT (150–200 Gauss), and 45–50 mT (450–500 Gauss)." It should be noted that the first "B window" includes the Earth's DC magnetic field, about 58 µT in Cambridge, MA, and has questionable validity. Higher amplitude "B windows" are not natural, and have definite therapeutic value. The B windows cited above are B values measured at the coils; B will obviously be lower in the tissues, and must be estimated by calculation.

Optimum current waveshapes and frequencies in PMF generation are fuzzy sets of parameters on which there is some little agreement. DC and steady AC excitation have been used, but pulsed DC in the frequency range from 1 to 1 kpps with variable duty cycles has also been found effective. Optimum pulse repetition rates (PRRs) appear to lie in the range of 1–15 pps overlapping a 10–50 pps range (Philipson 2015). In addition, current pulses may be switched on and off in bursts (squarewave, 0–1 gating) that is at a lower pps. For example, an AC carrier of say 60 Hz may be 0–1 modulated (gated) at say 6 pps, or the PMF current can be a full-wave rectified 30 Hz AC current that is 0–1 gated at 15 pps, etc. In terms of neuromuscular stimulation, evidence indicates that a fast current (B field) rise time is more effective therapeutically than a slower one.

There are a number of applications of magnetic field therapy (MFT), probably the most familiar is its use in expediting the healing of accidental bone fractures, tendon ruptures, and deep bruising. MFT also has been used to expedite healing in lumbar spine fusion surgeries, as well as promote healing and relieve pain in certain joint diseases. Also cited are more rapid graft healing, healing in myocardial ischemia and strokes (Curatronic® Ltd. 2015, Bassett 1993). Athanasiou et al. (2006) reported on an experimental study of accelerated skin wound healing in Wistar rats using PMFs. A 2 × 2 cm^2 of skin from the rat's back was surgically removed. $\mathbf{B}$ pulses of 1 ms duration, 12.5 mT peak magnitude, having a rise time of 0.1 µs, a fall time of 10 µs, and a frequency of 3 pps were used on the wound. A statistically significant acceleration of wound healing was observed for the first 9 days in the animals exposed to the PMFs. The majority of the treated rats had completed the healing process by day 18, while it took 22 days for the control group to heal.

In conclusion, it appears that the physiological effects of time-varying $\mathbf{B}$ fields on tissues at the molecular level are complex, and are just beginning to be understood. One manufacturer of PEMF therapeutic devices (Trio33® 2015) has made claims for "Major Benefits," including:

- Eliminates pain (acute and chronic)

- Directly dilates blood vessels

- Increases blood flow

- Enhances delivery and effect of medication

- Increases blood oxygen-carrying capacity

- Accelerates cellular metabolism

- Improves tissue vitality

- Stimulates cellular resistance to disease

- Regenerates body cells and bone structure

- Natural noninvasive alternative for pain relief

- May reduce need for medication

These benefits have been observed in various clinical studies in various degrees. They also include the absence of "any harmful side effects." Of course the degree each "Major Benefit" is expressed depends on many factors, including PMF field strength, pulse parameters (e.g., pulse rise time, fall time, frequency, duty cycle), nature of injury, individual anatomy and physiology, duration of treatment, etc.

A comprehensive review of the effects of PMFs (Shupak 2003) revealed that PMFs have been used experimentally to treat a wide variety of medical conditions other than bone injuries. These included:

- Orthopedic disorders (osteoporosis, Perthes' disease, hip arthroplasty)

- Joint disorders (rheumatoid arthritis, OA, rotator cuff tendonitis, lateral epicondylitis)

- Spinal fusions

- Venous leg ulcers

- Pelvic pain

- Nerves (sciatic nerve, peroneal nerve, median-ulnar nerve, endocrine ophthalmology)

- Neurological disorders (tinnitus, multiple sclerosis)

- Neuroendocrine system (cortisol secretion, melatonin levels)

- Cerebral ischemia (stroke)

- Coronary protection (cardiac stimulation, myocardial protection)

- Cancer (various studies)

- Psychophysiological regulation (human standing balance)

- Pain (various studies)

Most of the studies cited in Shupak (2003) used different stimulation parameters (peak **B**, d**B**/dt, **B**(t) waveshape [for example, half-sine, rectangular, trapezoidal, triangular], pulse width, pulse frequency, etc.) and generally got some level of satisfactory therapeutic results. The question we are left with, however, is what would be the optimum set of pulse parameters for a given medical condition? That is, what parameters would provide the maximum therapeutic effect? Also, what medications might expedite (or interfere with) various PMF therapies?

Note that the magnetic stimulation dose D is given in T/s (1 Tesla = 1 T = 10^4 Gauss). For a pulsed DC **B**: pk T × (pulse of duration (s) ÷ pulse period (s)) = ave T in a period. Total dose = ave T × No. of pulse periods given.

See the comprehensive analysis and summary of critical evidence for the effects of electrical bone stimulation (DC, capacitive coupled AC or pulses, and inductive coupling) since 1959 written by Griffin and Bayat (2011), also the evaluation of bone stimulation by various modalities by Wienke and Dayton (2011).

18.10 NI RESPIRATORY (PNEUMATIC) THERAPIES

18.10.1 Introduction

NI respiratory assistance devices may be grouped in two major categories: negative-pressure ventilators (NPVs) (e.g., the iron lung), and positive-pressure ventilators (PPVs) which include the CPAP and bi-level positive airway pressure (BPAP) systems. The NPV was first described by Scottish physician John Dalziel in 1832. A hand bellows-driven "Spirophore" was devised by a Dr. Woillez in Paris in 1876. The NPV *Iron Lung* was perfected in the early twentieth century to meet the demand of poliomyelitis victims with paralyzed respiratory muscles. They literally breathed for the patients by mechanically modulating the negative pressure inside the iron lung (outside the patient lying in it). As polio vaccines became widely administered, the use of NPV iron lungs declined: in 1959, there were 1200 people using iron lungs in the United States; this dropped to 39 by 2004 (Smithsonian 2015). Iron lungs evolved into the biphasic cuirass ventilation device, a wearable, rigid, plastic upper body shell which functions as a biphasic NPV.

For less severe problems than paralyzed respiratory muscles, NI PPV and ventilation procedures have been developed that use an airtight mask over the nose or nose and mouth to couple to a programmed pressure to the respiratory system. PPV systems are used primarily in cases of respiratory failure where blood PaO_2 is less than 8 kPa (60 mmHg), and/or the $PaCO_2$ is too high. Below we describe various PPV paradigms and their sometimes confusing acronyms.

18.10.2 CPAP and BPAP

The simplest PPV ventilation paradigm is CPAP. The patient breathes on his/her own into a fixed positive air pressure supplied into a face or nose mask. CPAP is used to treat obstructive sleep apnea (OSA) at home, and improve gas exchange in the lungs by keeping the alveoli dilated in ICU settings. A typical CPAP machine can deliver (manometer) pressures between 4 and 20 cmH_2O, however between 6 and 14 cmH_2O is used to treat sleep apnea, and permit normal sleep. (Note: 1 cmH_2O = 0.0142 psi = 980.6 $Dynes/cm^2$.)

Side effects from CPAP may include dizziness, sinus infections, bronchitis, dry eyes, dry mucosal tissue irritation, ear pain, and nasal congestion (Ayow et al. 2009). Some of these symptoms may be due to the CPAP air supply needing higher humidity.

Another PPV paradigm is called BPAP. BPAP provides the airway with alternating high- and low-positive pressures: High-positive pressure to aid inspiration, and a lower-positive pressure to facilitate exhalation.

BPAP is used to treat OSA, central sleep apnea (CSA), and severe COPD with accompanying low-blood O_2 saturation and high-blood pCO_2. There are three BPAP modes: (1) *Spontaneous* (**S**). In **S** mode, sensors detect when there is inspiratory effort, and trigger higher pressure. It then automatically cycles back to lower pressure when expiratory effort is sensed. (2) *Timed* (**T**) *mode*. In timed mode, the BPAP cycling is fixed at a set rate and amplitude. (3) *Spontaneous/Timed* (**S/T**) *mode*: As in **S** mode, the BPAP system switches to higher pressure when it senses inspiratory effort, then back again to timed (**T**) mode if it senses fewer than a set number of spontaneous breaths/minute.

BPAP is sometimes called variable positive airway pressure (VPAP). BPAP cycles consist of expiratory positive airway pressure (EPAP) and (higher) inspiratory positive airway pressure (IPAP). BiPAP® is a trade name of *Respironics Corporation* for their design of BPAP machines. Note that PPV airflow generators can have the option of adding humidity to the air, bronchodilators, or supplementary oxygen.

18.11 US MAY HELP TREAT AD

Accumulation of the amyloid-β (Aβ) peptide plaques in the brain (see Glossary) has been implicated in the pathogenesis of AD, a progressive and fatal CNS condition. Recently, an experimental, NIT for AD has been investigated in a mouse model (Leinenga and Götz 2015). Externally applied scanning ultrasound (SUS) radiation applied to the head was used after injecting the blood of the AD mice with lipid microbubble resonators. The lipid-shelled microbubbles had an octafluoropropane core, were from 1 to 10 μm diameter (mean diameter of 4 μm), and had a concentration of $1–5 \times 10^7$ microbubbles/mL.

Twenty mice, genetically modified to develop amyloid plaques in their brains (and AD), were given microbubble injections; then 10 AD mice were given five sessions of US over 6 weeks, and 10 AD (control) mice were given sham (placebo) treatments. The microbubble resonators were thought to disrupt the blood–brain barrier, apparently allowing molecules to enter the brain from the blood that activated microglial cells that destroy amyloid plaques. Following the US therapy, the 10 treated mice were compared with the 10 controls in three memory tasks: A Y-maze, a novel object recognition test, and an active place avoidance task. The 10 treated mice displayed improved performance over the AD control mice. In addition, Aβ plaques were reduced in the US-treated AD mice.

Leinenga and Götz pointed out that mice are not humans, and:

- The human brain is much larger and the skull is thicker, so higher US energy would be required to treat all areas of the brain. This may have negative consequences, such as causing damage to healthy brain tissue.

- There are concerns that the level of immune response might be too high. To avoid this, the researchers suggest that the treatment protocol could focus on ensonifying smaller skull sections at a time.

- The mice in their study already had plaques when the US therapy was started. They stated that they do not know at what point in human AD it would be appropriate to start treatment. They were concerned that US treatment given in early AD may damage brain tissue.

- Their study did not examine the long-term effects of the US treatment on mice.

Leinenga and Götz (2015) stated: "Our results revealed that SUS treatment engages microglia and promotes internalization of Aβ into microglial lysosomes, thereby reducing Aβ and plaque load in the APP23 transgenic mouse model of AD as well as restoring function in tests of spatial and recognition memory."

Clearly, further studies must be done on AD animal models with larger skulls, such as sheep or pigs, then primates, before any human studies are contemplated. There is much research to be done to demonstrate the long-term effectiveness of NI US on AD (Underwood 2015).

18.12 HEARING AIDS

18.12.1 Introduction

HAs are an excellent example of NI therapeutic devices. They attempt to restore a patient's hearing, including speech comprehension, to a "normal" level. They address a growing medical problem in an increasingly aging population. About 30 years ago, most HAs used analog electronics for sound amplification and filtering. Their properties (e.g., volume, frequency response) were adjusted using a small screwdriver or miniature switches. They often were plagued with high-frequency acoustic feedback if the earpiece came unseated. As you will see below, modern HAs now use DSP to condition the input sound to best match the patient's hearing characteristics, shaping the output sound spectrum to compensate for HLs and eliminating acoustic feedback.

HL may be characterized as: mild (adults): 26–40 dB HL; moderate: 41–54 dB HL; moderately severe: 55–70 dB HL; severe: 71–90 dB HL; or profound: ≥91 dB HL. The severity of a HL is the required dB increase in sound pressure level (SPL) above the normal level before a subject can detect it, at a given frequency. Note that frequencies >3 kHz contribute to ~25% of the audible speech cues required for recognition of spoken language. For example, the peak energy of the fricative /s/ spoken by a child or female talker falls between 6.3 and 8.3 kHz, and ranges in level between 57 and 68 dB SPL.

Modern HAs have many useful features, such as UHF RF (e.g., Bluetooth®) links to electronic sound sources such as cell phones, directional microphones, CD players, and TVs. Most HAs use disposable zinc-air batteries for power.

18.12.2 Human Hearing Characteristics

Normal human hearing can be characterized by a frequency response function. Human hearing is most sensitive in a frequency range between 2 and 4 kHz. Sensitivity drops off precipitously around 20 kHz, and is also slowly attenuated from 1 kHz down to 20 Hz. In 1933, Fletcher and Munson defined an objective measure of human hearing frequency response in their *equal loudness contours* which they plotted on linear-log coordinates. The vertical axis was the dB SPL of the perceived sinusoidal tone; the horizontal (log) axis was tone frequency. For example, at 30 Hz, the dB SPL for threshold hearing (0 phon) was given as ~60 dB. At maximum hearing sensitivity, the 0 phon curve was at ~−8 dB SPL at 3 kHz, and ~+10 dB SPL was required for hearing at ~16 kHz. The equal loudness contours have been remeasured and revised; the generally accepted version now being the 2003 ISO 226 revision. The ISO 226 curves differ significantly from the 1933 curves at LFs from 400 to 20 Hz, generally being higher at these LFs. One reason the equal loudness contours have maximum sensitivity in the 2–4 kHz range is the natural resonance of the ear canal (Villchur 2004).

There are many medical and physical causes of HL, including aging, which we will not cover here. Many persons with HL (*anacusis*) generally have lost high-frequency sensitivity in one or both ears. This can be described using a joint time–frequency (JTF) spectrogram of a test sentence with sound energy covering a 50 Hz–10 kHz frequency range. In moderate-to-severe high-frequency HL, all sound energy above, say, 3 kHz in the JTF spectrogram is inaudible, representing a considerable loss of information. Another way of describing severe losses is to plot the dB HL versus frequency for a subject given standard audiology tests. In one example, the dB HL dropped ~90 dB (10 dB loss to 100 dB loss) in an octave, beginning at 1 kHz (Alexander 2012). A 100 dB HL is too severe to compensate for with a simple high-frequency boost filter in the HA. One current practice is to use a frequency-lowering (FL) technique that moves the spectral content of high-frequency input sounds to the HA to a spectral region of the JTF spectrogram that is audible for the patient.

Equal loudness curves characterize the perceived frequency response of the human sound source–ear–middle ear–inner ear–brain perceptual system. The various types of HAs also impose their frequency responses on the sound perceptual system. HAs generally consist of (1) a sound input transducer (also known as microphone) which is coupled to (2) an electronic amplifier which has an associated frequency response. The amplifier drives (3) an output transducer (OT) (called the "receiver" by audiologists). The OT is also characterized by its electromechanical frequency response. The OT may be coupled to the ear canal through a (4) tube, or be inserted directly in the ear canal. The coupling tube also has a characteristic audio frequency response.

18.12.3 HAs, Frequency Compensation, and Frequency Flowering Technologies

The history of HAs goes back to seventeenth century where passive, inverse-horn ear trumpets were used by deaf persons. They were made from sheet metal, silver, wood, mollusk shells, or animal horns. Ear trumpets were very popular in the nineteenth century, even Ludwig van Beethoven used one when he started to go deaf. The advent of electronic amplification (first vacuum tubes in the early twentieth century, then transistors, then analog and digital integrated circuits) made the large, unwieldy ear trumpets, and other passive HAs obsolete. HAs in the 1930s were basically audio systems having a microphone, a vacuum tube amplifier with adjustable gain, and an output earphone. They could run on heavy batteries or line power.

Twenty-first-century HAs use analog and/or digital circuitry. Early HAs were generally analog and were worn on the body. The microphone, signal filtering unit, transistor amplifier, and batteries were housed in a module the size of a pack of cigarettes; wires ran from the module to one or two earphones clipped to the ear(s). As discrete transistors were replaced by integrated circuits, HA module sizes shrank to include the behind-the-ear (BTE) designs, and the various in-the-ear canal configurations. The BTE HAs generally had the microphone and the OT (receiver) on their body. The conditioned sound from the *OT* is conducted by a plastic tube to the ear canal, or in another design, wires carry the conditioned analog audio output of the HA to an OT imbedded in the ear canal, eliminating the frequency distortion inherent in the plastic tube.

Figure 18.4 illustrates the design of a typical, modern HA. The input transducer is generally an electret microphone; its analog output is sampled and converted to digital form by an ADC. Nonlinear amplitude compression (or expansion) is introduced at this stage. Next, the amplitude-compressed digital signal is acted on by a digital signal processor (DSP). The DSP shapes the

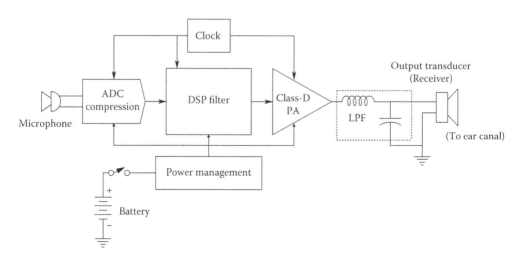

Figure 18.4 Block diagram of a modern hearing aid.

bandwidth of the digitized signal, which is next simultaneously amplified and converted back into analog (output) form by a Class-D power Amplifier (PA)/Low-pass Filter. This conditioned, amplified, analog signal drives the OT (also known as receiver). Also in the HA is a zinc-air battery and a Power Management IC, also a high-frequency clock oscillator that drives the ADC, the DSP, and the PA.

The HA OT can use an electrodynamic, moving-coil/permanent magnet design, or an electret or piezoelectric transducer.

Sophisticated digital HA designs now can use one of several DSP algorithms for FL to improve the comprehension of individuals with severe or profound HL at high frequencies (Simpson 2009, Galster et al. 2012). Simpson described five different ways of implementing FL in HA DSP. These include: (1) Vocoding. (2) Slow playback (SP) (not a real-time process). (3) Transposition. (4) Nonlinear frequency compression (NLFL). (5) Frequency shifting. We will summarize these techniques below.

Vocoding is a technique of speech processing in which the input signal is passed through an array of band-pass (BP) filters having abutting BP ranges. In doing FL, the n signal outputs of each of n BP filters ($y_1, y_2, ..., y_n$) are each modulated by narrowband noise that has been conditioned by passing white noise through n BP filters, each with pass bands lower than the BP filters used to derive the $\{y_n\}$ signals. The n outputs of the modulators, $\{z_n\}$, are then passed through corresponding BP filters with the same pass bands as used to condition the noise. The $\{w_n\}$ outputs of the final BP filter array are summed linearly and constitute the frequency-lowered output. This complicated scheme was studied experimentally in the 1960s and 1970s, but not put into practice in a HA device (Simpson 2009).

SP is a nonreal-time FL algorithm. It yields an HA output whose entire passband (e.g., 50 Hz–8 kHz) is shifted down by a fixed amount and lengthened in time. It has the advantage of retaining the harmonic relationship between frequency components of the input and the disadvantage of stretching the signal in time. This can cause the input and output signals to be desynchronized in time. In SP, epochs (adjoining intervals) of the input signal are digitized at an input sample frequency f_{si} and stored; simultaneously, the samples are converted to analog form at a slower clock speed, f_{so}, lowering the frequency of the entire output spectrum below that of the input spectrum. In one implementation of SP by AVR Sonovation [www.avrsono.com/index.html (Accessed 6/18/15)], if the input spectrum contains little sound energy above 2.5 kHz, then the input signals are amplified without the SP algorithm (Simpson 2009).

Frequency Transposition (FT) moves high-frequency sounds to lower frequencies and adds the transposed signal to an unprocessed lower frequency signal. In FT, the input sound spectrum is divided into a low-pass and a high-pass band. The high-frequency band contains frequencies inaudible to the subject. In one embodiment of an FT HA, the frequency dividing the LF and HF bands, f_x, can be manually selected by the clinician from 630 Hz to 6 kHz in one-third octave intervals. Frequencies below f_x are amplified but not transposed. Higher frequencies up to two octaves above f_x are analyzed by the HA electronics. "A narrow range of frequencies with the highest intensity levels within this range are selected, transposed by one octave, and overlapped with the lower frequency signal below the starting frequency $[f_x]$" (Simpson 2009). Simpson continued: "...this processing has the advantage of a more natural sound quality. In addition, the ratio between frequency components in the high-frequency transposed region is usually preserved." Simpson also commented that a major disadvantage of FT is that the addition of a transposed high-frequency signal can mask important, lower amplitude LF information. Transposed high-frequency background noise can also mask LF information. This disadvantage can be overcome by making the FT HA input adaptive, that is, enabling FT only when the input signal contains mostly high-frequency information.

Frequency Compression (FC) reduces the bandwidth of the output signal (sent to the OT). Linear frequency shifting is analogous to the Doppler effect from a receding sound source: All input frequency components are lowered by a constant factor. Linear shifting has the advantage of preserving spectral information because the ratios among the input frequency components are left unchanged. The relations between the frequencies of speech formant peaks remain constant. Nonlinear frequency compression (NLFC) reduces the high-frequency bandwidth of a speech signal by implementing increasing amounts of frequency lowering to relatively high-input frequencies. Advantages of NLFC include no overlap between the shifted and unshifted signals, and low- and mid-frequency information remains preserved as the whole first-formant frequency range is left unchanged by the processing. The Phonak Naida HA is a commercially available device that uses NLFC.

Spectral iQ is another input-adaptive FL algorithm, developed by Starkey Laboratories, Eden Prairie, MN, that identifies and classifies acoustic features of high-frequency source (input) sounds and uses this information to perform selective FL. Galaster et al. (2012) stated:

> Once appropriate high-frequency features are detected, Spectral iQ uses a sophisticated processing technique to replicate (or translate) those high-frequency features at a lower, audible frequency. ... new features are created in real time, resulting in the presentation of audible cues while minimizing the distortion that occurs with other technologies.

The Spectral iQ system remains inactive until its Special Feature Identification algorithm detects the presence of a high-frequency speech feature (frequency and amplitude), prompting the creation of a new lower (listener-audible) frequency feature. This cues the listener to the presence of high-frequency speech or music components. Galaster et al. (2012) continued:

> the dynamic nature of Spectral iQ retains the natural distribution of frequencies and comparatively broadband sound quality, while also avoiding the introduction of high-frequency noise that was not present in those lower frequency regions. This is accomplished by providing a complementary, audible cue when high-frequency speech sounds such as /s/ and /ʃ/ are present.

Many modern HAs now offer a UHF wireless feature for an alternate sound input. Radio-linked directional microphones, cordless phones, TV sound links, and FM radio music sound links can be sources.

18.12.4 Conclusions

Modern HAs have now evolved into miniature, sophisticated, digital-electronic, sound-conditioning systems that are typically worn BTE(s) designs. In one configuration, the conditioned sound from their OT is directed through a small, flexible plastic tube to inside the ear canal, thence to the eardrum. Other models place the OT directly in the ear canal and connect it to the HA electronics with wires; this eliminates frequency distortions caused by sound transmission through the tube. Still other miniature HAs are inserted directly into the ear canal (ITC).

Because most HL is above 2.5 kHz, most HA manufacturers have implemented some sort of optional DSP FL algorithm in their HA designs. The effectiveness of these algorithms is very patient dependent, but generally shows some sort of hearing improvement (Simpson 2009).

Finally, there is the question of HA prices (Barber 2005). Barber cited some factors that go into determining the prices of HAs. These include, but are not limited to

- Technology (R&D)
- Durability and reliability
- Personal fitting
- Professional costs
- The high cost of low volume
- Marketing costs
- Warrantee costs
- Free Trial costs
- Inflation
- Customization

The 10 factors summarized above were described in detail by Barber (2005).

Vance (2013) wrote an essay on this topic in which she cited a source that claimed it costs ~$250 to make an HA device that will be sold to an audiologist for ~$1000. HA manufacturers spend ~$75 per device on R&D and $250 on marketing, then chalk up $425 in profit. The retailers then mark up the price by $2000 to cover overhead and make a profit, resulting in a ~$3000 patient price tag. Such high costs for an electronic/audio system seem unreasonable when contrasted with the complexity and costs of modern laptop PCs. HA costs are generally not covered by Medicare/Medicaid insurance, so the patient is wise to shop around to minimize their cost/benefit ratio.

By visiting the Amazon.com pages on HAs, it is evident that there is an ongoing HA price war. Many models of advertised BTE and ITC HAs use DSP. One BTE model which has 12-band DSP claims to focus on voices and simultaneously reduce background noise. Sold by LifeEar Corp., it costs only ~$50 at Amazon. An ITC HA made by *easyuslife,* sold through Amazon, uses DSP and costs $70. Common to many Amazon-marketed HAs is a relatively high level of customer dissatisfaction. Some of this may come from the do-it-yourself nature of the sale; customers must fit and adjust their HAs themselves, and may have unwarranted high expectations of their performance. Other customer dissatisfaction may arise from shoddy overseas manufacturing processes. Many Amazon HA prices are ~1/10 that of similar HAs acquired through professional audiologists.

18.13 "SMART" WOUND DRESSINGS

Strictly speaking, a bandage over a wound, burn, or scald is not a therapeutic device. Its function is to keep dirt and bacteria out of the wound. However, you will see that the novel wound dressings described in this section do have a therapeutic value: They release a targeted antibiotic on infection-causing bacteria under them and also signal caregivers that the wound is infected (Just 2010, Zyga 2010, Zhou et al. 2010). Pathogenic bacteria in wounds (for example, *Pseudomonas aeruginosa, Staphylococcus aureus*) generally form a biofilm; a confluent community of adhering bacteria encased in an extracellular biopolymeric matrix (Thet et al. 2015).

One version of the "smart" wound dressing is made from nonwoven polypropylene fabric. Attached to the membrane are nanovesicles containing an antibacterial agent. One of the virulence factors of many pathogenic bacteria is that they secrete toxins or enzymes that damage the nanovesicle membranes and lyse them. When they rupture, the vesicles release the antibacterial agent and destroy the pathogenic bacteria; a very targeted antisepsis. Nonpathogenic, commensal skin bacteria (e.g., *Escherichia coli* and *Lactobacillus* spp. in the patient's microbiome) do not secrete enzymes that lyse the nanovesicles. Thet et al. (2015) reported on an improved, "smart" wound dressing made from a hydrated agarose film in which a fluorescent dye was placed inside the nanovesicles with the antibiotic. The dye is released when the vesicles are lysed by the pathogenic bacteria, signifying their presence. The UK researchers who are developing these smart dressings have patented them (Jenkins et al. 2015), and expect to have safety testing completed in the EU by 2017.

18.14 NEGATIVE-PRESSURE WOUND THERAPY

Negative-pressure wound therapy (NPWT) is an NI therapeutic means of expediting wound healing by applying a vacuum through a special, sterile, dressing sealed to the skin around the wound. A continuously or intermittently applied partial vacuum of ~-75–125 mmHg is used to draw out fluid (serum, pus) from the wound to prevent its accumulation and possible infection; the vacuum also increases blood flow under the dressing. NPWT devices may also support the delivery of fluids to the wound, for example, saline, antibiotics, etc.; intermittent removal of the used fluid supports cleaning and drainage of the wound bed. An example of an improved NPWT dressing is found in the US Patent Application EP1758837 B1 filed 6/20/05 by P.W. Watt et al. for *Systagenix Wound Management IP Co. BV.* The first company to have an NPWT product cleared by the US FDA was *Kinetic Concepts,* in 1995. *Worldwide Innovative Health Care* (WiCare) offers a mechanically operated Wound-Pump™ NPWT device (2013) (Domings 2016). Their Wound-Pump does not require line electric power (or batteries).

NPWT dressings have been used effectively for diabetic ulcers, burns, bedsores, deep wounds requiring effective drainage, etc. The best results have been seen in treating the diabetes-associated chronic leg wounds (Xie et al. 2010).

18.15 GENE EDITING WITH CRISPR-Cas9 AND CRISPR-Cpf1 AS A PROSPECTIVE THERAPY FOR GENETIC DISEASES

18.15.1 Genetic Disorders

There are many known and suspect human genetic disorders. They are caused by: (1) A point mutation (**P**), or any insertion/deletion entirely inside one gene. (2) Deletion of a gene (or genes) (**D**). (3) A whole extra chromosome (e.g., in Down syndrome), and/or missing chromosome (**C**). (4) Trinucleotide repeat disorders (**T**), where a gene is extended in length. In Table 18.3, some of the most common genetic disorders, the type of causative mutation, the chromosome involved, and the approximate prevalence in the population are listed.

Table 18.3: Some Common Genetic Disorders. Hundreds of Others Exist

Disorder	Cause	Chromosome	Prevalence
Color blindness	P	X	Red/green, males: 6.6%
Cri du chat	D	5p15	1:50,000
Cystic fibrosis	P	7q	1:2000
Down syndrome	C	21	~1:1000
Duchenne muscular dystrophy	D	Xp	1:7000
Hemophilia	P	X	1:10,000
Klinefelter syndrome	C	X	
Neurofibromatosis Type 2	—	17q11.2/22q11-13.1	1:60,000
Phenylketonuria	P	12q	1:12,000
Polycystic kidney disease	P	16(PKD1) or 4(PKD2)	1:2500
Prader–Willi syndrome	D, C	15 (q11-13)	$1:10^4$–1:25,000 newborns
Sickle-cell anemia	P	11p	1:625
Tay–Sachs disease	P	15 (HEXA gene)	1:30 Ashkenazi Jews

18.15.2 Correcting Chromosome Damage with Genetically Engineered CRISPR-Cas9 and CRISPR-Cpf1 Gene Editing Tools

First, we must ask if gene editing is/or can be a truly NIT. We begin by describing some recent successes using animal (mouse) models. Much more research must be done before CRISPR-based gene editing can become an approved tool to treat human genetic disorders.

In the past 4 years, much research has been done toward genome editing with the ultimate goal of correcting and/or eliminating the expression of certain genetic diseases and conditions in individuals and bloodlines. Use has been made of the CRISPR-Cas molecular systems originally found in certain bacteria which used them as an adaptive defense against invading bacteriophage viruses and plasmids. CRISPR stands for Clustered Regularly Interspaced Short Palindromic Repeats; Cas stands for CRISPR-associated systems (DNA nucleases).

Yin et al. (2014) reported on the successful use of the CRISPR-Cas9 molecular system to correct a *Fah* gene mutation in a mouse hepatocyte model of the human disease, *Hereditary Tyrosinemia, Type 1* (cf. Glossary). Delivery of components of the CRISPR-Cas9 system by hydrodynamic tail vein injection resulted in initial expression of the wild-type *Fah* protein in ~1/120 liver cells. Expansion of normal *Fah*-positive hepatocytes corrected the body weight-loss phenotype. The authors commented: "Our study indicates that CRISPR-Cas9-mediated genome editing is possible in adult animals and has potential for correction of human genetic diseases."

A report by Wu et al. (2013) showed that mice with a dominant mutation in their *Crygc* gene that causes cataracts could be rescued by coinjection into their zygotes of Cas9 mRNA and a single-guide RNA (sgRNA) targeting the mutant allele. Correction occurred by homology-directed repair (HDR). They found that the treated mice were fertile, and able to transmit the corrected allele to their progeny.

Mice carrying mutations in multiple genes were created by use of CRISPR-Cas injections into embryonic stem cells and zygotes (Wang et al. 2013). As many as five genes were disrupted (*Tet-1, -2, -3, Sry,* and *Uty-8* alleles) in mouse embryonic stem cells. The purpose of the study was to allow the one-step generation of animals carrying mutations in multiple genes, an approach that will greatly accelerate the *in vivo* study of functionally redundant genes and of epistatic gene interactions.

In a recent review paper, Hsu et al. (2014) described the development and applications CRISPR-Cas9 for genomic engineering. They stated: "...we describe the development and application of Cas9 for a variety of research or translational applications while highlighting challenges as well as future directions. Derived from a remarkable microbial defense system, Cas9 is driving innovative applications from basic biology to biotechnology and medicine."

Also, see the papers by Nuñez et al. (2016) and Wright et al. (2016) for more information on "tunable" genome engineering. Cradick et al. (2013) and Ran et al. (2013) have discussed the problem and solutions for off-target activity of CRISPR-Cas9 systems.

Recently, a different CRISPR-associated endonuclease, Cpf1, has been discovered and characterized (Ledford 2015, Zetsche et al. 2015). Zetsche et al. demonstrated "that Cpf1 mediates robust

DNA interference with features distinct from Cas9. Cpf1 is a single RNA-guided endonuclease lacking tracrRNA, and it utilizes a T-rich protospacer-adjacent motif. Moreover, Cpf1 cleaves [targeted] DNA via a staggered DNA double-stranded break." "Cpf1 contains a single identified nuclease domain, in contrast to the two nuclease domains present in Cas9."

Cpf1 is a single crRNA-guided endonuclease, unlike Cas9 which requires tracrRNA to process crRNA arrays. Zetsche et al. commented: "For example, the shorter ($\approx$42 nt) crRNA employed by Cpf1 has practical advantages over the long ($\approx$100 nt) guide RNA in Cas9-based systems because shorter RNA oligos are significantly easier and cheaper to synthesize." Cpf1 could provide an effective way to precisely introduce DNA into a target genome by nonhomology-directed repair mechanisms. Cpf1 needs only one RNA molecule to guide its cut of DNA, while the Cas9 endonuclease requires two guide RNAs. Also, Cpf1 leaves one DNA strand longer than the other, creating "sticky" ends that are easier to work with.

The reader might ask, can the use of CRISPR-Cas9 or CRISPR-Cpf1 for the repair of genomic damage causing human genetic diseases be an NIT? At present, the answer is yes and no. From the mouse studies described above, if *in vitro* fertilization is used, the therapy can be a *fait accompli* for F1 and subsequent generations if a zygote is used. Injection of an adult with the necessary CRISPR molecules is also possible; however, this is semi-invasive. In this case, the affected target cells must be self-replicating in order to reproduce the corrected gene(s), such as in liver cells and certain epithelial cells. The bottom line is that somehow the necessary CRISPR molecules must be presented to the genome containing the bad genes, either by injection to the body or by presentation to embryonic stem cells, or via a zygote. The problem of genome editing specificity must be solved (Ran et al. 2013).

18.16 CHAPTER SUMMARY

Section 18.2 presented a summary of certain NITs and therapeutic devices. We began by describing NI brain stimulation therapies using AC magnetic fields and electric currents applied to the scalp.

The use of US to treat OA was described in Section 18.3, and the use of ionizing radiations and LF, AC electromagnetic fields to fight tumors was described in Sections 18.4 and 18.5. TENS used to mitigate pain was described in Section 18.6. Section 18.7 described ICT, its theory and applications. Bone healing using pulsed electric and magnetic fields was considered in Section 18.8. The category of noninvasive pneumatic therapies (CPAP & BPAP) was covered in Section 18.9.

In Section 18.10, we reviewed the recent research on mouse models showing that US therapy could mitigate the physiological and behavioral symptoms of AD. Extending this therapy from mice to humans is the challenge.

In Section 18.11, we concluded this chapter by describing recent advances in HA technology (spectrum manipulation) using DSP.

The technology of modern HAs was examined in Section 18.12, and Section 18.13 described a prototype "smart" bandage that used microvesicles to deliver targeted antibiotics to certain pathogens, as well as signaling their presence with a fluorescent dye.

The prospects of enzymatic gene editing with bioengineered CRISPR complexes to cure certain genetic diseases were discussed in Section 18.14.

Bibliography

ACGS. 2015. *Association for Clinical Genetic Science*. Accessed 12/16/15 at: www.acgs.uk.com/about-us.aspx.

ACHE. 2014. *Cefaly for Migraine Prevention?* Online ACHE Newsletter. 2pp. Accessed 1/20/15 at: www.achenet.org/resources/cefaly_for_migraine_prevention/.

ACHRE. 1994. *Advisory Committee on Human Radiation Experiments*. Online US Government Report. Accessed 3/20/15 at: https://bioethicsarchive.georgetown.edu/achre/.

ACS. 2015. *Mammography*. 3pp online article. American Cancer Society. Accessed 10/19/15 at: www.cancer.org/treatment/understandingyourdiagnosis/examsandtestdescriptions/imagingradiologytests/imaging-radiology-tests-mammogram.

ADA. 2013. Economic cost of diabetes in the U.S. in 2012. *Diabetes Care*. 36(4): 1033–1046.

Adler, A. 2008. *Electrical Impedance Tomography: Image Algorithms and Applications*. 66pp BIOM5200 Class Notes. Accessed 3/17/16 at: www.sce.carleton.ca/faculty/adler/talks/2008/biom5200-Electrical-Impedance-Tomography.pdf.

Adler, F.H. 1933. *Clinical Physiology of the Eye*. Macmillan, NY.

Alcoholism. 2014. *Alcohol in Urine Test*. 2pp online article. Accessed 4/03/15 at: alcoholism.about.com/od/work/a/etg.htm.

Alexander, J.M. 2012. Frequency lowering in hearing aids. *2012 ISHA Convention Presentation*. March 29–31. 12pp. Accessed 6/12/15 at: www.islha.org/Resources/Documents/Alexander20201220Frequency%20Lowering.pdf.

AICR. 2013. *Cancer Mortality Compared to Other Diseases*. 3pp online information bulletin. Accessed 6/23/15 at: www.aicr.org/learn-more-about-cancer/infographics-mortality.html?gclid=CMG4zMz5pcYCFYU8gQod4hsAAw.

Alix-Panabières, C. and K. Pantel. 2013a. Circulating tumor cells: Liquid biopsy of cancer. *Clin. Chem.* 59(1): 110–118.

Alix-Panabières, C. and K. Pantel. 2013b. Real-time liquid biopsy in cancer patients: Fact or fiction? *Cancer Res.* 73(21): OF1–OF5. doi: 10.1158/0008-5472.CAN-13-2030.

Alix-Panabières, C. and K. Pantel. 2013c. Real-time liquid biopsy: Circulating tumor cells versus circulating tumor DNA. *Ann. Transl. Med.* 1(2): 2pp. Accessed 3/29/15 at: www.ncbi.nlm.nih.gov/pmc/articles/PMC4200637/pdf/atm-01-02-18.pdf.

Alqasemi, U., H. Li, G. Yuan, P. Kumavor, S. Zanganeh and Q. Zhu. 2014. Interlaced photoacoustic and ultrasound imaging system with real-time coregistration for ovarian tissue characterization. *J. Biomed. Opt.* 19(7): 8.

Anbar, M. 1998. Clinical thermal imaging today. *IEEE Eng. Med. Biol. Mag.* 17(4): 25–33.

Andersson, B. et al. 1998. Glucose concentration in parotid saliva after glucose/food intake in individuals with glucose intolerance and diabetes mellitus. *Eur. J. Oral Sci.* 106(5): 931–937.

Andor. 2014. *Diffuse Reflectance Imaging Sheds Light on Oral Cancer*. 2pp web article. Accessed 2/29/16 at: www.spectroscopynow.com/details/news/143b5501d2c/Diffuse-Reflectance-Imaging-sheds-light-on-Oral-Cancer.html?tzcheck=1,1,1,1,1,1,1,1&tzcheck=1.

Andor. 2015. *Raman Micro-Spectroscopy: A Diagnostic Aid to Skin Cancers*. 2pp web article. Accessed 7/11/15 at: file:///C:/Users/Owner/Downloads/Andor_Learning_Raman_micro-spectroscopy.pdf.

APACOR. 2013. *RAPYDTEST® for the Detection of Human Haemoglobin in Faeces*. 4pp sheet. Accessed 5/31/15 at: www.apacor.com/PDF/APA056-FaecalOccultBloodDipstick.pdf.

Appn. 2014. *Alere INRatio©2 Method and Sample Collection. IE.8.v4. Issue date 08.08.14*. 9pp. Accessed 12/17/14 at: www.appn.net.au/Data/Sites/1/appn/02implementation/technicalresources/inr/aler-einratio2methodandsamplecollection.pdf.

Anger, H.O. 1964. Scintillation camera with multichannel collimators. *J. Nuc. Med*. 5: 515–531.

Anguiano, A. et al. 2012. Spectral Karyotyping for identification of constitutional chromosomal abnormalities at a national reference laboratory. *Mol. Cytogenet*. 5(3): 6.

Arnold, M.A. and D.C. Klonoff. 1999. Noninvasive laser measurement of blood glucose in the eye: A bright idea or an optical illusion? *Editor. Diabetes Technol. Ther*. 1(2): 117–119.

Artyomov, E., A. Fish and O. Yadid-Pecht. 2007. Image sensors in security and medical applications. *Int. J. Inform. Theor. Appl*. 14: 114–127.

ASGE. 2013. Technology status evaluation report: Wireless capsule endoscopy. *Gastrointest. Endosc*. 78(6): 805–815. http://dx.doi.org/10.1016/j.gie.2013.06.026.

Athanasiou, A. et al. 2006. The effect of pulsed electromagnetic fields on secondary skin wound healing: An experimental study. *Bioelectromagnetics*. Published online by Wiley InterScience. 7pp. doi: 10.1002/bem.20303 Accessed 2/02/15 at: www.papimi.com/papimi%20studies/skin%20wound%20healing%mice/bioelectromagnetics_papimi.pdf.

Ayow, T.M., F. Paquet, J. Dallaire, M. Purden and K.A. Champagne. 2009. Factors influencing the use and nonuse of continuous positive airway pressure therapy: A comparative case study. *Rehabil. Nurs*. 34(6): 230–236. doi: 10.1002/j.2048-7490.2009.tb00255.x.

Ayub, M. and H. Bailey. 2012. Individual RNA base recognition in immobilized oligonucleotides using a protein nanopore. *Nano Lett*. 12(11): 5637–5643. doi: 10.1021/nl3027873.

Azevedo, F.A. et al. 2009. Equal numbers of neuronal and nonneuronal cells make the human brain an isometrically scaled-up primate brain. *J. Comp. Neurol*. 513(5): 532–541. doi: 10.1002/cne.21974.

Badawi, R. 1999. *Introduction to PET Physics*. Table of contents with hotlinks. Online tutorial. Accessed 6/30/15 at: depts.washington.edu/nucmed/IRL/pet_intro/.

Bakeev, K.A., R. Thomas, R. Chirmenti and M. Claybourn. 2013. The use of Raman spectroscopy in cancer diagnostics. *Spectroscopy*. 28(9): 6pp. Accessed 10/15/15 at: www.spectroscopyonline.com/use-raman-spectroscopy-cancer-diagnostics-0.

Baker, L. 2000. Blood test measures radiation damage. *The University of Buffalo Reporter*. 31(18): 3pp web article. Accessed 6/24/15 at: www.buffalo.edu/ubreporter/archive/vol31/vol31n18/n8.html.

Bandorski, D. et al. 2011. Review Article: Capsule endoscopy in patients with cardiac pacemakers, implantable cardioverter defibrillators, and left heart devices: A review of the current literature. *Diagn. Ther. Endosc*. 2011: Article ID 376053, 6pp. doi: 10.1155/2011/376053.

Barker, A.T. and I. Freeston. 2007. Transcranial magnetic stimulation. *Scholarpedia*. 2(10): 2936. 5pp. Accessed 11/29/14 at: www.scholarpedia.org/article/Transcutaneous_magnetic_stimulation.

Barnes Engineering Co. 1983. *Handbook of Infrared Radiation Measurement*. Barnes Engineering Co., Stamford, CT.

Barro, S. et al. 1998. Classifying multichannel ECG patterns with an adaptive neural network. *IEEE Eng. Med. Biol. Mag.* 17(1): 45–55.

Bartlett, J.M.S. and D. Stirling, Eds. 2003. *PCR Protocols, 226: (Methods in Molecular Biology, Vol. 226).* 2nd Ed. Humana Press, New York, NY, August 1, 2003. ISBN-10: 0896036278. 556pp.

Bartsch, H., C. Bartsch, W.E. Simon, B. Flehming, I. Ebels and T.H. Lippert. 1992. Antitumor activity of the pineal gland: Effect of unidentified substances versus the effect of melatonin. *Oncology* 49(1): 27–30. doi: 10.1159/0000227005.

Basel. 2006. *Fluorescence and Phosphorescence.* March 27, 2006. 15pp web tutorial. Accessed 1/04/15 at: https://physik.unibas.ch/Praktikum/VPII/Fluoreszenz/Flouresence_and_phosphorescence.pdf.

Bassett, C.A.L. 1993. Beneficial effects of electromagnetic fields. *J. Cell. Biochem.* 51(4): 387–393.

Bastiaans, M.J. 1997. Application of the Wigner distribution function in optics. In: *The Wigner Distribution—Theory and Application in Signal Processing.* W. Mecklenbrauker and F. Hlawatsch, Eds. Elsevier Science, Amsterdam, Netherlands. pp. 375–426.

Beach, R.D., F.v. Küster and F. Moussy. 1999. Subminiature implantable potentiostat and modified commercial telemetry device for remote glucose monitoring. *IEEE Trans. Instrum. Meas.* 48(6): 1239–1245.

Beck, B.R. et al. 2008. Do capacitively-coupled electric fields accelerate tibial stress fracture healing? *Am. J. Sports Med.* 36(3): 545–553. doi: 10.1177/0363546507310076.

Becker, R.P., C.A.L. Basset and C.H. Bachman. 1964. Bioelectric factors controlling bone structure. In: *Bone Biodynamics.* H. Frost, Ed. Little-Brown, NY. pp. 209–232.

Behrens, S.B., M.E. Deren and K.O. Monchik. 2013. A review of bone growth stimulation for fracture treatment. *Curr. Orthop. Pract.* 24(1): 84–91.

Bennett, T.J. 2013. *Scanning Laser Ophthalmoscopy.* 3pp web paper. Accessed 5/03/15 at: www.opsweb.org/page=SLO.

Benowitz, S. 2014. *Nanopore DNA Sequencing: New Approaches to an Old Challenge.* 2pp online research note. Accessed 3/20/15 at: www.genome.gov/27555652.

Berger, A.J. et al. 1999. Multicomponent blood analysis by near-infrared Raman spectroscopy. *Applied Optics.* 38(13): 2916–2926.

Bergholt, M.S. et al. 2013. (Review Article): Raman endoscopy for objective diagnosis of early cancer in the gastrointestinal system. *J. Gastroint. Dig. Syst. S* 1: 5pp. http://dx.doi.org/10.4172/2161-069X.S1-008.

Bertone, P. and M. Snyder. 2005. Advances in functional protein microarray technology. *FEBS J.* 272: 5400–5411.

BioSpace. 2015. *Urine Test for Early Stage Pancreatic Cancer Possible After Biomarker Discovery.* 2pp web paper. Accessed 8/04/15 at: www.biospace.com/News/early-stage-pancreatic-cancer-urine-test-possible/386505.

Bisset, G.S. et al. 1996. Perflubron as a gastrointestinal MR imaging contrast agent in the pediatric population. *Pediatr. Radiol.* 26(6): 409–415. doi: 10.1007/BF01387316.

Blank, T.B. et al. 1999. The use of near infrared diffuse reflectance for the noninvasive prediction of blood glucose. *IEEE LEOS Newsletter.* 13(5): 9–12. Accessed 4/21/15 at: photonicssociety.org/newsletters/oct99/article5.htm.

Blazek, K. et al. 1995. YAP multi-crystal gamma camera prototype. *IEEE Trans. Nucl. Sci.* 42(5): 1474–1482.

Blume, S.W. and J.R. Curtis. 2011. Medical costs of osteoporosis in the elderly Medicare population. *Osteoporos. Intl.* 22(6): 1835–1844.

Boeijinga, P.H. 2002. Objective markers of drug effects on brain function from recordings of scalp potential in healthy volunteers. *Dialogues Clin. Neurosci.* 4(4): 388–394. Accessed 4/30/15 at: www.ncbi.nlm.nih.gov/pmc/articles/PMC3181706/pdf/DialoguesClinNeurosci-4-388.pdf.

Bonnick, S.L. 1998. *Bone Densitometry in Clinical Practice: Application and Interpretation.* Humana Press, New York, NY.

Boopalan, P.R.J.V.C. et al. 2011. Pulsed electromagnetic field therapy results in healing of full thickness articular cartilage defect. *Int. Orthop.* 35: 143–148. doi: 10.1007/s00264-0100994-8.

Barber, S. 2005. *Hearing Aid "Sticker Shock" and Things to Consider When Purchasing.* 7pp web article. Accessed 6/18/15 at: www.nchearingloss.org/article_costofhearingaids.htm.

Boushey, C.J. et al. 1995. A quantitative assessment of plasma homocysteine as a risk factor for vascular disease. *JAMA.* 274(13): 1049–1057.

Bronstrup, A. et al. 1998. Effects of folic acid and combinations of folic acid and vitamin B12 on plasma homocysteine concentrations in healthy young women. *Am. J. Clin. Nutr.* 68: 1104–1110.

Browne, A.F. 1998. *A New Approach to Monitoring Glucose Concentration Based on Reflection of Polarized Light from a Liquid/Lens Interface and Detection by an Improved Closed-Loop Optical Polarimeter.* PhD dissertation. The University of Connecticut. Area: Biomedical Engineering. (R.B. Northrop, major advisor).

Brozek-Pluska, B. et al. 2012. Raman spectroscopy and imaging: Applications in human breast cancer diagnosis. *Analyst.* 137: 3773–3780.

Brownbill, R.A. and J.Z. Ilich. 2005. Measuring body composition in overweight individuals by dual energy X-ray absorptiometry. *BMC Med. Imaging.* 5(1): 7. doi: 10.1186/1471-2342-5-1.

Braig, J.R., D.S. Goldberger and S.B. Bernhard. 1997. *Self-Emission Noninvasive Infrared Spectrophotometer with Body Temperature Compensation.* US Patent No. 5,615,672. April 1, 1997.

Brauchle, E. and K. Schenke-Layland. 2013. Review: Raman spectroscopy in biomedicine— Non-invasive in vitro analysis of cells and extracellular matrix components in tissues. *Biotechnol. J.* 8: 288–297. doi: 10.1002/biot.201200163.

Brown, L.J. 1980. A new instrument for the simultaneous measurement of total hemoglobin, percent oxyhemoglobin, percent carboxyhemoglobin, percent methemoglobin, and oxygen content in whole blood. *IEEE Trans. Biomed. Eng.* 27(3): 132–138.

Browne, A.F. 1998. *A New Approach to Monitoring Glucose Concentrations Based on Reflections of Polarized Light from a Liquid/Lens Interface and Detection by an Improved Closed-Loop Optical Polarimeter.* PhD dissertation. The University of Connecticut, Storrs. Area: Biomedical Engineering (R.B. Northrop, advisor).

Bruce, J.N. 2014. *Glioblastoma Multiforme.* 11pp Medscape web article. Accessed 1/21/15 at: emedicine.medscape.com/article/283252-overview.

Brunoni, A.R. et al. 2012. Clinical research with transcranial direct current stimulation (tDCS): Challenges and future directions. *Brain Stimul.* 5(3): 175–193. doi: 10.1016/j.brs.2011.03.002.

Bukhari, I. 2013. *Early Detection of Alzheimer's—A Crucial Requirement.* 4pp online paper. Accessed 4/14/16 at: https://arxiv.org/ftp/arxiv/papers/1305/1305.2713.pdf.

Burmeister, J.J., M.A. Arnold and G.W. Small. 1998. Spectroscopic considerations for non-invasive blood glucose measure-ments. *IEEE LEOS Newsletter.* 12(2): 6–9.

Butler, N.R. and C.M. Marshall. 2004. *Uncooled Focal Plane Array Sensor.* US Patent No. 6,791,610. Issued September 14, 2004.

Cabib, D. et al. 1996. *Method for Simultaneously Measuring the Spectral Intensity as a Function of Wavelength for All of the Pixels in a Two-Dimensional; Scene.* US Patent No. 5,539,517. July 23, 1996.

Cabib, D. et al. 1998. *Spectral Bio-Imaging Methods for Biological Research, Medical Diagnosis and Therapy.* US Patent No. 5,784,162. July 21, 1998.

Calzón, F.S. and M.A. Llanos. 2013. Terapia de campo de tumores en el tratamiento del glioblastoma. Revisión sistemática. (*Tumor Treating Fields Therapy [TTF] for Glioblastoma. A Systematic Review of the Literature.*) Online report in Spanish. Agencia de Evaluación de Tecnologias Sanitarias de Andalucía. Accessed 1/21/15 at: www.juntadeandalucia.es/salud/servicios/contenidos/nuevaaetsa/up/AETSA_2012_lioblastoma.pdf.

Cancer. 2015. *Prostate Cancer: Survival Rates for Prostate Cancer.* 2pp online bulletin by the American Cancer Society. Accessed 6/23/15 at: www.cancer.org/cancer/prostatecancer/detailedguide/prostate-cancer-survival-rates.

Carroll, F.E. et al. 1991. Production of tunable, monochromatic X-rays by the Vanderbilt free-electron laser. *Proc. SPIE.* 3614: 8pp. Free-Electron Laser Challenges II, 139 (July 19, 1991). (Conf. Vol. 3614.)

Castle, J.R. and W.K. Ward. 2010. Amperometric glucose sensors: Sources of error and potential benefit of redundancy. *J. Diabetes Sci. Technol.* 4(1): 221–225.

Cavallerano, A.A. et al. 1994. *Optometric Clinical Practice Guideline: Care of the Patient with Age-Related Macular Degeneration.* American Optometric Association, St. Louis, MO.

Cave, D. 2015. Wireless video capsule endoscopy. *UpToDate®.* 2pp. Accessed 4/01/15 at: www.uptodate.com/contents/wireless-video-capsule-endoscopy.

Chandra, H., P.J. Reddy and S. Srivastava. 2011. Protein microarrays and novel detection platforms. *Expert Rev. Proteomics.* 8(1): 61–79.

Chang, T.W. 1983. Binding cells to matrixes of distinct antibodies coated on solid surface. *J. Immunol. Methods.* 65(1–2): 217–223. doi: 10.1016/0022-1759(83)90318-6.

Chao, C.-L. et al. 1999. Effect on short-term vitamin (folic acid, vitamin B6, and B12) administration on endothelial function induced by post-methionine load hyperhomocysteinemia. *Am. J. Cardiol.* 84: 1356–1361.

Cheing, G.L.Y. and C.W.Y. Hui-Chan. 2003. Analgesic effects of transcutaneous electrical nerve stimulation and interferential currents on heat pain in healthy subjects. *J. Rehabil. Med.* 35: 15–19.

Cherry, G. 2016. Flexible film may lead to phone-sized cancer detector. *Michigan News.* 3pp online news bulletin. Accessed 2/17/16 at: ns.umich.edu/new/multimedia/slideshows/23406-flexible-film-may-lead-to-phone-sized-cancer-detector.

Chin, T.J. and M. McGrath. 1998. Diagnoses of deep vein thromboses. *Australian Prescriber.* 21: 6pp.

CIRS. 2015. Tissue Simulation and Phantom Technology. Products. *CIRS.* Accessed 4/15/15 at: www.cirsinc.com/products/all.

Clayton, R.H., R.W.F. Campbell and A. Murray. 1998. Characteristics of multichannel ECG recordings during human ventricular tachyarrhythmias. *IEEE Eng. Med. Biol. Mag.* 17(1): 39–44.

Collins, C.M. et al. 2002. Numerical calculations of the static magnetic field in three-dimensional multi-tissue models of the human head. *Magn. Reson. Imaging.* 20: 413–424.

Collins, R.D. 1968. *Illustrated Manual of Laboratory Diagnosis: Indications and Interpretations.* J.B. Lippincott Co., Philadelphia, PA.

Cote, G.L. 2001. Noninvasive and minimally-invasive optical monitoring technologies. *J. Nutr.* 131: 1596S–1604S.

Courbet, A., D. Endy, E. Renard, F. Molina and J. Bonnet. 2015. Detection of pathological biomarkers in human clinical samples via amplifying genetic switches and logic gates. *Sci. Transl. Med.* 7(289): 289ra83. doi: 10.1126/scitranslmed.aaa.3601.

CPLFig. 2015. Figure illustrating the generation of left-handed circularly polarized light. Accessed 2/17/16 at: https://commons.wikimedia.org/wiki/File:Circular.Polarization.Circular.Polarized. Light_Circular.Polarizer_Creating.Left.Handed.Helix.View.svg (Figure is public domain.).

Cradick, T.J. et al. 2013. CRISPR/Cas9 systems targeting β-globin and CCR5 genes have substantial off-target activity. *Nucleic Acids Res.* 41(20): 9584–9592. doi: 10.1093/nar/gkt714.

Croce, R.A. Jr. et al. 2013. A miniaturized transcutaneous system for continuous glucose monitoring. *Biomed Microdevices.* 15(1): 151–160. doi: 10.1007/s10544-012-9708-x.

Cuneo, B.F. et al. 2013. *In utero* diagnosis of long QT syndrome by magnetocardiography. *Circulation.* 128: 2183–2191. doi: 10.1161/CIRCULATIONAHA.113.004840.

Cunningham, R.F. 2011. *Otoacoustic Emissions: Beyond Newborn Hearing Screening. Audiology Online* March 14, 2011. 5pp online article. Accessed 3/15/15 at: www.audiologyonline.com/articles/otoacoustic-emissions-beyond-newborn-hearing-838.

Curatronic® Ltd-. 2015. *Scientific Articles and Abstracts.* 6pp web article. Accessed 1/27/15 at: www.curatronic.com/scientific2.html.

Curran, L.J. 2000. Imaging system equips ophthalmologists with noninvasive detection method. *Vision Systems Design.* August: 30–32.

Daghigian, F. et al. 1993. Evaluation of a cerium doped lutetium orthosilicate (LSO) scintillation crystal for PET. *IEEE Trans. Nucl. Sci.* 40(4): 1045–1047.

Dähne, C. and D. Gross. 1987. *Spectrophotometric Method and Apparatus for the Non-Invasive [sic].* US Patent No. 4,655,225. April 7, 1987. (NIR transcutaneous measurement of blood glucose.)

Danne, T., K. Lange and O. Kodonouri. 2008. Real-time glucose sensors in children and adolescents with Type-1 diabetes. *Horm. Res.* 70: 193–202. doi: 10.1159/000151592 (Mini Review).

Davidson, M. 2015. *Optical Microscopy Primer: Fundamentals of Film Exposure.* 14pp online article. Accessed 11/24/15 at: micro.magnet.fsu.edu/primer/photomicrography/filmexposure.html.

Davies, A.M., U. Weinberg and Y. Palti. 2013. Tumor treating fields: A new frontier in cancer therapy. *Ann. N.Y. Acad. Sci.* 1291: 86–95. doi: 10.1111/nyas.12112.

D'Ambrosio, C. et al. 1998. The ISPA-tube and the HPMT, two examples of a new class of photodetectors: The hybrid photodetectors. *Nucl. Phys. B. (Proc. Suppl.)* 61B: 638–643.

D'Ambrosio, C. et al. 1999. Further developments on an ISPA-camera for γ-rays in nuclear medicine. *Nucl. Physics B. (Proc. Suppl.)* 78: 598–603.

Danino, T. et al. 2015. Programmable probiotics for detection of cancer in urine. *Sci. Transl. Med.* 7(289): 289ra84. doi: 10.1126/scitranslmed.aaa3519.

Davenport, L. 2014. *No Benefit From Ultrasound Screening in Dense Breasts*. 4pp web article. Accessed 2/07/16 at: www.medscape.com/viewarticle/836106#vp_2.

de Berardinis, E., O. Tieri, A. Polzella and N. Iuglio. 1965. The chemical composition of the human aqueous humor in normal and pathological conditions. *Exp. Eye Res.* 4: 179–186.

de Boer, J.F. et al. 1999. Polarization effects in optical coherence tomography of various biological tissues. *IEEE J. Sel. Top. Quantum Electron.* 5(4): 1200–1204.

de Kock, J.P. and L. Tarassenko. 1993. Pulse oximetry: Theoretical and experimental models. *Med. Bio. Eng. Comput.* 31: 291–300.

de Kock, J.P. et al. 1993. Reflectance pulse oximetry measurements from the retinal fundus. *IEEE Trans. Biomed. Eng.* 40(8): 817–823.

Deng, Z.-D., S.H. Lisanby and A.V. Peterchev. 2014. Coil design considerations for deep transcranial magnetic stimulation. *Clin. Neurophysiol.* 125(6): 1202–1212. http://dx.doi.org/10.1016/j.clinph.2013.11.038.

Diaz, L.A. and A. Bardelli. 2014. Liquid biopsies: Genotyping tumor DNA. *J. Clin. Oncol.* 32(6): 579–586. doi: 10.1200/JCO.2012.45.2011.

Dickson, H. 2010. The Analysis of Cadmium in Chocolate by Graphite Furnace Atomic Absorption Spectrometry. *Thermo Scientific Application Note 43034*. 2pp. Accessed 3/18/15 at: https://thermoscientific.com/content/dam/tfs/ATG/CMD/CMD%20Documents/AN-43034-Analysis-of-Cadmium-in-Chocolate-AA.pdf.

DiFiori, N. et al. 2013. Optoelectronic control of surface charge and translocation dynamics in solid-state nanopores. *Nat. Nanotechnol.* 8(12): 946–951. doi: 10.1038/nnano.2013.221.

Digitherm. 2015. *Digatherm Tablet*. 3pp online spec sheet. Accessed 7/6/15 at: vet.digatherm.com/products/.

Dilmanian, F.A. et al. 2000. Computed tomography of X-ray index of refraction using the diffraction enhanced imaging method. *Phys. Med. Biol.* 45: 933–936.

Ding, M. et al. 2000. Short-window spectral analysis of cortical event-related potentials by adaptive multivariate autoregressive modeling: Data preprocessing, model validation, and variability assessment. *Biol. Cybern.* 83: 35–45.

Doheny, K. 2015. *Breast Ultrasound vs. Mammography*. 4pp web article. Accessed 2/07/16 at: www.webmd.com/breast-cancer/news/20151228/breast-ultrasound-mammography-may-be-equally-effective-study.

Dougherty, D.M. et al. 2012. Comparing the detection of transdermal and breath alcohol concentrations during periods of alcohol consumption ranging from moderate to binge drinking. *Exp. Clin. Psychopharmacol.* 20(5): 373–381. doi: 10.1037/a0029021.

Domings, B. 2016. Building a better wound healer. *MIT Technology Review. Alumni Connection.* 119(1): 23.

Drake, A.D. and D.C. Leiner. 1984. A fiber Fizeau interferometer for measuring minute biological displacements. *IEEE Trans. Biomed. Eng.* 31(7): 507–511.

Durmus, N.G. et al. 2015. Magnetic levitation of single cells. *PNAS.* Pub. online June 29, 2015. E3661-E3668, at: www.pnas.org/cgi/doi/10.1073/pnas.1509250112.

Duteil, L., J.C. Bernengo and W. Schalla. 1985. A double wavelength laser Doppler system to investigate skin microcirculation. *IEEE Trans. Biomed. Eng.* 32(6): 439–447.

Dwight, H.B. 1969. *Tables of Integrals and Other Mathematical Data*, 4th Ed. MacMillan Co., London, UK.

Edgar, M., C. Dawes and D. O'Mullane, Eds. 2004. *Saliva and Oral Health*, 3rd Ed. British Dental Association, London, UK. ISBN: 0-904588-87-4.

Edic, P.M., G.J. Saulnier, J.C. Newell and D. Isaacson. 1995. A real-time electrical impedance tomograph. *IEEE Trans. Biomed. Eng.* 42(9): 849–859.

EGI. 2015. *Geodesic Sensor Nets.* 2pp online brochure. Accessed 7/16/15 at: www.egi.com/clinical-division/geodesic-sensor-nets; www.egi.com/clinical-division/clinical-division-clinical-products/ges-400-series.

Enejder, A.M.K. et al. 2005. Raman spectroscopy for noninvasive glucose measurements. *J. Biomed. Opt.* 10(3): 03114-1–03114-9.

Ercal, F.A. et al. 1994. Neural network diagnosis of malignant melanoma from color images. *IEEE Trans. Biomed. Eng.* 41(9): 837–845.

Everything.Explained.Today. 2015. *MRI Contrast Agent Explained.* 4pp web article. Accessed 10/23/15 at: everything.explained.today/MRI_contrast_agent/.

EyeWiki. 2015. *Optical Coherence Tomography.* 4pp web article. Accessed 3/26/16 at: eyewiki.aao.org/Optical_Coherence_tomography.

Falk, T.H., W.-Y. Chan, E. Sejdić and T. Chau. 2010. Spectro-temporal analysis of auscultatory sounds. Ch. 5. In: *New Developments in Biomedical Engineering.* D. Campolo, Ed. ISBN: 978-953-7619-57-2. pp. 93–104. Accessed 5/03/15 at: cdn.intechopen.com/pdfs-wm/9077.pdf.

Faraj, B.A. et al. 1981. Melanoma detection by enzyme-radioimmunoassay of L-dopa, dopamine, and 3-*o*-methyldopamine in urine. *Clin. Chem.* 27(1): 108–112.

Farimani, A.B., K. Min and N.R. Aluru. 2014. DNA Base detection using a single-layer MoS_2. *ACSNANO* 8(8): 7914–7922.

FDA. 2011. *510(k) Substantial Equivalence Determination Decision Summary.* (510(k) Number: k111731). FDA Market permission for Gamma Medica-Ideas Molecular Breast Imaging Software, June 20, 2011. Accessed 7/3/15 at: www.accesssdata.fda.gov/cdrh_docs/pdf11/K111731.pdf.

FDA. 2014. *510(k) Substantial Equivalence Determination Decision Summary.* (510(k) Number: k110212). 12pp. Accessed 12/17/12 at: www.accessdata.fda.gov/cdrh_docs/reviews/K110212.pdf.

FDA. 2015a. *Laser Products and Instruments.* 4pp online bulletin. Accessed 6/05/15 at: www.fda.gov/radiation-emittingproducts/radiationemittingproductsandprocedures/homebusinessandentertainment/laserproductsandinstruments/default.htm.

FDA. 2015b. *Medical Devices: How to Study and Market Your Device*. 7pp online bulletin. Accessed 6/05/15 at: www.fda.gov/MedicalDevices/DeviceRegulationandGuidance/HowtoMarketYourDevice/default.htm.

Feke, G.T., D.G. Goger, H. Tagawa and F.C. Delori. 1987. Laser Doppler technique for absolute measurement of blood speed in retinal vessels. *IEEE Trans. Biomed. Eng.* 34(9): 673–680.

Feldchtein, F.I. et al. 1998. Endoscopic applications of optical coherence tomography. *Opt. Express.* 3(6): 257–270.

Fellows, K.R. 1997. *The Design of a Non-Dispersive Spectrophotometer to Measure Oxyhemoglobin*. MS dissertation in Biomedical Engineering. University of Connecticut, Storrs. (R.B. Northrop, major advisor.)

Feng, J. et al. 2012. Nanoscale plasmonic interferometers for multispectral, high-throughput biochemical sensing. *Nano Lett.* 12(2): 602–609. doi: 10.1021/nl203325s.

Fernandes, M.P., S. Venkatesh, S. Narayanan and V.G. Prabitha. 2015. Diffuse reflectance image enhancement for cervical cancer detection—A review. *Int. J. Technol. Enhanc. Emerg. Eng. Res.* 3(5): 133–140.

Ferns, T. 2007. Respiratory auscultation: How to use a stethoscope. *Nurs. Times.* 103(24): 28–29.

Ferraro, J.A. 2000. *Clinical Electrocochleography: Overview of Theories, Techniques and Applications*. 13pp online paper. Accessed 2/19/15 at: www.audiologyonline.com/articles/clinical-electrocochleography-overview-theories-techniques-1275-1275.

Ferraro, J.A. and R. Tibbils. 1999. SP/AP area ratio in the diagnosis of Ménière's disease. *Am. J. Audiol.* 8(1): 21–27.

Fintek. 2015. *History of Fracture Healing with Electrical Stimulus*. 3pp web article. Accessed 10/25/15 at: www.fintek.ca/history-of-fracture-healing-with-electrical-stimulus/.

Fishbine, B. 2003. *SQUID Magnetometry. Los Alamos Research Quarterly*. Spring. 8pp. Accessed 3/27/15 at: www.lanl.gov/quarterly/q_spring03/pdfs/larq_4_03_squid.pdf.

Fitzgerald, R. 2000. Phase-sensitive X-ray imaging. *Physics Today.* 57(3): 23–26. http://dx.doi.org/10.1063/1.1292471.

Fjield, T., E.P. Harhen and P.D. Lopath. 2004. *Ultrasound Transducer Unit and Planar Ultrasound Lens*. US Patent No. 6,787,974 B2. September 7, 2004.

Fletcher, H. and W.A. Munson. 1933. Loudness, its definition, measurement and calculation. *J. Acoust. Soc. Am.* 5: 82–105.

Fliss, M. et al. 2000. Facile detection of mitochondrial DNA mutations in tumors and bodily [sic] fluids. *Science.* 287(5460): 2017–2019.

Follest-Strobl, P.C. et al. 1997. Homocysteine: A new risk factor for atherosclerosis. *Am. Fam. Physician.* 56: 1607–1612.

Forbat, L.N. et al. 1981. Glucose concentrations in parotid fluid and venous blood of patients attending a diabetic clinic. *J. Royal Soc. Med.* 74: 725–728.

Forbes, M., P. Guillermo, Jr. and B. Grolman. 1974. A noncontact applanation tonometer. *Arch. Ophthalmol.* 91(2): 134–140.

Foveon. 2010. *X3 Fill Light*. 2pp web article. Accessed 5/06/16 at: www.foveon.com/article. php?a=73.

Fox, M.D. 1978. Multiple crossed-beam ultrasound Doppler velocimetry. *IEEE Trans. Sonics Ultrason.* 25(5): 281–286.

Fox, M.D. and W.M. Gardiner. 1988. Three-dimensional Doppler velocimetry of flow jets. *IEEE Trans. Biomed. Eng.* 35(10): 834–841.

Fraden, J. 1989a. *Infrared Electronic Thermometer and Method for Measuring Temperature*. US Patent No. 4,485,730. January 10, 1989.

Fraden, J. 1989b. *Radiation Thermometer and Method for Measuring Temperature*. US Patent No. 4,845,730. August 8, 1989.

Fraden, J. 1993. *Balanced Infrared Thermometer and Method for Measuring Temperature*. US Patent No. 5,178,454. January 12, 1993.

Friedenberg, Z.B. and C.T. Brighton. 1966. Bioelectric potentials in bone. *J. Bone Joint Surg. Am.* 48(5): 915–923.

Friedenberg, Z.B., M.C. Harlow and C.T. Brighton. 1971. Healing of nonunion of the medial malleolus by means of direct current: A case report. *J. Trauma.* 11: 883–885.

Friedman, R.J. et al. 1985. Early detection of malignant melanoma: The role of physician examination and self-examination of the skin. *CA Cancer J. Clin.* 35(3): 130–151.

Fromow-Guerra, J. 2012. The evolution of confocal scanning laser ophthalmoscopy. *Retina Today.* Sept. 2012: 63–65. Accessed 5/03/15 at: retinatoday.com/pdfs/0912RT_F5_Fromow-Guerra.pdf.

Fujimoto, J.G. et al. 1995. Optical biopsy and imaging using optical coherence tomography. *Nat. Med.* 1: 970–972.

Fukada, E. and I. Yasuda. 1957. On the piezoelectric effect of bone. *J. Phy. Soc. Japan.* 12: 1158–1162.

Fye, W.B. 1999. Profiles in cardiology: Rudolf Albert von Koelliker. *Clin. Cardiol.* 22: 376–377. Accessed 4/29/15 at: onlinelibrary.wiley.com/doi/qo.1002/clc.4960220517/epdf.

Gaifulina, R., K. Lau, M. Rodriguez-Justo, C. Kendall and G.M. Thomas. 2014. Editorial. Light at the end of the tunnel: Application of Raman spectroscopy in colorectal cancer diagnosis. *Austin J. Clin. Pathol.* 1(5): 1021.

Galster, J.A. et al. 2012. Spectral iQ: Audibly improving access to high-frequency sounds. *Audiology Online.* 7pp. Accessed 6/13/15 at: www.audiologyonline.com/articles/spectral-iq-audibly-improving-access-778.

Garini, Y. et al. 1996. Spectral karyotyping. *Bioimaginoryg.* 4: 65–72.

Garini, Y., I.T. Young and G. McNamara. 2006. Spectral imaging: Principles and applications. *Cytometry Part A.* 69A: 735–747. doi: 10.1002/cyto.a.20311.

Germano, C.P. 1961. On the Meaning of "g" and "d" Constants as Applied to Simple Piezoelectric Modes of Vibration. Technical Paper TP-222. Gould, Inc. Piezoelectric Division, Bedford, OH.

Gerster, J., J. Kraus, M. Thürk and P. Seidel. 1998. Non-magnetic low noise pulse tube cryocooler for cooling high-T_c DC-SQUID gradiometers. *Proc. ICEC 17.* IOP Publishing, London. p. 97.

Gilham, E.J. 1957. A high-precision photoelectric polarimeter. *J. Sci. Instr.* 34: 435–439.

Gilles, C. et al. 2002. Human models as tools in the development of psychotropic drugs. *Dialogues Clin. Neurosci.* 4(4): 377–387. Accessed 4/30/15 at: www.ncbi.nlm.nih.gov/pmc/articles/PMC3181700/pdf/DialoguesClinNeurosci-4-377.pdf.

Glass, S.B. and Z.A. Shah. 2013. Clinical utility of positron emission tomography. *Baylor Univ. Med. Center Proc.* 26(3): 314–319. Accessed 10/19/15 at: www.ncbi.nih.gov/pmc/articles/PMC3684309/pdf/bumc0026-0314.pdf.

Glucometer. 2014. *Electrochemical Glucometers.* Class notes, Univ. of VA. 3pp. Accessed 12/19/14 at: faculty.virginia.edu/analyticalchemistry/Electrochem%20Gluc/Electrochem.html.

Goats, G.C. 1990. Interferential current therapy. *Br. J. Sports Med.* 24(2): 87–92.

Goldman, B.D. 1999. The circadian timing system and reproduction in mammals. *Steroids.* 64(9): 679–685.

Goldmann, H. 1957. Applanation tonometry. In: *Glaucoma: Trans. of Second Conf. Dec. 3–5, 1956. Princeton, NJ.* F.W. Newell, Ed. Madison Printing Co., Fort Worth, TX. pp. 167–220.

Goldman, Z.Z. 1987. *Human Auditory and Visual Continuous Evoked Potentials.* PhD dissertation in Biomedical Engineering. The University of Connecticut, Storrs. (R.B. Northrop, major advisor.)

Gong, J. and C.A. Glomski. 1997. *Method of Detecting a Mammal's Prior Exposure to Radiation or Radiomimetic Chemicals.* US Patent No. 5,691,157. November 25, 1997.

Gong, J. and C.A. Glomski. 2000. *Screening for Human Incubation with Radioactivity; Scanning Erythrocytes for Transferrin Receptors, and Comparing to Control Cell[s] That Have Not Been Incubated with Radio-Activity.* US Patent No. 6,132,981. October 17, 2000.

Gorski, D. 2015. "Liquid biopsies" for cancer screening: Life-saving tests, or overdiagnosis and overtreatment taken to a new level? *Science-Based Medicine.* 6pp blog. Accessed 1/28/16 at: www.sciencebasedmedicine.org/liquid-biopsies-for-cancer-life-saving-tests-or-overdiagnosis-and-treatment-taken-to-a new-level/.

Griffin, M. and A. Bayat. 2011. Electrical stimulation in bone healing: Critical analysis by evaluating levels of evidence. *Open Access J. Plastic Surg. (Eplasty)* 11: e34. Published online July 26, 2011. 51pp. Accessed 1/16/15 at: www.ncbi.nih.gov/pmc/articles/PMC3145421/pdf/eplasty11e34.pdf.

Griffith, W.C., S. Knappe and J. Kitching. 2010. Femtotessla atomic magnetometry in a microfabricated vapor cell. *Opt. Express.* 18(26): 27167–27172. http://dx.doi.org/10.1364/OE.18027167.

Griffiths, D.J. 2012. *Introduction to Electrodynamics*, 4th Ed. Addison-Wesley, Boston, MA. ISBN-10: 0-3218-5656-2.

Griffin, M. and A. Bayat. 2011. Electrical stimulation in bone healing: Critical analysis by evaluating levels if evidence. *ePlasty.* 11: 30pp.

Grin, C.M. et al. 1990. Accuracy in the clinical diagnosis of malignant melanoma. *Arch. Dermatol.* 126: 763–766.

Guerra, S. et al. 2012. Enhancing the accuracy of subcutaneous glucose sensors: A real-time deconvolution-based approach. *IEEE Trans. Biomed. Eng.* 59(6): 1658–1669. doi: 10.1109/TBME.2012.2191782.

Guyton, A.C. 1991. *Textbook of Medical Physiology*, 8th Ed. W.B. Saunders Co, Philadelphia, PA. ISBN: 0-7216-3087-1.

Hahn, C.E.W. 1998. Electrochemical analysis of clinical blood gases, gases and vapors. *Analyst.* 123: 57R–86R.

Halberg, L.I. and K.E. Thiele. 1986. Extraction of blood flow information using Doppler-shifted ultrasound. *Hewlett-Packard J.* 37(6): 35–40. June 1986. Accessed 1/02/15 at: www.hpl.hp.com/hpjournal/pdfs/IssuePDFs/1986-06.pdf.

Hall, H. 2015. *Willow Curve Device for Pain: Strong Claims, Weak Evidence.* 3pp blog article (10/20/15) on Science-Based Medicine website. Accessed 2/18/16 at: https://sciencebasedmedicine.org/willow-curve-device-for-pain-strong-claims-weak-evidence/.

Hall, D.A., J. Ptacek and M. Snyder. 2007. Protein microarray technology. *Mech. Ageing.* 128(1): 161–167.

Hall, G.L., Z. Hantos, F. Peták, J.H. Wildhaber, K. Tiller, P.R. Burton and P.D. Sly. 2000. Airway and respiratory tissue mechanics in normal infants. *Am. J. Respir. Crit. Care Med.* 162(4): 1397–1402. doi: 10.1164/ajrccm.162.4.9910028.

Hamamatsu. 2012. *Photomultiplier Tubes and Assemblies.* 76pp online catalog and spec. sheets. Accessed 11/16/15 at: https://www.hamamatsu.com/resources/pdf/etd/High_energy_PMT_TPMO0007E.pdf.

Han, F. et al. 1999. Pteridine analysis in urine by capillary electrophoresis using laser-induced fluorescence detection. *Analyt. Chem.* 71: 1265–1269.

Hanchanale, V.S., A.R. Rao and S. Das. 2008. Raman spectroscopy and its urological applications. *Indian J. Urol.* 24(4): 444–450. doi: 10.4103/0970-1591.39550.

Hanlon, E.B. et al. 2000. Prospects for *in vivo* Raman spectroscopy. *Phys. Med. Biol.* 45(2): R1–R59.

Hannaford, B. and S. Lehman 1986. Short time Fourier analysis of the electromyogram: Fast movements and constant contraction. *IEEE Trans. Biomed. Eng.* 33(12): 1173–1181.

Harding, J.R. 1998. Investigating deep vein thrombosis with infrared imaging. *IEEE Eng. Med. Biol. Mag.* 17(4): 43–46.

Harikumar, R., R. Prabu and S. Raghavan. 2013. Electrical impedance tomography (EIT) and its medical applications. *Int. J. Soft Comput. Eng.* 3(4): 193–198.

Hartmann, S. et al. 2015. Phantom of human adipose tissue and studies of light propagation and light absorption for parame-terization and evaluation of noninvasive optical fat measuring devices. *Opt. Photonics J.* 5: 33–67. http://dx.doi.org/10.4236/opj.2015.52005.

Hasse, B., B. Camin and W. Reimers. 2007. *Characterization of an X-Ray Collimator.* 2pp online report. Accessed 10/18/15 at: hasyweb.desy.de/science/annual_reports/2007_report/part1/contrib/49/20494.pdf.

Hawthorne, J.S. and M.H. Wojcik. 2006. Transdermal alcohol measurement: A review of the literature. *Can. Soc. Forensic Sci.* 39(3): 65–71.

Healy, M. 2015. Researchers genetically engineer *E. coli* bacteria to detect cancer and diabetes. *Los Angeles Times article* May 28, 2015. 1pp. Accessed 5/31/15 at: www.geneticliteracyproject.org/2015/05/28/researchers-genetically-engineer-e-coli-bacteria-to-detect-cancer-and-diabetes/.

Hecht, E. 1987. *Optics.* Addison-Wesley, Reading, MA.

Hecht, E. 2000. *Optics,* 2nd Ed. Addison Wesley, Reading, MA.

Heidary, M. et al. 2014. The dynamic range of circulating tumor DNA in metastatic breast cancer. *Breast Cancer Res.* 16: 421. 10pp. doi: 10.1186/s13058-014-0421-y.

Heintzelmann, D.L., R. Lotan and R.R. Richards-Kortum. 2000. Characterization of the auto-fluorescence of polymorpho-nuclear leucocytes, mononuclear leucocytes, and cervical epithelial cancer cells for improved spectroscopic discrimination of inflammation from dysplasia. *Photochem. Photobiol.* 71(3): 327–332.

Heise, H.M., L. Küpper and R. Marbach. 1999. Limitations of infrared spectroscopy for noninvasive metabolite monitoring using the attenuated total reflection technique. *IEEE LEOS Newsletter.* 13(5): 12–15. Accessed 4/21/15 at: photonicssociety.org/newsletters/oct99/leos1099.pdf.

Heitzer, E., M. Auer, P. Ulz, J. Geigl and M.R. Speicher. 2013. Circulating tumor cells and DNA as liquid biopsies. *Genome Med.* 5: 73. 11pp. doi: 10.1186/gm477.

Heitzer, E., P. Ulz and J.B. Geigl. 2015. Circulating tumor DNA as a liquid biopsy for cancer. *Clin. Chem.* 61: 12pp. doi: 10.1373/clinchem.2014.222679.

Herculano-Houzel, S. 2009. *(Review Article)* The human brain in numbers: A linearly scaled-up primate brain. *Frontiers in Human Neuro-science.* 3: Article 31. 11pp.

Herman, C. 2012. Emerging technologies for the detection of melanoma: Achieving better out-comes. *Clin. Cosmet. Investigational Dermatol.* 5: 195–212.

Hieber, L. et al. 2011. Chromosomal rearrangements in post-Chernobyl papillary thyroid carci-nomas: Evaluation by spectral karyotyping and automated interphase FISH. *J. Biomed. Biotechnol.* 2011: Article ID 693691. 7pp. http://dx.doi.org/10.1155/2011/693691.

Hochhauser, D. 2000. Relevance of mitochondrial DNA in cancer. *Lancet.* 356(9225): 181–182.

Homola, J. 2008. Surface plasmon resonance sensors for detection of chemical and biological samples. *Chem. Rev.* 108: 462–493.

Hong, H.-D. 1994. *Optical Interferometric Measurement of Skin Vibration for the Diagnosis of Cardiovascular Disease.* PhD dissertation in Biomedical Engineering. The University of Connecticut, Storrs. (M.D. Fox, major adviser).

Hong, H.-D. and M.D. Fox. 1993. Detection of skin displacement and capillary flow using an opti-cal stethoscope. *Proc. 19th Ann. Northeast Bioengineering Conf.* IEEE Press, NY. pp. 189–190.

Hong, H.-D. and R.B. Northrop. 1991. Ultrasonic phase-shift oxygen measuring system. *Proc. 17th Ann. Northeast Bioengineering Conf.* IEEE Press, NY. pp. 53–55.

Hopkins, G.W. 2006. *Tissue Spectroscopy for Glucose Measurement.* Hewlett-Packard Laboratory Report HPL-98-85(R.1). July 10, 2006. 55pp. Accessed 1/31/16 at: www.hpl.hp.com/techreports/98/HPL-98-85R1.pdf.

Hopkins Medicine. 2015a. *Frequently Asked Questions About TMS.* 2pp online information bulletin. Accessed 5/08/15 at: www.hopkinsmedicine.org/psychiatry/specialty_areas/brain_stimulation/ect/faq_ect.html.

Hopkins Medicine. 2015b. *Frequently Asked Questions About ECT.* 2pp online information bulletin. Accessed 5/11/15 at: www.hopkinsmedicine.org/psychiatry/specialty_areas/brain_stimulation/tms/faq_tms.html.

Horiba. 2011. Application Note: *In vivo* Raman Measurement of human skin. *Biology/Life Sciences RA04.* 4pp. Horiba Scientific. Accessed 4/23/15 at: www.horiba.com/fileadmin/uploads/Scientific/Documents/Raman/RA04.pdf.

Hørven, I. 1973. Dynamic tonometry. *Acta Ophthalomogica.* 51: 353–366.

Hørven, I. and Gjønnaess. 1974. Corneal indentation pulse and intraocular pressure in pregnancy. *Acta Ophthalomogica.* 91: 92–98.

Hørven, I. and H. Nornes. 1971. Crest time evaluation of corneal indentation pulse. *Arch. Ophthal.* 86: 5–11.

Howarth, D. et al. 1999. Scintamammography: An adjunctive test for the detection of breast cancer. *Med. J. Australia.* 170: 588–591.

HPJ. 1986. *Hewlett-Packard J.* 37(6): June 1986. 48pp. Accessed 1/02/15 at: www.hpl.hp.com/hpjournal/pdfs/IssuePDFs/1986-06.pdf.

Hsieh, Y.-S. et al. 2013. Dental optical coherence tomography. *Sensors.* 13: 8928–8949. doi: 10.3390/s130708928.

Hsu, P.D., E.S. Lander and F. Zhang. 2014. Development and application of CRISPR-Cas9 for genome engineering. *Cell.* 157: 1262–1278. http://dx.doi.org/10.1016/j.cell.2014.05.010.

Hsu, K.L. and L.K. Mahal. 2006. A lectin microarray approach for the rapid analysis of bacterial glycans. *Nature Protoc.* 1: 543–549.

Hu, S. and D.T. Wong. 2009. Lectin microarray. *Proteom. Clin. Appl.* 3(2): 148–154. doi: 10.1002/prea.200800153.

Huber, R., V. Parsa and S. Scollie. 2014. Predicting the perceived sound quality of frequency-compressed speech. *PLoS ONE.* 9(11): 13pp. e110260. doi: 10.1371/journal.pone.0110260.

Hughes, J. and D. Bates. 2003. Historical review: The carbon monoxide diffusing capacity (DLCO) and its membrane (DM) and red cell (Theta. Vc) components. *Respir. Physiol. Neurobiol.* 138(2–3): 115–142. doi: 10.16/j.resp.2003.08.004.

Hughes, M.S. and J.O. Anglen. 2010. The use of implantable bone stimulators in nonunion treatment. *Orthopedics.* 33(3): 15pp. doi: 10.3928/01477447-20100129-15.

Hurley, D.A. et al. 2001. Interferential therapy electrode placement technique in acute low back pain: A preliminary investigation. *Arch. Phys. Med. Rehab.* 82: 485–493.

Huttenberger, D. et al. 2008. Autofluorescence detection of tumors in the human lung-spectroscopical measurements *in situ*, in an *in vivo* model and *in vitro*. *Photodiagnosis Photodyn. Ther.* 5(2): 139–147. doi: 10.1016/j.pdpdt.2008.05.003.

ICAD. 2008. *Alzheimer disease plaques seen with conventional MRI in animal model for the first time.* 3pp news bulletin. Accessed 4/14/16 at: https://www.alz.org/national/documents/release_ICAD_072708_mri.pdf.

IDF6E. 2014. *Key Findings 2014. IDF Diabetes Atlas*, 6th Ed. Accessed 4/22/15 at: www.idf.org/diabetesatlas/update-2014.

Imaginis. 2015. *Endoscopy Procedure—What Is Endoscopy.* 3pp web article. Accessed 5/04/15 at: www.imaginis.com/endoscopy.

Inaguma, M. and K. Hashimoto. 1999. Porphyrin-like fluorescence in oral cancer. *Cancer.* 86(11): 2201–2211.

Indiegogo. 2016. *Quell: The World's First Pain Relief Wearable.* 18pp online information bulletin. Accessed 2/15/16 at: https://www.indiegogo.com/projects/quell-the-world-s-first-pain-relief-wearable#/.

IOF. 2015. *Facts and Statistics*. 8pp online paper. Accessed 3/24/16 at: www.iofbonehealth.org/facts-statistics.

IQI. 2015. Industrial Quality, Inc. Gaithersburg, MD. 2pp website. Accessed 6/26/15 at: www.topicway.com/companies/100192644/INDUSTRIAL-QUALITY-Inc-in-Gaithersburg-MD.htm.

ISEAPT. 2015. *Interferential Therapy*. 10pp web paper. Accessed 1/15/15 at: www.electrotherapy.org/modality/interferential-therapy.

ISCEV Standards. 2015. *Current ISCEV Standards*. 2pp online information sheet. Accessed 2/19/15 at: www.iscev.org/standards/.

Jacobson, B. and J.G. Webster. 1977. *Medicine and Clinical Engineering*. Prentice-Hall, NY.

Jahn, T.L. 1968. A possible mechanism for the effect of electrical potentials on apatite formation in bone. *Clin. Oryhop.* 56: 261–273.

Jain, H., D. Isaacson, P.M. Edic and J.C. Newell. 1997. Electrical impedance tomography of complex conductivity distributions with noncircular boundary. *IEEE Trans. Biomed. Eng.* 44(11): 1051–1060.

James, O.G., P.M. Doraiswamy and S. Borges-Neto. 2015. PET imaging of tau pathology in Alzheimer's disease and tauopathies. *Front. Neurol.* 6(38): 1–4. doi: 10.3389/fneur.2015.00038.

Jaszczak, R.J. 1988. Tomographic radiopharmaceutical imaging. *Proc. IEEE.* 76(9): 1079–1094.

Jayanthi, J.L. et al. 2012. Diffuse reflectance imaging: A tool for guided biopsy. *Proc. SPIE.* 8220: 822004. 9pp.

Jenkins, A.T., N.T. Thet and J. Mercer-Chalmers. 2015. *Wound Dressing*. US Patent No. US20150111243 A1. Pub. date: April 23, 2015. Also European Patent No. WO2013104876vA1, published July 18, 2013.

Jenkins, D. 1997. *ECG Library: A Brief History of Electrocardiography*. http://home-pages.enterprise.net/djenkins/ecghist/html.

Jenkins, D. 2009. A (not so) brief history of electrocardiography. 17pp web article. Accessed 4/29/15 at: www.ecglibrary.com/ecghist.html.

Johns, D.P. and R. Pierce. 2008. *Spirometry: The Measurement and Interpretation of Ventilatory Function in Clinical Practice*. 24pp online handbook. National Asthma Council, Ltd., Australia. ISBN: 0-646-26307-2. Accessed 6/01/15 at: www.nationalasthma.org.au/uploads/content/211-spirometer_handbook_naca.pdf.

Johns, H.R. and J.R. Cunningham. 1983. *The Physics of Radiology*, 4th Ed. C.C. Thomas, IL.

Jory, M.J., G.W. Bradbury, P.S. Cann and J.R. Sambles. 1995. A surface-plasmon-based optical sensor using acousto-optics. *Meas. Sci. Technol.* 6: 1193–1200.

Jossinet, J., P. Castello and F. Risacher. 1995. Multichannel impedance plethysmography discriminates leg arteries. EMBC95. Paper 1.2.6.19.

Just, V. 2010. Revolutionary medical dressing uses nanotechnology to fight infection. 3pp University of Bath Press Release, July 6, 2010. Accessed 2/29/16 at: www2.mpip-mainz.mpg.de/eu-projekte/bacteriosafe/pu/pressreleases/pressrelease_3.pdf.

Kaiser, N. 1979. Laser absorption spectroscopy with an ATR prism. *IEEE Trans. Biomed. Eng.* 26(10): 597–600.

Kalapatapu, R.K. 2015. *Electroconvulsive Therapy*. 6pp online Medscape paper. Accessed 5/11/15 at: emedicine.medscape.com/article/1525957-overview.

Kandel et al. 1991. *Principles of Neural Science*, 3rd ed. Appleton & Lange, Norwalk, CT.

Kandel, E. et al., Eds. 2012. *Principles of Neural Science*, 5th Ed. McGraw-Hill Education, NY.

Karachaliou, N., C. Mayo-de-las-Casas, M.A. Molina-Villa and R. Rosell. 2015. Editorial: Real-time liquid biopsies become a reality in cancer treatment. *Ann. Transl. Med.* 3(3): 36. 3pp. doi: 10.3978/j.issn.2305-5839.2015.01.16.

Katz, B. 1966. *Nerve, Muscle and Synapse*. McGraw-Hill, NY.

Katzir, N. et al. 1998. *Method for Classification of Pixels into Groups According to Their Spectra Using a Plurality of Wide Band Filters and Hardwire [sic] Therefore*. U.S. Patent No. 5,834,203. November 16, 1998.

Keeler, R. 2015. Ophthalmoscopes, Part 1 of 3. *College of Optometrists, online paper*. Accessed 5/03/15 at: www.college-optometrists.org/en/college/museyeum/online_exhibitions/optical_instruments/ophthalmoscopes/index.cfm.

Kelley, L.M. et al. 1997. Scanning laser ophthalmoscope imaging of age-related macular degeneration and neoplasms. *J. Ophthalmol. Photog.* 19: 89–94.

Kelly, R.G. and A.E. Owen. 1991. Microelectronic ion sensors: A critical survey. *IEE Proc.* 132: 227–236.

Kemp, D.T. 2002. Otoacoustic emissions, their origin in cochlear function, and use. *Br. Med. Bull.* 63: 223–241.

Kerr, L.T., K. Domijan, I. Cullen and B.M. Hennelly. 2014. Applications of Raman spectroscopy to the urinary bladder for cancer diagnosis. *Photonics Lasers Med.* 3(3): 193–224. doi: 10.1515/plm-2014-0004. May 2014.

Khedr, E.M. et al. 2015. Repetitive transcranial magnetic stimulation in neuropathic pain secondary to malignancy: A randomized clinical trial. *Eur. J. Pain.* 19(4): 419–527. doi: 10.1002/ejp.576.

Kim, Y. et al. 2016. Reconfigurable chiroptical nanocomposits with chirality transfer from the macro- to the nanoscale. *Nat. Mater.* Pub. online January 4, 2016. doi: 10.1038/nmat4525.

Kimball. 2014. *Transport Across Cell Membranes*. 10pp tutorial article dated April 17, 2014. Accessed 2/25/16 at: users.rcn.com/jkimball.ma.ultranet/BiologyPages/D/Diffusion.html.

Kimura, H. 2010. *Engineer Interview: Early Diagnosis Made Possible by Endoscope*. 17pp online paper. Accessed 5/04/15 at: www.olympus-global.com/en/common/pdf/factbook_medical06.pdf.

Kirson, E.D. et al. 2004. Disruption of cancer cell replication by alternating electric fields. *Cancer Res.* 64: 3288–3295.

Kitabayashi, H. et al. 2010. Development of high powered infrared LED. *SEI Tech. Rev.* 70: 71–74.

Kitson, S.L. et al. 2009. Clinical applications of positron emission tomography (PET) imaging in medicine: Oncology, brain diseases and cardiology. *Curr. Radiopharm.* 2: 224–253.

Klonoff, D.C. 2007. The benefits of implanted glucose sensors. *J. Diabetes Sci. Technol.* 1(6): 797–800.

Klonoff, D.C., J. Braig et al. 1998. Mid infrared spectroscopy for noninvasive blood glucose monitoring. *IEEE LEOS Newsletter.* 12(2): 13–14. Accessed 4/21/15 at: photonicssociety.org/newsletters/apr98/midinfrared.htm.

Koch, H. 2004. Recent advances in magnetocardiography. *J. Electrocardiol.* 37(Suppl. 2004): 117–122. doi: 10.1016/j.jelectrocard.2004.08.035.

Kodak. 2015. *Kodak CCD Primer #KCP-001*. 13pp online tutorial. Accessed 2/18/15 at: science.unit. it/~semicon/members/pavesi/ccdPrimerPart2.pdf.

Komen, S.G. 2015. *Accuracy of Mammograms*. 3pp web paper. Accessed 10/19/15 at: ww5.komen. org/BreastCancer/accuracyofMammograms.html.

Kominis, I.K., T.W. Kornack, J.C. Allred and M.V. Romalis. 2003. A subfemtotesla multichannel atomic magnetometer. *Nature Lett. Nat.* 422: 596–599. doi: 10.1038/nature01484.

König, F. et al. 1994. Laser-induced autofluorescence of prostate- and bladder tissue. *Proc. of OE/ LASE '94*, Los Angeles, CA. *Laser-Tissue Interactions*, Vol. V. Photochemical Mechanisms. *SPIE.* 2324: 284–291.

Kong, K., C. Kendall, N. Stone and I. Notingher. 2015. Raman spectroscopy for medical diagnostics— From *in-vitro* biofluid assays to *in-vivo* cancer detection. *Adv. Drug Deliv. Rev.* 89: 121–134. http:// dx.doi.org/10.1016/j.addr.2016.03.009.

Koo, T.-W., A.J. Berger, I. Itzkan and M.S. Feld. 1999. Reagent blood analysis by near infrared Raman spectroscopy. *Diabetes Technol. Ther.* 1(2): 153–157.

Korhonen, P. et al. 1996. Frequency response measurements on commercially available stetho-scopes. *Med. Biol. Eng. & Comput.* 34(Suppl. 1, Part 1): 91–92.

Kottmann, J., J.M. Rey, J. Luginbühl, E. Reichmann and M.W. Sigrist. 2012. Glucose sensing in human epidermis using mid-infrared photoacoustic detection. *Biomed. Opt. Express.* 3(4): 667–680.

Kraus, J.D. 1953. *Electromagnetics.* McGraw-Hill Book Co., NY.

Kronfeld, P.C. 1943. *The Human Eye in Anatomical Transparencies.* Bausch & Lomb Press, Rochester, NY.

Kuhl, D.E. and R.Q. Edwards. 1963. Image separation radioisotope scanning. *Radiology.* 80: 653–662.

Kumar, A.R. 2008. Current clinical applications of positron emission tomography. *Australian Prescr.* 31(5): 123–128.

Kumar, R., D. Halanaik and A. Malhotra. 2010. Clinical applications of positron emission tomography-computed tomography in oncology. *Indian J. Cancer.* 47(2): 100–119. doi: 10:4103/0019-509X.62997.

Kunnen, B. et al. 2014. Application of circularly polarized light for non-invasive diagnosis of cancerous tissues and turbid tissue-like scattering media. *J. Biophotonics.* 1–7(2014). doi: 10.1002/ jbio.201400104.

Kuzyk, P.R.T. and E.H. Schemitsch. 2009. The science of electrical stimulation therapy for fracture healing. *Indian J. Orthop.* 43(2): 127–131. doi: 10.4103/0019-5413.50846.

Kwok, S. et al. 1987. Identification of HIV sequences by using *in vitro* enzymatic amplification and oligomer cleavage detection. *J. Virol.* 61(5): 1690–1694.

Kwon, S.-Y., H.-D. Kwen and S.-H. Choi. 2012. Fabrication of nonenzymatic glucose sensors based on multiwalled carbon nanotubes with bimetallic Pt-M (M = Ru and Sn) catalysts by radiolytic deposition. *Hindawi J. Sci.* 2012. Article ID 784167. 8pp. doi: 10.1155/2012/784167.

Lab Training. 2012. *Gas Chromatography: Module 8. Types of Gas Chromatography Detectors*. 4pp online tutorial. Accessed 3/18/15 at: lab-training.com/landinggc-module-8/.

Lab Manager®. 2014. *Gas Chromatography System Manufacturer List*. Accessed 4/25/15 at: www. labmanager.com//vendor-list/2010/01/gas-chromatography-systems-manufacturer-list?fw1pk=2#. VTveISFViko.

Lacourse, J.R. and D.A. Sekel. 1986. A contact method of ocular pulse detection for studies of carotid occlusions. *IEEE Trans. Biomed. Eng.* 33(4): 381–385.

Langridge, S. 2010. Online measurement of oxygen: Review and new developments. Paper presented in *Session 5.1, ISA 55th Analysis Division Symposium 2010*, New Orleans, LA. 15pp. Accessed 3/27/15 at: file:///C:/Users/Owner/Downloads/Online-Measurement-of-Oxygen.pdf.

LaRocca, F., A.-H. Dhalla, M.P. Kelly, S. Farsiu and J.A. Izatt. 2013. Optimization of confocal scanning laser ophthalmoscope design. *J. Biomed. Opt.* 18(7): 076015-1-9.

Lawaczeck, R., V. Arkadiev, F. Diekmann and M. Krumrey. 2005. Monochromatic x-rays in digital mammography. *Invest. Radiol.* 40(1): 33–39.

L3 Cincinnati. 2015. *Infrared Cameras: MWIR Cooled Thermal Imagers*. Online brochure. Accessed 7/6/15 at: www.cinele.com/index.php?option=com_content&view=article&id=1011&Itemid=231.

Leach, W.M., Jr. 1996. A two-port analogous circuit and SPICE model for Salmon's family of acoustical horns. *J. Acoust. Soc. Am.* 99(3): 1459–1464.

Ledford, H. 2015. Bacteria yield new gene cutter. *Nature.* 526: 17. doi: 10.1038/nature.2015.18432.

Lee, J.K.T., S.S. Sagel, R.J. Stanley and J.P. Heiken, Eds. 2003. *Computed Body Tomography with MRI Correlation*, 4th Ed. Lippincott, Williams & Wilkins, Philadelphia, PA. ISBN: 978-0-7817-4526-0.

Lee, P.S., R.F. Majowski and T.A. Perry. 1991. Tunable diode laser spectroscopy for isotope analysis—Detection of isotopic carbon dioxide in exhaled breath. *IEEE Trans. Biomed. Eng.* 38(10): 966–973.

Lee, Y.H. et al. 2008. 64-channel second-order axial gradiometer system based on DROS for magnetocardiogram in a thin shielded room. *Physica C: Supercond.* 468(15–20): 1942–1945. September 15, 2008.

Lee, Y.H., K.K. Yu, J.M. Kim, H. Kwon and K. Kim. 2009. A high-sensitivity magnetocardiography system with a divided gradiometer array inside a low boil-off Dewar. *Supercond. Sci. Technol.* 22: 114003. doi: 10.1088/0953-2048/22/11/114003.

Lee, Y.U., S. Lee and J.-I. Youn. 2011. Optical spectroscopic analysis of muscle spasticity for low-level laser therapy (LLLT). *J. Opt. Soc. Korea.* 15(4): 373–379. http://dx.doi.org/10.3807/JOSK.2011.15.4.373.

Lee, Y.W. 1960. *Statistical Theory of Communication*. John Wiley and Sons, NY.

Lei, H., Z. Chongxun, H. Ying and C. Qun. 1997. Detecting myocardial ischemia with 2-D spectrum analysis. *IEEE Eng. Med. Biol. Mag.* 16(4): 33–40.

Leinenga, G. and J. Götz. 2015. Scanning ultrasound removes amyloid-β and restores memory in an Alzheimer's disease mouse model. *Sci. Transl. Med.* 7(278): 278ra33. 11pp. doi: 10.1126/scitranslmed.aaa2512.

Lennox, R.B. 2000. *Biosensor Device and Method*. U.S. Patent #6,107,180. August 22, 2000.

Leonard, A., J. Smurzynski, M.D. Jung and D. Kim. 1990. Evaluation of distortion product otoacoustic emissions as a basis for the objective clinical assessment of cochlear function. *Adv. Audiol.* 7: 139–148.

Leong, D.J. et al. 2013. Therapeutic ultrasound: Osteoarthritis symptom-modification and potential for disease modification. *J. Surg.* 1(2): 5pp. Accessed 6/11/15 at: www.avensonline.org/wp-content/uploads/2014/01/JSUR-2332-4139-01-0009.pdf.

Leunig, A., C.S. Betz, R. Baumgartner, G. Grevers and W.J. Issing. 2000. Initial experience in the treatment of oral leukoplakia with high-dose vitamin A and follow-up 5-aminolevulinic acid induced protoporphyrin IX fluorescence. *Eur. Arch. Otorhinolaryngol.* 257: 327–331.

Leunig, A. et al. 1996. Fluorescent imaging and spectroscopy of 5-aminolevulinic acid induced protoporphyrin IX for the detection of neoplastic lesions in the oral cavity. *Am. J. Surg.* 172(6): 674–677.

Liakat, S., K.A. Bors, L. Xu, C.M. Woods, J. Doyle and C.F. Gmachi. 2014. Noninvasive *in vivo* glucose sensing on human subjects using mid-infrared light. *Biomed. Opt. Express.* 5(7): 2394–2404. doi: 10.1344/BOE.5.002397.

Liley, D.J.T. 2001. Course Notes for Medical Imaging, HET 408, at Swinburn University of Technology, Australia.

Lima, V.C. et al. 2011. Simultaneous confocal scanning laser ophthalmoscopy combined with high-resolution spectral domain optical coherence tomography: A review. *J. Ophthalmol.* 2011: 743670. doi: 10.1155/2011/743670.

Lin, J.C. Ed. 2012. *Electromagnetic Fields in Biological Systems.* CRC Press, Boca Raton, FL. ISBN: 978-1-4398-5999-5.

Lipson, J. et al. 2009. Requirements for calibration in noninvasive glucose monitoring by Raman spectroscopy. *J. Diabetes Sci. Technol.* 3(2): 233–241.

Li, X. et al. 2011. Effect of low-intensity pulsed ultrasound on MMP-13 and MAPKs signaling pathway in rabbit knee osteoarthritis. *Cell. Biochem. Biophys.* 61: 427–434.

Lockwood, G.R., D.H. Turnbull, D.A. Christopher and F.S. Foster. 1966. Beyond 30 MHz: Applications of high-frequency ultrasound imaging. *IEEE Engr. Med. Biol. Mag.* 15(6): 60–71.

Lodish, H., A. Berk, S.L. Zipursky et al. 2000. *Active Transport by ATP-Powered Pumps. Sect. 15.5 in Molecular Cell Biology.* W.H. Freeman, NY.

Loo, C.K., K. Sainsbury, P. Sheehan and B. Lyndon. 2008. A comparison of RUL ultrabrief pulse (0.3 ms) ECT and standard RUL ECT. *Intl. J. Neuropsychopharmacol.* 11: 883–890. doi: 10.1017/S1461145708009292.

Love, S. 2015. *Ultrasound.* 3pp web article. Accessed 2/7/16 at: www.drsusanloveresearch.org/ultrasound.

Lu, Y. 2010. Research on models and methods of magnetocardiography. *Proc. IEEE 2nd Intl. Conf. on Networking and Digital Society (ICNDS)*, Wenzhou, China. pp. 368–371. doi: 10.1109/ICNDS.2010.5479444.

Lupski, J.R. et al. 2010. Whole-genome sequencing in a patient with Charcot-Marie tooth neuropathy. *N. Engl. J. Med.* 362(13): 1181–1191. doi: 10.1056/NEJMoa0908094.

MacDonald, L.R. et al. 2001. Pinhole SPECT of mice using LumaGEM gamma camera. *IEEE Trans. Nucl. Sci.* 48(3): 830–836.

Macedo, M.F. and M. de Sousa. 2008. Transferrin and the transferrin receptor: Of magic bullets and other concerns. *Inflamm. Allerg. Drug Targets.* 7(1): 41–52. doi: 10.2174/187152808784165162.

MacIntyre, N. et al. 2005. Standardisation of the single-breath determination of carbon monoxide uptake in the lung. *Eur. Resp. J.* 26(4): 720–735. doi: 10.1183/09031936.05.00034905.

Macovski, A. 1983. *Medical Imaging Systems.* Prentice-Hall, Inc., Englewood Cliffs, NJ.

Magis, D. et al. 2013. Safety and patients' satisfaction of transcutaneous supraorbital neurostimulation (tSNS) with the Cefaly device in headache treatment: A survey of 2,313 headache sufferers in the general population. *J. Headache Pain.* 14: 95.

Magnin, P.A. 1986. Doppler effect: History and theory. *Hewlett-Packard J.* 37(6): 26–31. June 1986.

Magnoni, S. et al. 2012. Tau elevations in the brain extracellular space correlate with reduced amyloid-β levels and predict adverse clinical outcomes after severe traumatic brain injury. *Brain.* 135: 1268–1280. doi: 10.1093/brain/awr286.

March, W.F. 1977. *Non-Invasive Glucose Sensor System.* US Patent No. 4,014,321. March 29, 1977.

March, W.F. 1984. Ocular glucose sensor. *Proc. 1984 IEEE/NSF Symp. on Biosensors.* IEEE Press, Los Angeles, CA. pp. 79–81.

March, W.F., B. Rabinovitch and R.L. Adams. 1982. Noninvasive glucose monitoring in the aqueous humor of the eye. Part 2: Animal studies and the scleral lens. *Diabetes Care.* 5(3): 259–265.

Marketech. 2015. *Scintillator Crystals.* Online brochure. Accessed 7/02/15 at: mkt-intl.com/materials/single-crystals-oprical-materials/scintillator-crystals/.

Markov, M.S. 2007. Pulsed electromagnetic field therapy and history, state of the art and future. *Environmentalist.* 27: 465–475. Accessed 1/27/15 at: www.curatron.com/pdf/PEMF-environmentalist.pdf.

Marmor, M.F. et al. 2011. ISCEV standard for clinical electro-oculography (2010 update). *Doc. Ophthalmol.* 122: 1–7. doi: 10.1007/s10633-011-9259-0.

Maron, S.H. and C.F. Prutton. 1958. *Principles of Physical Chemistry.* MacMillan Co., NY.

Marques, P.R. and A.S. McKnight. 2007. *Evaluating Transdermal Alcohol Measuring Devices.* National Highway Traffic Safety Administration (NHTSA). 96pp online Final Report. Accessed 5/25/16 at: file:///C:/Users/Owner/Downloads/810875%20(4).pdf.

Mascarenhas, P., B. Fatela and I. Barahona. 2014. Effect of diabetes mellitus type 2 on salivary glucose—A systematic review and meta-analysis of observational studies. *PLoS ONE.* 9(7): e101706. 15pp.

Mascarin, N.C. et al. 2012. Effects of kinesiotherapy, ultrasound and electrotherapy in management of bilateral knee osteoarthritis: Prospective clinical trial. *BMC Musculoskelet. Disord.* 13: 182.

Matlashov, A.N. et al. 2002. *Design and Performance of the LANL 158-Channel Magnetoencephalography System.* LANL Report LA-UR-02-3147. Accessed 3/27/15 at: http://lib-www.lanl.gov/cgi-bin/getfile?00852311.pdf.

Mavrogiorgou, P. et al. 2011. Are routine methods good enough to stain senile plaques and neurofibrillary tangles in different brain regions of demented patients? *Psychiatr. Danub.* 23(4): 334–339.

Mayo Clinic. 2012. Electroconvulsive therapy (ECT). *Definition*. (Also: *Why it's done, Risks, How you prepare, What you can expect*, and *Results*). Medical information on the Mayo Clinic website. Accessed 5/11/15 at: www.mayoclinic.org/tests-procedures/electroconvulsive-therapy/basics/definition/prc-20014161.

McCulloch, D.L. et al. 2015. ISCEV Standard for full-field clinical electroretinography (2015 update). *Documenta Ophrhalmologica*. 130: 1–12. doi: 10/1007/s10633-014-9473-7.

McCusik, V.A., S.A. Talbot and G.N. Webb. 1959. Spectral phonocardiography: Problems and prospects in the applications of the Bell spectrograph to phonocardiography. *Bull. Johns Hopkins Hosp.* 94: 187–198.

McDonald, B.M. 1992. *Two-Phase Lock-In Amplifier with Phase-Locked Loop Vector Tracking*. MS dissertation in Biomedical Engineering. The University of Connecticut, Storrs. (R.B. Northrop, Major Advisor.)

McDonald, B.M. and R.B. Northrop. 1993. Two-phase lock-in amplifier with phase-locked loop vector tracking. *Proc. Euro. Conf. Circuit Theory and Design*, Davos, Switzerland. August 30–September 3, 1003. pp. 997–1003.

McGirr, A. et al. 2015. Effectiveness and acceptability of accelerated repetitive transcranial magnetic stimulation (rTMS) for treatment-resistant major depressive disorder: An open label trial. *J. Affect. Disord.* 173: 216–220.

McKee, A.C. et al. 2009. Chronic traumatic encephalopathy in athletes: Progressive tauopathy following repetitive head injury. *J. Neuropathol. Exp. Neurol.* 68(7): 709–735. doi: 10.1097/NEN.0b013e3181a9d503.

MedlinePlus. 2013. *Tests for H. pylori*. 2pp online bulletin. Accessed 4/26/15 at: www.nlm.nih.gov/medlineplus/ency/article/007501.

Melzack, R. and P.D. Wall. 1965. Pain mechanisms: A new theory. *Science*. 150(3699): 971–979. doi: 10.1126/science.1503699.971.

Mendelson, Y. et al. 1990. Blood glucose measurement by multiple attenuated total reflection and infrared absorption spectroscopy. *IEEE Trans. Biomed. Eng.* 37(5): 458–465.

Mendonca, M.E. et al. 2011. Transcranial DC stimulation in fibromyalgia: Optimized cortical target supported by high-resolution computational models. *J. Pain*. 12(5): 610–617.

Merk Manual Home Edition. 2013. *Tropical Sprue*. 3pp online. Accessed 3/19/15 at: www.merkmanuals.com/home/digestive_disorders/malabsorption/tropical_sprue.html.

Merk Manual Professional Edition. 2014. *Celiac Disease*. 6pp online. Accessed 3/19/15 at: www.merkmanuals.com/professional/gastrointestinal_disorders/malabsorption_syndromes/celiac_disease.html.

Merk Manual Professional Edition. 2015. *Osteoporosis*. 12pp. Accessed 4/15/15 at: www.merkmanuals.com/professional/musculoskeletal-and-connective-tissue-disorders/osteoporosis/osteoporosis.

Messier, S.P., D.J. Gutekunst, C. Davis and P. DeVita. 2005. Weight loss reduces knee-joint loads in overweight and obese older adults with knee osteoarthritis. *Arthritis Rheum.* 52: 2026–2032.

Mhaskar, R., S. Knappe and J. Kitching. 2012. A low-power, high-sensitivity micromachined optical magnetometer. *Appl. Phys. Lett.* 101: 241105. 4pp.

Middleton, S. 2011. *GE Mammography Equipment: Senographe 2000D vs Senographe Essential*. 3pp online article. Accessed 6/29/15 at: info.blockimaging.com/bid/72292/GE-Mammography-Equipment-Senographe-2000D-vs-Senographe-Essential.

Minsky, M. 1988. Memoir on inventing the confocal scanning microscope. *Scanning*. 10: 128–138.

Misra, B.R. et al. 2015. Comparison of anticraving efficacy of right and left repetitive transcranial magnetic stimulation in alcohol dependence: A randomized double-blind study. *J. Neuropsychiatry Clin. Neurosci.* 27(1): e54–9. doi: 10.1176/appl.neuropsych.13010013.

Misra, U.K., J. Kalita and S.K. Bhoi. 2012. High frequency repetitive transcranial magnetic stimulation (rTMS) is effective in migraine prophylaxis: An open labeled study. *Neurol. Res.* 34(6): 547–551.

Mitchell, J.S. and Y. Wu. 2010. Surface Plasmon Resonance Biosensors for Highly Sensitive Detection of Small Biomolecules. Ch. 9. In: *Biosensors*. P.A. Serra Ed. INTECH, Croatia. pp. 151–168. Accessed 3/17/15 at: cdn.intechopen.com/pdfs-wm/6919.pdf.

Moghadasian, M.H. et al. 1997. Homocysteine and coronary artery disease. *Arch. Internal Med.* 157: 2299–2308.

Morita. 2011. *Veraviewepocs® 2D HD Pan/Ceph Low Dose, High Definition Images*. 20pp online brochure. Accessed 6/29/15 at: www.morita.com/usa/root/img/pool/pdf/product_brochures/Veraviewepocs_2D_L-337_0911_v8.pdf.

Moseley, P.T., J.O.W. Norris and D.E. Williams. 1991. *Techniques and Mechanisms Is Gas Sensing*. Adam Hilger, NY.

Mueller, H.H. 2015. What is tDCS? 9pp web paper. Accessed 5/13/15 at: drmueller-healthpsychology.com/tDCS.html.

Murali, N. 2015. *Nuclear Magnetic Resonance Principles*. 44pp online slideshow. Accessed 6/30/15 at: nmrwiki.org/wiki/images/1/17/NM_NMR_Basics.pdf.

Musselman, J., A. Solanky and W. Arnold. 2013. Increasing Accuracy of Blood-Alcohol Analysis Using Automated Headspace-Gas Chromatography. 4pp online Case Study. Accessed 4/03/15 at: www.perkinelmer.com/cmsresources/images/44-74508cst_gaschromaaincraccuracybloodalchlanaly.pdf.

Nanoptics. 2000. *Fiberoptic Tutorial*. 9pp online tutorial. Accessed 2/18/15 at: caps.ncbs.res.in/SmoS/common/optics/Nanoptics,%20Inc_,%20Fiberoptic%20Tutorial.htm.

National Instruments. 2014. STFT Spectrogram (Advanced Signal Processing Toolkit). *LabVIEW 2014 Advanced Signal Processing Toolkit, Part No. 372656C-01*. Accessed 3/26/15 at: zone.ni.com/reference/en-XX/help/372656C-01/lvasptconcepts/aspt_stft_spectrogram/.

NCI. 2014. *Mammograms*. 9pp online article. National Cancer Institute. Accessed 10/19/15 at: www.cancer.gov/types/breast/mammograms-fact-sheet.

Nelson, T.R. 1999. *Development of a Type 1 Nonlinear Feedback System for Laser Velocimetry and Ranging*. MS Dissertation on Biomedical Engineering. University of Connecticut (R.B. Northrop, major advisor).

Nemec, H. 1959. Interferential therapy: A new approach in physical medicine. *Brit. J. Physiother.* 12: 9–12.

Net Amps. 2015. Net Amps 400 series amplifiers. 2pp. Accessed 4/30/15 at: human.kyst.com.tw/uploads/pdfs140235312135806.pdf.

Nguyen, D.T., C. Jin, A. Thiagalingham and A.L. McEwan. 2012. A review on electrical impedance tomography for pulmonary perfusion imaging. *Physiol. Meas.* 33: 695–707. doi: 10.1088/0967-3334/33/5/695.

NIH. 2015. *Brain Research Through Advancing Innovative Neurotechnologies[SM] (BRAIN).* Online information bulletin. Accessed 5/14/15 at: braininitiative.nih.gov/index.htm.

Nichols, B.S. et al. 2015. A quantitative diffuse reflectance imaging (QDRI) system for comprehensive surveillance of the morphological landscape in breast tumor margins. *PLoS ONE.* 10(6): e0127525. 25pp. doi: 10.1371/journal.pone.0127525.

Niemeyer, G. 1995. Selective rod- and cone ERG responses in retinal degeneration. *Digital Journal of Ophthalmology.* www.djo.harvard.edu/meei/OA/NIEM-EYER/INDEX.html.

NIMH. 2015. *Brain Stimulation Therapies.* 7pp. web paper. Accessed 1/17/15 at: www.nimh.nih.gov/health/topics/brain-stimulation-therapies/brain-stimulation-therapies.shtml.

Noble, J.G. et al. 2000. The effect of interferential therapy upon cutaneous blood flow in humans. *Clin. Physiol.* 20(1): 2–7.

NOF. 2015. Are You at Risk? *National Osteoporosis Foundation.* 1p. Accessed 4/15/15 at: nof.org/articles/2.

Nonle, G. 2006. Interferential therapy: Could it be more effective than TENS in the management of MS-related symptoms? *Way Ahead.* 10(4): 8–10. Accessed 1/18/15 at: www.mstrust.org.uk/professionals/information/wayahead/articles/10042006_06.jsp.

Northrop, A.P. 1994. Comments on gas used for laparoscopy. Personal Communication, 9/94.

Northrop, R.B. 1980. *Ultrasonic Respiration/Convulsion Monitoring Apparatus and Method for Its Use.* US Patent No. 4,197,856. Issued April 15, 1980. Filed April, 10 1978.

Northrop, R.B. 1990. *Analog Electronic Circuits: Analysis and Application.* Addison-Wesley Pub. Co., Reading, MA. ISBN: 0-201-11656-1.

Northrop, R.B. 1997. *Introduction to Instrumentation and Measurements.* CRC Press, Boca Raton, FL. ISBN: 0-8493-7898-2.

Northrop, R.B. 2000. *Endogenous and Exogenous Regulation and Control of Physiological Systems.* Chapman & Hall/CRC, Boca Raton, FL. ISBN: 0-8493-9694-8.

Northrop, R.B. 2001. *Introduction to Dynamic Modeling of Neuro-Sensory Systems.* CRC Press, Boca Raton, FL. ISBN: 0-8493-0814-3.

Northrop, R.B. 2002. *Noninvasive Instrumentation and Measurement in Medical Diagnosis.* CRC Press, Boca Raton, FL. ISBN: 0-8493-0961-1.

Northrop, R.B. 2003. *Signals and Systems Analysis in Biomedical Engineering.* CRC Press, Boca Raton, FL. ISBN: 0-8493-1557-3.

Northrop, R.B. 2004. *Analysis and Application of Analog Electronic Circuits to Biomedical Engineering.* CRC Press, Boca Raton, FL. ISBN: 0-8493-2143-3.

Northrop, R.B. 2005. *Introduction to Instrumentation and Measurements,* 2nd ed. Taylor & Francis, Boca Raton, FL. ISBN: 0-8493-3773-9.

Northrop, R.B. 2010. *Signals and Systems Analysis in Biomedical Engineering,* 2nd Ed. CRC Press, Boca Raton, FL. ISBN: 978-1-4398-1251-8.

Northrop, R.B. 2011. *Introduction to Complexity and Complex Systems*. CRC Press, Boca Raton, FL. ISBN: 978-1-4398-3901-0.

Northrop, R.B. 2012. *Analysis and Application of Analog Electronic Circuits to Biomedical Instrumentation*, 2nd Ed. CRC Press, Boca Raton, FL. ISBN: 978-1-4398-6669-6.

Northrop, R.B. 2014. *Introduction to Instrumentation and Measurement*, 3rd Ed. CRC Press, Boca Raton, FL. ISBN-13: 978-1-4665-9677-1.

Northrop, R.B. and A.N. Connor. 2009. *Introduction to Molecular Biology, Genomics and Proteomics for Biomedical Engineers*. CRC Press, Boca Raton, FL. ISBN No.13: 978-1-4200-6119-2.

Northrop, R.B. and A.N. Connor. 2013. *Ecological Sustainability: Understanding Complex Issues*. CRC Press, Boca Raton, FL. ISBN: 978-1-4665-6512-8.

Northrop, R.B. and B.M. Decker. 1978. Assessment of cerebral hemodynamics by no-touch ocular pulse. In: *Proc. 6th New England Bioengineering Conf.* D. Jaron Ed. March 23–24, 1978. Univ. of Rhode Island, Pergamon Press, Kingston. pp. 105–108.

Northrop, R.B. and S.S. Nilakhe. 1977. A no-touch ocular pulse measurement system for the diagnosis of carotid occlusions. *IEEE Trans. Biomed. Eng.* 24(3): 139–148.

NorthShore. 2015. *Why It Is Done*. 2pp sheet on slit lamp exams. Accessed 5/03/15 at: www.northshore.org/healthresources/encyclopedia.aspx?DocumentHwid=tu6231&lid=57328#tu6233.

Novikova, T., A. Pierangelo, A. De Martino, A. Benali and P. Validire. 2012. Polarimetric imaging or cancer diagnosis and staging. *Opt. Photonics News.* 23(10): 26–33. doi: 10.1364/OPN.23.10.000026.

NTP Nomination History and Review. 3/96. *Melatonin*. CAS No. 73-31-4. URL: http://ntp-server-niehs.nih.gov/htdocs/Chem_Background/ExecSumm/Melatonin.html.

Nuñez, J.K., L.B. Harrington and J.A. Doudna. 2016. Chemical and biophysical modulation of Cas9 for tunable genome engineering. *ACS Chem. Biol.* 11(3): 681–688. doi: 10.1021/acschembio.5B01019.

Nuñez, P.L. 1981a. A study of the origins of the time dependencies of the scalp EEG: I-Theoretical basis. *IEEE Trans. Biomed. Engrg.* 28(3): 271–280.

Nuñez, P.L. 1981b. A study of the origins of the time dependencies of the scalp EEG: II-Experimental support of theory. *IEEE Trans. Biomed. Engrg.* 28(3): 281–288.

Oberman, L., D. Edwards, M. Eldaief and A. Pascual-Leone. 2011. Safety of the theta burst transcranial magnetic stimulation. *J. Clin. Neurophysiol.* 28(1): 67–74. doi: 10.1097/WNP.0b013e318205135f.

O'Connell, R.G. Jr. 1986. The role of Doppler ultrasound in cardiac diagnosis. *Hewlett-Packard J.* 37(6): 20–25. June 1986.

OCT. 2016. *Optical Coherence Tomography*. 3pp technical paper. Accessed 3/26/16 at: usri.ucdavis.edu/research/retinal/oct.

Ogata, K. 1970. *Modern Control Engineering*. Prentice-Hall, Englewood Cliffs, NJ.

Ohno, H. and Y. Hayashi. 1976. *X-Ray Tomographic Apparatus*. U.S. Patent No. 3,963,932. June 15, 1976.

Olson, H.F. 1940. *Elements of Acoustical Engineering*. D. Van Nostrand Co., Inc., NY.

Olympus. 2012. *Introduction to CMOS Image Sensors*. 8pp web tutorial. Accessed 5/5/15 at: www.olympusmicro.com/primer/digitalimaging/cmosimagesensors.html.

Olympus®. 2015. *Operation Manual: Instructions—EVIS EXERA II—Gastrointestinal Videoscope & Colonovideoscope*. 110pp online. Accessed 5/04/15 at: www.franksworkshop.com/equipment/documents/endoscopy/user_manuals/Olympus%20GIF%20180%20Gastrointestinal%20Videoscope%20-%20Instructions.pdf.

Onescu, V. and D. Erickson. 2013. High volumetric power density, non-enzymatic, glucose fuel cells. *Scientific Reports*. 3(1226): 6pp. doi: 10.10.38/srep01226.

Onibere, R. and A. Khanna. 2008. The role of electrical stimulation in fracture healing. *Internet J. Orthop. Surg*. 11(2): 15pp. Accessed 1/24/15 at: https://ispub.com/IJOS/11/2/11122.

Online Orthopedics. 2015. *Electrical Stimulation of Bone Healing*. 5pp web article. Accessed 1/24/15 at: www.orthopodsurgeon.com/electstim.html.

Oostendorp, T.F. et al. 2008. Modeling transcranial DC stimulation. *Transactions of the 30th Annual International Conference of the IEEE Engineering in Medicine and Biology Society*. Vancouver, BC, August 20–25. pp. 4226–4229. doi: 10.1109/IEMBS.2008.4650142.

Oostveen, E. et al. 2003. The forced oscillation technique in clinical practice: Methodology, recommendations and future developments. *Eur. Resp. J*. 22: 1026–1041. doi: 10.1183/09031936.03.00089403.

Orthopedia. 2015. *Orthosis*. 3pp web article. Accessed 1/16/15 at: orthopedia.wikia.com/wiki/Orthosis.

OSHA. 1999. *OSHA Technical Manual (OTM) Section III: Chapter 6. Laser Hazards*. 21pp. Accessed 6/05/15 at: https://www.osha.gov/dts/osta/otm/otm_iii/otm_iii_6.html#4.

Ozcan, J., A.R. Ward and V.J. Robertson. 2004. A comparison of true and premodulated interferential currents. *Arch. Phys. Med. Rehabil*. 85: 409–415.

Pacific Northwest X-Ray, Inc. 2015. X-Ray Grids Datasheets. Accessed 10/18/15 at: www.ppnwx.com/Parts/Grids/.

Padiyar, S.D., H. Wang, M.V. Gubarev, W.M. Wilson and C.A. MacDonald. 2000. Beam collimation using Polycapillary X-ray optics for large are diffraction applications. *Advances in X-Ray Analysis*. 43: 254–259. Accessed 1017/15 at: www.icdd.com/resources/axa/vol43/v43_034.pdf.

Pállas-Areny, R. and J.G. Webster. 1991. *Sensors and Signal Conditioning*. John Wiley & Sons, NY.

Papoulis, A. 1977. *Signal Analysis*. McGraw-Hill Book Co., NY.

Park, J.-W. et al. 2005. Magnetocardiography predicts coronary artery disease in patients with acute chest pain. *Ann. Noninvasive Electrocardiol*. 10(3): 312–323.

Parsa, V., S. Scollie, D. Glista and A. Seelisch. 2013. Nonlinear frequency compression: Effects on sound quality ratings of speech and music. *Trends Amplif*. 17(1): 45–68. doi: 10.1177/1084713813480856.

Patient. 2014. *Helicobacter Pylori and Stomach Pain*. 2pp online bulletin. Accessed 4/26/15 at: www.patient.co.uk/health/helicobacter-pylori-and-stomach-pain.

Patton, B., O.O. Versolato, D.C. Hovde, E. Corsini, J.M. Higbie and D. Budker. 2012. A remotely interrogated all-optical [87]Rb magnetometer. *Appl. Phys. Lett*. 101: 083502. http://dx.doi.org/10.1063/1.4747206. Accessed 4/06/15 at: arxiv.org/pdf/1208.1236.pdf.

Patwa, R. et al. 2014. Laser drilling for high aspect ratio holes and a high open area fraction for space applications. *LMF Session Paper #M1101, 33rd International Congress on Applications of Lasers and Electro-Optics*, San Diego, October 19–23, 2014. 7pp. Accessed 10/18/15 at: www.cla.fraunhofer.

org/content/dam/ccl-laser/en/documents/papers-micromachining/Laser%20drilling%20for%20 high%20aspect%20ratio%20holes%20and%20a%20high%20open%20area%20fraction%20for%20 space%20applications.

Penfield, J.G. and R.F. Reilly. 2007. What nephrologists need to know about gadolinium. *Nat. Clin. Pract. Nephrol.* 3(12): 654–668. doi: 10.10.38/ncpneph0660.

Peng, W.K. et al. 2012. Development of miniaturized, portable magnetic resonance relaxometry system for point-of-care medical diagnosis. *Rev. Sci. Instruments.* 83(9): 095115. 8pp. http://dx.doi. org/10.1063/1.4754296.

Peng, W.K. et al. 2014. Micromagnetic resonance relaxometry for rapid label-free malaria diagnosis. *Nat. Med.* 20(9): 1069–1075. doi: 10.1038/nm.3622.

Pentax Medical. 2015. Data sheet for EC-3490TLi Video Colonoscope RetroView™. Accessed 5/5/15 at: pentaxmedical.com/pentax/en/99/1/EC-3490TLi-Video-Colonoscope-RetroView/.

Perry, I.J. et al. 1995. Prospective study of serum total homocysteine concentration and risk of stroke in middle-aged British men. *Lancet.* 346: 1395–1398.

Peterchev, A.V. et al. 2010. ECT stimulus parameters: Rethinking dosage. *J. ECT.* 26(3): 159–174. doi: 10.1097/YCT.0b013e3181e48165.

Petridou, N. et al. 2012. Pushing the limits of high-resolution functional MRI using a simple high-density multi-element coil design. *NMR Biomed.* 26(1): 65–73. doi: 10.1002/nbm.3820.

Philips. 2014. *Atomic Absorption Spectrometry (F-AAS, GF-AAS, CV-AAS).* 1 p Online article. Accessed 3/18/15 at: www.innovationservices.philips.com/service-catalog/techniques/atomic-absorption-spectrometry-f-aas-cv-aas.

Philipson, B. 2015. *PEMF Technology, What Is It Actually? Frequency.* 2pp web paper. Accessed 1/30/15 at: www.pemft.com/pulsed-electro-magnetic-field-therapy-frequency-for-pemf.

Photonics. 2016. *Stretchable Thin Film Produces Circularly Polarized Light.* 2pp online article. Accessed 2/15/16 at: www.photonics.com/Article.aspx?AID=58195.

Physiopedia. 2015a. *Interferential Therapy.* 4pp web article. Accessed 1/19/15 at: www.physio-pedia. com/Interferential_Therapy.

Physiopedia. 2015b. *Transcutaneous Electrical Nerve Stimulation (TENS).* 3pp web article. Accessed 1/19/15 at: www.physio-pedia.com/Transcutaneous_Electrical_Nerve_Stimulation_%28TENS%29.

Pikkemaat, R., K. Tenbrock, S. Lehmann and S. Leonhardt. 2012. Electrical impedance tomography: New diagnostic possibilities using regional time constant maps. *Appl. Cardiopulm. Pathophysiol.* 16: 212–225.

Pimmel, R.L., R.A. Sunderland, D.J. Robinson, H.B. Williams, R.L. Hamlin and P.A. Bromberg. 1977. Instrumentation for measuring respiratory impedance by forced oscillations. *IEEE Trans. Biomed. Eng.* 24(2): 89–93.

Pinto, L.H. and P.J. Dallos. 1968. An acoustic bridge for measuring the static and dynamic impedance of the eardrum. *IEEE Trans. Biomed. Eng.* 15(1): 10–16.

Pinzani, P., F. Salvianti, M. Pazzagli and C. Orlando. 2010. Circulating nucleic acids in cancer and pregnancy. *Methods.* 50: 302–307. doi: 10.1016/j.ymeth.2010.02.004.

Pohlmann, A., S. Sehati and D. Young. 2001. Effect of changes in lung volume on acoustic transmission through the human respiratory system. *Physiol. Meas.* 22(1): 233–243. doi: 10.1088/0967-3334/22/1/326.

Poljakova, I. et al. 2013. Glucose sensing module—Is it time to integrate it into real-time perioperative monitoring? An observational pilot study with subcutaneous sensors. *Biomed. Pap. Med. Fac. Univ. Palacky Olomouc. Czech. Repub.* 157(4): 346–357. http://doi.org/10.5507/bp.2013.049.

Polydorides, N. and W.B. Lionheart. 2002. A Matlab toolkit for three-dimensional electrical impedance tomography; A contribution to the Electrical Impedance and Diffuse Optical Reconstruction Software Project. *Meas. Sci. Technol.* 13(12): 1871. doi: 10.1088/0957-0233/13/12/310.

Pope, P.A. 2015. Modulating cognition using transcranial direct current stimulation of the cerebellum. *J. Vis. Exp.* 96: e52302. 15pp. doi: 10.3791/52302.

Prakash, R.V. Ed. 2012. *Infrared Thermography*. InTech. ISBN: 978-953-51-0242-7. 246pp. March 15, 2012.

Prikryl, R. and H.P. Kucerova. 2013. Can repetitive transcranial magnetic stimulation be considered effective treatment option for negative symptoms of schizophrenia? *J. ECT.* 29(1): 67–74. doi: 10.1097/YCT.0b013e318270295f.

Proakis, J.G. and D.G. Manolakis. 1995. *Digital Signal Processing: Principles, Algorithms and Applications*, 3rd Ed. Prentice-Hall, Inc., Englewood Cliffs, NJ.

PTI. 2014. Specifications for PTI QuantaMaster™ 400 Steady State Spectrofluorometer. *Photon Technology International*. Accessed 4/20/15 at: www.pti-nj.com/products/Steady-State-Spectrofluorometer/QuantaMaster400/QuantaMaster400-Specifications.html.

Puertolas, D. et al. 1997. Biomedical applications of an imaging silicon pixel array (ISPA) tube. *Nucl. Instr. Methods Phys. Rsch.* 387: 134–136.

Puliafito, C.A., M.R. Hee, J.S. Schumann, J.G. Fujimoto and N.J. Thorofare. 1996. *Optical Coherence Tomography of Ocular Diseases*. SLACK, Inc., Thorofare, NJ. 376pp.

Qi, J.-X. 1990. Determination of Cu, Zn, Fe, Ca, Mg, Na and K in Serum by Flame Atomic Absorption Spectroscopy. *Agilent Technologies, AN AA093*. 3pp. Accessed 3/18/15 at: www.chem.agilent.com/Library/applications/aa093.pdf.

Quell. 2015. sheet. Accessed 2/15/16 at: http://quellrelief.com/product/.

Rabinovitch, B., W.F. March and R.L. Adams. 1982. Noninvasive glucose monitoring of the aqueous humor of the eye. Part 1: Measurements of very small optical rotations. *Diabetes Care.* 5(3): 254–258.

Rader, R.L. 1998. *A White Noise Processing Approach in the Analysis of the Pulmonary System*. MS Dissertation in Biomedical Engineering. University of Connecticut (R.B. Northrop, major advisor).

Radiometer America. 2011. *TCM 4/40 Monitoring Systems Operator's Manual*. Publication 201101. Edition C. Code No. 944-941. 174pp online. Accessed 4/4/26/15 at: www.radiometeramerica.com/~/media/files/radiometercomcloneset/rame/manuals/tcm/944-941c-tcm4-40-operators-manual—english.pdf.

Radiometer America. 2012. *The tcpCO$_2$ Handbook*. Accessed 4/26/15 at: www.radiometeramerica.com/~/media/files/radiometercomcloneset/rame/links/tcpco2handbook.pdf?la=en-US.

Radon, T.P. et al. 2015. Identification of a three-biomarker panel in urine for early identification of pancreatic adenocarcinoma. *Clin. Cancer Res.* 21: 3512–3521. August 1. doi: 10.1158/1078-0432. CCR-14-2467.

Rahman, Md. M. et al. 2010. A comprehensive review of glucose biosensors based on nanostructured metal-oxides. *Sensors.* 10: 4855–4886. doi: 10.3390/s100504855.

R.A.L.E. 2008. *The R.A.L.E. Repository. Hear Respiratory Sounds.* Accessed 3/26/15 at: www.rale.ca/Recordings.htm.

Raman, C.V. and K.S. Krishnan. 1928. A new type of secondary radiation. *Nature.* 121: 501–502.

Raman Products. 2001. *Holographic Notch Filters. Raman Products Technical Note No. 1050.* Accessed 4/24/14 at: www.sciencemadness.org/talk/files.php?pid=118496&aid=4850.

RamanRXN Systems. 2001. *Holographic Notch Filters.* 2pp tutorial paper, No. 1050. Accessed 7/11/15 at: file:///C:/Users/Owner/Downloads/1050%20(4).pdf.

Ramos, I.R.M., A. Malkin and F.M. Lyng. 2015. Current advances in the application of Raman spectroscopy for molecular diagnosis of cervical cancer. *BioMed Res. Int.* 2015: 9pp. Article ID 561242. http://dx.doi.org/10.1155/2015/561242.

Ran, F.A. et al. 2013. Double nicking by RNA-guided CRISPR Cas9 for enhanced genome editing specificity. *Cell.* 154: 1380–1389. http://dx.doi.org/10.1016/j.cell.2013.08.021.

Rantala, J.K. et al. 2011. A cell spot microarray method for production of high density siRNA tranfection microarrays. *BMC Genomics.* 12: 162. 14pp. doi: 10.1186/1471-2164-12-162.

Rao, R.P.V. et al. 1995. Parallel Implementation of the Filtered Back Projection Algorithm for Tomographic Imaging. 23pp web paper. Accessed 10/20/15 at: www.sv.vt.udu/xray_ct/parallel/Parallel_CT.html.

Rappaz, B. et al. 2008. Comparative study of human erythrocytes by digital holographic microscopy, confocal microscopy, and impedance volume analyzer. *Cytometry.* 73A: 895–903. doi: 10.1002/cyto.a.20605.

Rawlings, C.A. 1991. *Electrocardiography: Biophysical Measurements.* Spacelabs. ISBN-10: 0-962-74491-3.

Redhead, J.T. 1998. Otoacoustic emissions and recreational hearing loss. *Med. J. Australia.* 169(11): 587–588.

Reilley, C.N. and D.T. Sawyer. 1961. *Experiments for Instrumental Methods.* McGraw-Hill, NY.

Reisch, S., H. Steltner, J. Timmer, C. Renotte and J. Guttmann. 1999. Early detection of upper airway obstructions by analysis of acoustical respiratory input impedance. *Biol. Cybernetics.* 81: 25–37.

Rhodes, D.J. et al. 2011. Dedicated dual-head gamma imaging for breast cancer screening in women with mammographically dense breasts. *Radiology.* 258(1): 106–118. doi: 10.1148/radiol.10100625.

Rice, D. 1983. Sound speed in pulmonary parenchyma. *J. Appl. Physiol.* 54: 304–308.

Ricor. 2015. *Stirling Cooler.* US Patent No. 6,397,605 B1. June 4, 2002. N. Pundak, inventor.

Riederer, K.A.J. and J. Backman. 1998. Frequency response of stethoscopes. *Proc. Nordic Acoustical Meeting 1998 (NAM98).* Stockholm, Sweden. 4pp. Accessed 5/02/15 at: www.kar/fi/KARAudio/Publications/publications/nam98.pdf.

Rijpma, A.P. et al. 1999. Design for a fetal heart monitor for clinical use. *4th Intl. Conf. on Neuroscience and Neuroimaging.* Friedrich Schiller University, Jena, Germany.

Riley, D.E. 2005. *DNA Testing: An Introduction for Non-Scientists—An Illustrated Explanation.* 24pp web tutorial. Accessed 1/02/15 at: www.scientific.org/tutorials/articles/riley/riley.html.

Riley, H.D. 2007. Slit lamp illumination types, associated ocular conditions and slit lamp examination procedures. Indiana University School of Optometry Lecture Notes. Jan. 2007.

Rillahan, C.D. and J.C. Paulson. 2011. Glycan microarrays for decoding the glycome. *Annu. Rev. Biochem.* 80: 797–823. doi: 10.1146/annurev-biochem-061809-152236.

Rivera-Ruiz, M., C. Cajavilca and J. Varon. 2008. Einthoven's string galvanometer: The first electrocardiograph. *Tex. Heart J.* 35(2): 174–178.

Robinette, M.S. and T.S. Glattke. 2011. *Otoacoustic Emissions: Clinical Applications*, 3rd Ed. Thieme Medical Publishers, Stuttgart, Germany. ISBN: 1604066296.

Robson, J.L. 2010. *Horses in Color: The Role of Thermal Imaging in the Equine Industry*. 10pp online review paper. Accessed 10/21/15 at: www.irinfo.org/articleofmonth/pdf/3_1_2019_robson.pdf.

Rogalski, A. 2009. Infrared detectors for the future. *Acta Physica Polonica A.* 116(3): 389–406.

Romalis, M.V. 2008. *The Spin Exchange Relaxation Free (SERF) Magnetometer*. 6pp online tutorial paper. Accessed 4/7/15 at: physics.princeton.edu/romalis/magnetometer/.

Routh, H.F. 1996. Doppler ultrasound. *IEEE Eng. in Med. and Biol. Mag.* 15(6): 31–40.

Rowell, J.M. 1998. Squid applications. Ch. 6. In: *WTEC Panel Final Report on: Electronic Applications of Superconductivity in Japan.* J.M. Rowell, M.R. Beasley and R.W. Ralston, Eds. Int'l. Technol. Rsch. Inst., Baltimore, MD. pp. 37–43. July 1998. Accessed 3/28/15 at: www.wtec.org/loyola/scel96/06_01.htm.

Rowell, N.D. 2000. Gains made in macular degeneration treatment. *Photonics Spectra.* 34(12): 50–55.

Rubina, S. and C. Murali Krishna. 2015. Raman spectroscopy in cervical cancers. *J. Cancer Res. Ther.* 11(1): 10–17. doi: 10.4103/0973-1482.154065.

Rubin, M. 2015. Amyotrophic lateral sclerosis and other motor neuron diseases. *Merck Manual Professional Version.* 7pp. Accessed 4/29/15 at: www.merckmanuals.com/professional/neurologic-disorders/peripheral-nervous-system-and-motor-unit-disorders/amyotrophic-lateral-sclerosis-and-other-motor-neuron-disorders.

Russo, P. and A. Del Guerra. 2014. Solid-state detectors for small-animal imaging. Ch. 2. In: *Molecular Imaging of Small Animals: Instrumentation and Applications.* Springer Science + Business Media, NY. 61pp. doi: 10.1007/978-1-4939-0894-3_2.

Sackeim, H.A. et al. 2008. Effect of pulse width and electrode placement on the efficacy and cognitive effects of electroconvulsive therapy. *Brain Stimul.* 1(2): 71–83. doi: 10:1016/j.brs.2008.03.001.

Salehi, H.S., T. Wang, P.D. Kumavor, H. Li and Q. Zhu. 2014. Design of miniaturized illumination for transvaginal co-registered photoacoustic and ultrasound imaging. *Biomed. Opt. Express.* 5(9): 3074–3079. doi: 10.1364/BOE.5.003074.

Salenius, J.P. et al. 1998. Biochemical composition of human peripheral arteries examined with near-infrared Raman spectroscopy. *J. Vasc. Surg.* 24(7): 710–719.

Salisbury, D.F. 2001. Free-Electron Laser: Creating a new kind of X-ray machine. *Exploration.* October 9, 2001. Accessed 10/15/15 at: www.vanderbilt.edu/exploration/news/news_fel_monox.htm.

Sander, T.H., J. Preusser, R. Mhaskar, J. Kitching, L. Trahms and S. Knappe. 2012. Magnetoencephalography with a chip-scale atomic magnetometer. *Biomed. Opt. Express.* 3(5): 981–985.

Saxer, C.E., J.F. de Boer et al. 2000. High-speed fiber-based polarization-sensitive optical coherence tomography of *in vivo* human skin. *Opt. Lett.* 25(18): 1355–1357.

Schauenstein, K. and E. Schauenstein. 1998. Diagnostic relevance of non-specific tumor-associated immune dysfunctions. *Cancer J.* 11(3): 106–110.

Schlager, K.J. 1989. *Non-Invasive Near Infrared Measurement of Blood Analyte Concentrations.* US Patent No. 4,882,492. (Transcutaneous non-dispersive spectrophotometry used to sense blood glucose using 900–1800 nm light.)

Schmitt, J.M., G.-X. Zhou and J. Miller. 1992. Measurement of blood hematocrit by dual-wavelength near-IR photoplethysmo-graphy. *Proc. SPIE.* 1641: 150–161.

Scott, G. and J.B. King. 1994. A prospective, double-blind trial of electrical capacitive coupling in the treatment of non-union of long bones. *J. Bone Joint Surg.* 76(6): 820–825.

Scott, R.P.W. 2015. The Mechanism of Fluorescence. 2pp web paper. From: *Analytical Spectroscopy,* by R.P.W. Scott. Accessed 1/05/15 at: www.analyticalspectroscopy.net/ap2-2.htm.

Sealock, R., O. Rondon-Aramayo and D.V.H. Bengis. 1998. Energy and Position Sensitive Radiation Detectors. US Patent 5,783,829 A.

Sears, F.W. 1953. *Electricity and Magnetism.* Addison-Wesley Pub. Co., Inc., Cambridge, MA.

Sellmeyer, M.A. et al. 2013. Visualizing cellular interactions with a generalized proximity reporter. *PNAS.* 110(21): 8567–8572.

Seltzer, S.J. and M.V. Romalis. 2004. Unshielded three-axis vector operation of a spin-exchange-relaxation-free atomic magnetometer. *Appl. Phys. Lett.* 85(20): 4804–4806. doi: 10.10.63/1.1814434.

Semenov, S.Y. and D.R. Corfield. 2008. Microwave tomography for brain imaging: Feasibility assessment for stroke detection. *Intl. J. Antennas Propag.* 2008. Article ID 254830. 8pp. doi: 10.1155/2008/254830.

Semenov, S.Y. et al. 1996. Microwave tomography: Two-dimensional system for biological imaging. *IEEE Trans. Biomed. Eng.* 43(9): 869–877.

Semwogerere, D. and E.R. Weeks. 2005. Confocal microscopy. In: *Encyclopedia of Biomaterials and Biomedical Engineering.* 10pp. doi: 10.1081/E-EBBE-120024153. Accessed 1/08/15 at: www.physics.emory.edu/faculty/weeks//lab/papers/ebbe05.pdf.

Sergeev, A.M. et al. 1997. *In vivo* endoscopic OCT imaging of precancer and cancer states of human mucosa. *Opt. Express.* 1(13): 432–440.

Shao, J. et al. 2012. *In vivo* blood glucose quantification using Raman spectroscopy. *PLoS ONE.* 7(10): e48127. 6pp. doi: 10.1371journal.pone.0048127.

Sharma, A.K. and A. Sharma, Eds. 2001. *Chromosome Painting: Principles, Strategies and Scope (Vol. 23).* Springer. 179pp. ISBN-13: 978-9401038409.

Shivashankar, G.V. and A. Libchaber. 1997. Single DNA molecule grafting and manipulation using a combined atomic force microscope and optical tweezers. *Appl. Phys. Lett.* 71(25): 3727–3729.

Shotton, D.M. 1989. REVIEW: Confocal scanning optical microscopy and its applications for biological specimens. *J. Cell Sci.* 94: 175–206.

Shung, K.K. and M. Zipparo. 1996. Ultrasonic transducers and arrays. *IEEE Eng. Med. Biol. Mag.* 15(6): 20–30.

Shupak, N.M. 2003. Therapeutic uses of pulsed magnetic field exposure: A review. *The Radio Science Bulletin*. 307: 24pp. Accessed 2/04/15 at: www.nisancos.com/wp-content/uploads/2013/09/shupak2003.pdf.

Shybut, G. and B. Donley. 2012. *OsteoGen™ Surgically Implanted Bone Growth Stimulator*. 20pp web article. Accessed 1/24/15 at: www.biomet.com/trauma/getFile.cfm?id=3005&rt=inline.

Siever, D. 2013. *Transcranial DC Stimulation*. 7pp online review paper. Accessed 5/13/15 at: mindalive.com/default/assets/File/tDCS%20Neuroconnections%20article.pdf.

Signal Processing, S.A. 2015. *Background of Ultrasonic Doppler Velocimetry*. 2pp online tutorial paper. Accessed 6/02/15 at: www.signal-processing.com/intro_udv.html.

Simon, H.J. 1998. *Sensor Using Long Range Surface Plasmon Resonance with Diffraction Double Grating*. US Patent No. 5,846,843. December 8, 1998.

Simpson, A. 2009. Frequency-lowering devices for managing high-frequency hearing loss: A review. *Trends Amplif.* 13(2): 87–106.

Simren, M. and P.-O. Stotzer. 2006. Use and abuse of hydrogen breath tests. *Gut.* 55(3): 297–303. doi: 10.1136/gut.2005.075127.

Sinusas, K. 2012. Osteoarthritis: Diagnosis and treatment. *Am. Fam. Physician.* 85(1): 49–56.

Sirohi, R.S. and M.P. Kothiyal. 1991. *Optical Components, Systems, and Measurement Techniques*. Marcel Dekker, Inc., NY.

Skin Cancer Foundation. 2015. *Skin Cancer Facts*. 10pp web article. Accessed 5/06/15 at: www.skin-cancer.org/skin-cancer-information/skin-cancer-facts.

Smith, F.E. et al. 2006. Comparison of magnetocardiography and electrocardiography: A study of automatic measurement of dispersion of ventricular repolarization. *Europace.* 8: 887–893. doi: 10.1093/europace/eul070.

Smith, J., C. Fritz and J. Wolfe. 2000. A new technique for the rapid measurement of the acoustic impedance of wind instruments. *Seventh International Conference on Sound and Vibration*. Garmisch-Pertenkirchen, Germany, July 4–7, 2000. 6pp.

Smith, S.W., R.E. Davidson and C.D. Emery. 1996. Update on 2-D array transducers for medical ultrasound. *1995 IEEE Ultrasonics Symp. Proc. 1273*.

Smithsonian. 2015. *Whatever Happened to Polio? The Iron Lung and Other Equipment*. 4pp online article. Accessed 5/15/15 at: amhistory.si.edu/polio/howpolio/ironlung.htm.

Sodickson, L.A. and M.J. Block. 1994. Kromoscopic analysis: A possible alternative to spectroscopic analysis for noninvasive measurement of analytes *in vivo*. *Clin. Chem.* 40: 1838–1844.

Sodickson, L.A. and M.J. Block. 1995. Non-Spectrophotometric Measurement of Analyte Concentrations and Optical Properties of Objects. US Patent No. 5,434,412 A. July 18, 1995.

Soenksen, D.C. et al. 1999. *Method of Cancer Cell Detection*. US Patent No. 5,995,645. November 30, 1999.

Song, X., J. Heimburg-Molinaro, R.D. Cummings and D.F. Smith. 2014b. Chemistry of natural glycan microarrays. *Curr. Opin. Chem. Biol.* 18: 70–77. doi: 10.1016/j.cbpa.2014.01.001.

Song, X., J. Heimburg, D.F. Smith and R.D. Cummings. 2012. Glycan microarrays. *Methods Mol. Biol.* 800: 163–171. doi: 10.1007/978-1-61779-349-3_11.

Song, Y., Q. Hao, X. Kong, L. Hu, J. Cao and T. Gao. 2014a. Simulation of the recharging method of implantable biosensors based on a wearable incoherent light source. *Sensors.* 14: 20687–20701. doi: 10.3390/s141120687.

Sosnytskyy, V. et al. 2013. Magnetocardiography capabilities in myocardium injuries diagnosis. *World J. Cardiovasc. Diseases.* 3: 380–388.

Spears, C. 1999. Controversies in glaucoma care. *Rev. Ophthalmol.* 199: 89–99.

Spegazzini, N. et al. 2014. Spectroscopic approach for dynamic bioanalyte tracking with minimal concentration information. *Sci. Rep.* 4: 7013. 7pp. doi: 10.1038/srep07013.

Speicher, M.R., B.S. Gwyn and D.C. Ward. 1996. Karyotyping human chromosomes by combinatorial multifluor FISH. *Nat. Genet.* 12(4): 368–375.

Srinavasan, R., D.M. Tucker and M. Murias. 1998. Estimating the spatial Nyquist of the human EEG. *Behav. Res .Meth. Instrum. Comput.* 30(1): 8–19.

Stark, H., F.B. Tuteur and J.B. Anderson. 1988. *Modern Electrical Communications.* Prentice-Hall, Englewood Cliffs, NJ.

Stelletta, C. et al. 2012. Thermographic applications in veterinary medicine. In: *Infrared Thermography.* Dr. R.V. Prakash, Ed. InTech, Rijeka, Croatia. ISBN: 978-953-51-0242-7.

Stephen, M.M. et al. 2013. Diagnostic accuracy of diffuse reflectance imaging for early detection of pre-malignant and malignant changes in the oral cavity: A feasibility study. *BMC Cancer.* 13: 278. 9pp.

Sticker, M., C.K. Hitzenberger and A.F. Fercher. 2000. Direct extraction of phase information in differential phase contrast OCT. *Proc. SPIE.* 4241: *Saratov Fall Meeting 2000: Optical Technologies in Biophysics and Medicine II, 168.* May 4, 2001. doi: 10.1117/12.431517.

Stowell, S.R. et al. 2014. Microbial glycan microarrays define key features of host-microbial interactions. *Nat. Chem. Biol.* 10: 470–476. doi: 10.10.38/nchembio.1525.

Strasburger, J.F., B. Cheulkar and R.T. Wakai. 2008. Magnetocardiography for fetal arrhythmias. *Heart Rhythm.* 5(7): 1073–1076. doi: 10.1016/j.hrthm.2008.02.035.

Strommer, J. 1996. *Let's Play PET—Main Menu.* Online PET tutorial. Accessed 6/30/15 at: www. analchem.ugent.be/radiochemie/funct_beeldvorming/Let's_Play_PET_static/laxmi.nuc.ucla. edu_8000/lpp/lpphome.html.

Sugiro, F.R., D. Li and C.A. MacDonald. 2004. Beam collimation with polycapillary x-ray optics for high contrast resolution monochromatic imaging. *Med. Phys.* 31(12): 3288–3297.

Suki, B. and K.R. Lutchen. 1992. Pseudorandom signals to estimate apparent transfer and coherence functions of nonlinear systems: Applications to respiratory mechanics. *IEEE Trans. Biomed. Engrg.* 39(11): 1142–1150.

Sullivan, D.J., Jr. 2005. Hemozoin: A biocrystal synthesized during the degradation of hemoglobin. In: *Biopolymers for Medical and Pharmacological Applications.* A. Steinbüchel and R.H. Marchessault, Eds. 1145pp. Wiley-VCH. ISBN: 3-527-31154-8.

Sunshine, I. and P.I. Jatlow, Eds. 1982. *Methodology for Analytical Toxicology, V. II.* CRC Press, Boca Raton, FL.

Takatani, S. and J. Ling. 1994. Optical oximetry sensors for whole blood and tissue. *IEEE Eng. Med. Biol. Mag.* June/July: 347–357.

Takehana, S., M. Kaneko and H. Mizuno. 1999. Endoscopic diagnostic system using autofluorescence. *Diagn. Ther. Endosc.* 5: 59–63.

Tangerman, A. and E.G. Winkel. 2007. Intra- and extra-oral halitosis: Finding a new form of extra-oral blood-borne halitosis caused by dimethyl sulfide. *J. Clin. Periodontol.* 34(9): 748–755.

Tangerman, A. and E.G. Winkel. 2010. Extra-oral halitosis: An overview. *J. Breath Res.* 4(1): 017003. doi: 10.1088/1752-7155/4/1/017003.

Taplidou, S.A., L.J. Hadjileontiadis, T. Penzel, V. Gross and S.M. Panas. 2003. WED: An efficient wheezing-episode detector based on breath sounds spectrogram analysis. *Proc. 25th Ann. Int'l. Conf. of the IEEE EMBS.* Cancun, Mexico, September 17–21, 2003. pp. 2531–2534.

Tarr, R.V. and P.G. Steffes. 1993. *Noninvasive Blood Glucose Measurement System and Method Using Stimulated Raman Spectroscopy.* US Patent No. 5,243,983. September 14, 1993.

Tarr, R.V. and P.G. Steffes. 1998. The noninvasive measurement of D-glucose in the ocular aqueous humor using stimulated Raman spectroscopy. *IEEE LEOS.* 12(2): 10pp. Accessed 4/23/15 at: photonicssociety.org/newsletters/apr98/dgloucose.htm [sic].

Tascioglu, F. et al. 2010. Short-term effectiveness of ultrasound energy in knee osteoarthritis. *J. Int. Med. Res.* 38: 1233–1242.

Taylor, L. 2015. *DUI Breathalyzer Accuracy.* 3pp web article. Accessed 6/11/15 at: https://www.dui-central.com/evidence/breathalyzer-accuracy/.

Tel Aviv U. 2015. *Flame Emission Spectroscopy (FES).* 3pp online class notes. Accessed 5/30/15 at: www.tau.ac.il/~chemlaba/Files/Flame%20supplement.pdf.

Theranos. 2015. *Theranos Wellness Centers.* 10pp online address listing. Accessed 5/1715 at: https://theranos.com/centers Also see: https://theranos.com/test-menu.

Thet, N.T. et al. 2015. Prototype development of the intelligent hydrogel wound dressing and its efficacy in the detection of model pathogenic wound biofilms. *ACS Applied Materials & Interfaces.* (/journal/1944-8252), 2015. doi: 10.1021/acsami.5b07372.

Thevis, M., G. Opfermann and W. Schänzer. 2003. Urinary concentrations of morphine and codeine after consumption of poppy seeds. *J. Analyt. Toxicol.* 27: 53–56.

Tilson-Chrysler. 1994. Understanding heart sounds, Part 1. *Dynamic Chiropractic.* 12(11): 4pp. Accessed 5/03/15 at: www.dynamicchiropractic.com/mpacms/dc/article.php?id=41254.

Tiporlini, V. and K. Alameh. 2013. Optical magnetometer employing adaptive noise cancellation for unshielded magnetocardiography. *Univers. J. Biomed. Eng.* 1(1): 16–21. doi: 10.13189/ujbe.3013.010104.

Toennies, J.L., G. Tortora, M. Simi, P. Valdastri and R.J. Webster. 2009. Swallowable medical devices for diagnosis and surgery: The state of the art. *Proc. IMechE.* 224(Part C): 18pp. doi: 10.1243/09544062JMES1879.

Tonometers. 2017. *Tonometers.* The College of Optometrists. 4pp. Accessed 5/31/17 at: https://college-optometrists.org/the-college/museum/online-exhibitions/virtual-ophthalmic-instrument-gallery/tonometers.html.

Tope, W.D. et al. 1998. Protoporphyrin IX fluorescence induced in basal cell carcinoma by oral 5-aminolevulinic acid. *Photochem. Photobiol.* 67(2): 249–255.

Transferrin. 2001. *Iron Transport and Cellular Uptake*. 12pp online tutorial paper. Accessed 6/24/15 at: sickle.bwh.harvard.edu/iron_transport.html.

Transonic. 2012. *Theory of Operation: Laser Doppler Tissue Perfusion Technology: Laser Doppler Uses and Limitations*. 2pp online tech note. Accessed 7/10/15 at: www.transonic.com/resources/research/laser-doppler-theory-of-operation/.

Treatable. 2016. *Treatable Conditions*. 8pp web advertising claim. Accessed 2/18/16 at: https://willowcurve.com/conditions.

Tremper, K.K. 1984. Review Article: Transcutaneous PO$_2$ measurement. *Can. Anaesth. Soc. J.* 31(6): 664–677.

Tremper, K.K. and S.J. Barker. 1987. Transcutaneous oxygen measurement: Experimental studies and adult applications. *Int. Anesthesiol. Clin.* 25(3): 67–96. Accessed 3/27/15 at: www.experts.umich.edu/pubDetail.asp?id=23405832&o_id=34&t=pm.

Trio33. 2015. *Pulse Electromagnetic Field Therapy: Clinically Proven for Over 20 Years to Help*. 11pp web article containing abstracts of papers on PEMF therapy. Accessed 1/28/15 at: www.trio33.com/pdf/Clinical%20Studies.pdf.

Truax, B., Ed. 1999. *Handbook for Acoustic Ecology*, 2nd Ed. Online reference text in acoustics. Accessed 5/02/15 at: www.sfu.ca/sonic-studio/handbook/ ©Cambridge Street Publishing 1999.

Tu, Q. and C. Chang. 2012. (Review article.) Diagnostic applications of Raman spectroscopy. *Nanomedicine: Nanotechnol. Biol Med.* 8(5): 545–558. http://dx.doi.org/10.1016/j.nano.2011.09.013.

Tumer, T.O. et al. 2009. New two-dimensional solid state pixel detectors with dedicated front-end integrated circuits for X-ray and gamma-ray imaging. *IEEE Trans. Nucl. Sci.* 56(4): 2321–2329. doi: 10.1109/TNS.2009.2022939.

Turner Designs. 1998. *Technical Note: An Introduction to Fluorescent Measurements*. 15pp App. notes. Accessed 6/03/15 at: www.turnerdesigns.com/t2/doc/appnotes/998-0050.pdf.

Underwood, E. 2015. *Ultrasound Therapies Target Brain Cancers and Alzheimer's Disease*. 6pp online science article. Accessed 3/13/15 at: news.sciencemag.org/biology/2015/03/ultrasound-therapies-target-brain-cancers-and-alzheimer-s-disease.

UWashington. 2015. *Demonstrations: Heart Sounds and Murmurs*. Accessed 3/26/15 at: depts.washington.edu/physdx/heart/demo.html.

Vance, A. 2013. *Why Do Hearing Aids Cost More Than Laptops? 2pp Bloomberg consumer electronics essay*. Accessed 6/18/15 at: www.bloomberg.com/bw/articles/2013-06-06/why-do-hearing-aids-cost-more-than-laptops.

van de Velde, F.K. 2006. The relaxed confocal scanning laser ophthalmoscope. *Bull. Soc. Belge. Ophtalmol.* 302: 24–35. Accessed 5/03/15 at: www.ophthalmologia.be/download.php?dof_id=383.

Verdon, W. 2000. Director, Electrodiagnostic and Vision Function Clinic. http://spectacle.berkeley.edu/ucbso/vfc/.

Verhoef, P. et al. 1996. Homocysteine metabolism and risk of myocardial infarction: Relation with vitamins B6, B12 and folate. *Am J. Epidemiol.* 143(9): 845–859.

Victoria, G., B. Petrisor, B. Drew and D. Dick. 2009. Bone stimulation for fracture healing: What's all the fuss? *Indian J. Orthoped.* 43(2): 117–120. doi: 10.4103/0019-5413.50844.

Vieira, P., A. Manivannan, C.S. Lim, P. Sharp and J.V. Forrester. 1999. Tomographic reconstruction of the retina using a confocal scanning laser ophthalmoscope. *Physiol. Meas.* 20(1): 1–19. doi: 10.1088/0967-3334/20/1/001.

Villchur, E. 2004. *Elements of Effective Hearing-Aid Performance*. 6pp online paper. Accessed 6/15/15 at: www.audiologyonline.com/articles/elements-effective-hearing-aid-performance-1098.

Vo, N.N., L. Chen, X. Liu, W.K. Peng, Z.Y. Ming and J. Han. 2014. Highly integrated, low cost, palm-top sized magnetic resonance relaxometry system for rapid blood screening. *IFBME Proc.* (43): 558–561. (*15th Intl. Conf. on Biomedical Engineering*, Singapore, December 4–7, 2013). doi: 10.1007/978-3-319-02913-9_142.

VTT. 2015. *Cell Spot Microarray Technology*. 2pp online specifications. Accessed 4/19/15 at: www.vtt. fi/files/research/bic/cell_spot_microarray_technology.pdf.

Wagner, A. 2014. MRI imaging may identify a biomarker for early detection of Alzheimer's disease. 3pp abstract: *Detection of pre-symptomatic Alzheimer's disease using 7-Tesla MRI*. Accessed 4/14/16 at: www.dana.org/Media/GrantsDetails.aspx?id=116652.

Wallace, V.P. et al. 2000. Spectrophotometric assessment of pigmented skin lesions: Methods and feature selection for evaluation of diagnostic performance. *Phys. Med. Biol.* 45: 735–751.

Wang, H. et al. 2013. One-step generation of mice carrying mutations in multiple genes by CRISPR/Cas-mediated genome engineering. *Cell.* 153: 910–918. http://dx.doi.org/10.1016/j.cell.2013.04.025.

Wang, T., S. Nandy, H.S. Salehi, P.D. Kumavor and Q. Zhu. 2014. A low-cost photoacoustic microscopy system with a laser diode excitation. *Biomed. Opt. Express.* 5(9): 6pp. doi: 10.1364/BOE.5.003053.

Wang, X.-J. et al. 1999. Characterization of dentin and enamel by use of optical coherence tomography. *Appl. Opt.* 38(10): 2092–2096.

Ward, A.R. 2009. Electrical stimulation using kilohertz frequency. *Phys. Ther.* 89: 181–190. doi: 10.2522/ptj.20080060.

Ward, J.W. 1977. Automatic Acoustic Impedance Meter. U.S. Patent No. 4,009,707. March 1, 1977.

Wayne, J.D., D.K. Rex and C.B. Williams, Eds. 2003. *Colonoscopy: Principles and Practice*. Blackwell Publishing. 666pp. ISBN-10 1-4051-1449-5. Accessed 5/4/15 at: www.colonoscopy.ru/books/rar/Colonoscopy%20Principles%20and%20Practice.pdf.

Webb, R.H. 1996. Confocal optical microscopy. *Rep. Prog. Phys.* 59: 427–471.

Webb, R.H., G.W. Hughes and F.C. Delori. 1987. Confocal scanning laser ophthalmoscope. *Appl. Optics.* 26(8): 1492–9. doi: 10.1364/AO.26.001492.

WebMD. 2014. *Skin Cancer*. Melanoma/Skin Cancer Health Center. 10pp web article. Accessed 5/06/15 at: www.webmd.com/melanoma-skin-cancer/melanoma-guide/skin-cancer.

WebMD. 2015. *Heat and Cold Therapy for Arthritis Pain*. Arthritis Health Center. 4pp web article. Accessed 2/18/16 at: www.webmd.com/arthritis/heat-and-cold-therapy-for-arthritis-pain.

Webster, G.D. and H.C. Gabler. 2007. Feasibility of transdermal ethanol sensing for the detection of intoxicated drivers. *Annu. Proc. Adv. Automot. Med.* 51: 449–464.

Webster, J.G. 1992. *Medical Instrumentation: Application and Design*, 2nd Ed. Houghton-Mifflin Co., Boston.

Webster, J.G. 1998. *Medical Instrumentation: Application and Design*, 3rd Ed. John Wiley & Sons, NY.

West, J.B., Ed. 1985. *Best and Taylor's Physiological Basis of Medical Practice*, 11th Ed. Williams & Wilkins, Baltimore.

Whitehouse. 2014. *Fact Sheet: Over $300 Million in Support of the President's BRAIN Initiative*. 11pp online bulletin. Accessed 5/14/15 at: https://www.whitehouse.gov/sites/default/files/microsites/ostp/brain_fact_sheet_9_30_2014_final.pdf.

WHO. 2014a. Malaria. *WHO Media Centre Fact Sheet No. 94*. (Updated 12/2014). 7pp. Accessed 12/14/14 at: www.who.int/mediacentre/factsheets/fs094/en/.

WHO. 2014b. World Malaria Report 2014. World Health Organization. 142pp. Accessed 4/15/15 at: www.who.int/malaria/publications/world_malaria_report_2014/wmr-2014-no-profiles.pdf?ua=1.

Wienke, J.C. and P. Dayton. 2011. Bone stimulation for nonunions: What the evidence shows. *Podiatr. Today*. 24(9): 6pp. Accessed 10/25/15 at: www.podiatyrtoday.com/bone=stimulation-nonunions-what-evidence-reveals.

Williams, C.S. 1986. *Designing Digital Filters*. Prentice-Hall, Inc., Englewood Cliffs, NJ.

Willow Curve. 2016. *The Device*. 8pp sales brochure. Accessed 2/18/16 at: https://willowcurve.com/device.

Wingert, T.A., C.J. Bassi, W.H. McAlister and J.C. Galanis. 1995. Clinical evaluation of five portable tonometers. *J. Am. Optom. Assoc.* 66(11): 670–674.

Wodicka, G.B., K.N. Stevens, H.L. Golub, E.G. Cravalho and D.C. Shannon. 1989. A model of acoustic transmission in the respiratory system. *IEEE Trans. BioMed. Eng.* 36(9): 925–934.

Wojcik, M.H. and J.S. Hawthorne. 2007. Sensitivity of commercial ethyl glucuronide (EtG) testing in screening for alcohol abstinence. *Alcohol Alcohol.* 42(4): 317–320.

Wolfbeis, O.S., Ed. 1991. *Fiber Optic Sensors and Biosensors, Vol. 1*. CRC Press, Boca Raton, FL.

Wood, J.C. and D.T. Barry. 1995. Time-frequency analysis of the first heart sound. *IEEE Eng. Med. Biol. Mag.* March/April: 144–151.

Wood, J.C., A.J. Buda and D.T. Barry. 1992. Time-frequency transforms: A new approach to first heart sound frequency dynamics. *IEEE Trans. Biomed. Eng.* 39(7): 730–740.

Wordpress. 2008. *Infrared Absorbances for Common Functional Groups. Table 2*. 2pp online summary table of Organic Functional Groups. Accessed 6/04/15 at: https://chimiquefiles.wordpress.com/2008/11/ir-spectroscopy-table2.pdf.

Wright, A.V., J.K. Nuñez and J.A. Doudna. 2016. Biology and applications of CRISPR systems: Harnessing nature's toolbox for genome engineering. *Cell.* 164: 29–44. http://dx.doi.org/10.1016/j.cell.2015.12.035.

Wu, Y. et al. 2013. Correction of a genetic disease in mouse via use of CRISPR-Cas9. *Cell Stem Cell.* 13: 659–662. http://dx.doi.org/10.1016/j.stem.2013.10.016.

Xie, X., M. McGregor and N. Dendukuri. 2010. The clinical effectiveness of negative pressure wound therapy: A systematic review. *J. Wound Care.* 19(11): 490–495. doi: 10.12968/jowc.2010.19.11.79697.

XOS. 2008. *Polycapillary Focusing X-Ray Optics*. X-Ray Optical Systems, Inc., Datasheet & Info. Accessed 10/17/15 at: https://xos.com/industries/high-performance-x-ray-optics/optics/polycapillary-optics/x-tra-polycapillary-focussing-optics/.

Yaghoubi, M. et al. 2015. Confocal scan laser ophthalmoscope for diagnosing glaucoma: A systematic review and meta-analysis. *Asia Pac. J. Ophthalmol.* 4(1): 32–39.

Yamaguchi, M., M. Mitsumori and Y. Kano. 1998. Noninvasively measuring blood glucose using saliva. *IEEE Eng. Med. Biol. Mag.* 17(3): 59–63.

Yazdanfar, S., M.D. Kulkarni and J.A. Izatt. 1997. High resolution imaging of in vivo cardiac dynamics using color Doppler optical coherence tomography. *Opt. Express.* 1(13): 424–431.

Yeaw, J., W.C. Lee, M. Aagren and T. Christensen. 2012. Cost of self-monitoring of blood glucose in the United States among patients on an insulin regimen for diabetes. *J. Manag. Care Pharm.* 18(1): 21–32.

Yin, H. et al. 2014. Genome editing with Cas9 in adult mice corrects a disease mutation and phenotype. *Nat. Biotechnol.* 32(6): 551–553. doi: 10.1038/nbt.2884.

Young, P.R. 1996. *Mass Spectrometry—Background.* Organic Chemistry OnLine. Accessed 1/12/16 at: people.stfx.ca/tsmithpa/chem361/labs/spec/MS1.htm.

Young, S.S., D. Tesarowskiá and L. Viel. 1996. Frequency dependence of forces oscillatory mechanics in horses with heaves. *APS Abstracts.* 3: 0497A.

Yu, B., A. Shah, V.K. Nagarajan and D.G. Ferris. 2014. Diffuse reflectance spectroscopy of epithelial tissue with a smart fiber-optic probe. *Biomed. Opt. Express.* 5(3): 675–689. doi: 10.1364/BOE.5.000675.

Yu, C.M. and J.C. Koo. 2001. A High Performance Hand-Held Gas Chromatograph. *Lawrence Livermore National Laboratory. Preprint UCRL-JC-130439-TRV-1.* 8pp. (Article submitted to *9th International Conf.*, Amelia Island, FL. January 21–24, 2001.). Accessed 4/25/15 at: https://e-reports-ext.llnl.gov/pdf/244009.pdf.

Zeng, X. et al. 2015. Phase change dispersion of plasmonic nano-objects. *Sci. Rep.* 5: 12665. 7pp. doi: 10.1038/srep12665.

Zeng, D. et al. 2012. The effect of therapeutic ultrasound to apoptosis of chondrocyte and caspase-3 and caspase-8 expression in rabbit surgery-induced model of knee osteoarthritis. *Rheumatol. Int.* 32: 3771–3777.

Zeng, H. et al. 2008. Raman spectroscopy for in vivo tissue analysis and diagnosis, from instrument development to clinical applications. *J. Innovative Opt. Health Sci.* 1(1): 95–106. doi: 10.1142/S1793545808000054.

Zetsche, B. et al. 2015. Cpf1 is a single RNA-guided endonuclease of a Class 2 CRISPR-Cas system. *Cell.* 163: 759–771. http://dx.doi.org/10.1016/j.cell.2015.09.038.

Zhang, W., Y. Du and M.L. Wang. 2015. Noninvasive glucose monitoring using saliva nano-biosensor. *Sensing Biosensing Res.* 4: 23–29. http://dx.doi.org/10.1016/j.sbsr.2015.02.002.

Zhang, X. et al. 1998. Time-frequency scaling transformation of the phonocardiogram based of [on] the matching pursuit method. *IEEE Trans. Biomed. Eng.* 45(8): 972–979. doi: 10.1109/10.704866.

Zhao, J., H. Lui, D.I. McLean and H. Zeng. 2010. Real-time Raman spectroscopy for noninvasive in vivo skin analysis and diagnosis. In: *New Developments in Biomedical Engineering.* D. Campolo, Ed. ISBN: 978-953-7619-57-2. InTech, DOI: 10.5772/7603. Available from: https://www.intechopen.com/books/new-developments-in-biomedical-engineering/real-time-raman-spectroscopy-for-noninvasive-in-vivo-skin-analysis-and-diagnosis.

Zhou, J., A.L. Loftus, G. Mulley and T.A. Jenkins. 2010. A thin film detection/response system for pathogenic bacteria. *J. Amer. Chem. Soc.* 132(18): 6566–6570. doi: 10.1021/ja101554a.

Zyga, L. 2010. 'Smart' wound dressings could identify and destroy infection-causing bacteria. 3pp PhysOrg web article. Accessed 2/29/16 at: file:///C:/Users/Downloads/2010-05-smart-wound-infection-causing-bacteria.pdf.

Glossary

A

Absorbance (in spectrophotometry): If a beam of monochromatic light (photons) of wavelength λ having power $P_{in}(\lambda)$ is passed through a sample substance, the emerging ray will have, in general, power $P_{out}(\lambda)$ watts. The *transmittance* of the substance at wavelength λ is defined as $T(\lambda) \equiv P_{out}/P_{in}$, $0 \leq T \leq 1.0$. Also used to describe the selective molecular absorption of photons is the *absorbance*; $A(\lambda) \equiv -\log_{10}[T(\lambda)]$. The absorbance is also known as the *optical density* (OD). Graphs of $T(\lambda)$ and $A(\lambda)$ are also often plotted versus *wavenumber*, (ν) (the number of waves [cycles]/cm) in cm^{-1}, that is, $\nu = k/\lambda$ in cm^{-1}, where λ is in nm, and $k = 10^7$ (the ratio of cm to nm). (For example, 940 nm IR light has a wavenumber of $\nu = 10,638$ cm^{-1}.) The optical path length, the concentration, pressure, and temperature of the substance are noted in taking spectrophotometric measurements.

Adiabatic: When a gas is compressed under adiabatic conditions (as when a sound wave is propagating), its pressure increases and its temperature rises without the loss or gain of heat. Conversely, when a gas expands under adiabatic conditions, its pressure and temperature both decrease without the gain or loss of heat.

Amyloid-β: Aβ is formed by the sequential cleavage of the amyloid precursor protein (APP), a transmembrane protein of undetermined function. Aβ is a peptide of 36–43 amino acids that is crucially involved in Alzheimer's disease. Aβ molecules take a misfolded oligomeric form, leading to an autocatalytic (chain) reaction that forms plaques; the reaction is similar to that in a prion protein infection. The Aβ plaques are toxic to neurons in the brain. The roles of normal Aβ in the brain are pleiotropic, and are just beginning to be understood; Aβ has been shown to activate kinase enzymes, protect against oxidative stress, regulate cholesterol transport, function as a transcription factor, and may have an antimicrobial activity.

Apoptosis: Also known as *programmed cell death* (PCD). An internally, genetically regulated form of cell suicide which can be triggered by: (1) (external) injurious agents such as heat shock, free radicals, UV, or other ionizing radiation, various drugs and toxins. (2) Biological apoptosis-inducing factors including *tumor necrosis factor alpha* (TNF-α) which binds to the TNF receptor on the cell membrane. *Lymphotoxin* (TNF-β) which also binds to the TNF receptors. *Fas ligand* (FasL) which binds to a cell-surface receptor named Fas (also known as CD95). Programmed cell death is necessary in embryonic development, and in maintenance of healthy adult tissues such as the skin, the uterine lining, and epithelial cells in the alimentary canal, mouth, and nasal passages. Note that the therapeutic ultrasound used to treat osteoarthritis inhibits the apoptosis of chondrocytes.

Aptamer: Short, single-stranded oligonucleotide or peptide molecules that bind to a wide range of specific target molecule. Aptamers can be used in analytical microarrays to detect the presence of disease-related nucleic acids and proteins.

Auger effect: A physical phenomenon involving radionuclide atoms—an external, high-energy electron strikes an atom. This collision knocks out an inner (K)-shell electron, leaving a vacancy (K-shell ionization). Sometimes an upper (L)-shell electron drops to fill the inner shell vacancy. This transition is accompanied by the emission of a *photon*. For heavy atoms, the photon energy is in the x-ray region (called x-ray fluorescence). Sometimes, the energy is transferred to an outer shell electron as kinetic energy, ejecting it from the atom. This ejected electron is called an *Auger electron*.

B

Becquerel (Bq): The SI-derived unit of radioactivity. One Bq is defined as the activity of a quantity of radioactive material in which one nucleus decays per second. Its dimensions in SI base units are s^{-1}. 1 Bq = 2.7×10^{-11} Ci = 2.7×10^{-5} μCi. Ci = curie; 1 Ci = 3.7×10^{10} Bq. The absorbed dose of radioactivity is given in rads (100 erg $\cdot$ g^{-1}) or grays (Gy; J $\cdot$ kg^{-1}).

Beer–Lambert Law: By definition *optical transmittance* is given by: $T \equiv \Phi_e/\Phi_i = 10^{-A}$, where: Φ_i is the radiant flux incident on a uniform medium, Φ_e is the radiant flux exiting the medium, and A is the *absorbance* of the medium. The Beer–Lambert Law can be written for the case of a medium having spatially uniform attenuation as: $T \equiv e^{-\mu l} = 10^{-\mu_{10} l}$, where $A = \mu_{10}l$, l = the optical path length, and μ = optical attenuation coefficient (a function of λ).

Bilirubin (also known as hematoidin): The yellow breakdown product of normal heme catabolism, due to the body's clearance of aged erythrocytes containing hemoglobin. See Figure GL1 for the bilirubin molecule. Bilirubin is secreted in the bile and urine, and elevated levels may indicate certain diseases. It is responsible for the yellow color of bruises and the yellow discoloration in jaundice. It is also responsible for the brown color of feces due to its conversion to stercobilin, and the yellow color of urine due to urobilin. Typical normal adult bilirubin ranges from 0.3 to 1.9 mg/dL. Jaundice in the conjunctiva of the eyes is generally noted for bilirubin concentrations of greater than 2–3 mg/dL.

Figure GL1

Biotin (also known as Vitamin H, Vitamin B$_7$, or Coenzyme R): The biotin molecule is shown in Figure GL2.

Figure GL2

Biotinylation: The process of covalently attaching *biotin* to a protein, nucleic acid, or other molecules. The biotin molecule is small (MW = 244.31 g/mol), and is unlikely to disturb the natural function of the target molecule. Biotin, in turn, binds to streptavidin and avidin with very high affinity, and these ligands can be used to attach fluorescent tags to the target molecule.

Boil (also known as furuncle): A deep folliculitis or infection of hair follicles, generally caused by the bacterium *Staphylococcus aureus*.

Brewster's angle: In geometrical optics, the angle of incidence at which a ray of light with a particular polarization (linear, circular, elliptical, random) is perfectly transmitted through a transparent dielectric surface with no reflection. Brewster's angle is simply expressed as: $\theta_B = \tan^{-1}(n_2/n_1)$, where n_1 is the refractive index of the surrounding medium (e.g., air) and n_2 is the refractive index of the other medium (e.g., a lens).

C

Cal: Abbreviation for kilocalorie (1 kcal. = 1 Cal.)

Calorie (1 Calorie = 1000 calories): A unit of energy used in physiology and biochemistry. Amount of energy required to heat 1 kg of air-free water by 1°C (1 Cal. = 4.184 kJ).

Cancer mortality: Mortality from cancers is highly variable, depending on the cancer type, and how long it has been growing before detection and treatment. Statistics from the *American Institute for Cancer Research* give the worldwide mortality from all kinds of cancers in 2013 as ~7.6 million deaths/year. The percent fatality rate (chance of a person dying if they have the disease) is 60%. Contrast this with the 1.3 million deaths/year from tuberculosis worldwide (AICR 2013). Online information bulletins from the *American Cancer Society* give survival rates for the following cancer types: cervical cancer, colorectal cancer, liver cancer, lung cancer (nonsmall cell), melanoma skin cancer, ovarian cancer, pancreatic cancer, and prostate cancer (Cancer 2015).

Carbuncle: A skin abscess larger than a boil, usually draining pus onto the skin. Most commonly caused by *Staphylococcus aureus* or *Streptococcus pyogenes*. The infection is contagious and may spread to other areas of the body. Carbuncles may be found in persons with diabetes or immune disorders, or having poor hygiene or poor nutrition. Injury can trigger a carbuncle under the above conditions.

Cas9: CRISPR-associated protein 9 is an RNA-guided DNA endonuclease enzyme associated with the CRISPR-acquired immunity system in certain bacteria (e.g., *Streptococcus pyogenes*). *S. pyogenes* uses Cas9 to record the structures of certain invading bacteriophage DNA or plasmid DNA. This recording process is accomplished by unwinding foreign DNA and checking whether it is complementary to the 20 bp spacer template region of the guide RNA. If the DNA substrate is complementary to the guide RNA template, Cas9 cleaves the invading DNA, protecting the phage-infected bacterium. Cas9 has been used experimentally in DNA genetic engineering applications in vertebrates.

Chemiluminescence: The emission of light (luminescence) as the result of a chemical reaction. As an example, when H_2O_2 reacts with *luminol* in the presence of a catalyst such as iron from hemoglobin, a vibronic-state, exited molecule of *3-aminophthalate* (3-APA) is formed; this excited molecule decays back to ground-state 3-APA with the emission of photons. There are many examples of chemiluminescence: Fireflies use it to generate their signal flashing, it is used to detect contaminants in air, detection, and assay of biomolecules in systems such as ELISA and Western blots, DNA sequencing by pyro-sequencing, children's toys (glowsticks), etc. (Note that chemiluminescence is not fluorescence, where molecular absorption of shorter wavelength photons causes the emission of longer wavelength photons. For example, green fluorescent protein.)

[57]Cobalt nuclide: Used in nuclear medical diagnosis linked to vitamin B_{12}. [57]Co has a half-life of 271.8 days. Its decay type is electron capture. It emits the following gamma photons: 0.014 MeV (9.54%), 0.122 MeV (85.6%), 0.136 MeV (10.6%), 0.692 MeV (0.02%), and beta electrons with 0.692 MeV max.

Collagen: The main structural protein in the intracellular spaces of various connective tissues and bone in animals. A single collagen molecule (also known as tropocollagen) is used to form collagen aggregates, such as fibrils. It is ~300 nm long and 1.5 nm diameter, and is made up of three polypeptide strands, each of which has the conformation of a left-handed helix. These three LH helices are twisted together into a right-handed super helix stabilized by many hydrogen bonds. Many tropocollagens bind together to form a collagen fibril, and many fibrils form a fiber. The organic part of bone matrix is 90%–95% composed of Type I collagen.

Complex (vector) refractive index: *Refractive index* n is a dimensionless number defined as the ratio of the speed of light in vacuum (c_o) to the speed of light in a certain medium (v), that is, $n \equiv c_o/v$. The *complex refractive index* (vector) can be written: $\mathbf{n^*} = n + j\kappa$. This can be computed at a point, $\mathbf{n^*}(x, y, z)$. The real part n is the refractive index and indicates the phase velocity of light in the medium; the imaginary part, κ, is called the *extinction coefficient* or *mass attenuation coefficient,* and indicates the amount of attenuation when the EM wave propagates through the material.

Confocal optical microscopy: This is a technique for increasing the contrast (and resolution) of microscopic images, particularly in thick specimens. By excluding most of the light from the specimen that is not from the microscope's focal plane, the image has less haze and better contrast than that from a conventional light microscope, and represents a thin cross section lying within the specimen. Thus, it is possible to build a high-resolution, 3-D reconstruction of a volume within the specimen by assembling a series of thin slices taken along the vertical (normal) axis. By restricting the observed volume, the technique keeps overlying or nearby scatterers from contributing to the detected signal. The price for this is that the instrument must observe only one point at a time (in the scanning laser version) (cf. Webb 1996, Semwogerere and Weeks 2005). See Figure 17.11 for a schematic illustration of a basic, scanning laser, fluorescent confocal microscope. The **x–y** scanning raster is generated by two orthogonal rotating mirrors. The pixel **z** depth is selected by focusing the lens shown in Figure 17.10.

CRISPR: Acronym for **C**lustered **R**egularly **I**nterspersed **S**hort **P**alindromic **R**epeats. The CRISPR array molecule is part of a prokaryotic (bacterial) immune system. It consists of segments of prokaryotic DNA containing short repetitions of base sequences. Each repetition is followed by short segments of "spacer DNA" from previous exposures to an invading bacteriophage virus or plasmid. CRISPRs are found in ~40% of sequenced bacterial genomes and 90% of sequenced archaea, they provide a form of acquired immunity. CRISPR spacers recognize, cut, and destroy invading viral and plasmid DNA in a manner analogous to RNA interference in eukaryotic organisms. Since 2012, CRISPR has been used for genome engineering/editing in human cell cultures, baker's yeast, zebrafish, fruit flies, axolotls, monkeys, mice, human embryos, and certain plants

CRISPR-Cpf1: A DNA-editing technology that works analogously to the CRISPR-Cas9 enzymes. CRISPR-Cpf1 is potentially more efficient than CRISPR-Cas9 because it is a smaller and simpler endonuclease molecule than Cas9. Cas9 requires two RNA molecules to select the DNA cut site while Cpf1 needs one. Cas9 cuts both DNA strands in a DNA molecule at the same targeted position, leaving behind "blunt" ends. Cpf1 leaves one strand longer than the other, leaving "sticky" ends that are easier to work with. Cpf1 appears to be more able to insert new sequences at the cut site, compared to Cas9. Cpf1 is a single RNA-guided endonuclease that lacks tracrRNA. It utilizes a T-rich protospacer-adjacent motif. Cpf1 cleaves DNA via a staggered DNA double-stranded break. Cpf1 mediates robust DNA interference with features distinct from Cas9. Cpf1 was found in the bacterium *Staphylococcus aureus* (Ledford 2015, Zetsche et al. 2015).

C-type lectin: A type of carbohydrate-binding protein domain. C-type lectins require calcium for binding. Proteins that contain C-type lectin domains have a diverse range of functions, including, but not limited to cell–cell adhesion, immune response to pathogens, and apoptosis.

Cyanosis: The appearance of a blue or purple coloration of the skin and/or mucous membranes due to the blood flowing near the skin surface having low-oxygen saturation. One criterion for cyanosis is if greater than 2.0–5.0 g/dL of deoxyhemoglobin is present in the capillaries.

D

Dielectrophoresis: When a dividing cell (during cytokinesis) reaches the hourglass shape in the presence of a tumor-treating, low-frequency AC field (TTF), there is a nonuniform (internal) electric field at the junction between the dividing cells. This nonuniform field exerts a force on polar macromolecules and organelles that moves them toward the narrow neck, a process called dielectrophoresis. The process slows and even stops dividing cancer cell mitosis (Davies et al. 2013).

Diffusing capacity of the lungs for carbon monoxide (CO): (DLCO) (Also called transfer factor of the lungs for CO by the European community.) DLCO has the SI units of $mmol*min^{-1}*kPa^{-1}$. For CO, the pulmonary capillary CO tension is near zero, hence: DLCO = total CO uptake over time/PACO = $(\Delta[CO] \times V_A/\Delta t)/PACO$, where PACO = unit of CO driving pressure.

Diopter (in ophthalmology): A unit of measurement of the *optical power* of a lens; equal to the reciprocal if the lens' focal length in meters (i.e., 1/m). For example, a 5 diopter lens will bring parallel rays of light to focus at 0.2 m. Convex lenses have positive dioptric values; concave lenses, used to correct for myopia, have negative values. When two or more thin lenses are used together in close proximity, the net optical power P_{net} of the combination is approximately the sum of the optical powers of the individual lenses; that is, $P_{net} = P_1 + P_2 + P_3 + \cdots$.

Drusen: Drusen are tiny yellow or white accumulations of extracellular lipid particles build up between Bruch's membrane and the retinal pigment epithelium of the eye. "Hard" drusen are small, distinct, and separated from each other; "soft" drusen are larger and cluster closer together. Their edges are not as clearly defined as hard drusen. The presence of soft drusen increases the risk of age-related macular degeneration (AMD). Drusen of both kinds are easily seen with an ophthalmoscope. Most people over 40 have some hard drusen.

E

Edema: An abnormal accumulation of extracellular fluid in the body, causing swelling and "pitting." Grade + edema is mild and involves both feet and ankles. Grade ++ edema is moderate, and involves both feet and lower legs, hands and/or lower arms. Grade +++ is severe pitting edema, and can occur in feet, legs, arms, and face. Edema can also occur in internal organs, for example, the lungs and brain. For causes of edema, see Chapter 25 in Guyton (1991).

Electron capture (EC): A radiation process in which a proton-rich nuclide absorbs an inner atomic electron, thereby changing a nuclear proton to a neutron, and at the same time, causing the emission of an *electron neutrino*. The nuclide, now in an excited state, then transitions to its ground state. An outer orbital electron replaces the electron that was captured, and an x-ray photon is emitted. Electron capture may result in the *Auger effect* (see above), where an electron is ejected from the atom, and a positive ion is created. Sometimes, a γ-ray photon is emitted because the nucleus is also temporarily in an excited state. Following EC, the nuclide's atomic number is reduced by one; however, there is no change in atomic mass.

Endolymphatic hydrops (also known as Ménière's disease): Endolymphatic hydrops is caused by an excess of endolymphatic fluid in the inner ear (semicircular canals). Symptoms include spells of vertigo, nystagmus, tinnitus, and progressive deafness.

Epitope (also known as antigenic determinant): The part of an antigen molecule recognized by the immune system's antibodies, B-cells, and T-cells. It is the specific site on an antigen molecule to which the antibody binds.

Epistasis: A phenomenon where the effect of one gene is dependent on the presence of one or more *modifier genes*. Epistasis can be positive or negative; negative, synergistic epistasis is where deleterious random mutations cause a greater loss in organismal fitness than that caused by purely additive mutation effects.

Enkephalins: Pentapeptide neurohormones involved in regulating pain and nociception in the body. Enkephalins bind to the body's opioid receptors. There are two human enkephalins: *Met-enkephalin*, Tyr–Gly–Gly–Phe–*Met*, and *Leu-enkephalin*, Tyr–Gly–Gly–Phe–*Leu*. The receptors for enkephalins are the delta opioid receptors.

F

FISH (fluorescence in situ hybridization): FISH is a complex cytogenetic technique used to detect and localize the presence or absence of specific genomic DNA sequences on chromosomes. FISH uses fluorescent probes that bind only to those parts of a chromosome with which they show a high degree of sequence complementarity. Epifluorescent light microscopy is used to find out where the fluorescent probe is bound. FISH can also be used to detect and localize specific RNA targets.

Fluor: A unique fluorescent marker.

Fluorescence: When certain molecules (e.g., GFP) absorb short wavelength light (photon) energy such as UVA, violet or blue visible light, they radiate light at longer wavelengths (e.g., blue, green, yellow, orange, red) in a relatively narrow spectral band (Scott 2015). Fluorescence is used as a tool to tag specific molecules or entire organisms (see the tutorial on fluorescence, delayed fluorescence, and phosphorescence at Basel (2006)). As a photochemical reaction, a fluorescent molecule M_0 is in its ground state. It absorbs excitatory photon energy, $h\nu_{ex}$, which excites it to a higher-quantum state, M^*. M^* spontaneously decays to its ground state, emitting light $h\nu_{em}$ plus heat (longwave IR) from molecular vibrations. Thus, $M_0 + h\nu_{ex} \rightarrow M^* \rightarrow M_0 + h\nu_{em} + \text{heat}$.

Frequency compression: A nonlinear process in hearing aids that reduces both the input frequencies and bandwidth by a preset factor. Because the input spectrum is "squeezed" with *Frequency Compression*, operation in real-time requires a complex algorithm that maintains the critical information.

Frequency shifting (in hearing aids): A technical term specifically relating to the use of a mixer (multiplier or square-law device) to lower the input audio signal by a fixed frequency value. Frequency shifting does not reduce the bandwidth, it only downshifts the input signal spectrum in frequency. When the shifting frequency is greater than the input signal frequency, strong distortions are created.

G

Galectins: A class of proteins defined by their binding specificity for β-galactoside sugars (e.g., *N*-acetyllacto-samine [Galβ1-3GlcNAc or Galβ1-4GlcNAc]), which can be bound to proteins by either *N*-linked or *O*-linked glycosylation. There are 15 galectins found in mammals; galectins have also been found in birds, amphibians, fish, nematodes, sponges, and fungi.

Gamma (for film): When photographic black-and-white and color negative films are exposed to photon energy, there is, in general, a power-law relation between the photon input (log [exposure in lux-seconds]) and output (film optical density [OD]). Note that $OD \equiv Absorbance = -10\log_{10}(T)$, where T is the transmittance: $T \equiv P_{out}/P_{in}$, $0 \leq T \leq 1.0$, of the developed film. If we plot film OD (on the y-axis) versus log exposure (on the x-axis) for a transparency film, we see an increasing sigmoid curve with a linear center section. The slope of the linear center part of the curve gives us the film's γ, sic: $\gamma \equiv \Delta OD/\Delta\log(Exp) = (OD_2 - OD_1)/[\log(Exp2) - \log(Exp1)]$, where $\log(Exp2) > \log(Exp1)$; Davidson (2015).

Gate pain control theory (GPCT): GPCT claims that activation of neurons that do not transmit pain signals, called non-nociceptive sensory fibers, can interfere (inhibit) with signals from pain sensory fibers, thereby inhibiting pain. Afferent pain receptive neurons sending pain signals to the brain comprise at least two kinds of fibers: Fast, relatively thick, myelinated "Aδ" fibers that carry intense pain messages quickly, and small, unmyelinated, slow "C" fibers that carry longer-term, chronic, throbbing pain. Large-diameter, myelinated **Aβ** sensory neurons are non-nociceptive and inhibit the firing of afferent **Aδ** and **C** pain fibers. This modulation of pain transmission occurs in neurons located in the dorsal spinal cord in the *substantia gelatinosa* of Rolando. A highly schematic neural circuit of a (chronic) pain gate is shown in Figure GL3. The firing of the afferent *projection neurons* sends pain signals to the brain. The gating is effected by *inhibitory interneurons* acting on the *projection neurons.* When the **Aβ (L)** fibers fire, they stimulate the inhibitory interneurons, whose activity suppresses firing of the projection neuron carrying pain signals to the CNS. In the nongated scenario, the **Aβ** fibers are not active, and the firing of the slow pain **C (S)** fiber inhibits the inhibitory neuron, allowing the **C** fibers signals to stimulate the projection neuron (P). In terms of neural (Boolean) logic: $\mathbf{P} = \mathbf{S}\,\overline{\mathbf{L}} = \overline{\mathbf{S}\mathbf{L}} = \overline{\mathbf{S}}\mathbf{L}$. Pain gate theory was first proposed by Melzack and Wall (1965).

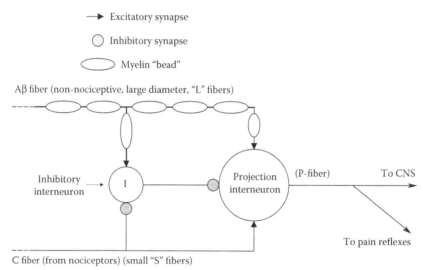

Figure GL3

Genetic disorders: The table below lists the most common genetic disorders. There are many more.

Disorder	Mutation Type	Chromosome
22q11.2 deletion syndrome	D	22q
Angelman syndrome	D, C, P	15
Canavan disease	—	17p
Charcot–Marie–Tooth disease	Many: see Lupski et al. (2010)	Many: see Lupski et al. (2010)

(Continued)

468

Disorder	Mutation Type	Chromosome
Color blindness	P	X
Cri du chat	D	5p
Cystic fibrosis	P	7q
Down syndrome	C	21-trisomy
Duchenne muscular dystrophy	D	Xp
Haemochromatosis	P	6
Hemophilia	P	X
Klinefelter syndrome	C	X
Neurofibromatosis	—	17q/22q/?
Phenylketonuria	P	12q
Polycystic kidney disease	P	16 (PDK1) or 4 (PDK2)
Prader–Willi syndrome	D, C	15
Sickle-cell disease	P	11p
Spinal muscular atrophy	D, P	5q
Tay–Sachs disease	P	15
Turner syndrome	C	X

(Table adapted from Wikipedia "List of genetic disorders," 21 Feb. 2017.)

Glioblastoma multiforme (GBM) (also known as Grade IV Astrocytoma): The most common and most aggressive malignant primary brain tumor. It involves brain glial cells, and accounts for 52% of all functional tissue brain tumor cases, and 20% of all intracranial tumors. GBM is rare; it has an incidence of two to three cases per 10^5 person life-years in North America and Europe. GBM is very difficult to treat due to several complicating factors:

- The tumor cells are very resistant to conventional therapies.

- Other brain cells are susceptible to damage due to conventional therapy.

- The brain has a very limited capacity for self-repair.

- Many drugs cannot cross the blood–brain barrier to act on the tumor.

Tumor-treating (AC) fields (TTF) have shown promise against GBM as an antimitotic therapy.

Glycan: Compounds consisting of a large number of monosaccharides linked glycosidically. Glycans usually consist solely of O-glycosidic linkages of monosaccharides. For example, cellulose and chitin are glycans. Glycans can be homo- or heteropolymers of monosaccharide residues, and can be linear or branched. Glycans can be found attached to proteins as in *glycoproteins* and *proteoglycans*. They are found on the external surface of cell membranes. O- and N-linked glycans are very common in eukaryotes.

Glycome: The glycome is the entire complement of sugars of an organism (compared to the *proteome*). It includes free sugar molecules, oligosaccharides, polysaccharides, and complex glycan molecules. The outer surface of cells has a sea of lipids with a fleet of sugar molecules attached to lipids and/or proteins. These cell-surface glycans are critical for communication between cells and the adhesion properties of cell surfaces.

Gram stain: One (binary) means of classifying bacteria. The Gram stain was named after the nineteenth-century Danish bacteriologist who developed it. The procedure is as follows:

- The bacteria are first stained with a purple dye, *crystal violet*.

- The stained preparation is then treated with alcohol or acetone. This dissolves the stain out of *Gram-negative* (G−) bacteria. The remaining blue bacteria are *Gram-positive* (G+).

- To visualize the G− bacteria, they are now treated with pink *safranin* stain.

The outer walls of G+ bacteria have an inner plasma membrane covered on the outside with a relatively thick peptidoglycan membrane. The G− bacterial outer wall consists of an inner plasma membrane, followed by a *periplasmic space*, outside of which is a peptidoglycan layer, covered with an *outer membrane* outer layer. Thus G− bacteria are encased in a triple outer layer.

Graphite furnace atomic absorption spectrometry (GFAAS): (also known as *electrothermal atomic absorption spectrometry* [ETAAS]). GFAAS instruments have the following five components: (1) A lamp light source that emits resonance line radiation. (2) An atomization chamber (graphite tube) in which the analyte sample (~20 μL) is vaporized. (3) A monochromator to select only one of the characteristic emission bands of the analyte. (4) A detector, generally a photomultiplier tube that measures the amount of photon absorption. (5) A signal-processing computer and spectrum display apparatus. GFAAS can detect trace metals at the ng/mL level (Philips 2014).

H

Half-life (biological): The time the concentration of a substance (drug, hormone, cytokine, radionuclide, amino acid, protein, circulating DNA or RNA molecule [or oligo], etc.) takes to decay to one-half of its initial concentration as the result of natural molecular breakdown by the liver, immune cells, etc., elimination through the urine, feces, breath, or cell metabolism, etc., also radioactive decay. If we assume first-order decay kinetics for the substance ($\dot{c} = -c/\tau$) , we can write the simple exponential expression for the decay: $C(t) = C_o\, e^{-t/\tau}$, assuming an initial concentration at $t = 0$ of C_o. By definition, at $t = T_{1/2}$, $C(T_{1/2}) = C_o/2$. Basic algebra tells us that $T_{1/2} = \tau \ln 2 = 0.693\, \tau$, where τ is the first-order decay time constant. If decay kinetics are of order >1, then $T_{1/2}$ is measured. The biological half-life for a substance can vary among individuals because of physiological differences in the decay mechanism.

Hemozoin: When hemoglobin from erythrocytes is digested by Malaria parasites (*Plasmodium* spp.), or by other blood-feeding organisms such as *Rhodnius* and *Schistosoma,* it is converted to free heme which is the nonprotein component of hemoglobin. A heme is a prosthetic molecule that contains a ferrous iron (Fe^{++}) atom located in the center of a heterocyclic porphyrin ring. Free heme is toxic to cells, so the parasite converts it into the insoluble, crystalline polymer called hemozoin. Hemozoin crystals form within the parasites, and when they die, hemozoin is released into the circulation. Thus, free hemozoin in the blood is an indicator of an ongoing or past malaria infection. Hemozoin polymer crystals are ~100 to 200 nm long and contain ~80,000 heme molecules. Hemozoin crystals are weakly magnetic, which offers a means for their detection and quantification.

Hereditary Type I Tyrosinemia: This hereditary disease results in the inability to metabolize the AA *tyrosine*. It is caused by a deficiency of the enzyme *fumarylacetoacetate hydrolase*. This condition is inherited in an autosomal recessive pattern. Worldwide, it affects about one person in 10^5, except in Quebec, Canada, the incidence is ~1 in 16,000. Type I tysosinemia typically is first seen in infancy as hepatomegaly and failure to thrive. The primary effects are progressive liver and kidney dysfunction. The urine has an odor of cabbage or rancid butter. *Fumarylacetoacetate hydrolase* catalyzes the final step in the metabolic degradation of tyrosine. Fumaryacetoacetate accumulates in liver cells and in proximal renal tubule cells, causing oxidative and DNA damage, leading to cell death and dysfunctional gene expression, which alters metabolic processes like protein synthesis and gluconeogenesis. There is also an increase of tyrosine in the body which causes neurodevelopmental and dermatological problems.

Hill function: The **n**th order Hill function is used to model the parametric variation of rate constants in CNLS models. They provide one means of introducing parametric feedback. *Rate constant saturation* is modeled by Hill functions of the form:

$$K_S = \frac{K_{So}[M]^n}{\beta + [M]^n},$$

where K_{So} and β are positive constants. [M] is the concentration of the regulating variable, M. **n** is an integer ≥ 1. $K_s \to K_{So}$ for $[M]^n \ll \beta$.

Rate constant suppression by the concentration of M is modeled by the decreasing Hill function:

$$K_N = \frac{K_{So}}{\beta + [M]^n}.$$

Here, $K_N \to 0$ as $[M]^n \to \infty$.

Holographic notch filter: A very narrowband, optical band-rejection filter. They are fabricated by recording interference patterns formed between two mutually coherent laser beams. The interference patterns are exposed and developed in a thick gelatinous film that typically is sandwiched between two glass plates. Since all layers are recorded simultaneously within a thick stack, the optical density of the filter notch is high and its spectral bandwidth is extremely narrow.

Holographic notch filters have revolutionized Raman spectroscopy by providing high attenuation of the Rayleigh line while passing light energy in the Stokes and anti-Stokes wavelengths with little attenuation. In one filter, the center of the stop-band was at ~527 nm, and the bandwidth at 50% attenuation of transmission was 11 nm with no sidelobes (Raman Products 2001).

I

Impedance matching: Matching the impedance of an electrical source of power to a load impedance will maximize the power dissipated in the load. Likewise, matching the acoustic impedance of a source of sound energy to an acoustic load impedance will transfer maximum acoustic power to the load. This principle is important in the design of stethoscopes and microphones. To illustrate impedance matching simply, consider an electrical Thevenin power source having an open-circuit voltage, V_S, and a series resistance, R_S. A load R_L is connected to the Thevenin source's terminals, and a current I flows from V_S through R_S and R_L. The power in R_L is simply $P_L = I^2 R_L$. To maximize P_L, we must maximize I by adjusting R_S. It is easy to show using Ohm's law that:

$$P_L = \frac{V_S^2}{(R_S^2/R_L + 2R_S + R_L)}.$$

To maximize P_L, we must minimize the denominator above. It is easy to show that this occurs when $R_S = R_L$. When this happens, $P_{Lmax} = V_S^2/4R_L$.

INR: A measure of a person's prothrombin formation (clotting) time in plasma, following the addition of *tissue factor* to the plasma sample. A normal INR is in the range of 0.8–1.2. An INR > 1.5 generally means poor clotting.

Instantaneous frequency: A pulse train can be defined as a series of unit impulses, $P_T(t) = \sum_{k=1}^{\infty} \delta(t - t_k)$, has an *instantaneous frequency sequence* associated with it given by: $R_T(t) = \sum_{k=2}^{\infty} r_k \delta(t - t_k)$, where $r_k = 1/(t_k - t_{k-1})$, k = 2, 3, 4, …, ∞. r_k is called the kth element of instantaneous frequency, and $[t_k]$ are the times pulses occur. An instantaneous frequency sequence can be written as a continuous function, $V_I(t)$:

$$V_I(t) = G \sum_{k=2}^{\infty} r_k [U(t - t_k) - U(t - t_{k+1})],$$

where $U(t - t_k)$ is a unit step function which occurs at $t = t_k$; by definition it is zero for $t < t_k$ and 1 for $t \geq t_k$. $V_I(t)$ thus is a stepwise series of voltages, each level of which is the instantaneous frequency of the preceding interspike interval. G is a constant.

Isobestic excitation wavelength: In spectroscopy, when trying to differentiate between two simultaneously occurring forms of an analyte (e.g., *oxyhemoglobin* and deoxyHb), it is the excitation wavelength at which the two analyte forms absorb (or transmit) equally.

J

Jaundice: Jaundice is a symptom of a high concentration of *bilirubin* (see above) in the blood and extracellular fluid. The normal concentration of bilirubin in blood plasma in normally <1.2 mg/dL. A concentration higher than ~3 mg/dL (>50 μmol/L) leads to jaundice. The main sign of jaundice is a yellowish discoloration of the skin and of the conjunctival membranes covering the sclera of the eye. There are three categories of jaundice: (1) Prehepatic/hemolytic, where the pathology is occurring before the liver. (2) Hepatic/hepatocellular, in which the pathology is located within the liver. (3) Posthepatic/cholestatic, in which the pathology is located after the conjugation of bilirubin in the liver.

K

Karyotype: A Karyotype describes the number of chromosomes, and what they look like under a light microscope. Features such as their length, the locations of the centromeres, banding patterns (G, R, C, Q, and T), any differences between the sex chromosomes, and other visible physical features. The field of cytogenetics includes the study of karyotypes.

L

Laminar flow: Laminar or streamline flow occurs when a fluid flows in parallel layers with no disruption between the layers. There are no crosscurrents, eddies, or swirls in the moving fluid. Laminar flow occurs for low *Reynolds numbers* and low-peak velocities.

Larmor frequency: All atomic nuclei have a spin; those with an odd number of neutrons and/or protons have a property called *magnetic dipole moment.* A magnetic moment is characterized by its alignment with an external magnetic field. These particular nuclei are also called dipoles because they have two poles (like N and S in a bar magnet). The atoms ^1H and ^{31}P are the examples of nuclei with an unpaired proton, while ^{14}N has both an unpaired neutron and proton. The atomic nucleus, like a top, will spin along an axis lying in the direction of the angular momentum vector for the nucleus. The spin of the nucleus can be related to the magnetic moment of the nucleus by the relation:

$$\mu = \gamma \mathbf{I},$$

where μ is the magnetic moment vector and γ is the proportionality constant called the *gyromagnetic moment.* $\mathbf{I}$ is the spin.

The nuclear magnetic moment will couple to an external magnetic field, $\mathbf{B}_0$. This coupling gives rise to a torque on the nucleus which causes precession around the magnetic field vector. (This is analogous to the circular precession in macroscopic tops, where the gravitational force couples with the mass of the spinning top.) In the atomic case, the Larmor or processional frequency refers to the rate of precession of the atomic magnetic moment around the external magnetic field vector. The Larmor frequency is given simply by the relation:

$$f_L = \gamma B_0,$$

where f_L is the Larmor frequency in MHz, γ is the gyromagnetic ratio in MHz/T, and B_0 is the strength of the static magnetic field in T.

The *gyromagnetic ratio* γ in MHz/T for some elements is given in the table below:

Atom	γ (MHz/T)
^1H	42.58
^{19}F	40.05
^{23}Na	11.26
^{31}P	17.24

Limit of detection (LOD): The lowest concentration of an analyte that can be reliably sensed by a measurement system. The LOD is generally set by noise and/or quantization accompanying the analyte signal.

Lorentz factor: Defined as:

$$\gamma = \frac{1}{\sqrt{1 - v^2/c^2}},$$

where c is the speed of light *in vacuo,* v is the object's relative velocity.

For example, when: $v/c = 0$, $\gamma = 1$; $v/c = 0.500$, $\gamma = 1.155$; $v/c = 0.999$, $\gamma = 22.366$.

Lugal: A molecule formed by attaching a luciferin molecule covalently with a sugar (galactose). In this form, the luciferin is "caged" and cannot react with the *luciferase enzyme* that produces light. The enzyme β-*galactosidase* splits the Lugal molecule into D-*luciferin* plus *galactose.* Once "uncaged," the enzyme *luciferase*, ATP, and O_2 react with the D-Luciferin to produce light (bioluminescence).

M

Magnetic susceptibility: The ratio of the magnetization within a material to the applied magnetic field strength; it is a tensor when these two quantities are not parallel; otherwise it is a simple, dimensionless number. Mathematically, it is: $\chi_v = M/H$, where M is the magnetization within the material in A/m and H is the applied external magnetic field strength in A/m. χ_v is the *volume* magnetic susceptibility. Also, the magnetic permeability μ of a substance is related to χ_v by: $\mu = (1 + \chi_v)\,\mu_o\ N/A^2$ or Henrys/m.

Malleolus: The bony prominences on each side of the human ankle. The medial malleolus is formed by the lower end of the tibia; the lateral malleolus is a protuberance on the lower end of the fibula.

Meninges: Three membranes directly under the skull that cover the outer surface of the brain. Specifically, the *dura mater* lies directly under the bone, then the *arachnoid,* and the thin *pia mater* covers the brain.

Mueller matrix: A matrix method for manipulating *Stokes vectors,* such as describing polarized light. A Mueller matrix is a 4×4 matrix. Any fully polarized, partially polarized, or unpolarized state of light can be represented by a Stokes vector, **S**, and any optical element (e.g., wave plate) by a Mueller matrix, **[M]**. When a beam of light in the Stokes state, $\mathbf{S}_i$, passes through an optical element, $\mathbf{[M_1]}$, we can write:

$$\mathbf{S}_o = \mathbf{[M_1]}\mathbf{S}_i.$$

If the beam passes through optical element $\mathbf{[M_1]}$ followed by element $\mathbf{[M_2]}$, then $\mathbf{[M_3]}$, then we can write:

$$\mathbf{S}_o = \mathbf{[M_3]}\mathbf{[M_2]}\mathbf{[M_1]}\mathbf{S}_i.$$

However, matrix multiplication is not commutative, so in general:

$$\mathbf{[M_3]}\mathbf{[M_2]}\mathbf{[M_1]}\mathbf{S}_i \neq \mathbf{[M_1]}\mathbf{[M_2]}\mathbf{[M_3]}\mathbf{S}_i.$$

N

Nevus: A mole on the skin, generally a benign lesion.

Nickase: A restriction endonuclease enzyme that introduces a specific break in one strand of a dsDNA segment. The break locus is determined by a 20 nt RNA guide sequence acting with the Cas9 endonuclease enzyme.

Noise-equivalent differential temperature (NEDT or NEΔT): The NEDT is the key figure of merit used to characterize the noise performance of midwave and longwave infrared (MWIR and LWIR) cameras. It is a signal-to-noise figure which represents the object temperature difference which would produce a signal equal to the camera's rms temporal noise. It thus represents approximately the minimum temperature difference which the camera can resolve. It is calculated by dividing the temporal noise by the response per degree (responsivity), and is usually expressed in units of millikelvins. The NEDT value is a function of the camera's f/number, its integration time, the temperature at which the measurement is made, and the sensor material. For a mathematical definition of NEDT (and how it is measured) for IR FPAs, see Rogalski (2009).

Nujol: A brand of mineral oil made by Plough, Inc., used in IR spectroscopy to suspend a powder of the analyte. It is a heavy, chemically inert paraffin oil; it has a density of 0.838 g/mL at 25°C and has a relatively simple IR spectrum, with major peaks in bands between 2950 and 2800, 1465 and 1450, and 1380 and 1370 cm^{-1}. The empirical formula of Nujol is not well defined because it is a mixture, but it closely follows the alkane formula $C_nH_{(2n+2)}$, where n is very large.

1/f noise: Where a time-varying stochastic process has a one-sided power spectral density model, S(f), of the form:

$$S(f) = \frac{\text{constant}}{f^\alpha} \text{ MSU/Hz, } 0 \leq f \leq \infty,$$

where $0.5 \leq \alpha \leq 1.5$, approximately.

1/f$^\alpha$ fluctuations are widely found in nature, science, and electronics.

O

Oligo: Abbreviation for oligonucleotide, a short, single-stranded DNA or RNA molecule.

Oncotic pressure (also known as colloid osmotic pressure): Osmotic pressure exerted by proteins (e.g., *albumin*) in a blood vessel's plasma that tends to pull water from intracellular volume into the circulatory system. The effect of oncotic pressure can be described by the Starling equation:

$$J_v = K_f \{[P_c - P_i] - \sigma[\pi_c - \pi_i]\},$$

where J_v is the net fluid movement between vascular and extravascular compartments. K_f is the filtration coefficient. $P_c =$ is the mean capillary hydrostatic pressure; $P_i =$ interstitial hydrostatic pressure; $\pi_c =$ capillary oncotic pressure; $\pi_i =$ interstitial oncotic pressure; $\sigma =$ reflection coefficient.

Optical density: See Absorbance above.

Orthoses: Examples of orthoses include powered exoskeleton (also known as bionic body) (controlled by EMGs) with force and position sensor feedbacks. Orthotic supports for damaged knees, feet, arms, elbows, wrists, etc. have been developed. Passive (nonpowered) orthoses include shoe inserts, the Kickstart Walking System®, muscle-operated artificial hand, and elastic lower limb replacements. In summary, an orthosis may be used to (Orthopedia 2015):

- Control, guide, limit, and/or immobilize an extremity, joint, or body segment

- Restrict movement in a specific direction

- Assist movement in a specific direction

- Reduce weight-bearing forces on a particular area

- Aid in rehabilitation or healing

- Directly or indirectly reduce pain

- Otherwise correct the shape and/or function of the body

Orthotics: A specialty branch of orthopedic medicine that is concerned with the design, construction, and application of *orthoses*, devices used to modify the structural and functional characteristics of the neuromuscular and skeletal system.

P

Paramagnetic: Paramagnetic materials have small, positive susceptibilities to external magnetic fields. These materials are slightly attracted by an external magnetic field; however, the material does not retain the induced magnetism when the external magnetic field is removed. Paramagnetic properties are the result of some unpaired electrons, and from the realignment of the electron orbits caused by the external magnetic field. Paramagnetic materials include the metal elements: Mg, Al, Mb, Li, Ta, Au, Cu, Pt, U, W, and Gd.

Paratope: The part of an antibody (Ab) which recognizes the molecular structure of an antigen (Ag). It is a small region of 15–22 AAs in the Ab's Fv region, and contains parts of the Ab's heavy and light chains. The paratope binds to the Ag's *epitope*.

Parenchyma: Parenchymas are the *functional* parts of an organ in the body. On the other hand, the *stromata* are the structural connective tissues of the organ. In the lungs, the parenchymas are alveolar tissues with respiratory bronchioles, alveolar ducts, and terminal bronchioles. Blood vessels may be included.

Pascal: SI pressure unit $= 1 \, N/m^2 = 1 \, kg/(m \, s^2)$.

Peptide: Peptides are short, linear chains of amino acids (AAs) linked by covalent peptide (amide) bonds. The linking bonds are formed when the carboxyl group of one AA reacts with the amino group of another. The shortest peptide consists of just two AAs (a *dipeptide*), and so on up to *icosapeptide* (20 AAs), and higher. A *polypeptide* is a long, continuous, unbranched peptide chain. Peptides are distinguished from proteins on the basis of size, and arbitrarily contain 50 or fewer AAs. Examples of hormones that are peptides include *glucagon, calcitonin, secretin, amylin,* etc.

Pfu DNA polymerase: A thermostable DNA polymerase derived from the hyperthermophylic archaeon, *Pyrococcus furiosus* used in high-fidelity PCR reactions. *Pfu* polymerase has superior thermostability and proofreading properties compared to *Taq polymerase*. Unlike *Taq polymerase, Pfu polymerase* possesses 3′–5′ exonuclease proofreading activity, meaning that it works its way along the DNA from the 5′ end to the 3′ end and corrects nucleotide misincorporation errors. Commercially available *Pfu polymerase* typically gives an error rate of 1 in 1.3 million base pairs. However, *Pfu* is slower acting and typically requires 1–2 min per cycle to amplify 1 kb of DNA at 72°C. *Taq* can be used in conjunction with *Pfu* to obtain some of the speed of *Taq* with the fidelity of *Pfu*. (*Pfu* is pronounced "Foo.")

pH: The measure of acidity of a solution: pH is defined as: $pH \equiv -\log_{10}(a_{H+}) = \log_{10}(1/a_{H+})$, where a_{H+} is the chemical activity coefficient of hydrogen ions in the sample solution. In general, the activity of an ionic species i is given by

$$a_i = \exp[(\mu_i - \mu_i^\theta)/RT,$$

where μ_i is the chemical potential of the species i under the conditions of interest, and μ_i^θ is the chemical potential of that species under some defined set of standard conditions. At low concentrations, $a_i \rightarrow$ concentration of i. pH can range from 0 (very acid) to 7 (neutral) to 14 (very basic). Normal physiological pH ranges from 7.34 to 7.45.

Phon: By definition, the number of phon of a tone of fHz is the dB SPL of a 1 kHz frequency that sounds just as loud. This implies that 0 phon is the limit of perception, and inaudible sounds thus have negative phon levels (at a given frequency). Equal loudness contours are a way of mapping the dB SPL of a pure tone of f Hz presented to a subject, to the perceived loudness level in phons. The phon is used as a unit of loudness level

Phon	40	50	60	70	80	90	100	110	120	130	140
Sone	1	2	4	8	16	32	64	128	256	512	1024

by the American National Standards Institute (ANSI); it *is not* an SI unit in metrology. The phon is related to the *sone* unit of loudness.

Pinned photodiode: A photosensor used in CMOS Active Pixel Sensors. It has $p + /n/p$ regions in it. It has a shallow $p+$ implant in an n-type diffusion layer over a p-type epitaxial substrate level "storage well." It *is not the same as* a PIN photodiode.

Platelets (also known as thrombocytes): Anucleate blood cells made by megakaryocytes in the bone marrow. Platelets are found only in the blood of mammals. They are biconvex discoids, ~2 to 3 μm diameter. Responding to chemical signals, the function of platelets is to stop bleeding at the site of damaged endothelium; they adhere and aggregate, forming a plug or clot. Normal platelets can respond to an abnormality on the vessel wall, producing abnormal platelet adhesion leading to a thrombosis inside the vessel, obstructing blood flow, causing downstream ischemia or infarction. Platelets are also biochemically activated by physical damage to endothelial tissues. They can initiate the complex synthetic pathway leading to the formation of a fibrin (red) clot. The ratio of the number of platelets to erythrocytes in the blood of a healthy adult is 1:10 to 1:20.

pO$_2$: Partial pressure of oxygen in mmHg (manometer pressure), in the blood, for example.

Poynting vector: The Poynting vector **S** gives the direction and intensity of the energy flux density in W/m^2 of a propagating electromagnetic field, including but not limited to light and radio waves. $\mathbf{S} \equiv (1/\mu_o)\mathbf{E} \times \mathbf{B} = c^2\varepsilon_o\mathbf{E} \times \mathbf{B}$. Let the EM wave be a harmonic, linearly polarized plane wave traveling through free space in the direction of **k**. Thus:

$$\mathbf{E} = \mathbf{E}_0\cos(\mathbf{k} \cdot \mathbf{r} - \omega t)$$

$$\mathbf{B} = \mathbf{B}_0\cos(\mathbf{k} \cdot \mathbf{r} - \omega t).$$

Using the equation for **S**, we find: $\mathbf{S} = c^2\varepsilon_o \mathbf{E}_0 \times \mathbf{B}_0 \cos^2(\mathbf{k} \cdot \mathbf{r} - \omega t)$ (Hecht 1990).

Polycythaemia: An excess of erythrocytes in the blood (a hematocrit >55%).

Primer (in DNA PCR reaction): A short, single strand of DNA, about 18–24 bases long, that is used as a starting point for PCR DNA synthesis. It is required for DNA replication because the DNA polymerase enzymes that catalyze this process can only add new nucleotides to an existing strand of DNA. The Primer is hybridized to a target DNA strand, which is then copied by a polymerase. The primer's DNA base sequence selects that complementary portion of the target DNA to be copied.

Protein: A biological macromolecule that consists of one or more long chains of amino acid residues. The words *protein, polypeptide,* and *peptide* can be ambiguous and overlap in meaning. Protein generally refers to the complete biological molecule in a stable, 3-D configuration, while peptide is generally reserved for a short AA oligomer often lacking a 3-D structure. The boundary between the two is fuzzy, and usually lies around 20–30 AA's. Proteins have many physiological and structural functions in life. Their primary molecular structures are coded by genes in the genome. *Secondary, tertiary,* and *quaternary* protein structures involve protein folding and the formation of linking hydrogen bonds and/or –S–S– bonds, and the action of chaperone proteins and protein enzymes. A protein with quaternary structure is a complex of two or more tertiary proteins; the examples include hemoglobin, DNA polymerase, and various transmembrane ion channels.

Q

Quarter-wave plate (in optics): A quarter-wave plate (QWP) is one type of wave plate (another is a half-wave plate). A QWP allows the conversion of a beam of linearly polarized light (LPL) to a beam of circularly polarized light. It consists of a carefully adjusted thickness of a *birefringent material* such that light associated with the larger index of refraction, n_2, is retarded by a phase of 90° ($\lambda/4$) with respect to that associated with the smaller, orthogonal index, n_1. When the plane of the incident LPL makes a 45° angle to the QWP's n_2 axis, it can be shown that the emergent beam is circularly polarized (CP). If the incident beam is CP with the correct alignment, the emergent beam will be LPL.

R

Raynaud's phenomenon: Excessively reduced blood flow in the extremities caused in response to cold or emotional stress. It also can be a chronic condition caused by connective tissue disorders such as systemic lupus erythematosus.

Redox reactions: An important two-part chemical reaction consisting of a *reduction reaction*, in which *electrons are gained* in the product (or equivalently, protons [H^+] are lost). Sic:

$$\text{Oxidant} + ne^- \rightarrow \text{Product} \quad \text{or} \quad \text{Oxidant} \rightarrow H^+ + \text{Product}.$$

In the *oxidation reaction, electrons are lost* from the product (or equivalently, protons are gained). Sic:

$$\text{Reductant} \rightarrow \text{Product} + ne^- \quad \text{or} \quad H^+ + \text{Reductant} \rightarrow \text{Product}.$$

A simple example of a redox reaction is:

$$H_2 + F_2 \rightarrow 2HF.$$

This reaction can be written as the sum of an oxidation reaction and a reduction reaction:

$$H_2 \rightarrow 2H^+ + 2e^- \, (\text{oxidation})$$

$$F_2 + 2e^- \rightarrow 2F^- (\text{reduction}).$$

A useful form of redox is seen in electrochemical cells consisting of two half-cells. An example is the zinc/copper battery. The Zn anode (electron source) is immersed in a $ZnSO_4$ solution, separated from the copper metal cathode immersed in a $CuSO_4$ solution, separated from the $ZnSO_4$ by a porous ceramic disk through which only SO_4^- anions flow to the Zn anode half-cell. That is, negative charge is carried inside the battery by sulfate ions. The overall reaction is:

$$Zn(s) + CuSO_4(aq) \rightarrow ZnSO_4(aq) + Cu(s).$$

Breaking this redox reaction into ionic form gives:

$$Zn + Cu_{++} \rightarrow Zn^{++} + Cu.$$

This ionic reaction can be written as two half-cell reactions:

$$Zn \rightarrow Zn^{++} + 2e^- (\text{oxidation of zinc})$$

$$Cu^{++} + 2e^- \rightarrow Cu \, (\text{reduction of copper}).$$

The chemical energy of this reaction is harvested as electrical work. The electrons leave the Zn anode through a Cu wire, pass through a lamp, and enter the Cu cathode where the Cu is reduced. The heat produced by the lamp filament represents the work from the galvanic cell or battery.

Another redox pair of reactions occurs in the measurement of blood glucose (bG) ($C_6H_{12}O_6$) with an electrochemical cell (two half-cells) using glucose oxidase (GOD) enzyme. In step 1:

$$bG + GOD_{ox} \rightarrow Gluconolactone + GOD_{red}.$$

Gluconolactone is an oxidized form of glucose. The pair of redox reactions is:

$$2e^- + GOD_{ox} \rightarrow GOD_{red} \text{ (reduction)}$$

$$G \rightarrow gluconolactone + 2e^- \text{ (oxidation)}.$$

The second step involves electron transport by the mediator, *ferrocene monocarboxylic acid* ($Fecp_2R$), to the working electrode. The reactions are:

$$GOD_{red} + 2Fecp_2R^+ \rightarrow GOD_{ox} + 2Fecp_2R + 2H^+$$

$$2Fecp_2R \leftrightarrow 2Fecp_2R + 2e^- \uparrow.$$

These reactions take place in the Freestyle® glucometer test strips. Rather than measure the cell EMF (which varies as the reactants are consumed), a constant potential (160 mV) is applied to the cell, and the *polarographic current* flowing between the working and reference electrodes is measured (Glucometer 2014) and is proportional to the glucose concentration.

Renal glucosuria: A rare condition in which blood glucose molecules are excreted in the urine, regardless of [bG]. It occurs because the renal tubules have lost the ability to resorb filtrate glucose. The condition is thought to be inherited as an autosomal recessive trait.

Reynolds number: The Reynolds number R_e is defined as the ratio of inertial to viscous forces in fluid flow. The Reynolds number R_e for a circular vessel carrying a moving fluid is generally defined as: $R_e = \rho v D_H/\mu$, where ρ is the density of the fluid (kg/m^3), v is the *mean velocity* of the fluid (m/s), D_H is the hydraulic diameter of the vessel (m), and μ is the dynamic viscosity of the fluid (s N/m^2 = Pa s). R_e is dimensionless. Laminar flow occurs for low R_es, turbulent flow happens for high R_es.

S

SELFOC® lenses: In 1968, *Nippon Sheet Glass Co., Ltd.* developed a lens for fiber-optic applications that has a radial, parabolic, refractive index distribution in the end of a glass rod or fiber. This distribution enables self-focusing on the flat end surface to enable the transmission of images and light. Selfoc lenses are distributed by the *Go!Foton Co.*

Shoulder–hand syndrome (SHS) (also known as Steinbrocker syndrome and reflex sympathetic dystrophy syndrome): A neuromuscular condition characterized by shoulder pain, swelling, stiffness, limited joint motion, swelling of the hand, and decalcification of the underlying bones. SHS sometimes occurs following the myocardial infarction, other causes (CVA, head trauma), or can be idiopathic.

Sone: A unit of how loud a sound is perceived. Loudness S in sones (for P > 40 phon) is given by

$$S = \{10^{(P-40)/10}\}^{0.30103} \cong 2^{(P-40)/10} \text{sones}.$$

The loudness level in phons (for S > 1) is given by

$$P = 40 + 10 \log_2(S) \text{phons}.$$

As an example, consider a very loud sound at the threshold of pain at 100 Pa sound pressure. The SPL in dB *re* 20 µPa is 134, and the loudness in sone is ~676. The sone is a non-SI unit. See *phon* above.

Sound Pressure Level (SPL): The dB SPL or acoustic pressure level is a logarithmic measure of the effective sound pressure of a sound relative to a reference pressure. dB SPL, denoted L_p, and measured in dB above a standard reference level is given by

$$L_p = 10 \log_{10}\left(\frac{P_{rms}^2}{p_o^2}\right) = 20 \log_{10}\left(\frac{p_{rms}}{p_o}\right) \text{ dB(SPL)},$$

where P_{rms} is the root mean square sound pressure, measured in Pa and p_o is the reference sound pressure level, in Pa. The commonly used p_o in air is 20 μPa (RMS), or 0.0002 dynes/cm^2.

Spectral karyotyping (the SKY technique): Spectral karyotyping is a technique that uniquely color-codes the chromosome pairs of a genome using fluorescently labeled complementary DNA probe molecules. Because there are a limited number of spectrally distinct fluorophores, a combinatorial labeling technique is used to generate the many different colors required. Spectral differences generated by combinatorial labeling are captured and analyzed by using an interferometer attached to a fluorescence microscope. Image processing software then assigns a pseudo-color to each spectrally different combination, allowing the visualization of the individually colored chromosomes. The SpectraCube® imaging system provides one means of spectral karyotyping (Garini et al. 1996). Spectral karyotyping is used to detect constitutional chromosomal abnormalities causing clinical abnormalities (Anguiano et al. 2012).

Stokes vector: A 4-D vector describing the polarization state of electromagnetic radiation. $S_0 = I$, the total intensity of the beam of polarized light. Three orthogonal Stokes vector magnitudes in spherical coordinates are:

$$S_1 = pI \, \cos(2\psi)\cos(2\chi)$$

$$S_2 = pI \, \sin(2\psi)\cos(2\chi)$$

$$S_3 = pI \, \sin(2\chi),$$

where I is the total beam intensity, p is the degree of polarization ($0 \leq p \leq 10$). In terms of the *Poincaré sphere,* pI is the sphere's radius, the S_0, S_1, S_2, and S_3 vectors and the angles ψ and χ are shown in Figure GL4.

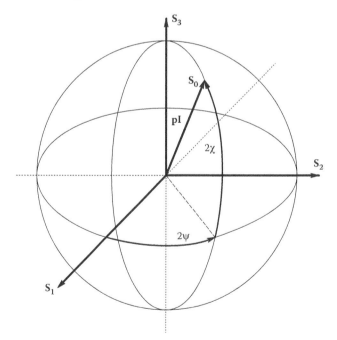

Figure GL4

Stroma: The part of a tissue or organ that has a connective and structural role; it consists of all the parts which do not perform the specific functions of the organ. The cells that stromal tissues are composed of serve as a matrix in which the other cells are imbedded.

Superluminescent diode: An SLD or SLED is an edge-emitting semiconductor light source based on superluminescence. It combines the high power and brightness of laser diodes with the low coherence of conventional LEDs. Its emission band is 5–100 nm wide. SLDs find application in designs that require high-intensity and spatial coherence and a broad, smooth optical output spectrum. Applications include optical coherence tomography, white light interferometry, optical sensing, and fiber-optic gyroscopes.

T

Taq polymerase: A thermostable DNA polymerase originally derived from the thermophylic bacterium, *Thermus aquaticus*. *T. aquaticus* lives in hot springs and hydrothermal vents. *Taq*'s optimum temperature range for activity is 75–80°C, with a half-life of greater than 2 hours at 92.5°C, 40 min at 95°C, and 9 min at 97.5°C. *Taq* lacks 3′–5′ exonuclease proof-reading activity. This results in a relatively low-DNA replication fidelity (error rate 1 in 9000). *Pfu* DNA polymerase possesses a proofreading activity and is used for high-fidelity amplification (see above).

Tau proteins: Proteins that stabilize microtubules of neurons in the brain; found in axons, peri-karya, and dendrites. Also found in lesser amounts in CNS astrocytes and oligodendro-cytes. Pathologies (such as traumatic brain injury), and dementias such as *Alzheimer's disease* and *Parkinson's* are associated with tau proteins that have become defective and no longer stabilize neuronal microtubules. The human tau proteins are the result of alter-nate splicing from a single gene (MAPT on chromosome 17). There are six isoforms of tau proteins in the human brain; each has a distinguishing feature. Using PET, workers have shown that there is a four- to eightfold higher level of damaged, phosphorylated tau protein in the brains of Alzheimer's disease patients compared to that of age-matched healthy brains (James et al. 2015). The hyperphosphorylated tau proteins form tangles of "paired helical filaments" (PHFs) in the brain characteristic of Alzheimer's disease. Also, tau PHFs occur in cases of repetitive head injury (McKee et al. 2009). At least seven tau pathology PET radiotracers have been developed and used in clinical studies (James et al. 2015).

Technetium (99mTc) sestamibi (also known as Cardiolite®): An injected drug which is a coor-dination complex consisting of the artificial radioisotope technetium-99 m bound to six (sesta = 6) methoxyisobutylisonitrile (MIBI) ligands. ^{99m}Tc has a half-life of 6 hours, and emits 140 keV gamma rays. ^{99m}Tc is made by cyclotron bombardment of molybdenum, converting it to radioactive ^{99}Mo, which in turn decays with a half-life of 2.75 days to ^{99m}Tc.

Technetium (^{99m}Tc) sestamibi (see Figure GL5) is used for medical imaging tests for cardiac blood flow, parathyroid tumors, and breast cancer (by scintimammography).

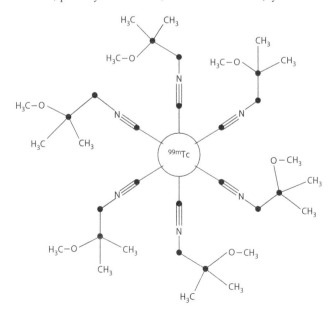

Figure GL5

Thermal noise (also known as Johnson or Nyquist noise): Thermal noise arises from the random motion of electrons in a resistive conductor. The thermal noise voltage from a resistor, or the resistive component of an impedance, is largely white, and has a power density spectrum given by

$$S_N(f) = 4\,kTR \text{ MSV/Hz}, \; 0 \leq f \leq \infty,$$

where k = Boltzmann's constant (1.380×10^{-23} J/K), T is Kelvin temperature, and R is the resistance in ohms.

The Thevenin equivalent for a thermal noise voltage is a resistor R in series with a noise source voltage with an RMS value of $e_n = [4kTR\Delta f]^{\frac{1}{2}}$. Δf = the noise bandwidth in Hz. A Norton equivalent noise model thus consists of a conductance $G = 1/R$ in parallel with and ideal noise current source, $i_n = [4kTR\Delta f]^{\frac{1}{2}}/R = [4kTG\Delta f]^{\frac{1}{2}}$ RMS amps. For a detailed description of noise and its sources in analog circuits, see Northrop (2012), Chapter 9.

Thrombin (also known as fibrinogenase, thrombase, blood coagulation factor IIa, β-thrombin, etc.): A serine protease that converts soluble fibrinogen into insoluble strands of fibrin, as well as catalyzing many other chemical reactions related to blood clotting.

Thromboplastin: A complex plasma protein that aids blood coagulation by catalyzing the conversion of prothrombin to thrombin. It is found in brain, lungs, and blood platelets. The thromboplastin reagent consists of *tissue factor, phospholipids,* and $CaCl_2$.

Time–frequency analysis (TFA): Signal analysis algorithms that allow the creation of a *Joint time–frequency* (JTF) *spectrogram,* generally from a sound signal. The JTF spectrogram is a 3-D plot displaying signal frequencies on the vertical axis, time on the horizontal axis, and signal intensity as color or gray shading. The sound signal can be physiological in origin, or from an ultrasound process such as sonar or Doppler ultrasound. TFA can be performed by a computer using one of the following algorithms: *short-term Fourier transform, Gabor transform, Wigner transform, Wigner–Ville transform, Binomial transform, Choi–Williams transform.* (See Section 3.2.3 in this book.)

Tissue factor (also known as platelet tissue factor, factor III, thromboplastin, or CD142): Is a cell-surface glycoprotein found in subendothelial tissues and leukocytes necessary for the initiation of thrombin formation from the zymogen, prothrombin.

Tomography: A type of 3-D imaging by sectioning using of any kind of penetrating wave and a computer. For example, in medical diagnosis, x-rays are used to make CT or CATScan tomograms, γ-rays make SPECT tomograms, RF waves are used in magnetic resonance imaging to make fMRI tomograms, laser scanning confocal microscopy makes LSCM tomograms, ultrasound transmission tomography (UTM), optical coherence tomography makes OCT tomograms, etc.

Trans-activating CRISPR RNA (tracrRNA): A small trans-encoded RNA that is a component of the CRISPR-Cas systems of bacteria and archaea. In bacteria, CRISPR-Cas works in three steps. First, a copy of the invading nucleic acid (from a phage) is integrated into the CRISPR locus. Next CRISPR RNAs (crRNAs) are transcribed from this CRISPR locus. Third, the crRNAs are then incorporated into effector complexes, where the crRNA guides the complex to the invading nucleic acid, and the Cas proteins degrade this nucleic acid. There are several pathways for CRISPR activation, one of which requires a tracrRNA which plays a role in the maturation of crRNA. tracrRNA is complementary to and base-pairs with a pre-crRNA, forming an RNA duplex. This is cleaved by RNase III, an RNA-specific ribonuclease, to form a crRNA/tracrRNA hybrid. This hybrid acts as a guide for the endonuclease Cas9, which cleaves the invading nucleic acid, leaving "blunt" ends.

Transferrin: Iron-binding blood plasma glycoprotein that controls the level of free iron in blood and other biological fluids. The liver is the main site of transferrin synthesis, but other organs, such as the brain, also make it. The main role of transferrin is to deliver iron (Fe^{++}) from absorption centers in the duodenum and macrophages to all tissues. It plays a key role where erythropoiesis and active cell division occur. The receptor helps to maintain iron homeostasis in cells by regulating iron concentrations. An increased plasma transferrin level is often seen in patients suffering from iron anemia. Transferrin and its receptor have been shown to diminish tumor cells by using the receptor to attract antibodies (Macedo and de Sousa 2008).

Transmittance (optical): See Absorbance above.

Type 1 control system: A single-loop feedback system that contains an integrator (1/s) in the feedback path. A Type 1 system has zero steady-state error.

U

Urobilinogen: A colorless by-product of bilirubin (cf. above) reduction. It is formed in the intestines by the microbiome acting on bilirubin. About half the urobilinogen formed is resorbed and taken up by the portal vein to the liver, where it enters the circulation and is excreted by the kidneys. *Elevated urine urobilinogen* levels may be an indication of hemolytic anemia (excessive breakdown of erythrocytes), a large hematoma, restricted liver function, hepatic infection, cirrhosis, or poisoning. *Low urine urobilinogen* levels have a number of causes: complete obstructive jaundice; treatment with broad-spectrum antibiotics which destroy the gut microbiome; Congenital enzymatic jaundice; treatment with drugs that acidify urine, such as ammonium chloride or ascorbic acid (vitamin C).

V

Vector cross product: A vector cross product is used to describe *Coriolis acceleration,* $\mathbf{a}_c$, and certain electromagnetic phenomena in MRI. The Coriolis acceleration vector acting on m can be shown to be given by

$$\mathbf{a}_c = 2(\mathbf{v} \times \mathbf{\Omega}) = -2(\mathbf{\Omega} \times \mathbf{v}),$$

where a reference plane (say the $\mathbf{x}$–$\mathbf{y}$) is rotating with angular velocity $\mathbf{\Omega}$ r/s. A point mass m is moving on the rotating plane with a linear velocity $\mathbf{v}$. The angular velocity vector $\mathbf{\Omega}$ is perpendicular to the rotating plane; its direction is given by the right-hand screw rule.

The magnitude of the acceleration is given by: $\mathbf{a}_c = 2\mathbf{v}\,\mathbf{\Omega}\,\sin\theta$. Figure GL6 illustrates two cases of finding $\mathbf{a}_c$: In (A), the vectors are orthogonal, and the platform is the XY plane which is rotating CCW (seen from above) with velocity ω r/s. The angular velocity vector, $\mathbf{\Omega}$, is found by multiplying a unit vector $\mathbf{k}$ which lies along the +z-axis (perpendicular to the XY plane) by ω, that is, $\mathbf{\Omega} = \omega\mathbf{k}$. The direction of $\mathbf{k}$ is given by the RH screw rule, that is, it is the direction a normal wood screw would advance is rotated if turned CCW, *viewed from above the XY plane.* (Note that this is CW rotation if viewed from the bottom (slot end)). Now if we rotate the mass velocity vector $\mathbf{v}$ into ω through angle θ, an RH screw would advance along the positive y-axis, giving the direction of $\mathbf{a}_c$ shown. In Figure GL6-B, the vector $\mathbf{v}$ does not lie in the XY plane. When it is rotated into $\mathbf{\Omega}$, the RH screw rule points $\mathbf{a}_c$ in a direction perpendicular to the plane formed by $\mathbf{v}$ and $\mathbf{\Omega}$. In both cases, the magnitude of $\mathbf{a}_c$ is still given by $\mathbf{a}_c = 2\mathbf{v}\,\mathbf{\Omega}\,\sin\theta$.

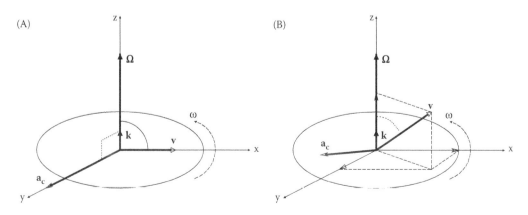

Figure GL6

Some general vector cross product identities are:

$$\mathbf{A} \times \mathbf{B} = |\mathbf{A}| \, |\mathbf{B}| \sin(\theta)\mathbf{k},$$

where θ is the angle between vectors $\mathbf{A}$ and $\mathbf{B}$, and $\mathbf{k}$ is a unit vector perpendicular to the plane containing $\mathbf{A}$ and $\mathbf{B}$ in the direction given by the thumb using the right-hand screw rule.

$$|\mathbf{A} \times \mathbf{B}| = |\mathbf{A}| \, |\mathbf{B}| \, |\sin(\theta)|, \quad \sin(\theta) \equiv \sqrt{1 - \cos^2(\theta)}$$

$$\mathbf{A} \times \mathbf{B} = -\mathbf{B} \times \mathbf{A}$$

$$\mathbf{A} \times (\mathbf{B} + \mathbf{C}) = \mathbf{A} \times \mathbf{B} + \mathbf{A} \times \mathbf{C}$$

$$(k\mathbf{A}) \times \mathbf{B} = k(\mathbf{A} \times \mathbf{B})$$

$$\mathbf{A} \cdot (\mathbf{B} \times \mathbf{C}) = \det(\mathbf{ABC})$$

$$\mathbf{A} \times (\mathbf{B} \times \mathbf{C}) = \mathbf{B}(\mathbf{A} \cdot \mathbf{C}) - \mathbf{C}(\mathbf{A} \cdot \mathbf{B})$$

$$(\mathbf{A} \times \mathbf{B}) \times (\mathbf{C} \times \mathbf{D}) = \det(\mathbf{ABD})\mathbf{C} - \det(\mathbf{ABC})\mathbf{D}.$$

Consider three orthogonal *unit vectors*: $\mathbf{i}_x$, $\mathbf{j}_y$, and $\mathbf{k}_z$:

$$\mathbf{i} \times \mathbf{j} = \mathbf{k} = -\mathbf{j} \times \mathbf{i}$$

$$\mathbf{j} \times \mathbf{k} = \mathbf{i} = -\mathbf{k} \times \mathbf{j}$$

$$\mathbf{k} \times \mathbf{i} = \mathbf{j} = -\mathbf{i} \times \mathbf{k}.$$

Also:

$$\mathbf{i} \times \mathbf{i} = \mathbf{j} \times \mathbf{j} = \mathbf{k} \times \mathbf{k} = \mathbf{0},$$

because $\sin 0 = 0$.

3-D cross products can be written in *matrix notation*. Note that the vectors need not lie in the x–y, x–z, or y–z planes. Representing the two vectors as sums of their orthogonal components:

$$\mathbf{A} = a_1\mathbf{i}_x + a_2\mathbf{j}_y + a_3\mathbf{k}_z$$

$$\mathbf{B} = b_1\mathbf{i}_x + b_2\mathbf{j}_y + b_3\mathbf{k}_z.$$

We can write:

$$\mathbf{A} \times \mathbf{B} = \begin{vmatrix} \mathbf{i}_x & \mathbf{j}_y & \mathbf{k}_z \\ a_1 & a_2 & a_3 \\ b_1 & b_2 & b_3 \end{vmatrix}$$
$$= \mathbf{C} = \mathbf{i}_x(a_2b_3 - a_3b_2) - \mathbf{j}_y(a_3b_1 - a_1b_3) + \mathbf{k}_z(a_1b_2 - a_2b_1).$$

Vector dot product: Vectors $\mathbf{A}$ and $\mathbf{B}$ lie in a plane. By definition: $\mathbf{A} \cdot \mathbf{B} \equiv |\mathbf{A}||\mathbf{B}|\cos(\theta)$, a scalar. θ is the angle between $\mathbf{A}$ and $\mathbf{B}$.

Vernix caseosa: Vernix is a waxy or cheese-like white substance that coats the skin of fetuses *in utero* in the second and final trimesters of pregnancy; it is secreted by sebaceous glands. In total, 12% of the dry weight of vernix is branched-chain fatty acid-containing lipids, cholesterol, and *ceramide*.

Vernix is thought to serve several purposes: It moisturizes and lubricates the infant's skin, facilitating its passage through the birth canal. It also serves to conserve heat and protect delicate newborn skin from injury. It may also have an antimicrobial effect and form a physical barrier to bacteria. Vernix also acts as an electrical insulator, making electrical recording of the fetal ECG difficult.

Voxel: A value characterizing a 3-D object (e.g., position, color, density) representing regularly sampled volumes that are not homogeneously filled. The position of a voxel is inferred based upon its position relative to other voxels. Alternately, a voxel is a unit of graphic information that defines a point in 3-D space.

W

Warfarin (also known as Coumadin, Jantoven, Marevan, Uniwarfarin): An anticoagulant drug normally used to inhibit the formation of thromboses and thromboembolisms, the formation of clots in blood vessels and their migration elsewhere where they do harm by restricting normal blood flow (e.g., brain, lungs, coronary circulation). Warfarin dosing is monitored by measurement of a patient's anticoagulation factor (INR). Note that common aspirin also inhibits clot formation.

Wavenumber (cm^{-1}): See Absorbance above.

White noise: An idealized approximation to a stationary random process having a "flat" power density spectrum given by

$$S(f) = hMSU/Hz \text{ (constant)}, 0 \leq f \leq \infty.$$

A white noise assumption is often used to approximate the midspectrum behavior of the density spectra of certain electronic systems, that is, between some f_{lo} and f_{hi}.

Wolff's Law: A theory developed by nineteenth-century German anatomist and surgeon, Julius Wolff. The theory states that bones in a healthy person will adapt to the loads under which they are placed. As a result of chronic bone loading, the bone remodels itself to be stronger to resist the loading.

Z

Zygote: A eukaryotic cell formed by a fertilization event between two gametes (viz., egg and sperm). It is the earliest developmental stage in multicellular organisms.

Zymogen: An inactive enzyme precursor.

Index

Printed and bound by CPI Group (UK) Ltd, Croydon, CR0 4YY

01/11/2024

01782600-0014